P9-CFX-276

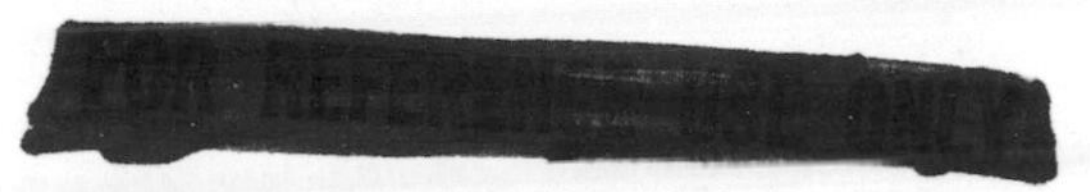

Medical reference works

1679–1966

a selected bibliography

John B. Blake

Charles Roos

editors

MEDICAL LIBRARY ASSOCIATION

Chicago · 1967

Medical Library Association Publication No. 3

Manufactured in the United States of America
Library of Congress catalog card number 67-30664

INTRODUCTION

The first two editions of the Medical Library Association's *Handbook of Medical Library Practice* included extensive and significant bibliographies. The first edition of 1943, edited by Janet Doe, contained a bibliography of 458 historical works compiled by Gertrude L. Annan and "An Annotated List of Reference Books" numbering 603 titles, compiled by Eileen R. Cunningham. Mrs. Cunningham, Miss Annan, and Mary E. Grinnell prepared the combined bibliography of 1,965 titles in the 1956 second edition, edited by Janet Doe and Mary Louise Marshall. Both editions were published by the American Library Association.

The third edition of the *Handbook*, now in preparation, will not contain a bibliography of reference works. The increased size of both the narrative text and the bibliography (the latter having grown to over 2,700 titles) plus the desirability of being able to revise the two sections at differing intervals have persuaded the Board of Directors of the Medical Library Association that publication should be as two separate titles. The completely rewritten chapters of text will retain the title and edition numbering of the earlier two editions, while the bibliography here begins a new career under its own title.

The skill and long hours of work of the staff of the National Library of Medicine and in particular of the two editors in expanding and revising this bibliography are a contribution from which medical librarians and all of the health professions should benefit greatly. To survey the world's bioscientific, medical, and allied health literature and select and organize from it an annotated list of the major works useful in gaining access to publications or frequently needed data is a service which can be fully appreciated only by those who have had to struggle without such a helpful guide. There are many specialized or partial medical bibliographies, as this volume reveals, but none, at least in the English language, gives as broad yet selective a picture of the medical reference tools as this. In making this compilation possible, the National Library of Medicine once again has demonstrated its leadership in service to the nation.

The Medical Library Association is proud to publish *Medical Reference Works, 1679–1966*. By so doing, the Association believes that it is furthering its important goal of improving library service to the health professions.

Stanley D. Truelson, Jr.
Chairman, Publication Committee
Medical Library Association

PREFACE

This work is a revision of "A Bibliography of the Reference Works and Histories in Medicine and the Allied Sciences," published in the Medical Library Association's *Handbook of Medical Library Practice*.[1] It continues the structure and content of the earlier work except that handbooks and treatises in the basic sciences and clinical medicine have only rarely been included.

The reference tools listed in this bibliography are those believed to be useful in answering a wide variety of questions in bio-science libraries large or small. Occasionally, however, items have been listed because of their intrinsic bibliographical interest. A number of basic references considered of special usefulness to the smaller medical library have been marked with an asterisk.

With respect to contents and editorial practice the following are to be observed:

1. In general only those indexes and abstracts are included which had a life span of 1 year or more.
2. Bibliographies of publications of single institutions are not included (except for the U. S. National Institutes of Health).
3. Some subjects are documented much less fully than others, notably Anthropology, Sociology, Zoology.
4. Bibliographies based on a single journal are not included.
5. Abstract sections in journals have been entered only when they have distinctive titles.
6. A minimum of cross references was used in the text. This type of direction is to be found in the index.
7. All material cited was examined in whole or in part; thus some relevant material not available for examination was not included.
8. The subject index for the most part has been based on concepts expressed in titles and subtitles.
9. All indexes, abstracts and bibliographies are arranged by subject (or class) unless otherwise stated. Similarly all have international coverage unless otherwise indicated.

The historical sections are of necessity highly selective. Insofar as the nature of the available material allowed, those works were listed which appeared to be particularly useful from a biographical or bibliographical point of view. With very few exceptions local histories, journal articles, and individual biographies have not been included.

The major part of the bibliography is a cooperative undertaking by members of the Reference Section of the National Library of Medicine. Material was

[1] Medical Library Association. *Handbook of Medical Library Practice*. 2 ed. Janet Doe and Mary Louise Marshall, ed. Chicago, American Library Association, 1956.

selected and annotated by nearly all staff members. Their names and the approximate areas covered are: Howard Drew, military medicine; Muriel Dury, nutrition and cardiovascular diseases; Stephen Kim, Oriental language entries in all fields; John Littlepage, the behavioral sciences; Virginia MacDonald, neoplasms; Betty Manson, periodicals; Elizabeth Moseley, directories and dictionaries in all fields; Charlotte Moulton, pharmacology; Jaroslav Nemec, Slavic entries in all fields; Robert Newburn, dentistry; Genevieve Schiffmann, pharmacy, pharmacology and other aspects of the drug literature; Marjory Wright, basic sciences.

Edith Blair had a special responsibility for medical education and related areas, and in addition reviewed and edited entries in all fields. The author and subject index was compiled by Mary Virginia Clark, who also provided extensive editorial assistance. Extensive general editorial assistance was also provided by Frances Hasemeier. Alvin Barnes, Joseph Forrest and James Keeling helped locate difficult references. Lena Ceccone typed the manuscript and proofed entries.

May G. Hardy of the History of Medicine Division of the National Library of Medicine bore the major burden of searching out references, verifying bibliographic data, comparing editions, tracking down reprint editions, and preparing annotations for the historical sections. Josephine Crosby and Margaret Donovan typed the entries.

Suggestions for inclusions and editorial advice were given by an advisory Editorial Committee of the Medical Library Association, Gertrude L. Annan, Frances Jenkins, Mildred C. Langner, and Joseph H. Roe, Jr.; by successive chairmen of the Publication Committee, Lee Ash and Stanley D. Truelson, Jr.; and by Alfred Brandon, who in addition was primarily responsible for signaling material useful for the smaller medical library.

CONTENTS

MEDICINE, GENERAL

Indexes and Abstracts 1–111
International 1–71
Regional and National 72–111
Reviews 112–127
Bibliographies 128–175
International 128–135
Manuals of Bibliography 136–143
Regional and National 143.1–175
Translations 176–178
Theses 179–185
Congresses 186–194
Dictionaries 195–317
Abbreviations 195–197
Etymology 198–208
Syndromes 209–214.1
General Medical 215–317
Polyglot 304–317
Periodicals 318–339
Histories 329–339
Directories 340–407
International 340–342
National 343–407
Encyclopedias 408–413

HISTORY OF MEDICINE

Bibliographies and Indexes 414–436
Historiography 437–440
Source Collections 441–443
Biographies 444–456
Dictionaries and Chronologies . 457–460
Comprehensive Histories 461–471
Shorter Histories 472–480
Pictorial Histories 481–486
History by Periods 487–512
National Histories 513–739
Special Topics in History 740–832
Art and Medicine 740–760
Bookplates 761
Famous Persons 762–768
Homeopathy 769–773
Jews 774–778
Literature and Medicine 779–784
Music and Medicine 785
Numismatics 786–788
Paleopathology 789–792
Philately 793–796
Primitive Medicine, Magic, and Folklore 797–804
Quackery 805–809
Religion and Medicine 810–820
Research 821–822
Symbolism, Medical 823–825
Women in Medicine 826–832

SPECIAL SUBJECTS

Aerospace and Submarine Medicine 833–850
Allergy 851–854.1
Anatomy 855–908.1
Cytology 899–902
Congenital Anomalies and Other Abnormalities 902.1–904.1
Histology 904.2–908.2
Anthropology 909–911
Biology 912–957
Biophysics 958–963
Botany and Agriculture 964–993
Chemistry and Biochemistry . . . 994–1098
Enzymes 1093–1098
Circulatory System 1099–1137
Communicable Diseases 1138–1267
General 1138–1155
Anthrax 1155.1
Bilharziasis 1156–1160
Botulism 1160.1
Brucellosis 1161–1163
Cholera 1164–1165
Coccidioidomycosis 1166–1166.1
Dengue 1166.2
Filariasis 1167–1168
Foot-and-Mouth Disease 1168.1
Hepatitis, Infectious 1169
Histoplasmosis 1170–1171
Influenza 1172–1174
Leishmaniasis 1175–1178
Leprosy 1179–1187
Leptospirosis 1188–1191
Malaria 1192–1198
Plague 1199–1205
Poliomyelitis 1206–1209
Psittacosis 1209.1–1209.2
Rickettsial Diseases 1210–1213
Salmonellosis 1214–1216
Smallpox 1217–1220

- Staphylococcal Infections ... *1221–1223*
- Toxoplasmosis ... *1224–1225*
- Trypanosomiasis ... *1226–1229*
- Tuberculosis ... *1230–1250*
- Tularemia ... *1251*
- Venereal Diseases ... *1252–1265*
- Yellow Fever ... *1266–1267*

Dentistry ... *1268–1346*
Dermatology ... *1347–1360*
Diagnosis ... *1361–1364*
Education, Medical ... *1365–1378*
Endocrinology ... *1379–1397*
- Diabetes ... *1392–1397*

Films ... *1398–1401*
Gastroenterology ... *1402–1408*
Genetics ... *1409–1423*
Gerontology ... *1424–1432*
Hospitals ... *1433–1463*
Legal Medicine ... *1464–1480*
Libraries, Medical ... *1481–1537*
- Manuals ... *1481–1488*
- Collections—Catalogs ... *1489–1502*
- Collections—Periodicals ... *1504–1517*
- Selection tools ... *1518–1525*
- Classification schemes ... *1526–1532*
- Directories ... *1533–1537*

Microbiology ... *1538–1582*
- Immunology ... *1569–1572*
- Mycology ... *1573–1582*

Microscopy ... *1583–1589*
Military Medicine ... *1590–1652*
Musculoskeletal System ... *1653–1681*
- Orthopedics ... *1664.1–1681*

Neoplasms ... *1682–1723*
Neurology and Psychiatry ... *1724–1877*
- Brain and Spinal Cord ... *1838.1–1848*
- Hypnosis ... *1849–1850*
- Mental Deficiency ... *1851–1858*
- Psychopharmacology ... *1859–1865*
- Senses and Sense Organs ... *1865.1–1877*

Nosology ... *1878–1887*
Nursing ... *1888–1913*
Nutrition ... *1914–1937*
- Vitamins ... *1930–1937*

Obstetrics and Gynecology ... *1938–1986*
Ophthalmology ... *1987–2033*
- Blind ... *2025–2028*
- Optometry ... *2029–2033*

Otorhinolaryngology ... *2034–2056*
Parasitology ... *2057–2078*
- Entomology ... *2070–2078*

Pathology and Clinical Pathology ... *2080–2107*
Pediatrics ... *2108–2139*
Pharmacy and Pharmacology ... *2141–2245*
- Antibiotics ... *2218–2224*
- Pest Control ... *2225–2228*
- Toxicology ... *2229–2245*

Physical Education and Sports Medicine ... *2246–2254*
Physical Medicine and Rehabilitation ... *2255–2268*
Physiology ... *2269–2288*
Psychology ... *2289–2340*
Public Health ... *2341–2418*
- Environmental Health ... *2385–2396*
- Occupational Health ... *2397–2414*
- Social Welfare ... *2414.1–2415*
- Vital Statistics ... *2415.1–2418*

Radiology ... *2419–2459*
- Nuclear Medicine ... *2448.1–2459*

Reproduction, Fertility, etc. ... *2460–2472*
Research in Progress ... *2473–2486*
Respiratory System ... *2487–2490*
Science ... *2490.1–2527*
Sociology ... *2528–2537.1*
Surgery ... *2538–2610*
- Surgical Specialties ... *2576–2593*
  - Burns ... *2576*
  - Cardiac Surgery ... *2576.1–2578*
  - Neurosurgery ... *2579–2581*
  - Pediatric Surgery ... *2582*
  - Plastic Surgery ... *2582.1–2588*
  - Thoracic Surgery ... *2589*
  - Transplantation ... *2590*
  - Traumatic Surgery ... *2591–2593*
- Anesthesia ... *2593.1–2610*

Therapeutics ... *2610.1–2624*
Urology ... *2624.1–2638*
Veterinary Medicine ... *2639–2667*
Writing, Preparation of Manuscripts, etc. ... *2668–2676.1*
Zoology ... *2677–2703*

Index p. *280–343*

MEDICINE, GENERAL

INDEXES AND ABSTRACTS, INTERNATIONAL

Entries in this section index the literature of more than one country and cover the "standard" medical journals to a greater or lesser extent. Inclusion of books, reports, theses and other monographic material and coverage of nonmedical sources are indicated in the annotations.

Current

1★

Abstracts of world medicine; a monthly critical survey of periodicals in medicine and allied sciences. London, 1, 1947– . British Medical Association.

Monthly. Two volumes a year. A selection from more than 1600 periodicals. v. 39 (Jan.–June 1966) lists 1265 references, most with abstracts. Minimum time lag (1966) 5 months. Infrequent critical comments. After June 1952 absorbed no. 2452.

2

Actualidades e utilidades médicas. Lisboa, 1, 1927– .

Currently 3 times a year; originally annual. 1963 contains approximately 280 abstracts primarily from foreign journals.

3

Archivio di medicina mutualistica. Rassegna bibliografica. Roma, 1, 1956– . Istituto Nazionale per l'Assicurazione contro le Malattie.

Annual. 1964 contains in excess of 200 abstracts. Includes books.

4

Bibliography of medical reviews. Bethesda, 1, 1955– . U.S. National Library of Medicine.

Currently an annual cumulation of entries published in the *Bibliography of medical reviews* section of *Index medicus.*

From 1955–Aug. 1961 BMR listed some review articles not listed in *Current list of medical literature* or *Index medicus*; from Sept. 1961 to Feb. 1965 review articles continued to be selected from some non-*Index medicus* titles but these articles were also listed in *Index medicus.*

v. 6, *Cumulation, 1955–1961* (i.e. 1960) cumulates (with numerous omissions) v. 1–5 and the reviews for 1960.

5

Bulletin signalétique. Paris, 1, 1940– . France. Centre National de la Recherche Scientifique.

Abstracts of articles, theses and books. Currently in 23 sections. Sections 12–17, monthly; sections 19–23 quarterly. Minimum time lag 6 months. Annual cumulated author and subject indexes about two years late.

v. 1–16, 1940–55, as *Bulletin analytique.* v. 1–21, 1940–60, issued in 3 major parts; the subjects corresponding to the current sections 12–17 were in pt. 2, Science biologique; subjects currently in sections 19–23 were in pt. 3.

The following sections are of special interest to medicine:

5.1 Sect. 12. Biophysique; biochemie; chimie analytique biologique. 22, 1961– .
5.2 Sect. 13. Sciences pharmacologiques; toxicologie. 22, 1961– .
5.3 Sect. 14. Microbiologie; virus; bactériophages; immunologie; génétique. 22, 1961–.
5.4 Sect. 15. Pathologie générale et expérimentale. 22, 1961– .
5.5 Sect. 16. Biologie et physiologie animales. 22, 1961– .
5.6 Sect. 17. Biologie et physiologie végétales. 22, 1961– .
5.7 Sect. 19–23 (in one v.) Sciences humaines. 19. Philosophie. Sciences religieuses. 20. Psychologie. Pédagogie. 21. Sociologie. Ethnologie. Sciences du langage. 22. Histoire des sciences et des techniques. 23. Esthétique. Archéologie. Arts.

6★★

Cumulated index medicus. Chicago, etc., 1, 1960– . U.S. National Library of Medicine

Annual. Cumulation of the monthly issues of no. 11. v. 1–5, 1960–64, published by the American Medical Association. Supersedes nos. 28 and 34.

Contains *List of journals indexed* (published separately as no. 326) and with 1966 also *Medical subject headings* (MESH) (published separately as no. 1531).

7

Current contents; your weekly guide to the chemical, pharmaco-medical and life sciences. Philadelphia, 1, 1958– . Institute for Scientific Information.

Reproduces tables of contents of more than 700 journals, many in advance of publication date. Minimum time lag (1966) 1 week. Lists over 150,000 articles a year. Alphabetical journal list, author index, and address directory in each issue. List of journals covered in Jan. 5, 1965, issue.

8

Current medical references. [1]- ed. Los Altos, Calif., Lange Medical Publications, 1959– .

3 ed., 1963, 666 p. English language references only. Includes books.

9★

Excerpta medica. Amsterdam, 1947– . Excerpta Medica Foundation.

127,154 abstracts published in 1966. In 1964, 120,673 abstracts from 2728 journals of which 1011 were not *Index medicus* titles. 1717 of the 2373 *Index medicus* journals were abstracted by *Excerpta medica*. Minimum time lag 5 months. In 1964, 81 Soviet biomedical journals were abstracted. Currently in 24 sections. For list of journals indexed see no. 319.

9.1 Sect. 1. Anatomy, anthropology, embryology and histology. 1, 1947– . 5502 abstracts in 1964.

9.2 Sect. 2A. Physiology. 18, 1965– ; 2B. Biochemistry. 18, 1965– ; 2C. Pharmacology and toxicology. 18, 1965– . v. 1–17, 1948–64 as Section 2. *Physiology, biochemistry and pharmacology*. 10,708 abstracts in 1964.

9.3 Sect. 3. Endocrinology. 1, 1948– . 2754 abstracts in 1964.

9.4 Sect. 4. Medical microbiology, immunology and serology. 8, 1955– . v. 1–7, 1948–54 as *Medical microbiology and hygiene*. Continued in part as Section 17. 6677 abstracts in 1964.

9.5 Sect. 5. General pathology and pathological anatomy. 1, 1948– . 4346 abstracts in 1964.

9.6 Sect. 6. Internal medicine. 1, 1947– 6409 abstracts in 1964.

9.7 Sect. 7. Pediatrics. 1, 1947– . 3927 abstracts in 1964.

9.8 Sect. 8A. Neurology and neurosurgery. 1, 1948– . 5000 abstracts in 1966. v. 1–18, 1948–65, as *Neurology and psychiatry*.

9.8 Sect. 8B. Psychiatry. 1, 1948– . 3000 abstracts in 1966. v. 1–18, 1948–65, as *Neurology and psychiatry*.

9.9 Sect. 9. Surgery. 1, 1947– . 7000 abstracts in 1966.

9.9 Sect. 9B Orthopedic surgery. 1, 1956– 2000 abstracts in 1966. v. 1–10, 1956–65, as *Orthopedics and traumatology*.

9.10 Sect. 10. Obstetrics and gynaecology. 1, 1948– . 5088 abstracts in 1964.

9.11 Sect. 11. Oto-, rhino-, laryngology. 1, 1948– . 4154 abstracts in 1964.

9.12 Sect. 12. Ophthalmology. 1, 1947– . 2792 abstracts in 1964.

9.13 Sect. 13. Dermatology and venereology. 1, 1947– . 3807 abstracts in 1964.

9.14 Sect. 14. Radiology. 1, 1947– . 4528 abstracts in 1964.

9.15 Sect. 15. Chest disease, thoracic surgery and tuberculosis. 1, 1948– . 3129 abstracts in 1965. v. 1–2, 1948–49, as *Tuberculosis;* v. 3–8, 1950–55, *Tuberculosis and pulmonary diseases;* v. 9–18, 1956–65, *Chest diseases*.

9.16 Sect. 16. Cancer. 1, 1953– . 6726 abstracts in 1964.

9.17 Sect. 17. Public health, social medicine and hygiene. 1, 1955– . 6009 abstracts in 1964. Supersedes in part Sect. 4.

9.18 Sect. 18. Cardiovascular diseases and cardiovascular surgery. 1, 1957– . 3842 abstracts in 1965. v. 1–9, 1957–65, as *Cardiovascular diseases*.

9.19 Sect. 19. Rehabilitation and physical medicine. 1, 1958– . 2405 abstracts in 1964. v. 1–6, 1958–63, as *Rehabilitation*.

9.20 Sect. 20. Gerontology and geriatrics. 1, 1958– . 2014 abstracts in 1964.

9.21 Sect. 21. Developmental biology and teratology. 1, 1961– . 6607 abstracts in 1964. v. 1–2, 1961–62, as *Abstracts of human developmental biology* (without Section designation); v. 3–4, 1963–64, as *Human developmental biology* (Sect. 21)
Supplement: *Abstracts of human developmental biology. Supplement to v. 1, 1961. Teratology; abstracts and titles of papers on congenital malformations.* Published as a separate: *Teratology; abstracts and titles of papers on congenital malformations collected from the 1962 medical literature.* Amsterdam, 302 p. 2006 references, most with abstracts.

9.22 Sect. 22. Human genetics. 1, 1963– . 3091 abstracts in 1964.

9.23 Sect. 23. Nuclear medicine. 1, 1964– . 3423 abstracts in 1964.

9.24 Sect. 24. Anesthesiology. 1, 1966– .

10

I hsueh wen chai [Medical digest] Peking, 1958– . Chung Kuo I Hsueh K'o Hsueh Yuan Ch'ing Pao Yen Chiu So [Chinese Academy of Medical Sciences. Information Office] Peking.

Chinese language abstracts of foreign language periodical articles. Frequency varies.

10.1 Sect. 1. Nei k'o hsueh [Internal medicine] 1958– .
10.2 Sect. 2. Wai k'o hsueh [Surgery] 1958– .
10.3 Sect. 3. Yao hsueh [Pharmacy] 1958– .
10.4 Sect. 4. Wei sheng hsueh [Public health] 1962– .
10.5 Sect. 5. Hsin hsieh kuan chi ping [Cardiovascular disease] 1964– .
10.6 Sect. 6. Chieh heu ping yu hu hsi hsi ping [Tuberculosis and respiratory diseases] 1964– .
10.7 Sect. 7. Fu ch'an k'o hsueh [Obstetrics and gynecology] 1964– .
10.8 Sect. 8. Erh k'o hsueh [Pediatrics] 1964– .
10.9 Sect. 9. Yen k'o hsueh [Ophthalmology] 1964– .
10.10 Sect. 10. Erh pi yen hou k'o hsueh [Otorhinolaryngology] 1964– .
10.11 Sect. 11. K'ou ch'iang i hsueh [Oral medicine] 1964– .
10.12 Sect. 12. Pi fu hsing ping hsueh [Dermatology] 1964– .
10.13 Sect. 13. Liu hsing ping hsueh chuan jan ping hsueh [Epidemiology and infectious diseases] 1964– .
10.14 Sect. 14. Chi sheng ch'ung ping [Parasitology] 1964– .
10.15 Sect. 15. Fang she hsueh [Radiology] 1964– .

11★★

Index medicus. Washington, 1, 1960– . U.S. National Library of Medicine.

Monthly. In 1966 indexed approximately 170,000 articles from 2300 biomedical journals. Minimum time lag 3 months. Cumulated annually as no. 6.

Monthly issues include as separate section *Bibliography of medical reviews* (since March 1965). Cumulated annually as no. 4.

January issue has *List of journals indexed* (LJI) (listed separately as no. 326). Additions, deletions, and title changes are noted in subsequent issues.

Recent United States publications, consisting of reproductions of catalog cards for selected current titles, included through December 1965.

Continues no. 28.

For a list of subject headings used see no. 1531.

11.1

Internal medicine digest. Northfield, Ill., 1, 1966– .

Abstracts, mainly from the English language literature.

12

International medical digest; a monthly abstract journal of current literature. Hagerstown, Md., W. F. Prior Co., Inc., 1, 1920– .

600 abstracts a year mainly from English language journals. From 1962 contains section "Drug notes," information on drug toxicity Minimum time lag 4 months.

Some volumes have added title on spine: Practice of medicine. Tice or Tice-Sloan.

13

Kongresszentralblatt für die gesamte innere Medizin und ihre Grenzgebiete. Berlin, 1, 1912– . Deutsche Gesellschaft für innere Medizin.

Currently 12 volumes a year, 3 issues a volume and a 4th index issue (delayed about a year). A recent volume listed approximately 1150 references, most with abstracts. Includes some books. Minimum time lag 5 months.

v. 1-11, 1912-14, as *Zentralblatt für die gesamte innere Medizin und ihre Grenzgebiete (Kongresszentralblatt)*.

See also no. 37.

14

Medical digest; a monthly summary of the world's medical literature. Northfield, Ill., etc., v. 1, 1955– .

In 1965 about 1200 abstracts. No indexes.

15

Medical review of reviews. Delhi, 1, 1939– .

Monthly. Abstracts. 1963 contained approximately 350 abstracts. Includes book reviews. Minimum time lag 3 months.

16

Meditsinskiĭ referativnyĭ zhurnal [Medical abstract journal] Moskva, 1, 1957– . Ministerstvo Zdravookhraneniia SSSR.

Monthly. Lists some 30,000 references annually, most with abstracts. Includes books. Listing limited to material of practical value to the Russian practitioner. In 1962 abstracted 1397 biomedical serials. Foreign literature, especially English, formed the greatest percentage of entries. In 1962 abstracted 88 Soviet periodicals compared to 72 abstracted in *Die Medizin die Sowjetunion*, 81 in *Excerpta medica*, and 115 indexed in *Index medicus* in 1964.

Supersedes no. 109.

1957–59 in four sections; 1960–62, ten sections; 1963– , thirteen sections. All sections commenced in 1957 unless otherwise indicated. Section titles translated from the Russian.

16.1 Sect. 1.
Internal diseases; endocrinology; climatotherapy; physiotherapy and medical gymnastics.

16.2 Sect. 2.
Tuberculosis. 1957–59 in Sect. 4.

16.3 Sect. 3.
Medical microbiology. 1960– .
Virology. 1960– .
Medical parasitology. 1960– .
Epidemiology. 1957–59 in Sect. 4.
Infectious diseases. 1957–59 in Sect. 1.
Antibiotics. 1960– .

16.4 Sect. 4.
Surgery. 1957–59 in Sect. 2.
Traumatology and orthopedics. 1957–59 in Sect. 2.
Neurosurgery. 1957–59 in Sect. 2.
Urology. 1957–59 in Sect. 2.

16.5 Sect. 5.
Diseases of children. 1957–59, in Sect. 3.

16.6 Sect. 6.
Oncology. 1957–59 in Sect. 2.
Medical radiology. 1957–59 in Sect. 2.
Roentgenology. 1957–59 in Sect. 2.

16.7 Sect. 7.
Hygiene and sanitation. 1957–59 in Sect. 4.
Radiation hygiene. 1960– .
Organization of public health. 1957–59 in Sect. 4.
History of medicine. 1957–59 in Sect. 4.
Forensic medicine. 1957–59 in Sect. 4.
Medical technology. 1960– .

16.8 Sect. 8.
Ophthalmology. 1957–59 in Sect. 2.

16.9 Sect. 9.
Neuropathology and psychiatry. 1957–59 in Sect. 1.

16.10 Sect. 10.
Obstetrics and gynecology. 1957–59 in Sect. 3.

16.11 Sect. 11.
Skin and venereal diseases. 1957–62 in Sect. 1.

16.12 Sect. 12.
Stomatology. 1957–59 in Sect. 2; 1960–62 in Sect. 8.

16.13 Sect. 13.
Otorhinolaryngology. 1957–59 in Sect. 2; 1960–62 in Sect. 8.

17

Minerva medicobibliografica; indici trimestrali della letteratura medica chirurgica e specialistica mondiale. Torino, 1, 1953– .

Approximately 40,000 references a year. Titles listed as indexed include a considerable number not indexed in *Index medicus*. Entries for 1964 first appear in the Apr./June issue of 1964.

No author indexes or annual subject index.

18

Mises à jour de médecine pratique. Paris, 1, 1957– .

Monthly. 1964 contained in excess of 500 abstracts. Some issues bimonthly.

18.1

Novye knigi za rubezhom. Ezhemesiachnyi kritiko-bibliograficheskiĭ zhurnal. Seriia B. Biologiia, meditsina, sel'skoe khoziaistvo [New books abroad. A monthly critico-bibliographical journal. Series B. Biology, medicine, agriculture] Moskva, 1, 1957– .

Signed reviews of foreign books. Each issue contains between ten and fifteen reviews of books on medicine.

18.2

Physicians' basic index. Kettering, Ohio, 1, 1966– . Charles F. Kettering Memorial Hospital.

Monthly. In 1966 indexes 131 English language journals of interest to the practitioner. Time lag 1 month.

19

Přehled světové zdravotnické literatury [A survey of world literature on health] Praha, 1, 1954– . Ústav pro zdravotnickou dokumentaci.

Monthly. Index to foreign medical literature received in Czechoslovak libraries. Titles in original language and Czech or Slovak translation. In excess of 40,000 entries a year, most with abstracts. Semiannual author index beginning 1964.

20

Progressos da medicina. Rio de Janeiro,

1, 1952– . Indústria Química e Farmacêutica Schering, S. A.

Annual. More than 500 abstracts in 1964.

21

Referativnyĭ zhurnal [Abstract journal] Moskva, 1953– . Akademiia nauk SSSR, Institut nauchnoĭ informatsii.

Currently covers over 25 fields of which the following are of interest to medicine. Some sections are published as separates.

21.1 Biogeografiia; meditsinskaia geografiia [Biogeography; medical geography] 1960–62.
Continued by no. 21.9.

21.2 Biologiia [Biology] 1954– .
24 issues per year. Originally about 70,000 abstracts annually, now more than 120,000.

21.3 Biologicheskaia khimiia [Biological chemistry] 1955– .
24 issues per year. More than 35,000 abstracts in 1963. Author index to each issue.

21.4 Farmakologiia. Toksikologiia [Pharmacology. Toxicology] 1963– .
24 issues per year. 350–500 abstracts per issue. Annual indexes.

21.5 Issledovanie kosmicheskogo prostranstva [Research in cosmic space] 1964– .
12 issues per year. About 400 abstracts each issue. The section "Cosmonautics. Safety and biological problems of space flights" contains between 15 and 35 abstracts an issue.

21.6 Khimiia [Chemistry] 1953– .
24 issues per year. More than 50,000 abstracts in 1954; more than 99,000 in 1960. Author, formula, patent, and subject indexes.

21.7 Khimiia. Biologicheskaia khimiia [Chemistry. Biological chemistry] 1955–62.
24 issues per year. More than 35,000 abstracts a year. Author index to each issue.
1953–54 included in no. 21.6.
Continued by no. 21.3.

21.8 Kibernetika [Cybernetics] 1964– .
12 issues per year. About 500 abstracts each issue. Contains abstracts on theoretical and technical cybernetics. Author index to each issue.

21.9 Meditsinskaia geografiia [Medical geography] 1963– .
12 issues per year. 200–500 abstracts each issue. No indexes. Continues no. 21.1.

21.10 Obshchie voprosy patologii. Onkologiia [General problems of pathology. Oncology] 1963– .
24 issues per year. 250–450 abstracts per issue. No indexes.

22

Revista de resumenes. Havana, 1, 1965– . Cuba. Ministerio de Salud Publica.

Monthly. 934 entries, Jan.–Mar. 1966, most with abstracts.

23

Was gibt es Neues in der Medizin? Hanover, 1, 1948/50– .

Annual. Abstracts. German language journals only (German, Austrian, Swiss). No author index.

24

World-wide abstracts of general medicine. New York, 1, 1958– . Excerpta Medica Foundation.

Monthly. Selected abstracts of papers in general practice. About 350 abstracts in 1965. Minimum time lag (1965) 3 months. No author or subject indexes.

Supplement (1966) *Urology*: Installment 1–6: A new programmed course; 7–12: A basic systems program.

Noncurrent

Discontinued since 1950

Of the indexes discontinued during this period, nos. 29 and 34 are of special importance. The *Index-catalogue* is perhaps the most comprehensive index to the world literature of medicine ever published. The first series, edited by John Shaw Billings, covers literature published up to the date of each volume. Beginning in 1941 the Army Medical Library (now the National Library of Medicine) began publication of the *Current list of medical literature* to achieve greater current coverage. The index is relatively difficult to use, however. To fill in the hiatus between the *Index-catalogue* and *Index medicus* or to provide an author approach to articles in journals many users will find the *Quarterly cumulative index medicus* the tool of choice. The latter, however, covers only through 1956, leaving the *Current list of medical literature* to cover the period 1957–59.

Books not found in the *Index-catalogue* may sometimes be most quickly identified by searching general library catalogs such as those of the Library of Congress, British Museum, or Bibliothèque Nationale.

25
Annata clinica e terapeutica. Roma, 1949–1956?

Annual. Supersedes *Annata terapeutica* and *Annata diagnostica* (not listed).

Subtitles: Clinica nuova. Supplemento annuale di aggiornamento clinico e terapeutico; supplemento annuale di Clinica nuova. With 1956: Recentia medica. Supplemento annuale di aggiornamento . . . ; supplemento annuale di Recentia media.

26
Bibliographia medica latina. Roma, 1–2, 1954–56.

v. 1: 13,190 entries; v. 2: 13,696.

27
British abstracts. A. III. Anatomy, biochemistry, experimental biology, experimental medicine, microbiology, pathology, pharmacology and physiology. London, 1938–53. Supported by the Chemical Society, the Society of Chemical Industry, the Physiological Society, the Biochemical Society, etc.

1953 listed 31,200 references, most with abstracts.

1938–44, as *British chemical and physiological abstracts.*

A. III. 1938, as *Physiology and biochemistry*; 1939–44, *Physiology and biochemistry (including anatomy)*; 1945–48, *Physiology, biochemistry, anatomy*; 1948–51, *Physiology, biochemistry, anatomy, pharmacology, experimental medicine.*

Continues no. 1007 and indirectly no. 1005.1.
Continued by no. 918.

28★★
Current list of medical literature. Washington, 1–36, 1941–59. U.S. National Library of Medicine.

Monthly. In three parts: Register of articles, which lists tables of contents of each journal; Subject index; and Author index. Semiannual cumulative indexes. In 1959, 1620 biomedical journals were indexed and 107,021 individual articles listed. A 1954 survey showed that 56 percent of all material published was less than one year old; 93 percent of the American material appeared within six months.

Recent United States publications, a separate section consisting of reproductions of National Library of Medicine catalog cards for current titles, is included in the issues for 1957–59.

Recent book acquisitions of the Army Medical Library issued as a supplement, v. 1–8, 1941–45.

Issued Jan. 1941–Apr. 1952 by the Army Medical Library; May 1952–Sept. 1956 by the Armed Forces Medical Library.

Each volume since 1950 contains a *List of journals indexed* (published separately in 1956 and 1959)

Superseded by no. 11.

28.1
General practice clinics. Washington, 1–10(2), 1943–Feb. 1953; Mar. 1953–56. Washington Institute of Medicine.

Through 1945 bimonthly; 1946–48 quarterly; 1949–56 monthly.

Through 1953 general abstract journal; 1954–56 limited to abstracts of reports of unpublished papers delivered at current medical meetings in the United States and abroad.

v. 1–7, 1943–50, published separately; v. 8–10 (2), 1951–Feb. 1953, in *International record of medicine and general practice clinics*, v. 164–166(2), 1951–Feb. 1953; Mar. 1953–56 published without voluming in *International record . . .* v. 166(3)–169, Mar. 1953–1956.

Supersedes no. 38.1.

Continued as *Advanced reports from current medical meetings, IRM*, v. 170(1–11) Jan.–Nov. 1957 (not listed).

29★★
Index-catalogue of the Library of the Surgeon General's Office, National Library of Medicine. Washington [ser. 1] 1–16, 1880–95; ser. 2, 1–21, 1896–1916; ser. 3, 1–10, 1918–32; ser. 4, 1–11 (Mh–Mn) 1936–55; ser. 5, 1–3 (v. 1, Authors, v. 2–3, Subjects) 1959–61.

Ser. 1–4 index a total of about 3,000,000 journal articles, books, and pamphlets and cover the earliest literature through 1950. Ser. 5 indexes, for the most part, the monographs (including theses) received by the Library during the period from about 1927 through 1950 and contains approximately 120,000 references. Some author entries in series 5 are entered under subject in ser. 3 or 4 and *vice versa.*

Ser. 3, v. 6–10, 1926–32, contains no subject periodical material later than 1925. Monographs and theses are included up-to-date. 1926–1932 material was, however, included in the 4th series through the M2 volume.

Special features: 1. Congresses and supplement, ser. 4, v. 3–4 (see no. 192) 2. Bio-bibliography of 16th century medical authors (A-Alberti) By Claudius F. Meyer. 52 p. Supplement to ser. 4, v. 6.3. Military medicine, ser. 4., v. 11, p. 289–1226 (also issued as a separate). 4. List of abbreviations for serial publications, *passim.*

Ser. 1, 1–ser. 3, 10, 1880–1932, as *Index-catalogue of the Library of the Surgeon General's Office, U. S. Army;* ser. 4, 1–10, 1936–48, as *Index-catalogue of the Library of the Surgeon-General's Office, U.S. Army (Army Medical Library)*; ser. 4, 11, 1955, as *Index-catalogue of the Library of the Surgeon General's Office, U.S. Army (Armed Forces Medical Library).*

Regarding the coverage of the 1st series, Billings wrote " . . . permit me to call attention to the fact that this is not a complete medical bibliography, and that anyone who relies upon it as such will commit a serious error. It is a Catalogue of what is to be found in a single collection. . ." (*Index-catalogue,* ser. 1, v. 1, p.v.). Elsewhere Billings estimated that at the time of the 1st series the library contained about 75 percent of all that had been published in medical journals. In the same paper he indicated that he would rely on the work of Ploucquet (no. 133) and Reuss (no. 2492) for indexing the journal literature prior to 1800. (Medical libraries, in Rogers, F. B., *Selected papers of John Shaw Billings,* [Chicago] Medical Library Association, 1965, p. 82–83.)

29.1

Indice bibliografico. Sección 4. Medicina. México, D. F., 1–3, 1962–64. Instituto Politécnico Nacional de México. Centro de Investigación y de Estudios Avanzados.

Bimonthly. Lists contents of journals under journal title.

In two parts: 1. Medicina. Ciencias Básicas; 2. Medicina clínica, higiene y medicina social.

30

J.A.M.A. clinical abstracts of diagnosis and treatment. New York, 1955–57. American Medical Association.

Annual. Selected abstracts from the "Medical literature abstracts" section of *JAMA.* No author index.

30.1

Medizinischer Literaturnachweis. Deutsche und ausländische Bücher, Zeitschriften und Zeitschriftenaufsätze aus den Beständen der Deutschen Staatsbibliothek. Berlin, 1–13, 1952–64. Deutsche Staatsbibliothek.

Monthly. In several sections. In excess of 4000 references a month. Monthly author and subject indexes.

31

Medical abstracts. Philadelphia, 1–3, 1955/56–57.

Monthly. Abstracts of articles selected from over 200 journals. Intended for the practicing physician.

32

Nippon naika shōnika chūo zasshi [Abstracts of internal medicine and pediatrics from Japanese journals] Tokyo, 1–9, 1936–44; [new ser.] 1–18, 1952–61.

Numbered abstracts of articles from 163 Japanese journals (1960). Includes reports of association meetings and symposia.

33

Progresos en la practica medicoquirurgica. Buenos Aires, 1945–50?

Abstracts. 7–15 issues a year, each on a special subject or group of subjects. No cumulative author indexes.

1945–46 as *Progresos anuales en la practica medicoquirurgica.*

34★★

Quarterly cumulative index medicus. Chicago, 1–60, 1927–56. American Medical Association.

Authors and subjects in one alphabet. Includes some form entries, e.g., biographies, obituaries. The volume for 1956 indexes 933 biomedical journals.

Main index preceded by author and classified list of new books and *List of journals indexed.*

Full title entry in the vernacular under author; abbreviated, inverted, translated, or otherwise altered titles appear under subject.

v. 1 includes literature for 1926.

Quarterly through v. 44, 1948, with semiannual cumulations; semiannual with v. 45, 1949.

1927–31 jointly sponsored by the Army Medical Library and the American Medical Association.

Continues nos. 36 and 38.

Superseded by no. 11.

For a list of subject headings used see no. 1530.

35

Quarterly review of medicine. Washington, 1–9, 1943–52. Washington Institute of Medicine.

Approximately 200 selected abstracts per volume.

Absorbed no. 1350 in 1950.

v. 7–8, 1950–51, as *Quarterly review of internal medicine and dermatology;* v. 9(3–4), Aug.–Nov. 1952, in *International record of medicine and general practice clinics*, v. 165 (8, 11), Aug., Nov. 1952.

v. 8, 1951: Incorporating the *International record of internal medicine and dermatology* (original article section); v. 9, 1952: Incorporating the *International record of medicine* (original article section).

Discontinued 1920–1949

Of the items discontinued during this period nos. 36, 38, and 39 are of special importance. The *Index medicus* was founded in 1879 by John Shaw Billings and Robert Fletcher of the Library of the Surgeon General's Office, U.S. Army, to provide more current coverage of the literature indexed in the *Index-catalogue* and to provide an author approach to articles in the periodical literature. It will generally be the tool of choice as an author approach to the periodical literature published between 1880 and 1927.

35.1

Excerpta medica. Leipzig, etc. 1–36? 1891/92–1927?

Abstracts.

Subtitle: Kurze monatliche Journalauszüge aus der gesammten Fachliteratur zum Gebrauch für dem praktischen Arzt.

36★

Index medicus; a quarterly classified record of the current medical literature of the world. Washington, etc., ser. 1, 1–21, Jan. 31, 1879–Apr. 1899; ser. 2, 1–18, 1903–20; ser. 3, 1–6(5), 1921–June 1927. Carnegie Institution of Washington.

Books and theses listed by authors under subjects, followed by author listing of articles.

Entries are in the vernacular.

Journals devoted to chemistry, pharmacy, veterinary medicine, and dentistry are not fully indexed.

Includes some form headings: bibliography, biography (including obituaries), periodicals, etc.

Ser. 1, v. 1, no. 1, indexes principally literature for 1878 with a few earlier references. The last volume of ser. 1 indexes the literature for 1899. Ser. 2, v. 1 commences with the literature for late 1902 and the last volume of the 3rd series indexes the literature through late 1926.

Ser. 1 published by various commercial publishers or by the editors, J.S. Billings and Robert Fletcher.

Ser. 1–2 as *Index medicus; a monthly record . . .*

May–Dec. 1895 issued as a single number out of chronological sequence as v. 18, no. 5, following April 1896.

Includes: Bibliography of public hygiene, by J. S. Billings, 1: 164–8; 272–6; 370–2; 419–20; 468, 1879; Notes and queries in v. 1 and 2.

See also no. 42.

36.1

Index universalis. Dissertationum originalium artis medicinae e libellis periodicis extractus. Igaku gencho sakuin. Mukden, 1–16, 1924–39. Collegium Medicinae Manjurici.

v. 1–6, 1924–29, author arrangement under subjects; with v. 7, 1930 alphabetical by journal title with contents listed under issue number. No indexes.

36.2

International medical and surgical survey. New York, 1–9, 1920–25. American Institute of Medicine.

Abstracts. Various subsections: Surgery; Gynecology and obstetrics; Pediatrics; Medicine; Ophthalmology, otology and rhinolaryngology; Gastro-enterology; Roentgenology and radiotherapy; Urology and venerology, etc.

In later years subsections as: *International survey of surgery, International survey of gynecology and obstetrics*, etc.

Annual combined indexes to subsections.

37

Jahresbericht innere Medizin. Berlin, 1–14, 1912–31.

Annual cumulation of references of no. 13.

[v. 1–3] 1912–20, as *Bibliographie der gesamten inneren Medizin und ihrer Grenzgebiete.* [v. 4–9] 1921–26, as *Jahresbericht über die gesamte innere Medizin und ihre Grenzgebiete.*

[v. 1–2] 1912–13, has subtitle: Auf Grund des Zentralblattes für die gesamte innere Medizin und ihre Grenzgebiete (Kongresszentralblatt). [v. 3] 1920, Auf Grund des Kongresszentralblattes . . . [v. 4–14] 1921–31, Bibliographisches Jahresregister des Kongresszentralblattes . . .

38

Quarterly cumulative index to current medical literature. Chicago, 1–12, 1916–26. American Medical Association.

Intended for the general practitioner, not a complete index to the literature. 1926 indexed only 326 periodicals.

Authors and subjects in one alphabet. Titles of foreign language articles translated into English.

Cumulated annually 1916–25; semiannually 1926.

Main index preceded by author and classified list of new books, list of publishers, and recent government publications of interest to the medical profession (arranged by Department).

Merged with no. 36 to form no. 34.

38.1

Review of medicine, surgery and obstetrics-gynecology. Washington, 1–7, 1936–43. Washington Institute of Medicine.

Monthly. Abstracts.

1936-Mar. 1938, as *Medical survey;* Apr.-July/Aug. 1938, *International surveys of recent advances in medicine;* Sept. 1938-May 1941, *International review of recent advances in medicine.*

Superseded by no. 28.1.

39

Schmidt's Jahrbücher der in- und ausländischen gesammten Medicin. Leipzig, 1–336, 1834–1922.

2 volumes a year divided into three principal sections: 1. Periodical abstracts: Auszüge aus sammtlichen in- und ausländischen med. Journalen; with v. 69, 1851, Auszüge. 2. Book reviews: Kritik der in- und ausländischen medicinischen Literatur; with v. 69, 1851, Kritiken; v. 209, 1886, Bücheranzeigen; v. 315, 1912, Bücherbesprechungen. 3. Bibliography: Medicinische Bibliographie des in- und Auslands (from v. 57, 1848) (previously divided by country).

The abstract and bibliography sections arranged by subject; the book review section arranged by country through v. 69, 1851, thereafter at random. Each section separately numbered consecutively through each volume with references indexed by author. Abstracts number around 200 in the earlier volumes and later as high as 2100; reviews number from 50 to 200 a volume irrespective of date. Occasional original and review articles.

v. 1–40, 1834–43, as *Jahrbücher* . . . v. 41–80, 1844–54, *Carl Christian Schmidt's Jahrbücher.*

Discontinued 1879–1919

40

Anuario internacional de medicina y cirugía; revista semestral. Madrid, ser. 1, 1–21, 1865–84; ser. 2, 1–59, 1885–1914.

v. 59, 1914, contains in excess of 400 abstracts. Selective author index.

Ser. 1, v. 1–21, 1865–84, as *Anuario de medicina y cirugía practicas;* ser. 2, 1–14, 1885–91, *Anuario de medicina y cirugía; revista semestral.*

41

Annali universali di medicina e chirurgia. Milano, 1–286, 1817–88.

Abstracts. Includes books and theses.

With v. 236, 1876, abstracts issued as a separate volume: *Parte revista.*

Cumulative, separately published author and subject indexes, 1814–30 (indexes no. 55 below), 1831–40, 1841–50, 1851–60 and 1861–70.

v. 1–230, 1817–74, as *Annali universali di medicina.*

Continues no. 55.

42

Bibliographia medica (Index medicus). Recueil mensuel. Classement méthodique de la bibliographie internationale des sciences médicales. Paris. 1–3, 1900–02. Institut de Bibliographie.

Monthly. Indexes the literature from 1900 through the fall of 1902. Lists books and journal articles by author, at random, under detailed subject breakdowns; books listed first. Some form headings used, e.g., périodiques, biographie et nécrologie, etc.

Intended by the publishers to be a continuation of *Index medicus* (no. 36) (suspended during this period), it bridges the hiatus with the exception of the literature for late 1899. Editors state that between 50,000 and 60,000 titles a year will be indexed.

Annual author index, but only an abbreviated subject index. Special annual index to biographies and obituaries.

43
Index medicus novus; Inhaltsangabe der periodisch erscheinenden medicinischen Literatur aller Länder. Wien, 1–2, June 15, 1899-Feb. 10–25, 1900.

Abbreviated coverage of the literature during period when no. 36 was not published. No annual author or subject indexes.

No. 1–6, 1899 as *Die medicinische Weltliteratur.*

44
International catalogue of scientific literature. London, 1–14, 1901–16. International Council. By the Royal Society of London.

Annual. Of 17 sections, A–R, the following are of interest to medicine: D. Chemistry; L. General biology; M. Botany; N. Zoology; O. Human anatomy; P. Physical anthropology; Q. Physiology; R. Bacteriology.

Each volume in two parts, author catalog and subject catalog.

Continues no. 2400.

45
Jahrbuch für praktische Aerzte. Berlin. 1–16, 1877–92.

v. 16 contains in excess of 1000 abstracts. Includes books.

v. 1–2, 1877–78, has subtitle: Fortsetzung von Grävell's Notizen.

Continues no. 62.

46
Jahresbericht über die Leistungen und Fortschritte in der gesammten Medicin. Berlin, [1]-51, 1866–1916.

References listed under subjects, then selectively abstracted.

[v. 1], 1866, has subtitle: Fortsetzung von Canstatt's Jahresbericht; v. 37–51, 1902–16, Fortsetzung von Virchow's Jahresbericht.

Virchow was editor, [v. 1]-36, 1866–1901.

General register, v. 1–25, 1866–90. Subjects only.

Continues no. 61.

47
Medicinische Bibliographie und Anzeiger zum Centralblatt für die gesammte Medizin. Leipzig, 1–11, 1883–93.

Includes books.

48
Monthly abstract of medical sciences. Philadelphia, 1–6, 1874–79.

Continues American edition of no. 63.

v. 1, 1874, had subtitle: Supplement to the Medical news and library.

49
Quarterly compendium of medical science. Philadelphia, 1–56, 1868–89.

1869 contained about 700 abstracts, approximately half from American and half from European sources.

1868–1882 as *Half-yearly compendium of medical science.*

No author index.

Also numbered in 4 series.

50
Retrospect of medicine. London, 1–123, 1840–1901.

2 volumes a year. v. 123, 1901, contains approximately 350 abstracts.

Half title: *Braithwaite's retrospect*, v. 12–123, 1845–1901.

v. 1–12, 1840–45, as *Retrospect of practical medicine and surgery.*

Cumulated index, 1840–65.

51
Revue des sciences médicales en France et à l'étranger. Paris, 1–52, 1873–93.

Quarterly. Abstracts. Includes theses.

52
Zentralblatt für die medizinischen Wissenschaften. Berlin, 1–53, 1863–1915.

Weekly. Abstracts of some 15–30 articles per week. In the earlier volumes the articles were few but extensively reviewed or discussed.

Discontinued before 1879

Listed below are a number of indexes which provide an author (as well as subject) approach to articles before the period covered by *Index medicus*. Readers interested will find a fairly comprehensive list of early indexes in no. 434 of this bibliography. Callisen (no. 60) is useful for author entries of its period as, of course, are other author directories and biographical dictionaries which list publications (e.g. Eloy) (no. 451).

53
Allgemeine medizinische Zeitung mit Be-

rücksichtigung des neuesten und interessantesten der allgemeinen Naturkunde. Leipzig, etc., 1798–1832.

Contains review sections, by subject or country, listing new journals, articles in journals, books and theses with annotations or long discussions. Occasionally lists journal titles with review of contents. 1798–99 contains a supplement, *Intelligenzblatt der Medizinischen National-Zeitung für Deutschland*, which lists new books and the titles and contents of journals (this section not indexed).

1798–99, as *Medizinische National-Zeitung für Deutschland;* 1800, *Allgemeine medizinische Annalen des Jahres 1800;* 1801–30, *Allgemeine medizinische Annalen des Neunzehnten Jahrhunderts.*

Annual index entitled: *Repertorium der Allgemeinen . . . Supplementenband* for 1801–1810, 1821–25 contains essentially the same information in the same format as the original, together with a combined index (*Generalrepertorium*) to the original for the period covered by the supplements and to the supplements themselves.

54

Allgemeines Repertorium der medizinisch-chirurgischen Journalistik des Auslandes in vollständigen, kurzgefassten Auszügen. Berlin, 1–21, 1830–35.

Arranged by journal title and issue with review of contents.

v. 1–4, 1830, as *Neueste medizinisch-chirurgische Journalistik des Auslandes* . . . 1834–35 also as n. s., 1–6.

55

Annali di medicina straniera. Milano. 1–4, 1814–16.

Superseded by no. 41.

56

Annual record of homeopathic literature. New York, 1870–75.

Principally extracts from 22 homeopathic journals (1875).

57

Bollettino delle scienze mediche. Bologna, 1–12, 1829–35.

Pubblicato per cura della Società Medico-Chirurgica di Bologna.

Abstracts. Includes books and proceedings of societies. No annual author indexes. v. 12, 1835, has subject index to v. 7–12.

58

British and foreign medical review. London, 1–25, 1836–48.

Includes books, reports, new journals.

United with no. 65 to form no. 59.

59

British and foreign medico-chirurgical review. London, 1–60, 1848–78.

Includes books, reports, new journals.

Formed by union of nos. 58 and 65.

60

Callisen, Adolph C. P. Medicinisches Schriftsteller-Lexicon der jetzt lebenden Aerzte, Wundärzte, Geburtshelfer, Apotheker, und Naturforscher aller gebildeten Völker. Copenhagen, Altona, 1830–45. 33v.

Author catalog listing 90,597 works under 36,307 authors. In addition, lists under title 5375 anonymous works including pharmacopeias and 3029 collected works—a total of 99,001 entries. Authors in two alphabets: v. 1–21, 1830–35; v. 26–33, 1838–45.

Gives brief biographical data and then lists publications (articles and monographs) in chronological order. Authors are numbered sequentially in each volume as are works listed. Reviews of works cited are frequently referenced. Some American works cited as published were in fact not printed.

v. 22–23 (p. 1–138), consists of a title list of anonymous monographs, reports, etc.

v. 23 (p. 139–) - v. 25, consists of a title list of serials (journals, society publications, and collected works of more than one author), giving bibliographic data and frequently full or selected contents of individual volumes from beginning to date. List includes nonmedical serials.

v. 26–33, 1838–45, have subtitle: Nachtrag. Enthaltend: Berichtigungen, Ergänzungen, die neuere Literatur, und die seit 1830 verstorbenen medicinischen Schriftsteller.

Reprinted Nieuwkoop, De Graaf, 1962–65.

61

Canstatt's Jahresbericht über die Fortschritte der gesammten Medicin in allen Ländern. Würzburg, 1841–65.

Literature reviews with articles, books, theses listed under subject by author and summarized or discussed in order of listing. A sample year (1862) contained about 4300 abstracts.

1841 in 2 volumes; 1842–43 in 4 volumes;

1844–65 in 7 volumes; each volume on a separate discipline of medicine and separately numbered. The seven sections entitled: 1. Physiologische Wissenchaften. 2. Allgemeine Pathologie. 3. Specielle oder local-Pathologie. 4. Specielle Nosologie. 5. Heilmittellehre. 6. Thierheilkunde. 7. Staats-Arzneikunde. These, and their subsections, are sometimes listed as separate publications, i.e., *Jahresbericht* or *Canstatt's Jahresbericht über die Fortschritte der Staats-Arzneikunde, Jahresbericht über die Fortschritte in der Chirurgie und Geburtshülfe in allen Ländern*; etc.

1841–48, as *Jahresbericht über die Fortschritte der gesammten Medicin in allen Ländern*; 1849–50, *C. Canstatt's . . .*

Combined author and subject indexes to the seven volumes.

Continued by no. 46.

62

Graevell's Notizen für praktische Ärzte über die neuesten Beobachtugen in der Medicin. Berlin, 1–9, 1848–56; n.s. 1–20, 1857–76.

v. 1 had in excess of 1000 numbered abstracts of articles and books.

v. 1–9, 1848–56, as *Notizen . . .*

Continued by no. 45.

63

Half-yearly abstract of the medical sciences. London, 1–58, 1845–73.

v. 58 contained 289 abstracts. Includes books.

Also an American edition, published in Philadelphia. American ed. continued by no. 48.

64

The Medical intelligencer; or monthly compendium of medical, chirurgical knowledge; being a review of the contents of the various transactions of learned societies and of the monthly and quarterly journals, English and foreign; forming a concentrated record of medical literature. London, 1–4, 1819–23.

Journals listed by title, with review of contents. Includes book reviews and lists of new books. Selectively reviews a number of non-medical periodicals. Journals reviewed are almost exclusively British or French. Author and subject index to reviews.

65

Medico-chirurgical review. London, 1–4, 1820–24; n.s. 1–47, 1824–47.

Primarily a review of books. No annual author index.

v. 1–4, 1820–24, as *Medico-chirurgical review and journal of medical science*; 1827–44, as *Medico-chirurgical review and journal of practical medicine.* United with no. 58 to form no. 59.

66

Neues Repertorium der gesammten deutschen medicinisch-chirurgischen Journalistik. Leipzig, [1]–21, 1827–47.

Through 1840, German journals listed by title and issue number with selective review of contents. Foreign material, introduced in 1840, listed under subject arrangement, with review. From v. 19, 1845, all material listed under subject.

Monthly through 1844. Irregular 1845–47.

Also in separately numbered series: 1–10, 1827–36; n.s. 1–8, 1837–44; 1–3, 1845–47.

1827–28 annual subject indexes only. Author-subject indexes (General-Register) for other years. Some years have *Supplement-Heft.*

At end of some volumes, *Intelligenz-Blatt und Bibliographie zum allgemeinen Repertorium der gesammten deutschen medizinisch-chirurgischen Journalistik*, consisting of announcements of new publications.

v. 1–18, 1827–44, as *Allgemeines Repertorium . . .*

With v. 14–21, 1840–47, has subtitle: Mit Berücksichtigung des neuesten und wissenswürdigsten aus der ausländischen medizinisch-chirurgischen Journal-Literatur.

67

Nuovo giornale della più recente letteratura medico-chirurgica d'Europa. Milano, 1–11, 1791–96.

Long reviews and extracts of selected books, 15–60 per volume.

68

Repertorisches Jahrbuch für die Leistungen der gesammten Heilkunde. Leipzig, etc., 1–10, 1832–41.

Brief summary of "results" of research; articles and books. Works by 800–1000 authors cited per volume.

v. 1–5, 1832–36, as *Die Leistungen und Fortschritte der Medizin in Deutschland*; v. 6, 1837, *Jahrbuch für die Leistungen der gesammten Heilkunde.* With v. 6, 1837, in two parts: pt. 1, *Die Heilkunde Deutschlands*; pt. 2, *Die Heilkunde des Auslandes.* v. 6, pt. 1, has added t.p., *M. J. Bluff's Uebersicht der Leistungen und Fortschritte der Medicin. Band 9. Sechster Jahrgang, im erweiterten Umfange fortgesetzt von Dr. J. J. Sachs.* v. 6–10, pt. 2, has added t.p., *Uebersicht der vorzüglichsten*

Ergebnisse aus der medicinischen Literatur des Auslandes.

v. 1–6, ed. by M. J. Bluff; v. 7–10, by J. J. Sachs.

69

Summarium des neuesten aus der gesammten Medicin. Leipzig, 1828–31.

3 v. a year (numbered 1–3 for each year; no over-all volume numbers).

1831 contained 1346 numbered abstracts or annotations.

Annual author and subject index for 1828; no indexes 1829–30; 1831, author and subject indexes for each volume.

1828–29 ed. by L. H. Unger and F. A. Klose; 1830 ed. by D. W. H. Busch, L. H. Unger, F. A. Klose; 1831 by D. W. H. Busch and F. L. Meissner.

Superseded by 69.1.

69.1

Summarium des neuesten und wissenswürdigsten aus der gesammten Medicin zum Gebrauche für practische Aerzte und Wundärzte. Leipzig, 1–12, 1832–35; ns 1–24, 1836–43.

3 v. a year. 1843 contained 1299 numbered abstracts or annotations.

Author and subject indexes for each volume.

v. 1–2, 1832, as *Summarium des neuesten aus der in- und ausländischen Medicin*; v. 3–9, 1832–34 . . . *zum Gebrauche praktischer Aerzte* (t.p. of v. 3; issue titles of v. 3, without *zum* . . . .

v. 1–6, 1832–33, ed. by A. F. Haenel; v. 6–9, 1833–34, ed. by W. Friedrich.

Continues no. 69.

70

Wissenschaftliche Uebersicht der gesammten medicinisch-chirurgischen Literatur, 1803–41. In Bibliothek der praktischen Heilkunde. Berlin, 12–86, 1804–43.

Annual review of articles, books, dissertations, new journals. Review section arranged by subject, with references reviewed, varying from 300–1500, listed at end and in numbered sequence. Author index to reviews.

The *Bibliothek* published in 2–3 volumes a year, the *Uebersicht* generally appearing in the second volume; only one volume published for 1840 and 1841. v. 77–86, 1837–43, as *C. W. Hufeland's Bibliothek . . .*

71

A year-book of medicine, surgery, and their allied sciences. London, 1859–64. New Sydenham Society.

Items listed by author at random under subject; then reviewed. Includes books.

INDEXES AND ABSTRACTS, REGIONAL AND NATIONAL

Current

The national indexes, both current and noncurrent, index many minor journals not indexed by the international indexes and hence may be of interest to those wishing to cover in greater depth the medical publications of any given area. Local epidemiology or local medical history are among the subjects covered in this type of index which may not be found elsewhere.

Brazil

72

Bibliografia brasileira de medicina. Rio de Janeiro, etc., 1, 1937/38– .

v. 7, 1958 (published in 1962) lists 3617 references. Includes books and theses.

v. 1–4, 1937/38–1952 [Pt. 1] assuntos, as *Indice-catalogo medico brasileiro.*

v. 1–7, 1937–1958 edited or prepared by Jorge de Andrade Maia.

Bulgaria

73

Abstracts of Bulgarian scientific literature. Medicine and physical culture. Sofia, 1, 1958– . Bulgarian Academy of Sciences. Centre for Scientific Information and Documentation.

Quarterly. Approximately 800–1000 abstracts a year from about 45 Bulgarian journals.

Continues *Abstracts of Bulgarian scientific literature. Biology and medicine* (not listed).

China

74

Science abstracts of China. Medicine. Chung kuo k'o hsueh wen chai. I hsueh. Peking, 1, 1963– . Institute of Scientific and Technical Information of China.

596 English abstracts from the Chinese literature through v. 2, no. 3, 1964.

Colombia

75

Indice medico colombiano. Medellin, 1, 1961– .

Quarterly with annual "Acumulación". The 1962 "Acumulación" lists 1043 references from the Colombian literature.

Czechoslovakia

76
The annual of Czechoslovak medical literature. Praha, 1, 1956– . Státní lékařská knihovna (National Medical Library)

6000–8000 entries a year. Consists of 3 parts: 1. Almanacs and books; 2. Journals; and 3. Works of Czechoslovak authors published abroad. Entries in original language with English translation; most with English abstracts or annotations. Comprehensive coverage of almanacs and books. Only the important journals are indexed (72 in 1957; 77 in 1958; 50 in 1959; and 49 in 1960 and 1961). Not as comprehensive as no. 77.

Items in pt. 3 do not include abstracts or annotations.

No author index prior to 1959.

77
Bibliographia medica Čechoslovaca. Praha, 1, 1947– . Státní ústav pro zdravotnickou dokumentační a knihovnickou službu.

Annual. The most comprehensive index to Czechoslovak books and articles. No abstracts or annotation. Includes works of Czechoslovak authors published abroad. 1958, published in 1963.

Denmark

78
Index medicus danicus. Copenhagen, 1948/49– . Danish Medical Association in collaboration with the Copenhagen University Library, Scientific and Medical Department.

Currently twice a year. About 1500 abstracts a year from Danish medical literature, including works published abroad by Danes, works relating to Denmark, and translations into Danish.

Voluming began in 1950 as v. 1. v. 3, 1954/57– , published as *Danish medical bulletin. Bibliographical supplement.* 1948/49 published in 1955 in author arrangement. For earlier references see history of the *Index* in 1948/49 volume.

Finland

79
Medicina fennica; bibliography of Finnish medicine. Helsinki, 1, 1925– . Sŏmalainen Lääkäriseura Duodecim.

Annual. Abstracts, mostly in English, of literature published in Finland or published abroad by Finnish authors. Author arrangement.

v. 34, 1962, published in 1964, contains about 900 references, most with abstracts.

Hungary

80
Hungarian medical bibliography. Bibliographia medica Hungarica. Budapest, 1961– . National Medical Library and Center for Documentation.

Annual. Books and articles by Hungarian authors published in Hungary or elsewhere irrespective of language, and papers by non-Hungarians in Hungarian periodicals. All entries given in English translation. 1961 contains 3904 entries.

81
Magyar orvosi bibliográfia. Budapest, 1, 1957– . Orvostudományi Dokumentációs Központ.

Monthly. Includes books, congress proceedings, dissertations.

India

82
Index to Indian medical periodicals. New Delhi, 1, 1959– . Directorate General of Health Services. Central Medical Library.

Semiannual. Indexes approximately 118 journals. Pt. 1, Subject index; pt. 2, Author index.

Japan

83
Igaku chuo zasshi. Japana centra revuo medicina. Tokyo, 1, 1903– .

Abstracts most medical and paramedical Japanese journals including those in other languages published in Japan and Japanese territories (1107 in July 1964, including 116 non-Japanese). Author and subject indexes for each volume.

Publication suspended Oct. 1944–Feb. 1956.

84
Japan science review. Medical sciences. Tokyo, 1, 1953– . Science Council of Japan and the Ministry of Education, Japan.

Quarterly. About 10,500 articles a year from approximately 260 journals of which 87 are *Index medicus* titles. Each issue has two sections: 1. Bibliography; 2. Abstracts. Approximately 800 abstracts a year. Beginning in 1962 each volume lists Japanese medical associations, schools, and institutes. Author index.

Lithuania

84.1
Lietuviškoji medicinine bibliografija [Lithuanian medical bibliography] Vilnius, 1959– . Lietuvos TSR Sveikatos Apsaugos Ministerija, Valstybinė Mokslinė Biblioteka.

Literature (including books and dissertations) by Lithuanians published in and outside Lithuania. Includes material about Lithuanian medicine.

v. 1 (1959) covers 1940–57; v. 2 (1963) 5,117 entries, 1958 to 1960; v. 3 (1965) 6,209 entries, 1961 to 1963.

T.p. also in Russian: *Litovskaia meditsinskaia bibliografiia.*

Philippines

85
The Philippine index medicus. Manila, 2, 1917/44– .

v. 1, 1900/16, is a projected volume; v. 3, covers 1945/51.

Poland

86
Polska bibliografia lekarska [Polish medical bibliography] Warszawa, 1925/26– . Główna Biblioteka Lekarska.

Annual. 1959 published in 1966 contained more than 9,200 entries. Includes books. Author and subject entries in a single alphabetical arrangement. Suspended publication 1928–37 and 1939–44.

1925/26 and 1926/27 published by Warszawski Kalendarz Lekarski, 1938 (tom 1–3) by Wydawnictwo Biblioteki Centrum Wyszkolenia Sanitarnego.

1938 quarterly (last quarter not published)

86.1
Przegląd piśmiennictwa lekarskiego polskiego [Survey of Polish medical literature] Warszawa, 1879–1926. Warszawskie Towarzystwo Lekarskie.

Annual. Most entries annotated. 1924 published in 1933; 1926 in 1929.

87
Przegląd piśmiennictwa lekarskiego polskiego [Survey of Polish medical literature] Warszawa, 1, 1963– . Główna Biblioteka Lekarska.

Monthly. Author index of Polish medical journals. Subject index for each issue.

87.1
Warsaw. Państwowy Zakład Wydawnictw Lekarskich. Katalog wydawnictw PZWL [Catalog of publications of the Government Publishing House of Medical Literature] Warszawa, 1950– .

Annual. Includes monographs, textbooks, society publications, health education pamphlets, scripta for students, and translations. Also contains a list of journals issued by the agency. Beginning 1952, each entry abstracted.

Title varies slightly.

Portugal

87.2
Bibliografia médica portuguesa. Lisboa, 1, 1940/44– .

v. 16, 1962/63 contained 2502 references. Voluming begins with v. 4, 1948. From 1945 sponsored by Instituto de Alta Cultura, Centro de Documentaçâo Científica.

Rumania

88
Rumanian medical review. Bucharest, 1957– . Medical Publishing House and Board of Health. Documentation Center.

Quarterly. In English. Includes summaries of selected articles and reviews of medical essays, texbooks, and treatises by Rumanian scientists. Each issue contains about 15 to 20 reviews. Issued also in French with title: *L'information médicale roumaine.*

Spain

88.1
Indice medico español. Valencia, 1965– .

Quarterly. Author arrangement. Index to Spanish periodicals received in the Hemerotica of the Faculty of Medicine of Valenica. The first two issues listed 1,279 numbered entries.

Switzerland

89
Bibliographia medica Helvetica. Basel, 1, 1943– .

v. 12–13, 1954–55, contain 10,725 entries. Includes books. Pt. A. Index; Pt. B. Text.

U.S.S.R.

90
Meditsinskaia literatura SSSR; sistematicheskiĭ ukazatel' knig i zhurnal'nykh stateĭ

[Medical literature of the USSR; systematic index to books and papers published in periodicals] Moskva, 1931– . Ministerstvo zdravookhraneniia SSSR. Gosudarstvennaia tsentral'naia nauchnaia meditsinskaia biblioteka.

The most comprehensive current index to the Soviet medical literature. 1962 (pt. 1) indexed 445 Soviet serials.

1962 (pt. 1 of 2 pts.) published in 1965 (894 p.)

Time lag 2–4 years. Some years may not have been published.

1941–44 volume as *Sovetskaia literatura po meditsine.*

Continues no. 108.

91

Revista de referate din literatura sovietica de specialitate. Bucureşti, 1956– . Academia Republicii Populare Romine, Institutul de Studii Romino-Sovietic.

6 times a year. Selected abstracts of articles from the Soviet literature. In Rumanian. Published in the following series: Biologie, Chirurgie, Igiena si organizare sanitara; Medicina generala; Stiinte medico-biologice; Zootehnie si medicina veterinara. Annual author index.

91.1

Sovetskie knigi po meditsine; katalog dlia zaiavok [Soviet medical books; a catalog for orders] Moskva, Mezhdunarodnaia kniga, 1960 (?)–

Announcement of books planned for publication by Gosudarstvennoe izdatel'stvo meditsinskoĭ literatury (Medgiz).

1964 lists 489 annotated entries with bibliographic data, including number of copies printed and price.

Venezuela

92

Bibliografia medica venezolana. Caracas, 1, 1946– . Ministerio de Sanidad y Asistencia Social.

3 ed. lists 5367 references in a single author-subject alphabetical arrangement; chronological subarrangement under author. Includes lists of 119 books published 1952–58; of abbreviations of the 100 reviews and journals cited; of titles of scientific films produced in the country; of doctors deceased 1952–58.

1 ed., 1946, 705 p. (Publicaciones de la Fundación Biogen, no. 4); 2 ed., 1955, 1041 p.; 3 ed., 1960, 494 p., by Ricardo Archila.

Yugoslavia

93

Medical bibliography. Belgrade, 1, 1964– . Institute for Military Medical Documentation.

Annual? Selective list of articles on medicine from Yugoslavian medical journals. v. 1, 1964, which covers the literature for 1963, contains about 400 references. No special emphasis is given to military medicine.

94

Medicinska knjiga. Katalog medicinskih knjiga [Catalog of medical books] Beograd-Zagreb, 1, 1946– .

Covers medicine, pharmacy and related subjects. Entries frequently annotated. List of periodicals published in Yugoslavia is included.

Title varies slightly.

2 ed. (1955, 1041 p.), covering literature to time of publication, probably supersedes the 1 ed. (705 p.) 3 ed. (1960, 494 p.) lists 5367 references, 1952–58.

INDEXES AND ABSTRACTS, REGIONAL AND NATIONAL

Noncurrent

Belgium

94.1

Archiva medica belgica. Bruxelles, 1–14, 1946–59/60. Association des Sociétés Scientifiques Médicales Belges.

Bimonthly.

In two principal sections: *Bibliographia medica belgica*, abstracts; and *Activités scientifiques des sociétés associées*, a current contents type listing of Belgian medical society serials.

Brazil

95

Annuario medico brasileiro. Rio de Janeiro, 1–12, 1886–97.

Periodical articles, books, theses and reports. Some entries extensively annotated. Includes annual summaries of activities of selected medical institutions. No author index.

Cuba

96

Trelles y Govín, Carlos M. Biblioteca cientifica Cubana. Tomo segundo. Ciencias medicas. Ingenieria. Matanzas, 1919. 505 p.

Includes books, theses. Gives birth and death dates of authors. Some annotations. Engineering p. 380–401. The remainder of the text consists largely of additional medical references in the form of appendices.

Germany

96.1
Geist und Kritik der medicinischen und chirurgischen Zeitschriften Deutschlands für neunzehnte Jahrhundert. Breslau, etc., 1–9, 1798–1806.

Each year in 2 pts. Journals arranged by title and issue with selective review of contents. Cumulative subject indexes for each series of 3 volumes.

1798–1800 as *Geist und Kritik . . . für Aerzte und Wundärzte;* 1801–06 has original title, for most years, as added title.

Voluming differs on t.p. and added t.p.

97
Systematisches Repertorium der gesammten medicinischen Literatur Deutschlands, Marburg, 1825(?)–29.

Abstracts. Includes books. Title on spine: *Busch's systematisches . . .*

Italy

98
Annuario bibliografico italiano delle scienze mediche ed affini. Roma, etc. 1–11, 1916–26.

v. 1, 1916, has *Supplemento.*

99
Bibliografia italiana. Medicina. Roma, 1–16, 1928–43. Consiglio Nazionale delle Ricerche.

1941 contained 6996 entries, most with abstracts.

1928 as *Bibliografia scientifico-tecnica italiana. Gruppo 7. Biologia-Medicina;* 1929–40, *Gruppo B. Medicina.*

99.1
Bibliografia italiana di medicina interna, 1922–28. In Archivio di patologia e clinica medica, 1–8, 1921/22–29.

Annual. 1928 lists 2731 entries from 98 journals. Author index.

99.2
Bibliografia italiana delle scienze mediche. Bologna, 1–2, 1858–59.

Abstracts.

100
Bibliografia medica italiana; riassunto di lavori originali italiani relativi alle scienze mediche. Torino, [1]–3, 1891–93.

101
Bibliografia medico-biologica; rassegna mensile dei libri e della stampa periodica italiana di medicina e biologia. Roma, 1–7, 1939–45.

1939 listed 5212 references, most with abstracts.

102
Rassegna della letteratura medica italiana contemporanea. Napoli, 1, 1892.

Lists in excess of 600 references, most with abstracts.

Japan

103
Abstracts of Japanese medicine. Amsterdam, 1–2, 1960–62. Excerpta Medica Foundation.

Monthly. About 6500 abstracts a year. Beginning in 1963 abstracts of Japanese literature were incorporated in the various sections of *Excerpta medica.*

104
Nippon iji zasshi sakuin [Periodical index of Japanese medical literature] Tokyo, 1892–1918.

105 (not used)

U. S. S. R.

106
Abstracts of Soviet medicine. Amsterdam, 1–5, 1957–61. Excerpta Medica Foundation.

Monthly. About 5000 abstracts a year. Beginning in 1962 abstracts of Soviet literature were incorporated in the various sections of *Excerpta medica.*

107
Die Medizin der Sowjetunion und der Volksdemokratien im Referate. Berlin, 1–11, 1954–64. Dokumentations-Zentrum

für medizinische wissenschaftliche Literatur.

1964, 72 Russian, 38 Polish, 46 Czech, 25 Rumanian, 27 Hungarian, 13 Bulgarian and 1 Chinese journal.

108
Nauchnaia literatura SSSR; sistematecheskiĭ ukazatel' knig i zhurnal'nykh stateĭ, 1928. Meditsina [Scientific literature of the USSR; a systematic index of books and papers published in periodicals, 1928. Medicine] Moskva, Ogiz RSFSR, 1931. [739] 76 p.

11,000 titles, most with annotations.

Continued by no. 90.

109
Sovetskoe meditsinskoe referativnoe obozrenie [Soviet medical abstract review] Moskva, 1948–56.

Abstracts in 15 series, 2 to 4 issues per year for each series. Includes books and dissertations.

Continued by no. 16.

110
Tsentral'nyĭ referativnyĭ meditsinskiĭ zhurnal [Central medical abstract journal]. Moskva, Medgiz, 1928–41.

Monthly. Selective annotated list of books and articles in the Russian language published in the USSR, with abstracts of the more important titles. From 1932 to 1941 it also included abstracts of foreign literature. In 1938 reorganized into four series: 1. Theoretic medicine. 2. Internal disease. 3. Surgery. 4. Microbiology, sanitation, public health.

The only medical abstracting tool in Russian before World War II. Irregular in scope and arrangement. Ceased publication in 1941.

From 1928 to 1935 as *Tsentral'nyĭ meditsinskiĭ zhurnal.*

United States

111
Index to original communications in the medical journals of the United States and Canada . . . classified by subjects and authors. Comp. by Wm. D. Chapin. New York, 1877–78.

Annual. Indexes 65 journals. Citations include month but not volume and page numbers.

REVIEWS

It was considered of use to attempt to distinguish reviews from indexes and abstracts, both here and throughout the special subjects. No doubt the distinction is often tenuous, particularly in the older literature. Special subject reviews are listed under the appropriate subject.

Many of the current English language and polyglot reviews are indexed in nos. 4 and 11 and elsewhere.

112★★
Advances in internal medicine. Chicago, etc., Year Book Medical Publishers, 1, 1942– .

Biennial.

113 (not used)

114★★
Annual review of medicine. Palo Alto, etc., 1, 1950– .

Review articles with bibliographies.

115
Annual review of medicine. 1, 1962– . In Medical world news, 4, 1963– .

Consists of succinct review of progress in various specialties. 1965 included: new legislation (Federal and state), reports from 15 countries, new drugs of 1965, etc.

116
The British encyclopaedia of medical practice . . . Medical progress, London, Butterworths, 1939– .

Annual.

1939–40 as: *Surveys and abstracts.*

117
Cyclopedia of medicine, surgery and specialties. Review service. Philadelphia, Davis, 1936–62.

Annual. 1936–51 as *Revision service* (1941 as *Service volume*)

118
Ergebnisse der inneren Medizin und Kinderheilkunde. Berlin, 1–65, 1908–45; n.F. 1, July 1949– .

Annual.

119
Ergebnisse der medizinischen Grundlagenforschung. Stuttgart, 1, 1956– .

Triennial.

120
Kiso igaku saikīn no shinpo [Recent advances in basic medicine] Tokyo, 1, 1956– .

121
Medical annual; a yearbook of treatment and practitioner's index. London, [1] 1883/4– .

Title varies slightly. Absorbed 2617.1.

122
Medical progress; a review of medical advances, New York, 1952– .

123
Naika saikin no shinpo [Recent advances in internal medicine] Tokyo, 1, 1956– .

Irregular.

124
Quoi de nouveau en pratique médicale? Paris, 1, 1922– .

Annual. v. 1–34, 1922–56, as *Année médicale pratique: médicine, obstétrique, spécialités.*

125
Recent advances in medicine (Beaumont and Dodds) 14 ed. Ed. by D. N. Baron, et al. London, Churchill, 1964. 440 p.

Designed for the general medical reader, and for specialists with interests in current medical practice outside their subject.

Chapter bibliographies (omitting titles of articles). No over-all author index.

1 ed., 1924; 13 ed., 1952.

Translated into Spanish, Italian, Rumanian.

126
The scientific basis of medicine. Annual reviews. London, 1951/52– . British Postgraduate Medical Federation.

[v. 1–8] 1951/52–58/59, as *Lectures on the scientific basis of medicine.*

127★
Year book of medicine. Chicago, Year Book Medical Publishers, 1901– . (The practical medicine year books).

Abstracts, with editorial comment.

1901–32 as *General medicine.*

1901–05 as Practical medicine series of year books; 1906–32, Practical medicine series.

BIBLIOGRAPHIES

International

Published since 1900

128
Bloomfield, Arthur L. A bibliography of internal medicine; selected diseases. Chicago, University of Chicago Press, 1960. 312 p.

Attempts to list every reference of fundamental importance in the development of the literature on auricular fibrillation, coronary occlusion, Stokes-Adams disease, subacute bacterial endocarditis, periarteritis nodosa, pernicious anemia, chlorosis, leukemia, Hodgkin's disease, diabetes mellitus, diabetes insipidus, Addison's disease, Graves' disease, myxedema, tetany, hyperparathyroidism, gout, Bright's disease, bronchial asthma, scurvy, trichinosis. Includes excerpts from publications and annotations.

129
Stern, Neuton S. Rare diseases in internal medicine. Springfield, Thomas, 1966. 572 p.

Consists of 1089 abstracts of journal articles.

Published before 1900

Listed below are some of the better known bibliographies which attempted to index the whole of medicine published up to their day, or for limited time spans. They remain essential for a comprehensive coverage of the earliest literature. A study of these indexes reveals changing patterns in the history of medical bibliography and of medical literature as a whole.

Nos. 130 and 133 are renowned in the history of medical bibliography.

130
Haller, Albrecht von. Bibliotheca medicinae practicae qua scripta ad partem medicinae practicam facientia a rerum initiis ad A. MDCCLXXV recensentur. Basileae, Schweighauser, 1776–88. 4 v.

v. 1. to 1533; v. 2. 1534–1647; v. 3. 1648–85; v. 4. 1686–1707.

Books (libri) of v. 1 are entitled; Graeci, Arabes, Arabistae, Instauratores; books of other volumes are named after Schools (Chemici, Schola Hippocratica), century (Seculum XVII only) or representative physician of a given period. Within chapters subarrangements are by person (entered under the date of his thesis or first known writing) or by form, such as journal (diaria) with selected contents, theses, language, or country. Essentially a chronological arrangement (by year or more inclusive time spans). Contains brief biographical information and frequent descriptive or critical comments on works cited. Journal citations are primarily to the *Philosophical Transactions of the Royal Society* (London).

Author index in v. 4. No subject index. Addenda, no. 132.1

See also by the same author nos. 866, 970, 2556.

131
Lipenius, Martinus. Bibliotheca realis medica, omnium materiarum, rerum, et titulorum, in universa medicina occurentium. Francofurti ad Moenum, 1679. 492, [42] p.

Covers from the beginning of printing. Arranged alphabetically by detailed subjects. Subject arrangement includes some title entries for collected works and serials and some form entries (consilia, dictionaries, theses, etc.) Occasionally indexes parts of books.

132
Manget, Jean J. Bibliotheca scriptorum medicorum veterum et recentiorum. Genève, Perachon & Cramer, 1731. 4 pt. in 2 v.

Biographic notes, synopsis of contents, or lengthy quotations from books and periodical articles cited are frequently given. Not so comprehensive as no. 130.

132.1
Murr, Christoph G. von. Adnotationes ad bibliothecas Hallerianas botanicam, anatomicam, chirurgicam et medicinae practicae. Erlangae, Palm, 1805. 67 p.

Additions and corrections to nos. 130, 866, 970, 2556.

133
Ploucquet, Wilhelm G. Literatura medica digesta sive repertorium medicinae practicae, chirurgiae atque rei obstetriciae. Tubingae, apud J. G. Cottam, 1808–09. 4 v. Cont. et suppl. I. Tubingae, apud auctorem, 1813. 226 p.

Subject index to books and periodicals. Frequently indexes in detail selected monographs or books dating from the beginning of printing.

Supersedes the earlier edition, *Initia bibliothecae medico-practicae et chirurgicae*, 1793–97, with its continuation and supplement, 1799–1803 (not listed separately).

No author index.

134
Sprengel, Kurt. Kritische Uebersicht des Zustandes der Arzneykunde in dem letzten Jahrzehend. Halle, 1801. 547 p.

Review of principal publications, 1790–1800, arranged by subject under each year. Author and subject indexes.

135
——. Literatura medica externa recentior seu enumeratio librorum . . . qui extra Germaniam ab anno inde 1750 impressi sunt. Lipsiae, 1829. 630 p.

8243 numbered entries. Includes books, theses, and periodical titles.

Manuals of Bibliography

Published since 1900

The items listed below are for the most part bibliographies of medical bibliography. They frequently provide some discussion of the nature and utility of the items included, rather than mere listing of references.

136
Academia Republicii Populare Romîne. Biblioteca. Ghid de documentare în stiinţele medicale. [Bucharest] 1959. 131 p.

137
Gnucheva, Vera V. Putevoditel' po inostrannoĭ bibliografii meditsinskoĭ literatury (1945–1956) [Guide to foreign bibliographies of medical literature (1945–1956)] Leningrad, Gos. publich. biblioteka im. M.E. Saltykova-Shchedrina, 1957. 108 p.

213 publications listed.

138
——. Putevoditel' po meditsinskim spravochnikam [Guide to medical reference books] Leningrad, Gos. publich. biblioteka im. Saltykova-Shchedrina, 1959. 111 p.

299 annotated references, 1949–58.

139
Kricker, Gottfried. Die Schrifttumsnachweise der Medizin: Übersicht über Handbücher, Bibliographien, Referatenblätter und sonstige Literaturquellen. 3 ed. Leipzig, Barth, 1944. 105 p.

992 annotated citations.

140
Malclès, Louise N. Les sources du travail bibliographique. T. 3. Bibliographies spécialisées (sciences exactes et techniques). Genève, 1958. 575 p.

Lists principal monographs, treatises, and bibliographies in the history of science, the physical and biological sciences, the preclinical sciences, and medicine and its specialties.

140.1
Trenkov, Khristo Iordanov. Meditsinskata bibliografiia v pomoshch na nauchnite rabotnitsi [Medical bibliography; an aid to scientific workers] Sofiia, Durzhavno izd-vo "Nauka i izkustvo", 1956. 114 p.

A textbook of medical bibliography. Describes principal reference tools published in Europe and the United States.

140.2
Zamkova, Zinaida N. Bibliografiia v nauchnoĭ i prakticheskoĭ rabote vracha [Bibliography for a physician's scientific and practical work] Moskva, Medgiz, 1963. 159 p.

Primarily Russian but includes some foreign literature.

Published before 1900

141
Hahn, Lucien. Essai de bibliographie médicale; étude analytique des principaux répertoires bibliographiques concernant les sciences médicales; de leur utilité dans les recherches scientifiques. Paris, Steinheil, 1897. 206 p.

142
Rothe, Immanuel V. Handbuch für die medizinische Litteratur . . . Leipzig, 1799. 664 p.

Includes books, theses, dictionaries, biographies.

143
Young, Thomas. An introduction to medical literature, including a system of practical nosology, intended as a guide to students, and an assistant to practitioners. 2 ed. London, 1823. 658 p.

Includes books, journal articles, and selected theses. Author and subject indexes. Occasional comments on references.

BIBLIOGRAPHIES

Regional and National

Brazil

143.1
Índice-catálogo médico Paulista 1860–1936. Organizado pelo . . . Jorge de Andrade Maia. S. Paulo, 1938. 640 p.

Dictionary catalog of material published (with a few exceptions) in the state of St. Paulo. Includes books, theses.

Bulgaria

144
Bulgarska Akademiia na naukite. Tsentralna biblioteka. Bibliografiia na bulgarskata meditsinska knizhnina, 1944-1956. Compiled by L. Karaminova-Tsatcheva, S. Danev, and B. Bojilov. Sofiia, 1963. 562 p.

9791 references to the Bulgarian literature published in Bulgaria and abroad. Table of contents and subject index in English and Bulgarian. Title pages in English and Bulgarian.

Colombia

144.1
Asociación Colombiana de Facultades de Medicina. Indice de la literatura médica colombiana, 1890–1960. Recopilada por . . . Beatriz Cespedes J., et al. Bogotá, Ediciones Tercer Mundo, 1965. 305 p.

7528 entries from 58 periodicals.

Denmark

145
Preisler, Oscar C. S. Bibliotheca medica Danica; fortegnelse over den danske mediciniske literatur fra de aeldste tider til 1913. Lyngby, 1916–19. 7 v.

v. 7 Registerbind.

145.1
Winther, Mathias. Bibliotheca Danorum medica; sive, Plenus conspectus litterarum medicarum et hisce affinium in Dania, Norvegia, Holsatia usque ad annum 1832. Hafniae, Sumptibus Librariae Wahlianae, Typis Graebii & Filii, 1832. 304 p.

Alphabetical subject bibliography. Includes books and articles. Occasionally cites reviews. No index of authors.

East Africa

145.2
Langlands, B. W., comp. Bibliography of the distribution of disease in East Africa. Makerere, Uganda, Makerere University College, 1965. 184 p. (Makerere Library publ. no. 3)

1335 entries through 1963. Arranged by region: East Africa (general), Kenya, Uganda, Tanganyika and subregions with diseases and citations listed under geographic entities.

Ecuador

146
Rolando L., Carlos A. Bibliografia medica ecuatoriana. Guayaquil, 1953. 387, 55 p.

Estonia

147
Norman, Herbert. Eesti meditiiniline bibliografia. Bibliographie médicale estonienne. Tartu, 1932–33. 217, 128 p.

v. 1, 1918–30, 4415 items; v. 2, 1931–32, 2373 items. Author arrangement.

Finland

148
Hjelt, Otto E. A. Finlands medicinska bibliografe, 1640–1900, systematiskt ordnad. Helsingfors, Helsingfors Centraltryckeri, 1905. 497 p.

Includes books and articles by Finnish authors, and by foreign authors published in Finland. Indexes of authors and translators, with dates and brief identifications of Finnish authors. No subject index.

149
Suomen Lääketieteellinen Bibliografia 1901–1955. Ed. by H. M. Kauppi. Helsinki, Societas Medicorum Fennica Duodecim, 1960. 759 p.

14,895 references by Finnish physicians in and outside of Finland. Excludes writings by nonphysicians and popular works for laymen.

Germany

149.1
Engelmann, Wilhelm. Bibliotheca medico-chirurgica et anatomico-physiologica. Alphabetisches Verzeichniss der medizinischen, chirurgischen, geburtshülflichen, anatomischen und physiologischen Bücher, welche vom Jahre 1750 bis zu Ende des Jahres 1847 in Deutschland erschienen sind . . . Sechste gänzlich umgearbeitete Auflage der Bibliotheca medico-chirurgica von [Theodor-Christian Friedrich] Enslin. Leipzig, Engelmann, 1848. 740 p.

149.2
——. Supplement-Heft. Enthaltend die Literatur vom Jahre 1848 bis Ende des Jahres 1867. Leipzig, Engelmann, 1868. 350 p.

150
Pfeiffer, Louis. Universal-Repertorium der deutschen medizinischen, chirurgischen und obstetrizischen Journalistik des 19. Jahrhunderts. Cassel, Krieger, 1833. 2 v.

References from 34 journals. Subjects include place names and a few personal names. Author indicates intent to supplement no. 133.

Ghana

150.1
Hughes, H. H. Medical bibliography of the Gold Coast 1900–1951. Accra, Govt. Print. Dept., 1953. 27, 2 p.

380 entries listed by author. Includes reports. Addendum of 33 entries covering 1950–53.

Great Britain

151
British medical book list. London, 1, 1950– . British Council, Medical Department.

Monthly. Lists books, pamphlets, new journals, official publications, brochures, and reports from voluntary organizations. Arranged alphabetically by author.

Hungary

151.1
Katona, András. Altalános belgyógyászat (nephrologia, allergologia, toxicologia, néhány fertözöbetegség) magyar bibliográfiája (1945–1960) [Hungarian bibliography of general internal medicine (nephrology, allergology, toxicology and some infectious diseases) 1945–1960] Budapest, Országos Orvostudományi Könyvtár és Dokumentációs Központ, 1966. 243 p.

2383 references. Some German and English titles cited.

Iran

152
Nadjmabadi, Mahmoud, comp. A bibliography of printed books in Persian on medicine and allied subjects. v. 1, Titles of books. Tehran, 1964. 922 columns.

Text in Persian.

Israel

153
Jerusalem. S. Syman Public Health Library. Israel medical bibliography. Jerusalem 1948/59- .

Includes papers by Israeli authors published in Israel or abroad and a selection of theses of the Hadassah medical and dental schools.

1948/59 (published in 1964) 13,907 entries; 1960/61, 4077 entries. Nadia Levenberger, comp.

Italy

154
Dieci anni di bibliografia medica italiana, 1947–1956. Torino, Minerva Medica, 1958. 77 p. (Minerva medicobibliografica, anno 6, Supplemento al no. 1, April 1958).

Author list. Subject index.

155–156 (not used)

Poland

157
Wykaz oryginalnych prac lekarskich polskich za czas od r. 1831 do 1890 włacznie [Register of original Polish medical works from the period of 1831 to 1890, inclusive] Warszawa, Kowalewski, 1896. 1015 p.

Continues and, in part, supplements no. 622. Over 12,000 items. Includes books. Coverage does not include medical botany, pharmacy, veterinary medicine, or balneology.

158 (not used)

U.S.S.R.

159
Gnucheva, Vera V. Bibliografiia sovetskoĭ meditsinskoĭ bibliografii (1917–1957 gg.) [Bibliography of Soviet medical bibliographies (1917–1957)] Leningrad, Gos. publich. biblioteka im. M. E. Saltykova-Shchedrina, 1958. 118 p.

Selective annotated list of 412 bibliographies.

160
Mul'tanovskiĭ, M. P. Russkaia meditsinskaia pechat'; bibliograficheskie materialy 1792–1929 [Russian medical publications; bibliographic materials, 1792–1929] Leningrad, Gos. izd-vo, 1930. 80 p.

921 entries, chiefly in Russian. In 3 parts: bibliographies of medicine in general; bibliographies of medical specialties; other bibliographic materials (periodical indexes, indexes to society publications, publisher's catalog, journals devoted to announcement of new books, and catalogs published by medical libraries).

161
Nevskiĭ, V. A. Meditsina v Tadzhikistane; bibliograficheskiĭ ukazatel' literatury po istorii i sovrem. sostoianiiu meditsiny i zdravookhraneniia v Tadzhik. SSR [Medicine in Tadzhikistan; bibliographic index to literature on the history and current status of medicine and public health in the Tadzhik SSR] Pod red. V. S. Vail'. Stalinabad, Ministerstvo zdravookhraneniia Tadzhik. SSR, 1959. 381 p.

4329 references to books, journal and newspaper articles, collected works, and dissertations published in Russian or Tadzhik from about 1700 to 1957.

162
Růžička, Karel. Bibliografie referátů uveřejněných v letech 1945–1950 v československém odborném tisku o sovětských publikacích lékařských a zdravotnických [Bibliography of reviews published from 1945 to 1950 in the Czechoslovak professional periodicals on the Soviet medical and health literature] Praha, 1952. 248 p.

About 2500 reviews.

163 (not used)

164
U. S. National Library of Medicine. Guide to Russian medical literature. Ed. by Scott Adams and Frank B. Rogers. Washington, 1958. 88 p. (Public Health Service. Publication no 602).

165
Zamkova, Zinaida N. Otechestvennaia meditsinskaia bibliografiia [National medical bibliography] Moskva, 1962. 2 pts. in 1 v.

GEORGIAN SSR

166
Tbilisskiĭ gosudarstvennyĭ meditsinskiĭ institut. Nauchnaia literatura Gruzii. Meditsina, 1921–1947gg.; bibliograficheskiĭ spravochnik [Scientific literature of Georgia. Medicine, 1921–1947; bibliographic reference book] Sostavili E. A. Vachnadze i T. B. Dzhaparidze-Iosidze. Tbilisi, Gruzmedgiz, 1951. 493 p.

7196 references to works by Georgian authors published in and outside Georgia.

In Georgian and Russian. Does not cover physiology. Includes list of Georgian periodicals.

United States

167
Guerra, Francisco. American medical bibliography 1639–1783; a chronological and critical and bibliographical study of books, pamphlets, broadsides, and articles in periodical publications relating to the medical sciences: medicine, surgery, pharmacy, dentistry, and veterinary medicine; printed in the present territory of the United States of America during the British dominion and the Revolutionary War. New York, L. C. Harper, 1962. 885 p. (Yale Univ. School of Medicine. Dept. of the History of Medicine. Publication no. 40)

Must be used with caution: title transcriptions inaccurate and newspaper index so incomplete as to be misleading. Chiefly useful as finding tool.

168
U. S. National Institutes of Health. Office of Research Information. National Institutes of Health scientific directory 1965 and annual bibliography 1964. Bethesda, 1965. 208 p. (Public Health Service. Publication no. 1290. Bibliography Series no. 58)

Arranged by institute and division, with the directory and bibliography entries combined at the laboratory or branch level within each institute or division.

169★
U. S. National Library of Medicine. Early American medical imprints: a guide to works printed in the United States, 1668–1820. By Robert B. Austin. Washington, 1961. 240 p.

Lists monographs and serial titles, alphabetically by author. 2105 items, with locations. Chronological index.

170
U. S. Public Health Service. Public Health Service numbered publications; a catalog, 1950–1962. Washington, 1964. 190 p. (Public Health Service. Publication no. 1112. Bibliography Series no. 55, June 1964)

170.1
——. Supplement no. 1, 1963–1964. Washington, 1965. 114 p. (Public Health Service. Publication no. 1112. Suppl. no. 1, 1963–1964. Bibliography Series no. 55)

Viet-Nam

171
Noyer, B. Bibliographie analytique des travaux scientifiques en Indochine, 1939–1940–1941 (sciences medicales et veterinaires). Hanoi, Imprimerie d'Extrême-Orient, 1943. 48 p.

More than 800 citations, some with annotations.

Published by the Conseil des Recherches Scientifiques de l'Indochine.

172
Viet-Nam. Centre National de la Recherche Scientifique. Bulletin analytique des travaux scientifiques publiés au Viet-Nam. v. 1, 1942/62. Sect. 1. Médecine et sciences affiliées. By Nguyên-Hii'u and Vũ-Văn-Nguyên. Saigon, Service de Documentation, 1964. 160 p.

1494 entries, most with annotations. Indexes 11 serials and lists without annotation doctoral theses presented at Hanoi and Saigon. Omits military medicine. Does not index *Revue medico-chirurgicale des forces armées d'extrême-orient* (1952–55) published by the French in Viet-Nam.

Continues no. 171.

Yugoslavia

173
Grmek, Mirko D. Hrvatska medicinska bibliografija; opis tiskanih knjiga i članaka s područja humane i veterinarske medicine

i farmacije, koji se odnose na Hrvatsku [Bibliographia medica Croatica; descriptio librorum articulorumque de humana, veterinaria medicina pharmaceuticeque spectantium ad Croatiam] Zagreb, 1955– .

Lists publications by Croatians, printed in Croatia, or relating to Croatia. Pt. 1, Books, 1470–1875, 230 p. 1003 references arranged by author with brief biographical data and annotations. Locates copies. Includes many Latin dissertations.

174
Jeremić, Risto. Bibliografija srpske zdravstvene književnosti 1757–1918 [Bibliography of Serbian medical literature, 1757–1918] Beograd, 1947. 223 p.

Lists 4748 books and articles written by Serbs or other nationals in Serbia. Includes serials of the Serbian Medical Association, hospital reports, congress proceedings, etc. Chiefly in Serbian, but includes some works in other languages.

175
Ristić, V. K. Medicinska bibliografija FNR Jugoslavije, 1944–1953 god [Medical bibliography of the Federation of National Republics of Yugoslavia, 1944–1953] Beograd-Zagreb, Medicinska knjiga, 1955. 357 p.

Indexes 56 Yugoslav periodicals and serials.

TRANSLATIONS

Indexes and Abstracts

176★
U. S. National Library of Medicine. Bibliography of medical translations. Washington, [1]-3, 1959–66.

Irregular. Subject arrangement of translations selected by the Clearinghouse for Federal Scientific and Technical Information, U. S. Department of Commerce, from its *Technical Translations*. Each issue contains an author index, original source index, and a directory of sources.

v. 1, Jan. 1959–June 1962, prepared by the U. S. Department of Commerce, Office of Technical Services.

Collections

177
Federation proceedings. Translation supplement; selected translations from medical-related science. Washington, 1963-66. Federation of American Societies for Experimental Biology, under contract with the National Library of Medicine.

Bimonthly. Contains approximately 300 translations a year and lists approximately 300 unpublished translations of articles selected exclusively from the Russian and East European research literature. Includes occasional notices of other sources of foreign literature available in the English language.

Comprises pt. 2, *Federation proceedings*, v. 22–25, 1963–66.

Directories

178
Translators and translations: services and sources in science and technology. New York, 1, 1959– . Special Libraries Association.

Lists individuals and commercial translating firms; data include: names, addresses, telephone numbers, subject and language proficiencies; describes pools and other sources of translation information; cites bibliographies and lists of translated literature.

2 ed. 1965.

THESES

There is no current comprehensive index to medical theses. Listed below are a few publications which include theses of a medical and paramedical interest. There are similar lists for other countries (France, Switzerland, etc.), and individual universities publish their own lists.
Older dissertations are indexed in the *Index-catalogue* and a number of other indexes listed in the present work. The inclusion of theses in these is generally noted in the annotations. Nos. 184 and 185 are two of the most comprehensive older lists of theses.

Current

179
American doctoral dissertations. Ann Arbor, University Microfilms, Inc. etc., 1, 1933/34– .

Annual. Currently a complete listing of all doctoral dissertations accepted by American and Canadian universities. Compiled from commencement programs issued by universities.

Lists a number of dissertations not included in no. 180.

Same subject coverage as no. 180.

Issued as no. 13, Index, of each volume of *Dissertation abstracts*, v. 16, 1955/56– (except v. 18, no. 7, Index, 1957/58). Issues for 1955/56 and 1956/57 combined with index to *Dissertation abstracts*, v. 16 and 17.

1933/34–1954/55 as *Doctoral dissertations accepted by American universities*; 1955/56–1962/63 as *Index to American doctoral dissertations*.

180

Aslib. Index to theses accepted for higher degrees in the universities of Great Britain and Ireland. London, 1, 1950/51– .

Includes M.D., Ph.D., M.A. and other theses in the basic, biological, and health sciences.

181

Dissertation abstracts; abstracts of dissertations and monographs in microfilm. Ann Arbor, University Microfilms, Inc., 1, 1938– .

Monthly. Currently a compilation of abstracts of doctoral dissertations submitted to University Microfilms, Inc. by more than 140 institutions.

Includes Ph.D. theses in the basic biological and health sciences.

v. 1–11, 1938–51 as *Microfilm abstracts;* a collection of abstracts of doctoral dissertations and monographs available in complete form on microfilm.

182

Jahresverzeichnis der deutschen Hochschulschriften. Leipzig, etc. 1885– .

Includes theses in medicine and allied sciences. Arranged by university.

183

Moscow. Gosudarstvennaia biblioteka SSSR im. V. I. Lenina. Katalog kandidatskikh dissertatsiĭ postupivshikh v biblioteku im. V. I. Lenina i Gosudarstvennuiu tsentral'nuiu nauchnuiu meditsinskuiu biblioteku [Index to candidate dissertations received in V. I. Lenin Library and in the National Central Scientific Medical Library] Moskva, 1957?– .

Medicine is usually Chapter 11. 1962 volume listed over 2000 medical dissertations.

Noncurrent

184

Doering, Sebastian J. L. Critisches Repertorium der auf in- und ausländischen höhern Lehranstalten vom Jahre 1781 bis 1800 herausgekommenen Probe- und Einladungsschriften aus dem Gebiete der Arzneygelahrtheit und Naturkunde. Erste Abtheilung, enthaltend das Verzeichniss der Schriften von 1781 bis 1790. Herborn, Hohe-Schulbuchhandlung, 1803. xvi, 412 p.

2794 theses and other academic publications, with summaries and critical notes and references to reviews. Index of the 70 academies and universities covered, with citations arranged by year. Index of authors; subject indexes in Latin and German.

185

Heffter, Johann K. Museum disputatorum physico-medicum tripartitum. Zittaviae Lusatorum, Apud J J. Schoepsium, 1756–64. 2 v.

18,498 European theses of the 16th–18th centuries listed.

Each vol. in 3 parts, the first and main part an alphabetical list under praeses, the second an index of subjects, and the third an index of respondents; theses without praeses are listed in the first part under authors.

v. 1. reissued 1763.

CONGRESSES

No. 188 is probably the most comprehensive current list of medical congresses and meetings published. Since it is not exhaustive the other lists are useful as supplementary tools. No. 186 is believed to be the only frequently issued publication listing material published by congresses. Individual journals are, of course, a source of information for congresses in special fields.

Current

186

Annual international congress calendar. Belgium, 1960/61– . Union of International Associations.

Chronological list of scheduled international

congresses, meetings, symposia, etc. Date, place, address of organizing body, theme, estimated number of participants, concurrent exhibition (if any) and plans for publishing are indicated; subject and geographical indexes. Approximately 10 percent of the items are of medical interest.

Monthly supplements in: *International associations; monthly review of international organizations and meetings.* Bruxelles.

187
Bibliographical current list of papers, reports, and proceedings of international meetings. Brussels, 1, 1961– . Union des Associations Internationales, Brussels.

Monthly. An average of 10 items of medical interest each issue.

188
JAMA reference directories. Meetings in the United States. [Meetings outside the United States] In Journal of the American Medical Association, 183, 1963– .

Meetings in the United States are published in full in the first issue of *JAMA* for each month; meetings outside in the second issue.

Before 1963 published without distinctive titles.

189★
Scientific meetings, describing future meetings of technical, scientific, medical and management organizations and universities. New York, 1, Spring 1957– . Special Libaries Association.

Three times a year. The basic issue appears in January with supplements in May and September. Alphabetical and chronological listings.

190★
U. S. Library of Congress. General Reference and Bibliography Division. World list of future international meetings. Washington, 1959/62– .

Monthly. In two parts: pt. 1, Science, technology, agriculture, medicine; pt. 2, Social, cultural, commercial and humanistic. Issues for March, June, September, and December list all international meetings scheduled for the ensuing 3 years. Intervening issues list new meetings, and changes. Arranged chronologically. Includes subject, sponsor and geographical indexes.

Supersedes no. 194.

190.1
What goes on [series]

Monthly. Information on meetings, postgraduate courses, and in the New York–New Jersey publication, medical programs on radio and television. Usually gives speakers and titles of addresses. Issued in the following [sections]:

Alaska, Arizona, Colorado, Idaho, Montana, Neveda, New Mexico, Oregon, Utah, Washington, Wyoming. Published from the Offices of the Rocky Mountain Medical Journal. 1959?– .

Connecticut, Maine, Massachusetts, New Hampshire, Rhode Island, Vermont. Postgraduate Medical Institute. 1954?– .

New York, New Jersey. Medical society of the State of New York. 1958?– .

In North Carolina, South Carolina and Virginia. Duke University Medical Center. 1965?– .

In Texas medicine and dentistry. Compiled by the University of Texas. Graduate School of Biomedical Sciences at Houston. 1958?– .

Noncurrent

191
Bishop, William J. Bibliography of international congresses of medical sciences. Bibliographie des Congrès internationaux des sciences médicales. Springfield, Ill., Thomas, 1958. 238 p.

Lists 363 individual congresses.

192
Congresses. Tentative chronological and bibliographical reference list of national and international meetings of physicians, scientists, and experts. In Index-Catalogue of the Library of the Surgeon General's Office (U. S. Army Medical Library) [now National Library of Medicine]. Washington. ser. 4, v. 3, 1938. 295 p. Suppl. 1, Index-Catalogue, ser. 4, v. 4, 1939. p. 29–51.

Lists 1811 individual congresses, but many are nonmedical.

See no. 29.

192.1
Paris. Université. Faculté de médecine. Bibliothèque. Catalogue des congrès, colloques et symposia intéressant les sciences médicales et biologiques. 2 ed. By Janine Samion-Contet. [Paris, 1963] 623 p.

Congresses listed under 1293 key words and then chronologically. Includes publications in journals.

193
Stümke, Hans. Bibliographie der interna-

tionalen medizinischen Kongresse und Verbande. Leipzig, Harrasowitz, 1939. 281 p. Added t.p.: Bibliographie der internationalen Kongresse und Verbande in der Preussischen Staatsbibliotek . . . Bd. 1. Medizin.

Includes a number of national and regional congresses and meetings of other organizations. Lists more than 338 individual congresses.

194
U. S. National Science Foundation. List of international and foreign scientific and technical meetings. Washington, Oct. 1952–Jan. 1959.

Superseded by no. 190.

DICTIONARIES

Abbreviations

195
Medical abbreviations; a cross reference dictionary. Comp. by the Special Studies Committee of the Michigan Occupational Therapy Association. [Ann Arbor] 1961. 241 p.

Pt. 1, abbreviations; pt. 2, meaning of abbreviations; includes list of symbols.

196★
Peyser, Alfred. Pars pro toto; breviarium medicum internationale. Stockholm, Almqvist & Wiksell, 1950. 196 p.

Abbreviations currently employed in English, German, Danish, French, Spanish, Italian, Swedish, and Latin, also those of international significance. Indicates language of origin and subject field of terms.

197
Steen, Edwin B. Dictionary of abbreviations in medicine and the related sciences. Philadelphia, Davis, 1960. 102 p.

List of medical abbreviations alphabetically arranged. Includes various societies, organizations, and government agencies having a relationship to medicine. Includes a limited number of journal abbreviations.

Etymology

198
Agard, Walter R., and Howe, Herbert M. Medical Greek and Latin at a glance. 3 ed. New York, Hoeber, 1955. 96 p.

Contains about a thousand Greek and Latin words used in forming scientific terms; intended for the medical undergraduate. Gives verb roots, prefixes, and suffixes; lists of combining forms arranged according to body system.

199
Bollo, Louise E. Introduction to medicine and medical terminology. Philadelphia, Saunders, 1961. 356 p.

Written for the student. Principles of medical terminology and disease classification, with lists of prefixes and suffixes and stems connected with selected diseases; includes alphabetical list of medical words and stems.

200
Flood, Walter E. Scientific words; their structure and meaning. New York, Duell, Sloan and Pearce, 1960. 220 p.

Glossary listing about 1150 roots, prefixes, and suffixes entering into the formation of scientific terms; meaning of each element and its origin given.

201
Frenay, Sister Mary Agnes Clare. Understanding medical terminology. 3 ed. St. Louis, Mo., Catholic Hospital Association [1964] 246 p.

Each chapter devoted to a specialty; gives anatomical, diagnostic, operative, and symptomatic terms, abbreviations.

202
Harned, Jessie M. Medical terminology made easy. Chicago, Physicians' Record Co., 1951. 275 p.

Groups words around anatomic system with use in sample case records. List of abbreviations, medical equivalents of lay terms.

203★
Jaeger, Edmund C. A source-book of medical terms. Springfield, Ill., Thomas, 1953. 145 p.

An alphabetical list of word elements, combining forms, prefixes and suffixes, with emphasis on etymology. Gives basic principles for the construction of synthesis of words. Occasional historical information and illustrations.

204★
Pepper, Oliver H. Medical etymology; the history and derivation of medical terms for students of medicine, dentistry, and nursing. Philadelphia, Saunders, 1949. 263 p.

Divided into preclinical and clinical subjects and dentistry. Greek and Latin derivations indicated and explained.

205
Roberts, Ffrangcon. Medical terms, their origin and construction. 4 ed. London, Heinemann, 1966. 96 p.

Discusses word derivation and construction; lists Greek and Latin combining forms, English meaning, and examples. Intended for medical students and other health workers. Index.

206★★
Skinner, Henry A. The origin of medical terms. 2 ed. Baltimore, Williams & Wilkins, 1961. 447 p.

4000 terms; includes illustrations and biographical sketches.

207
Smith, G. I., and Davis, P. E. Medical terminology: a programmed text. New York, Wiley, 1963. 1 v. (various pagings)

Main part consists of medical term column with answer column opposite; contains sections on prefixes and suffixes and review sheets. Intended for students in medicine and related fields.

208
Wain, Harry. The story behind the word; some interesting origins of medical terms. Springfield, Ill., Thomas, 1958. 342 p.

More than 5700 medical terms; includes biographies.

Syndromes

209
Aimes, Alexandre. Maladies et syndromes rares ou peu connus; description clinique, repertoire des signes et liste des noms propres. 3 ser. Paris, Masson, 1964. 333 p.

Arranged by medical specialty; includes one or more citations of the literature.

210★★
Durham, Robert H. Encyclopedia of medical syndromes. New York, Hoeber, 1960. 628 p.

Gives clinical manifestations, pathologic findings, etiology, clinical course, and treatment; includes synonyms and one or more citations to the literature. Less inclusive than no. 213.

211
Fejgin, Mieczyslaw, ed. Leksykon zespołów i objawów chorobowych. Współautorzy: Zbigniew Bochenck and others. Wyd. 1, Warszawa, Państwowy Zakład Wydawn. Lekarskich, 1959. 253 p.

Dictionary of approximately 2000 eponyms; origin usually given. Latin name, often with French or English equivalent, and a short explanation in Polish. In most cases the source of information is cited (journal article or book).

212
Gorlin, Robert J., and Pindborg, Jens J. Syndromes of the head and neck. New York, McGraw-Hill [1964] 580 p.

Includes about 150 symptom complexes involving oral structures. Gives manifestations, laboratory aids, and differential diagnosis. Bibliographies.

213★
Leiber, Bernfried, and Olbrich, Gertrud. Wörterbuch der klinischen Syndrome. 3 ed. München, Urban & Schwarzenberg, 1963. 966 p.

Alphabetical listing of syndromes; for each gives synonyms, definitions, original investigator, symptoms, etiology, differential diagnosis, and citations to the literature. Contains synonym index and extensive symptom index.

214
Purjész, Béla. A belgyógyászat és határterületeinek syndromái [The syndromes of internal medicine and its related subjects] Budapest, Medicina Könyvkiado, 1965. 992 p.

214.1
Unghváry, László. Taschenbuch der Krankheitssyndrome. Budapest, Akadémiai Kiadó, 1966. 354 p.

Synonyms, definitions, and symptoms for some 1100 syndromes. No references.

Translation of *Betegség-syndromák zsebkönyve* (1962)

General Medical

Only English–foreign language, foreign language–English general medical dictionaries and those wholly in a given language (e.g., German-German) are listed below. Subject dictionaries are listed under subject. For the most part older medical dictionaries have not been listed.

Afrikaans

215
Mönnig, Hermann O. Voorlopige geneeskundige woordelys. In medewerking met. F. Z. van der Merwe [en] J. D. Louw. 3 ed. Pretoria, Suid-Afrikaanse Akademie vir Wetenskap en Kuns, 1956. 256 p.

South African equivalents for English medical (and some nonmedical) terms.

Arabic

216
Sharaf, Mohammad. An English-Arabic dictionary of medicine, biology, and allied sciences. Cairo, Government Press, 1928. 971 p.

At head of title: Ministry of Education, Egypt. Cover has 1929.
See also no. 309.

Bulgarian

217
Arnaudov, Georgi D. Meditsinsko-farmatsevticheski naruchnik. 2 ed. Sofiia, Nauka i izkustvo, 1951. 831 p.

Medico-pharmaceutical terms and names of drugs in Latin followed by the Bulgarian equivalent, which is defined or described. Country of origin is given for foreign drugs. At end of volume are lists of Bulgarian and Russian terms with Latin equivalent.

218
Meditsinski entsiklopedichen rechnik. Sofiia, Lekarska kooperatsiia. 1, 1949- .

Encyclopedic medical dictionary in Bulgarian. Many Latin equivalents given. Includes eponyms and brief biographies.

219(not used)

Chinese

220
Cousland, Philip Brunelleschi. Kao shih i hsüeh tz'u hui [Cousland's medical lexicon] 12 ed. T'ai-pei, Wu chou ch'u pan shê, 1960. 588 p.

English-Chinese dictionary revised to include names of new drugs and current terms in dentistry, hematology, parasitology, and immunology. Chinese terms given in Chinese characters. Includes list of special characters, abbreviations used in prescriptions, tables of weights and measures.

221
Ho, Huai-tê, and T'ien, Li-chih. O ying chung i hsüeh tzŭ hui [Russian-English-Chinese medical dictionary. 1 ed.] Peiping, Jên-min-wei-shêng-chu'u-pan-shê, 1954. 714 p.

Russian terms followed by equivalents in English and Chinese (in Chinese characters); covers medicine and allied fields including pharmacy; contains section on Russian drug terms; supplement includes list of Russian prefixes and suffixes.

222
La, ying, chung wên tui chao i hsüeh ming t'zŭ hui pien. Latin-English-Chinese dictionary of medical terms. Hong Kong [Shih yung-k'o, chu-pan-she, 1961] 761 p.

Chiefly Latin terms followed by the English and Chinese translation in the simplified characters. Includes some dental and botanical terms.

Czech

See no. 313.

Danish

223
Secher, Knud I. A. Klinisk ordbog. 6 ed., by Martin Kristensen, København, Høst, 1962. 600 p.

Dano-Norwegian dictionary; includes word derivations, abbreviations, eponyms, and brief biographical data.

Dutch

224
Coëlho, Maurice B. Praktisch verklarend zakwoordenboek der geneeskunde . . . 10 ed. by G. Kloosterhuis. Den Haag, Van Goor, 1966. 664 p.

225
Haan, Henri R. M. de, and Dekker, W. A. L. Groot woordenboek der geneeskunde; encyclopedia medica. Leiden, Stafleu, 1955-1960. 4 v.

Comprehensive. Basic terms in chemistry, physics, and biology. Includes non-Dutch medical terms and for many Dutch terms gives Latin, German, English, French and other synomyms. Contains abbreviations and brief biographical information.

226
Hoolboom-Van Dijck, S. J. M. Geenee-

skundig handwoordenboek. Leiden, Stafleu & Zoon, 1963. 799 p.

Short definitions; includes abbreviations and eponyms.

227
Pinkhof, H. Vertalend en verklarend woordenboek van uitheemse geneeskundige termen. 5 ed., by G. J. Schoute. Haarlem, 1963. 613 p.

Short definitions; includes new terms and abbreviations; contains brief biographies.

228
Schuurmans Stekhoven, Willem. Geneeskundig woordenboek: Engels-Nederlands, Nederlands-Engels. 2 ed. Met medewerking van W. M. Corbet en C. Visser. Amsterdam, De Bussy, 1955. 284 p.

Equivalent terms; includes list of abbreviations.

English

229
Blakiston's Illustrated pocket medical dictionary. 2 ed. New York, Blakiston Division, McGraw-Hill, 1960. 985 p.

Abridged edition of no. 230.

230★
Blakiston's New Gould medical dictionary, a modern comprehensive dictionary of the terms used in all branches of medicine and allied sciences, including medical physics and chemistry, dentistry, pharmacy, nursing, veterinary medicine, zoology and botany, as well as medicolegal terms; with illustrations and tables. Ed. by N. L. Hoerr and Arthur Osol. 2 ed. New York, Blakiston Division, McGraw-Hill, 1956. 1463 p.

Gives derivations and pronunciations; includes abbreviations, eponyms, brief biographical information, tables of arteries, bones, nerves, enzymes, isotopes, phobias, etc.

231
Butterworths medical dictionary. Ed. by Sir Arthur S. MacNalty. London, Butterworth, 1965. 1663 p.

Comprehensive; includes brief biographies, eponyms, and abbreviations. Appendix: anatomical nomenclature, tables of weights and measures, and pharmaceutical specialties list.

First published in 1961 as *British medical dictionary.*

Preface has brief history of medical dictionaries.

232
Brown, J. A. C. Pears medical encyclopedia. Rev. ed. New York, Arco, 1963. 508 p.

Intended for nurses. Frequently extensive discussion of terms.

233
Dorland, William A. N. American pocket medical dictionary. A dictionary of the principal terms used in medicine, nursing, pharmacy, dentistry, veterinary science, and allied biological subjects. 20 ed. Philadelphia, Saunders, 1959. 698 p.

Abridged from Dorland's *Illustrated medical dictionary.*

234★★
——. Illustrated medical dictionary, including modern drugs and dosage, by Austin Smith, and fundamentals of medical etymology, by L. W. Daly. 24 ed. Philadelphia, Saunders, 1965. 1724 p.

Comprehensive; contains terms used in medicine and related sciences, with pronunciations and derivations, etc. 1 ed. 1900.

235
Dunglison, Robley. A dictionary of medical science. [1]-23 ed. Philadelphia, etc., 1833–1903.

Includes biographies; bibliographies for some name and subject entries. Some patent medicines listed under proprietors' names.

1 ed. has title *A new dictionary of medical science and literature*; 1839–1866 ed. have title *Medical lexicon.*

1874–1900 ed. revised by Richard J. Dunglison; 1903 ed. rev. by Thomas L. Stedman.

235.1
Parr, John A. Parr's concise medical encyclopedia. Amsterdam, Elsevier, 1965. 514 p.

Intended for the layman.

236
The Putnam medical dictionary. By Norman B. Taylor and A. E. Taylor. New York, Putnam, 1961. 933 p.

For students, nurses, and allied personnel.

237
Stanton, Isabel Alice. A dictionary for medical secretaries. Springfield Ill., Thomas, 1960. 175 p.

Definitions of principal terms. No abbreviations.

238★★
Stedman, Thomas L. Medical dictionary; a vocabulary of medicine and its allied sciences, with pronunciations and derivations. 21 ed. Baltimore, Williams and Wilkins, 1966. 1836 p.

Comprehensive standard medical dictionary. Gives etymological word list; includes eponyms, brief biographical information. Anatomical terms revised according to new nomenclature, *Nomina anatomica parisiensia*; pharmaceutical preparations official in the U.S., British, and international pharmacopeias.

1–17 ed., 1911–49, have title *Practical medical dictionary*; title varies slightly. 14–15 ed. by S. T. Garber; 16–17 ed. by N. B. Taylor.

239
Taber, Clarence W. Cyclopedic medical dictionary, including a digest of medical subjects: medicine, surgery, nursing, dietetics, physical therapy, treatments, drugs, etc. 9 ed. Philadelphia, Davis, 1964. 1339 p.

240
Thomson, William A. R. Black's medical dictionary. 6 ed. London, Black, 1965. 1013 p.

Combines dictionary features with those of an abridged encyclopedia. Contains notes on causes, symptoms and treatment of diseases. 1–21 ed., 1906–53, by John Dixon Comrie. United States edition published under the title *The Macmillan medical cyclopedia*, New York, 1959. 1012 p.

French

241
Garnier, Marcel, and Delamare, Valéry. Dictionnaire des termes techniques de médecine. 18 ed., by Jean Delamare. Paris, Maloine, 1965. 1087 p.

Standard French medical dictionary; includes derivations from the Greek and Latin, names of diseases, anatomical and laboratory terms.

242★★
Lépine, Pierre. Dictionnaire français-anglais, anglais-français des terms médicaux et biologiques. Paris, Éditions Médicales Flammarion, 1952, 829 p.

243
Nouveau Larousse médical illustré. Paris, Larousse, 1952. 1214 p.

A semipopular, profusely illustrated encyclopedic dictionary. Includes the allied sciences. No biographic data.

Finnish

244
Pesonen, Niilo, and Ponteva, E. Lääketieteen sanakirja. 2 ed. Porvoo, Söderstrom, 1963. 469 p.

English-German-Latin in one alphabet with Finnish equivalents.

German

245
Abderhalden, Rudolf. Medizinische Terminologie; Wörterbuch der gesamten Medizin und der verwandten Wissenschaften. Basel, Schwabe, 1948. 1214 columns.

Includes list of eponyms with biographical data.

246★★
De Vries, Louis. German-English medical dictionary. New York, McGraw-Hill, 1952. 586 p.

40,000 terms.

247
Der Gesundheits Brockhaus; Volksbuch vom Menschen und der praktischen Heilkunde. 2 ed., by H. Mommsen-Frankfurt. Wiesbaden, F. A. Brockhaus, 1964. 812 p.

Encyclopedic type dictionary including practical information as well as clinical medicine; illustrated. Includes pharmaceutical terms.

248
Gfrörer, Dieter. Medizinisches Wörterbuch. Stuttgart, Medica Verlag, 1961. 356 p.

Includes eponyms. Appendix: tables of arteries, muscles, nerves.

249
Goulden, William O. German-English medical dictionary. London, Churchill, 1955. 513 p.

English equivalents of about 50,000 medical expressions; essential chemical, dental, and veterinary terms included.

250★
Lang, Hugo. Lang's German-English dictionary of terms used in medicine and the allied sciences with their pronunications. 4 ed., by M. K. Meyers. Philadelphia, Blakiston, 1932. 926 p.

56,500 medical terms.

251★★
Lejeune, Fritz. German-English, English-German dictionary for physicians. Stuttgart, Thieme, 1951–53. 2 v. v. 1, German-English, 1348 p.; v. 2, English-German, 1737 p.

Over 43,000 terms. Pocket-sized.

252
Pschyrembel, Willibald. Klinisches Wörterbuch mit klinische Syndrome. Berlin, de Gruyter, 1964. 980 p.

Derivations, illustrations.

253
Schoenewald, Friedrich S. German-English medical dictionary. Philadelphia, Blakiston, 1949. 241 p. English-German medical dictionary. Philadelphia, Blakiston, 1951. 242 p.

Illustrates varying shades of meaning of a word or expression by giving suitable examples of its use.

254
Unseld, Dieter W. Medizinisches Wörterbuch der deutschen und englischen Sprache. 4 ed. Stuttgart, Wissenschaftliche Verlagsgesellschaft M.B.H., 1964. 489 p.

Compact dictionary of equivalent terms. Added t.p. in English.

255
Volkmann, Herbert. Medizinische Terminologie; Ableitung und Erklärung der gebräuchlichen Fachausdrücke aller Zweige der Medizin und ihrer Hilfswissenschaften. 35 ed., by Kurt Hoffman. Berlin, Urban & Schawarzenberg, 1951. 1130 columns.

Early editions as W. Guttmann's *Medizinische Terminologie*.

256
Zetkin, Maxim, and Schaldach, Herbert, ed. Wörterbuch der Medizin. 2 ed. Berlin, Verlag Volk und Gesundheit, 1964. 1087 p.

Comprehensive. Includes new medical words, names and chemical composition of drugs, derivations, eponyms, brief biographies.

Greek

256.1
Castelli, Bartolomeo. Lexicon medicum Graeco-Latinum, novissime retractatum et auctum. Patavii, Ex Typographia Seminarii, apud T. Bettinelli, 1792. 2v.

First ed., Messina, 1598, mainly based on the works of Hippocrates and Galen; revised and enlarged in successive editions by Emanuel Stupanus, Adrian Ravestein, Jakob P. Bruno, and others into a comprehensive lexicon of Greek and Latin medical terms, including early modern coinages as well as classical words, and reflecting the development of the standard medical terminology. Entries either in transliterated or Latinized Greek or in Latin (usually with reference from Greek) followed by equivalents or roots in Greek type and definitions and illustrative citations in Latin. Includes an alphabetical list of Latin terms with equivalents in Arabic, Hebrew, Greek, French, and Italian.

Also entitled *Castellus renovatus* and *Amaltheum Castello-Brunonianum.*

257
Christomopoulos, Geōrgios D. Angloellēnikon lexikon iatrikēs horologias [English-Greek dictionary of medical terminology] 1 ed. Athenai, Oikonomidēs, 1954. 300 p.

Greek equivalents of 20,000 English terms; includes list of abbreviations, tables of weights and measures and conversion formulas, components of medical preparations, lists of muscles, nerves, and arteries.

258
Tsoukas, Andreas G., and Psaltēs, I. A. Mega angloellēnikon iatrikon lexikon [Large English-Greek medical dictionary] 2 ed. Athenai, Parisianos, 1957. 3 v.

Comprehensive; includes abbreviations, brief biographies, eponyms.

Hawaiian

258.1
Handy, Edward S. C. et al. Outline of

Hawaiian physical therapeutics. Honolulu, Bishop Museum, 1934. 51 p. (Bernice P. Bishop Museum. Bulletin no. 126).

Glossary of Hawaiian medical terms p. 25–38.

Hebrew

259
Academy of the Hebrew Language, Jerusalem. Dictionary of anatomical terms, Hebrew-Latin. Jerusalem, 1957. 304, 53 p. (Its Specialized Dictionaries, 4).

Alternate columns of Hebrew and Latin terms arranged by body part; Hebrew and Latin indexes.

260
Masie, Aaron M. Sefer ha-munahim li-refuah ule-mada e ha-teva. Dictionary of medicine and allied sciences, Latin-English-Hebrew. Ed. by S. Tchernichowsky. Jerusalem, 1934. 787 p.

Latin and English terms are in one alphabet with Hebrew in opposite column.

Hungarian

261
Lee-Delisle, Dora. 4000 orvosi müszó; angolul-magyarul, magyarul-angolul. New York, Stechert-Hafner, 1957.

4000 common medical terms.

Indonesian

262
Ramali, Ahmad, and Pamoentjak, K. S. Kamus kedokteran arti dan heterangan istilah. Djakarta, Kjambatan, 1953. 327 p.

Terms are given in Indonesian, Latin, or language of origin, with equivalents or definitions in Indonesian.

Italian

263★
Arcieri, John P. Italian-English medical dictionary. Rome, Tip. Consorzio Nazionale, 1931. 194 p.

Index of terms arranged by organs and regions of the body.

264★★
Dizionario medico. Diretto dal Prof. Emanuele Lauricella. Venezia, Istituto per la Collaborazione Culturale, 1960-61. 2 v.

About 120,000 terms. Includes abbreviations, brief biographies, derivations, illustrations. Appendix: Paris Nomina anatomica.

265
Ferrio, Luigi. Terminologia medica. 4 ed., by Carlo Ferrio. Torino, Unione tipografico-editrice torinese, 1961. 926 p.

Comprehensive. Some derivations; includes eponyms.

266
Helder, M. P. Dizionario medico: italiano-inglese, inglese-italiano. Torino, Lattes, 1952. 543 p.

Over 30,000 English words defined in Italian. Italian-English part brief.

267
Marconi, Ruggero, and Zino, Elena, ed. Dizionario inglese-italiano per le scienze mediche. 2 ed. Torino, Minerva medica, 1958. 564 p.

40,000 English terms.

268
Marino, Vincenzo. Dizionario medico fraseologico: italiano-inglese, inglese-italiano. (Frasi tipiche del linguaggio medico). Roma, Abruzzini Editore, 1960. 387 p.

Equivalent terms, followed by phrases illustrating use in the practice of medicine.

See also no. 308.

Japanese

269
Aoyagi, Yasumasa, ed. Wa-Ra-Ei-Doku-Futsu taishō igaku dai jiten [Japanese-Latin-English-German-French medical terminology] Ed. by Yasumasa Aoyagi et al. 1 ed. Tokyo, Kanehara, 1957. 1259 p.

Comprehensive dictionary including many eponyms. Transliterated Japanese term followed by Japanese characters and equivalent term in one or more other languages; definitions in Japanese characters; includes identifying biographical information.

270
Ishikawa, Mitsuteru, ed. Ei-Wa-igo dai jiten [English-Japanese medical dictionary] 1 ed. Osaka, Nippon Rinshōsha, 1955. 1350 p.

Patterned after the 22 ed. of Dorland. Equivalent terms and definitions in Japanese characters. Includes abbreviations, eponyms, with brief biographies, tables of muscles, nerves, arteries, and veins; some anatomical illustrations.

271
Katō, Katsuji, ed. Igaku Ei-Wa dai jiten. Integrated English-Japanese medical dictionary. Tokyo, Nanzando, 1960. 1718 p.

150,000 terms; contains new terms in medicine, nuclear physics, radiation and space medicine; includes eponyms, abbreviations, brief biographies. Definitions in Japanese characters.

272
Nanzando's medical dictionary. Ed. by T Ogawa et al. 1 ed. Tokyo, 1954. 1353 p.

Comprehensive. Japanese terms are followed by equivalents in English, Latin, German, or other language, with definition in Japanese characters. Includes terms in pharmacology, brief biographies, eponyms. Has a predominantly English index section.

273
Ōya, Zensetsu. Ei-wa igaku jiten [English-Japanese medical dictionary] Tokyo, Kanehara, 1963. 1611 p.

Comprehensive. Includes biological, dental, pharmaceutical, and veterinary terms. Gives abbreviations, eponyms.

274
Satō, Kazuo, ed. Igaku shigaku jiten, Wa-Ei-Doku-Ra. Medico-dental dictionary, Japanese-English-German-Latin. Tokyo, Nippon Daigaku Shigakubu Dosokai, 1958. 1790 p.

Transliterated Japanese term followed by equivalent in Japanese characters, with English, German, and Latin synonyms.

275
Watanabe, Yoshitaka. Shōkōmei jiten [Dictionary of terms in symptomatology] 1 ed. Urawa, Chūgai Isho, 1955. 577 p.

English terms followed by Japanese definitions in Japanese characters. Contains primarily terms used in diagnosis, eponyms, syndromes, and tests. Extensive Japanese-English index.

Korean

276
Lee, W. C., and Choi, K. D., ed. English-Korean medical dictionary. Seoul, Eul-Yoo Pub. Co., 1958. 484 p.

English terms with Korean equivalents in Korean characters. Appendix includes list of abbreviations, with English and Korean meanings, list of medicines with Latin or English names, tables of weights and measures.

Latin

277
Motherby, George. A new medical dictionary or general repository of physic. 5 ed., by George Wallis. London, 1801. 811 p.

Latin-English. English index. Occasionally long definitions with historical and contemporary clinical descriptions and theories of diseases including therapy. Some entries have bibliographies. 1 ed., 1775.

278
Parr, Bartholomew. The London medical dictionary. London, 1809. 2 v. 786, 744 (156) p.

Latin-English. Some definitions include history of subject and references. English index.

Malayan

279
Gimlette, John D. A dictionary of Malayan medicine. Ed. by H. W. Thomson. London, Oxford Univ. Press, 1939. 259 p.

A guide to Malayan medical practices and customs as well as a language dictionary. Under the Malayan names of plants and herbs are given the names in English and Latin, their descriptions, their uses and legends in Malay folk medicine. Under the names of organs are found the many vernacular terms and their connotations. Brief classified index in English.

Norwegian

280
Evang, Karl, ed. Norsk medisinsk ordbok. 4 ed. Oslo, Sem & Stenersen, 1955. 348 p.

Contains about 13,500 terms. For each gives numerical key to international morbidity nomenclature which appears at end of text.

Polish

281
Jedraszko, Sabina. Słownik lekarski; angielsko-polski i polsko-angielski. Wyd. 2 Warszawa, Państwowy Zakład Wydawn. Lekarskich, 1961. 797 p.

Polish equivalents of English terms in medicine, dentistry, and pharmacy, including lay terms, with some definitions. Includes many new terms. Contains list of abbreviations and list of Latin words and abbreviations used in treatment, tables of weights and measures. Small Polish-English section with equivalents.

282
Tomaszewski, Wiktor. Słownik lekarski angielsko-polski i polsko-angielski [English-Polish and Polish-English medical dictionary] 2 ed. Edinburgh, Livingstone, 1953. 304 p.

An appendix of genetic and cytologic terms, prefixes and suffixes, abbreviations, weights and measures, notes on prescription writing, illustrations of instruments with names, and other useful features.

Portuguese

283
Fortes, Hugo. Diccionário de têrmos médicos; inglês-português. 2 ed. Rio de Janeiro, Editôra Científica, 1958. 702 p.

Portuguese equivalents of English terms in medicine and related fields; English pronunciations indicated.

See also no. 307.

284
Pinto, Pedro. Diccionário de têrmos médicos. 7 ed. Rio de Janeiro, Editôra Científica, 1958. 507 p.

Short definitions.

Russian

285★
Jablonski, Stanley. Russian-English medical dictionary. Ed. by Ben S. Levine. New York, Academic Press, 1958. 423 p.

English equivalents of Russian terms in medicine and peripheral sciences; lists abbreviations with emphasis on organizations.

286
Karpovich, Eugene A. Russian-English biological and medical dictionary. Rev. ed. New York, Technical Dictionaries Co., 1960. 400 p.

About 35,000 Russian entries in biology, botany, zoology, medicine and agriculture, with English equivalents.

287
Mul'tanovskiĭ, Mikhail P., and Ivanova, A. English-Russian medical dictionary. Moscow, State Pub. Office for Medical Literature, 1958. 635 p.

37,000 terms including terms used in agriculture and chemical technology. Includes abbreviations.

Serbian

288
Kostić, Aleksandar [et al.] ed. Medicinski leksikon za lekare i studente. Beograd, Medicinska knjiga, 1957. 641 p.

Includes basic terms in allied fields. Anatomical terms are based on the Basle nomenclature. Includes eponyms.

Slovenian

289
Černič, Mirko. Slovenski zdravstveni besednjak. Ljubljana, Državna založba Slovenije, 1957. 707 p.

About 15,000 terms in medicine and related sciences. Includes some derivations, eponyms, brief biographies, names and descriptions of drugs, diseases and operations.

Spanish

290
Braier, Léon. Diccionario enciclopédico de medicina. 2 ed. Buenos Aires, Lopez Libreros, 1964. 1593 p.

Includes new words, pharmaceutical terms, and biographical sketches. Word derivation is given in most cases followed by definition. Appendix: lists of eponyms, tests, reactions, syndromes, polyglot dictionary in Spanish, German, French, English, and Italian of more than 1,000 commonly used terms.

291
Cardenal Pujals, León. Diccionario terminológico de ciencias médicas. 8 ed. Barcelona, Salvat, 1963. 1304 p.

Includes new words, identifying biographical information, tables of muscles, nerves, arteries, and veins. Supplement: short lists of German, French, Italian, English, and Portuguese medical terms with Spanish equivalents.

292
Garnier, Marcel, and Delamare, Valéry. Diccionario de los términos téchnicos usados en medicina. 10 ed., with the collaboration of Joaquín Pi y Arsuaga, et al. Madrid, Bailly-Baillière, 1955. 1422 p.

Includes Greek and Latin derivations, names of diseases, anatomical and laboratory terms.

293★★
Goldberg, Morris. English-Spanish chemical and medical dictionary; comprising terms employed in medicine, surgery, dentistry, veterinary medicine, biochemistry, biology, pharmacy, allied sciences, and related scientific equipment. New York, McGraw-Hill, 1947. 692 p.

40,000 terms, with brief definitions.

294★★
——. Spanish-English chemical and medical dictionary. New York, McGraw-Hill, 1953. 609 p.

Companion volume to no. 293.

295
McElligott, Maurice C. Spanish-English medical dictionary. London, Lewis, 1946. 249 p.

Over 15,000 terms.

296★
Ruiz Torres, Francisco. Diccionario inglés-español, español-inglés de medicina. 3 ed. Madrid, Editorial Alhambra, 1965. 714 p.

English-Spanish section contains 50,000 words; includes idiomatic phrases, list of Latin and English abbreviations with Spanish meanings.

See also no. 306.

Swedish

297
Engström, Einar. Svensk-engelsk teknisk ordbok. 6 ed. Stockholm, Svensk trävarutidining förlaget, 1961. 543 p.

298
Wernstedt, Wilhelm E. Medicinsk terminologi. 4 ed. Stockholm, Nordiska Bokhandeln, 1959. 612 p.

299
Wrete, Martin. Kortfattad medicinisk ordbok. Stockholm, Svenska Bokförlaget, 1962. 247 p.

Primarily for students.

Tagalog

300
Sytamco, José Reyes. English-Spanish-Tagalog medical dictionary. Diccionario médico inglés-español-tagalog. Taláhuluganang Inglēs-Kastilā-Tagalog sa panggagamót. Rev. ed. Maynilá, 1961. 1023 p.

Includes many nonmedical terms.

Turkish

301
Noyan, Fazil, and Gürson, Cihad T. Küçük tip termimleri kilavuzu. Istanbul, Ismail Akgün Matbaasi, 1947. 272 p. (I.U.T.B. Tip Fakültesi. Talebe Cemiyeti Yayinlari, no. 23)

Turkish with equivalents in English, French, and German.

Urdu

302
Cornelius, A. W. Hospital conversation with vocabulary and phrases in Roman Urdu. Mussoorie, U.P., Mussoorie Book Society, 1943. 60 p.

English with Urdu equivalents.

Zulu

303
A handbook to aid in the treatment of Zulu patients. Natal, 1958. 131 p.

Includes lists of hospitals, health centers in Natal that admit Zulus.

Polyglot

304
Arnaudov, Georgi D. Meditsinska terminologiia na shest ezika. Latinum, Bulgarski, Russkiĭ, English, Français, Deutsch [Medical terminology in six languages. Latin, etc.] Sofiia, Meditsina i fizkultura, 1964. 1112 p.

Over 10,000 Latin medical terms (including eponyms and anatomical terms) with equivalents in Bulgarian, Russian, English, French and German.

Added title page and cover title: *Terminologia medica polyglotta.* Title page also includes titles in other languages.

305★
Clairville, Alexandre L. Dictionnaire polyglotte des termes médicaux. 2 ed. Paris, S.I.P.U.C.O., 1953. 1152 p.

Main portion in French includes over 14,000 numbered terms, with English, German, and Latin cited for each. Keys to the other languages refer to French numbered term.

306
——. Version española. By Edwin Velez and Antonio Galvan. Paris, S.I.P.U.C.O., 1952. 351 p.

307
——. Versâo brasileira. Tr. by Bernardo Radunski. Paris, S.I.P.U.C.O., Rio de Janeiro, Freitas Bastos, 1953. 351 p.

308
——. Versione italiana. By A. Calciati. Paris, S.I.P.U.C.O., 1955. 320 p.

309
——. Version arabe. By Munshid Khātir et al. Damascus, 1956. 960 p.

Arabic version has alternate columns of French and Arabic terms, and also refers to the number of the term in the original volume.

310
Del Guercio, Louis R. M., ed. The multilingual manual for medical interpreting. New York, Pacific Printing Co., 1960. 160 p.

Contains sections in French, Spanish, German, Italian, Polish and Russian of 100 questions usually asked on medical history forms. The question appears first in English followed by the language of the section with phonetic pronunciation of that language. Subject index with reference to number of question.

311★★
Elsevier's medical dictionary in five languages: English/American, French, Italian, Spanish and German. Comp. and arr. on an English alphabetical base, by A. Sliosberg. Amsterdam, Elsevier, 1964. 1588 p.

312
Foster, Frank P. An illustrated encyclopedic medical dictionary; being a dictionary of the technical terms used by writers on medicine and the collateral sciences, in the Latin, English, French, and German languages. New York, Appleton, 1888–93. 4 v. in 12 pts. 3095 p.

All 4 languages in one alphabet, with definitions, sometimes lengthy, in English; includes botanical and pharmaceutical terms.

313
Kábrt, Jan, and Valach, Vladislav. Stručný lékařský slovník. 3 ed. Praha, Státní zdravotnické nakl., 1965. 368 p.

An abridged medical dictionary giving about 18,000 terms in one alphabet in Latin, Greek, Czech, English, and French. Non-Czech words have Czech equivalents; Czech terms have Latin equivalents. Intended for students and workers in medical and health fields; includes words commonly used in chemistry, pharmacology.

314
Kostić, Aleksandar. Medicinski rečnik. Beograd, Medicinska knjiga, 1956. 762 p.

Contains Latin, English, German, French, and Serbian sections of terms (some nonmedical) with a section of 3800 eponyms, totaling 41,000 terms in all. Latin section gives origin of word, followed by equivalent term in English, German, French and Serbian. Other sections give equivalents. Includes some abbreviations.

315
Meyboom, Frederika. Quaestionarium medicum in English, French, Italian, Spanish, Portuguese, German, Dutch, Norwegian, Swedish, Finnish, Polish, Russian, Greek, Chinese, Japanese, Malay, Esperanto. New York, Elsevier, 1961. 213 p.

475 questions and directions used by the physician or hospital staff.

316
Parry, S. Chalmers. Polyglot medical questionnaire in twelve languages, with digital system of communication. London, Lewis, 1953. 62 p.

With no language in common with patient, doctor points to numbered question and patient looks it up in his language and answers yes or no; 191 questions in 12 languages.

317★
Veillon, Emmanuel [et al.] Medical dictionary. Dictionnaire médical. Medizinisches Wörterbuch. London, Lange, Maxwell and Springer, 1950. 3 pts.

Pt. 1, English-French-German, 496 p. Pt. 2, Français-allemand-anglais, 435 p. Pt. 3, Deutsch-english-französisch, 476 p.

Each part alphabetized according to key language with equivalents in others; 25,000 terms. Also available in a Swiss edition (Bern, Huber, 1950).

PERIODICALS

Only international or national lists of periodicals are included here. Holdings of specific libraries or union lists are entered under Libraries, Medical. Subject lists are entered under subject.

318
Akademiia nauk SSSR. Biblioteka. Sistematicheskiĭ katalog otechestvennykh periodicheskikh i prodolzhaiushchikhsia izdaniĭ po meditsine, 1792–1960 [Classified index of national periodicals and serials in the field of medicine, 1792–1960] Sost. E. N. Chernova. Leningrad, 1965. 495 p.

Classified list of medical serials in Russian published in Russia and the USSR and available in the collection of the Academy of Sciences of the USSR.

2191 entries (some repetitions) with full bibliographic data, arranged alphabetically by the title under subject.

Alphabetical and geographical index.

319
Excerpta medica. List of journals abstracted. Amsterdam, Excerpta Medica Foundation, 1964. 188 p.

Lists 2728 current journals in the medical and related sciences, indicating title abbreviations and countries of origin. Includes separate list of Japanese titles translated into English.

320
Fernandez, Alicia de. Venezuelan medical and related periodicals, libraries and societies. Caracas, Bibliotecaria Jefe, Ministerio de Sanidad y Asistencia Social, 1963. 9 p.

321
Japan. National Diet Library. Directory of Japanese scientific periodicals, 1962. 229 p.

Gives transliterated title, title in Japanese characters, translation of title and full bibliographical information. 2241 titles.

321.1
Levit, Moiseĭ Markovich. Meditsinskaia periodicheskaia pechat' Rossii i SSSR (1792–1962) [Medical periodicals of Russia and of the USSR (1792–1962)] Moskva, Gos. izd-vo medits. lit., 1963. 243 p.

971 titles alphabetically arranged with basic bibliographic data. Titles of special importance annotated. History of medico-legal periodicals (p. 7–42). Subject and geographic indexes.

322
List bio-med; biomedical serials in Scandinavian libraries. Göteborg, 1965. 212 p.

Annual. Union list of approximately 5,500 titles for Denmark, Finland, Norway, and Sweden.

323
Nippon Igaku Toshokan Kyōkai. Igaku zasshi sōgō mokuroku [Union list of medical periodicals in the medical libraries of Japan] 4 ed. Tokyo, 1961–63. 2 v. 420, 262 p.

[pt. 1] 1961, ōbun hen [periodicals in foreign languages]; [pt. 2] 1963, wabun zasshi hen [periodicals in the Japanese language]

1–3 ed., 1932–42, in one v. each.

324 (not used)

325
Periodica medica; Titelabkürzungen medizinischer Zeitschriften. 4 ed. By Walter Artelt, Edith Heischkel, Carl Wehmer. Stuttgart, Thieme, 1952. 280 p.

List, with abbreviations, of 12,624 publications. Includes proceedings of state and municipal societies and department of health publications.

326★★
U.S. National Library of Medicine. List of journals indexed in Index medicus. Washington, 1960– .

With 1966 consists of full title, abbreviated title, subject, and geographic listings of journals.

Also published in no. 6.

1962 not published separately.

327★★
Vital notes on medical periodicals. Chicago, 1, 1952– . Medical Library Association.

Quarterly. Lists new journals which began after 1949. Indicates changes in title, mergers, and titles suspended or discontinued.

328★★
World medical periodicals. 3 ed. New York, World Medical Association, 1961. 407 p.

Alphabetical list of over 5800 journals by title. Entry includes name and address of publisher and abbreviation of title. Principal international abstracting and indexing journals are given in the appendix. Indexed by subject and by country. 1 ed., 1952; 2 ed., 1957.

Histories

329
Brunn, Walter von. Das deutsche medizinische Zeitschriftenwesen seit der Mitte des 19. Jahrhunderts. Riedel-Archiv, Sonderheft, 1925. 50 p.

Selective list of German medical periodicals arranged chronologically under each subject. Genealogies of the periodicals and names of editors are given in most cases. No title index. Continues no. 338.

330
Brunn, Walter A. L. von. Medizinische Zeitschriften im neunzehnten Jahrhundert. Beiträge zur Geschichte der allgemein-medizinischen Fachpresse. Stuttgart, Thieme, 1963. 95 p.

Historical survey. List of journals (p. 76–89) gives title, period of publication, frequency, relations to other journals (supersessions, mergers, etc.), important editors, and brief descriptions of selected journals, mostly European. Bibliography: p. 90–95.

331
Delprat, Constant C. De geschiedenis der Nederlandsche geneeskundige tijdschriften van 1680–1857. Amsterdam, Ellerman, Harms, 1927. 302 p.

Chronological bibliography of 83 periodicals, with notes on editors, title changes, scope, and contents. No title index.

332
Ebert, Myrl. Rise and development of the American medical periodical, 1797–1850. In Bulletin of the Medical Library Association, 40:243–76, 1952.

Discussion of the most important journals, with a chronologic list and title index.

333
Garrison, Fielding H. The medical and scientific periodicals of the 17th and 18th centuries, with a revised catalogue and checklist. In Bulletin of the Institute of the History of Medicine, 2:285–343, 1934.

Historical survey and lists. 17th century items are in two chronological lists, medical and scientific; 18th century medical periodicals and transactions are classified by subject, subdivided by decade. The entire checklist is arranged in 21 sections, including an alphabetic index of medical journals in sections 1–10. Supplemented by David A. Kronick, The Fielding H. Garrison list of medical and scientific periodicals . . . Addenda and corrigenda, Bulletin of the History of Medicine, 32:456–74, 1958.

334
Guitard, Eugène H. Deux siècles de la presse au service de la pharmacie, et cinquante ans de "L'Union pharmaceutique." Histoire et bibliographie des périodiques intéressant les sciences, la médecine et spécialement la pharmacie en France et à l'étranger (1665–1860). 2 ed. Paris, La Pharmacie centrale de France, 1913. 315 p.

Pt. 1 (p. 1–151) describes important journals and annuals and the publications of academies, societies, etc., including data on the editors and publishing bodies.

335
Kronick, David A. A history of scientific and technical periodicals: the origins and development of the scientific and technological press, 1665–1790. New York, Scarecrow Press, 1962. 274 p.

336
LeFanu, William R. British periodicals of medicine, a chronological list. In Bulletin of the Institute of the History of Medicine, 5:735–61, 827–46, 1937; 6:614–48, 1938.

1362 entries in two parts (1684–1899 and 1900–1938), from entire British empire. Title index for each part.

Supplemented by Shadrake, A. M., British medical periodicals, 1938–61, *Bull Med Libr Ass* 51:181–96, 1963.

337
Neelameghan, Arashanapalai. Development of medical societies and medical periodicals in India, 1780 to 1920. Calcutta, Oxford Book Co., 1963. 120 p. (IASLIC [Indian Association of Special Libraries and Information Centres] Special publication no. 3)

Includes histories of societies and journals, classified and alphabetical lists, and list of union catalogs of periodical publications in Indian libraries.

338
Sudhoff, Karl. Das medizinische Zeit-

schriftenwesen in Deutschland bis zur Mitte des 19. Jahrhunderts. In Münchener medizinische Wochenschrift 50:455-63, 1903.

Includes chronologic checklist with detailed information. Continued by no. 329.

339
Wickersheimer, Ernest. Index chronologique des périodiques médicaux de la France (1679-1856). In Le Bibliographe moderne, courier international 12:58-96, 1908.

Lists 358 journals, reviews, and annuals and 112 periodical publications of medical societies alphabetically by cities and chronologically under cities. General chronologic index. Also issued separately in 1910.

DIRECTORIES

With few exceptions only international and national directories have been listed.

International

Physicians

340
World Medical Association. U.S. Committee. International medical directory. New York, 1, 1965- .

Gives names and addresses of a limited number of English-speaking physicians in 63 countries and addresses of national medical associations. Intended for use of members of the "allied health team".

Organizations

341
Annuaire des organisations internationales; yearbook of international organizations. Brussels [etc.], 1, 1948-

Main section gives data on aims, members, officers, meetings, publications of nongovernmental organizations; smaller sections related to United Nations, European community, and other intergovernmental organizations. Subject indexes in English and French. 9 ed., 1962-63.

342
Council for International Organizations of Medical Sciences. Directory; repertoire. [3 ed.] Paris, Conseil des Organisations Internationales des Sciences Médicales, 1961. 192 p.

Gives structure of the Council for International Organizations of Medical Sciences followed by list of international members. Data include address, chief officers, founding date, and list of national societies. In English and French.

National

Physicians (and allied personnel)

Directories limited to a specialty for which there is a subject heading (i.e. Dentistry, Nursing, etc.) are entered under the appropriate heading. Regular and substantial inclusion of allied professions and institutions in the directories listed below has been indexed in the subject index and not cross-referenced in the text.

Although some older and discontinued directories are listed, no attempt was made to include all.

Argentina

343
Argentine Republic. Consejo Nacional de Investigaciones Científicas y Técnicas. Centro de Investigaciones Científicas y Técnicas. Centros de investigación científica y docencia en los ramos basicos de la medicina. Buenos Aires, 1963. 161 p.

Universities and institutes in biomedical fields, with address, name of director and number on staff; includes lists of personnel with indication of specialty and title.

Australia

344
Medical directory of Australia. Sydney, 1, 1935- .

Alphabetical listing of physicians with brief professional information, followed by geographical listing. Includes data on hospitals, medical personnel, public health officials, medical school faculties, and medical societies and their members. Data given for Tasmania, the territories, and Pacific Islands.

11 ed., 1964.

Austria

345
Ärztliches Jahrbuch für Österreich. Wien, 1-10? 1906-15?

Physicians with occasional brief professional

information. Includes pharmacists, medical societies, etc.

346
Handbuch für die Sanitätsberufe Österreichs, Wien, 1, 1950?– .

Geographical listing of physicians, dentists, and pharmacists. Specialists are listed with address and telephone number. Other lists include university clinics and hospitals, teaching staffs of medical schools. 3 ed., 1963.

Belgium

347
Annuaire médical belge. (Congo Belge et Grand-Duché de Luxembourg). Bruxelles, 1, 1897?– .

Listing of physicians, pharmacists and hospitals, alphabetically and by localities. Brief professional information for physicians. Lists of specialists included. Kept current by four annual supplementary bulletins.

Canada

348★
Canadian medical directory. Toronto, Current Publications, 1, 1955– .

Brief professional information given in alphabetical list; geographical list of names. Also includes information on medical, nursing, and public health schools, associations and specialist societies, medical libraries. 10 ed., Seccombe House, 1964.

Chile

349
Chile. Servicio Nacional de Salud. Guía medica nacional; sección profesiónes médicas y paramedicas. 2 ed. Santiago, 1962. 162 p.

Alphabetical listing by surname of physicians and surgeons; gives address and specialty.

China

350
Chinese medical directory. Peking, 1928–41.

Czechoslovakia

351
Zdravotnická ročenka československá. Praha, 1, 1929– . Ministerstvo veřejného zdravotnictví a tělesné výchovy.

Annual. Describes the status of health in Czechoslovakia (organization of public health, budget, health legislation, physicians, medical education, hospitals, pharmacies, spas, control of food and drugs, social security benefits, etc.). Contains a geographically arranged list of approved pharmacies and a directory of physicians licensed to practice.

To 1938 was also published in German under the title: *Medizinische Jahrbücher für die Čechoslovakische Republik.*

Denmark

352
Denmark. Sundhedsstyrelsen. Fortegnelse over autoriserede laegertandlaeger, dyrlaeger m. fl. i Danmark. København, [1] 1879– .

Annual. Alphabetical listing of physicians, dentists, and veterinarians, with year of birth and examination; brief address given for some individuals. Kept current by supplements.

1879–1908 issued by the Department under its former name, Sundhetskollegium. None published, 1880–86.

Egypt

353
Annuaire médical egyptien. Cairo, 1, 1900– .

Geographical listing of physicians and surgeons; gives brief professional data. Oculists and dentists are listed separately. Other information includes medical legislation, public health officials, university medical faculties and names of hospitals.

50 ed., 1951/60.

Finland

354
Lääkärit hammaslääkärit, sairaalat; läkare-tandläkare sjukhus. Helsinki, [1] 1963– . Lääkintöhallitus Medicinalstyrelsen.

Alphabetical listings of physicians and dentists; gives brief professional data. Includes a list of hospitals. Captions in Finnish and Swedish.

Continues *Suomen laakarien ja hammaslaakarien luttelo* (not listed).

France

355
Almanach général de médecine, de pharmacie pour la France, l'Algerie et les colonies. Paris, 1–51?, 1827–81?

Latest issues listed by Département. No combined index. Includes physicians, medical schools and faculties, hospitals, etc.

Earlier volumes as: *Almanach général de médecine pour la ville de Paris.*

356
Annuaire médical et pharmaceutique de la France. Paris, 1–65, 1849–1913.

Contains medical and pharmaceutical legislation, medical societies of Paris and the provinces, governmental medical establishments, lists of military medical personnel, and a list of physicians, public health officers and pharmacists of France, arranged by geographic location.

357
Annuaire médical, ou almanach des medecins, chirurgiens, etc. Paris, Croullebois, 1, 1809.

Includes information on leading medical and pharmaceutical schools of France, with names of chief professors, lists of physicians, pharmacists, and health officials of Paris, hospitals of Paris, marine hospitals, laws dealing with medicine, necrology.

358
Guide Rosenwald, médical et pharmaceutique. Paris, 1, 1887– .

Annual. Geographical and alphabetical listing of physicians and pharmacists, with very brief professional information. Medical specialists are listed by specialty. Also included is information on public health and social welfare, lists of medical associations, faculties of medical schools, membership of academies of medicine, surgery, and pharmacy, lists of public and private hospitals. Data on physicians, pharmacists, hopitals, and medical schools are also given for overseas areas.

Germany

Provincial medical directories are now published in lieu of a national directory for West Germany. These are not listed.

359
Reichs-Medizinal-Kalender für Deutschland. Theil 2. Leipzig, Thieme, 1–58?, 1880–1937?

Directory of physicians.
1928–36 as *Ärztliches Handbuch und Ärzteverzeichnis;* 1937, *Verzeichnis der deutschen Ärzte und Heilanstalten.*

Great Britain

360
Medical directory. London, 1, 1845– .

Annual (in 2 v.). Alphabetical list of physicians registered with the General Medical Council and practicing in Great Britain, the Commonwealth, or elsewhere. For each physician gives address, professional data, and publications. Each is also entered in a local list. Includes universities, colleges, medical schools, hospitals, and miscellaneous information for England, Wales, Scotland, and Eire. Officials of governmental departments, professional societies, and institutions are given. 1845–46 as *London medical directory;* 1847–69, *London and provincial medical directory.*
1964 ed. contains 90,492 names.

361
Medical register. London, 1, 1859– . Printed and published under the direction of the General Medical Council.

Annual (in 2 parts). Lists names, addresses, and qualifications of medical practitioners in the United Kingdom, Commonwealth, and elsewhere. Inclusion in this list constitutes for physicians a legal right to practice.

362
Royal College of Physicians of London. A catalogue of the fellows, licentiates and extra-licentiates. [London] 1693–[1854?]

Title varies. Continued by no. 363.

363
——. List of the fellows and members. London [1871?–]

Presidents of the College, committees, and other information. List arranged by date of admission, with geographic list, including overseas members and name index. Continues no. 362.

Hong Kong

364
Hong Kong. Medical and Health Department. Register of medical and surgical practitioners, 1964. Hong Kong, Young, 1964. [93] p.

Alphabetical list of physicians and surgeons, with brief professional data. Published as special supplement to Hong Kong Government Gazette, no. 15, March 20, 1964.

India

365
The Indian medical directory. Banga [1945?–]

Arranged by state. Gives physicians with addresses and type of practice, health officials, hospitals and dispensaries, medical schools, and for some states, chemists, pharmaceutists, and suppliers of medical equipment, 1958/59 ed., 583 p.

366
National register of scientific and technical personnel in India. New Delhi, 1950–54. India. Council of Scientific and Industrial Research.

v. 2, pts. 1–3, Medical personnel. Alphabetical list of medical graduates. Brief professional information. Separate listings for medical licentiates and dentists.

Ireland

367
Irish medical and hospital directory. Dublin, 1, 1946?– .

24 ed., 1964. Lists physicians with brief professional data including publications. Also includes directory of dentists, physiotherapists, ophthalmologists, and chiropodists.

Earlier editions have title: *Irish medical directory and hospital year book.*

368
Medical register of Ireland. Dublin [1, 194?–]

Annual. Alphabetical listing of medical practitioners, with brief professional information.

Continues the *Medical register of Eire* (not listed).

369
Irish medical directory. By Henry Croly. Dublin, 1843–46?

Annual. Arranged by county. Physicians, with brief professional information. Hospitals by types (lying-in, fever, etc.)

370
Irish medical directory. Dublin, 1883–96?

Physicians with professional data, medical societies, hospitals, medical regulations. Drugs and medicines with prices.

371
Medical directory for Ireland. London, Churchill, 1851–56?

Physicians with brief professional information, obituaries, meetings of medical societies, etc.

Israel

371.1
Midrakh Harefui Jisraeli, 1959. Israel medical directory, 1959. Rev. b'hogith havad ham'rakhdi shel hasidroth harefuoth b'jisrael makhaladotta haparasomim. Haifa, Israel Medical Association, 1959. 327 p.

Alphabetical listing of physicians with address and license number; includes names of medical societies and hospitals. In Hebrew.

Italy

Several provincial and other local medical directories are published such as *Guida sanitaria del Piemonte*, *Milano sanitaria* but these have not been listed.

372
Roma sanitaria. Roma [1, 195?–]

Pharmacists, dentists, and physicians, listed by specialty; inclusive alphabetical list, with address, also a register of physicians by surname, giving brief professional information. Also gives public health officials, international, national and local medical and related associations, professional schools, lists of hospitals, and nursing homes.

Japan

373
Igaku kenkyūsha meibo [Japanese medical researchers directory] Tokyo, 1962/63– .

About 7,500 researchers classified by specialties, by schools, institutes, and associations, by gojūon order, by directors of medical associations.

Edited by Takamichi Tsusaki and Hiromasa Kita.

374
Igaku nenkan; igaku, shigaku, yakugaku, hoken eisei no nenji soran [Medical year book; annual review in medicine, dentistry, pharmacology, and public health] Tokyo, 1963– . Ishiyaku Shuppan Kabushiki Kaisha.

Covers entire field of medicine, 1956–61. Includes major events, statistics, list of hospitals, schools, associations, lists of films, drug manufacturing companies and medical journals.

Continues *Ishiyaku nenkan*, 1954 (not listed).

Luxemburg

See Belgium

Mexico

374.1
Directorio medico mexicano. Mexico, D.F., 1–3? 1924–36?

Lists physicians, dentists, veterinarians (addresses only) societies, schools (with brief history) hospitals, pharmacies, medical periodicals (with history) etc. *Indice terapéutico* lists common drugs under disease state. Geographical arrangement.
2 ed. 1927–28.

374.2
Libro azul medico mexicano, 1945–46. Mexico, D.F. [1946] 279 p.

Lists about 1300 physicians throughout the country and about 275 dentists in Mexico City and Guadalajara. Gives brief professional information. Geographic arrangement.

374.3
Mexico. Secretaria de Salubridad y Asistencia. Directorio de profesionistas de la medicina y actividades conexas que han registrado su titulo. Mexico, D.F., 1947. 228 p. Suplemento. Mexico, D.F. 1947. 5 p.

Alphabetical arrangement by profession: physician-surgeon, dentist, pharmacist, veterinarians, nurses, etc. Information limited to address and registration number.

Netherlands

375
Geneeskundig jaarboekje voor Nederland en Rijksdelen Overzee. v. 2. Rotterdam, 1862– .

Biennial. Geographic listing of practicing and nonpracticing physicians, specialists, and midwives. Also alphabetical listing, with year of diploma and address. Includes information on medical organizations, institutions, and hospitals with address and list of official personnel.
Title varies.

New Zealand

375.1
New Zealand medical register. Wellington, 1914?– . New Zealand Medical Council.

Brief professional information.
Earlier years also as: *Register of medical practitioners.*
1914– Extract from *New Zealand gazette.*

Panama

375.2
Directorio medico Panameño. Panama, 1956– .

1965 listed physicians with professional information and regulations for the practice of medicine.

Poland

376
Spis fachowych pracowników· słuzby zdrowia; zatwierdzony i zalecony do użytku służbowego przez Ministerstwo Zdrowia i Opieki Społecznej. Warszawa, Pánstwowy Zakład Wydawn. Lekarskich, 1, 1961– .

Separate alphabetical listings of physicians, dentists, and pharmacists. Brief professional information. 2 ed., 1964.

Portugal

377
Annuario medico de Portugal; continental, insular e ultramarino. Lisboa, 1946– .

Geographical lists of physicians, pharmacists, midwives, dentists, oculists. For physicians gives addresses, telephone numbers and specialization. Physicians are also listed by specialty. Includes lists of hospitals, clinics, public health services, pharmaceutical specialities.

Spain

378
Diccionario biográfico médico mundial. Barcelona, 1, 1958– .

Alphabetical listing of contemporary medical men in Spain and Spanish speaking countries of the world. Gives full biographical and professional information, including bibliographies and some portraits.

Sweden

379
Sweden. Medicinalstyrelsen. Läkare och Tankläkare; läkar-och tandläkartjänster; apotek och apoteksföreståndare. Stockholm, 1852?– .

Very brief information.
In addition to physicians, dentists and pharmacists gives governmental medical personnel (including armed forces), medical school faculties and institutes, staffs of hospitals and clinics (including dental).
1852–1957 as *Förteckning på* [after 1920? *över*] *Svenske läkare . . .*

From the 1860's through 1956 veterinarians included.

Through 1857 published by Sundhets Kollegium.

Switzerland

380

Schweizerisches mediziniches Jahrbuch. Basel, 1, 18– .

Annual. In German and French. Alphabetical and geographical listing of physicians, dentists, pharmacists, and veterinarians in Switzerland and Liechtenstein. Data for physicians include date of diploma, specialty, address and telephone number. Includes list of specialists. Other lists give hospital and public health services, health and social welfare organizations, medical associations, medical school faculties, and medical journals published in Switzerland.

Union of South Africa

381

Medical directory of South Africa; die mediese gids van Suid-Afrika. Durban, 1, 1960– .

Alphabetical listing of physicians with address, brief professional information. Also lists medical schools and faculties and hospitals. 2 ed., 1963.

382

Register of medical practitioners, interns and dentists for the Republic of South Africa. Pretoria, 1, 1924– .

Title varies slightly; 1947– title also in Afrikaans.

U.S.S.R.

383

Directory of biomedical institutions in the Union of Soviet Socialist Republics. Washington, 1, 1958– .

Alphabetical listing of about 1569 institutions, with name of director and chief staff members when known. 1 ed. by D. P. Gelfand has title *A directory of medical and biological research institutes of the USSR;* 2 ed. by Mordecai Hoseh, 1965.

384

Russia. Ministerstvo vnutrennykh del. Meditsinskiĭ departament. Rossiiskiĭ meditsinskiĭ spisok, izdannyĭ Meditsinskim departamentom Ministerstva vnutrennykh del na . . . god. S. Petersburg, 1809–1916.

Brief professional information. Includes physicians, veterinarians, dentists, and pharmacists.

384.1

Spisok meditsinkikh vracheĭ, Jan 1, 1924. Moskva, Izd. Narodnogo Komissariata zdravookhranenii͡a R.S.F.S.R., 1925. 827 p.

[pt. 1] Women doctors; [pt. 2] men doctors.

United States

CURRENT

Physicians

385

American Academy of General Practice. Membership directory with constitution and by-laws. Kansas City, Mo., 1949–

Officers, commissions and committees, and members listed alphabetically by name and geographically by state and city.

386

American College of Physicians. Directory. Philadelphia, 1, 1923– .

Brief personal and professional information for each member. Geographic arrangement; name index. Issued biennially with supplement in alternate years.

v. 1–2, as *Yearbook.*

387

American College of Surgeons. Directory. Chicago, 1953– .

Triennial with annual supplements. Gives officers and geographical and alphabetical lists of fellows; brief professional information includes specialty, school attended, societies and specialty boards to which certified. Issued as *Yearbook*, 1913–52. Cumulative necrology.

388

American Medical Association. Directory, officials and staff. Chicago [1, 1960?]–

Somewhat irregular; currently issued semiannually. Includes general officers and trustees, Woman's auxiliary officers and committee chairmen, members of the House of Delegates, commission, committee, and council members, scientific section officers, editorial boards of specialty journals, executives of state and county medical societies, editors of society journals and bulletins. The *American medical directory* prior to 1961 included this type of information.

389★★

American medical directory; a register of

legally qualified physicians. Chicago, 1906– . American Medical Association.

Revised irregularly since 1942. 23 ed., 1965, published in 3 parts: Pt. 1, alphabetical list of physicians of the United States, Isthmian Canal Zone, Puerto Rico, Virgin Islands, certain Pacific Islands, and U.S. physicians in foreign countries. Contains list of chief American scientific medical societies and United States and foreign medical schools. Pt. 2, separate listings of physicians in the Air Force, Navy, Public Health Service, Veterans Administration, followed by a geographical register of physicians arranged alphabetically within each state and city. Brief data give name, address, date of birth, graduation date and name of school, date of licensing, society memberships, specialty, and type of practice. Pt. 3, explanatory notes and guide to the codes and key numbers in the geographical register.

Through 1958 data given included state medical practice acts, personnel of state, county, and city health departments, officers of state medical societies, hospitals, list of residencies and fellowships, list of hospitals approved for internship, medical libraries, and medical journals. Data on Canadian physicians included through 1958.

390
American men of medicine. Farmingdale, N.Y., Institute for Research in Biography, 1, 1945– .

1961 (768 p.) contains personal and professional data on more than 10,000 physicians and surgeons.

1945 as *Who's important in medicine.*

391★★
Directory of medical specialists holding certification by American Specialty Boards. Chicago, Advisory Board of Medical Specialties, 1, 1939– .

Complete biographical data. Brief professional information arranged by state and city under each board. Also includes officers, history, and certification requirements for each board. v. 12, 1965/66, Marquis-Who's Who, 1965, 2375 p.

391.1
JAMA reference directories. AMA officials and executive staff, state medical associations, and examinations and licensure. In Journal of the American Medical Association, 163, 1963– .

Published regularly in the last issue of each month, and occasionally in the other issues. Includes dates for examinations by the Educational Council for Foreign Medical Graduates; the National Board of Medical Examiners; the basic science boards; the state boards of medical examiners; and the medical specialty boards.

Organizations

392
American Association of Medical Clinics. Directory. Charlottesville, Va., 1, 1952– .

Alphabetical listing of member and associate clinics by name; gives address, telephone number, founding date, professional staff, and population served. 7 ed., 1964/65.

393
American Medical Association. Committee on Voluntary Health Agencies. Handbook for medical societies and individual physicians on national voluntary health agencies. 3 ed. Chicago, 1962. 96 p.

Pt. 1 describes the purpose, organizational pattern, financing programs, and key personnel of national voluntary health agencies; pt. 2 gives explanatory paragraph on voluntary agencies of medical interest.

394
——. Council on Medical Service. Listing of group practices in the United States. Chicago, 1, 1959– .

Geographical listing, giving name and address.

395
A directory of information resources in the United States: physical sciences, biological sciences, engineering. Washington, [1] 1965– . U.S. National Referral Center for Science and Technology.

Arranged alphabetically by organization name. Data given include address, telephone number, and description of activities.

396★
Encyclopedia of associations. v. 1, National organizations of the United States. v. 2, Geographic-executive index. v. 3, New associations. Detroit, Gale Research Co., 1, 1956– .

v. 1 of 4 ed. lists over 12,500 organizations by key word under subject field. Data given include address, name of director or secretary, members, staff, and activities. Alphabetical and keyword index. Includes sections on health and social welfare. v. 2 covers material in v. 1. v. 3 appears periodically in loose-leaf form to supplement material between editions.

1–2 ed. as *Encyclopedia of American associations.*

397★
The Foundation directory. New York, Russell Sage Foundation, 1, 1960– .

2 ed., 1964, lists 6007 foundations alphabetically under state, with purpose and activities, financial data, and officers. Includes medicine and related fields.

397.1
JAMA reference directories. Organizations of medical interest. In Journal of the American Medical Association, 163, 1963– .

Published regularly in the second issue of each month, and occasionally in other issues. Gives number of members; names of officials; addresses; places and dates for meetings and annual conventions. Limited to the United States.

398
Roster of executives of state medical associations and county medical societies and editors of state journals and county medical society bulletins. Chicago, [1] 195?– . American Medical Association, Council on Medical Services.

Geographical arrangement; for societies lists secretaries and address; for journals lists editors and addresses. Beginning in 1963 included in no. 388.

399
Wasserman, C. S., and Wasserman, Paul. Health organizations of the United States and Canada. A directory of voluntary associations, professional societies and other groups concerned with health and related fields. Ithaca, N.Y., Graduate School of Business and Public Administration, Cornell University, [1] 1961– .

Alphabetical listing of organizations with address, name of director or secretary, purpose, membership, finances, meetings, and publications. Also listed by state and subject field. 2 ed., 1965, has title *Health organizations of the United States, Canada and internationally.*

NONCURRENT

Nos. 401 and 403 are the most comprehensive periodically published sources for older data. Some local and regional directories, periodical in character, antedate them, but they have not been listed. Additional biographical information will be found in the history sections. See especially nos. 651–658.

399.1
American Homoeopathic Biographical Association. Biographical cyclopaedia of homoeopathic physicians and surgeons. Chicago, 1893. 172 p.

400
American physicians and surgeons. A biographical directory of practicing members of the medical profession in the United States and Canada, including supplements in which are listed and classified the leading hospitals, sanitariums and health resorts of both countries. Minneapolis, The Midwest Co., 1931. 1737 p. Prepared by James C. Fifield.

Physicians listed by state and locality. Professional data, including publications (without source).

401
Butler, Samuel W. The medical register and directory of the United States, systematically arranged by states: comprising names, post office address, educational and professional status of more than fifty thousand physicians; with lists of medical societies, colleges, hospitals and other medical institutions, with abstracts of medical laws of each state, notices of mineral springs, etc. 1–2 ed. Philadelphia, Office of the Medical and Surgical Reporter, 1874–77.

No comprehensive name index.

402
Flint's medical and surgical directory of the United States and Canada. New York, Flint, 1897. 1026 p.

402.1
Herringshaw, Thomas W., ed. The American physician and surgeon blue book. A distinct cyclopedia of 1919. Five thousand medical biographies. Chicago, American Blue Book Publishers, 1919. 478 p.

403
Polk's medical and surgical directory of

the United States. Detroit, Polk, 1–14?, 1886–1917?

List of physicians arranged by state, with college of graduation and date. Also lists existing and extinct medical schools, medical societies, hospitals, and other medical institutions, synopsis of laws relating to medicine. Index to physicians and medical officers of the United States Army and Navy, and a list of medical journals published in the United States. Title varies: 1886, *Medical and surgical directory of the United States*; 1890–96, *Medical and surgical register of the United States and Canada*; 1904–14/15, *Polk's medical register and directory of North America*; 1902, 1917, *Polk's medical register and directory of the United States and Canada.*

404
The standard medical directory of North America; including a directory of practicing physicians in the United States of America, Canada, Cuba, Mexico and Central America. 1902–[03/4] Chicago, Englehard, 1901–[02]

Includes medical laws, hospitals, list of drugs with prices.

405
Who's who among physicians and surgeons. Ed. by J. C. Schwartz. New York, 1, 1938. 1336 p.

Professional data, selected works.

406
Who's who in American medicine, 1925. Ed. by L. Thompson and W. S. Downs. New York, Who's Who Publications, 1925. 1820 p.

Professional information, selected works, outstanding contributions to medicine, awards.

Uruguay

406.1
Guía oficial del club médico del Uruguay. Montevideo, 19 ?– .

Lists physicians, hospitals, clinics (with personnel), Faculty of Medicine, governmental medical agencies and personnel.

15 ed., 1938; 16 ed., 1940.

406.2
Servicio Científico de Publicaciones Medicas del Uruguay. Guía medica especializada del Uruguay . . . 1958. Montevideo [1958] 180 p.

Brief professional information.

Yugoslavia

407
Adresar zdravstvenih ustanova FNRJ [Directory of health establishments of the Federal National Republics of Yugoslavia] Beograd, Savremena administracija, 1961. 592 p.

Includes hospitals, dispensaries, pharmacies, spas, medical schools. Gives name and address of the organization and name of director. In earlier volumes advertisements for medical colleges give faculty, fees, etc.

ENCYCLOPEDIAS

Encyclopedias intended for the layman have not been listed.

408
Bol'shaia medisinskaia entsiklopediia. 2 ed., by A. N. Bakulev. Moskva, Medgiz, 1956–64. 35 v.

409
Cyclopedia of medicine, surgery, specialties. 3 ed. Philadelphia, Davis, 1950– . 14 v.

410
Enciclopedia medica italiana. Firenze, Sansoni, 1950–59. 10 v. Aggiornamento. Venezia, Istituto per la collaborazione culturale, 1961. 2 v.

Long articles; no biographies. v. 10 is index.

411
Enciclopedia Salvat de ciencias médicas. Barcelona, Salvat, 1955–60. 5 v. Apendice. Barcelona, Salvat, 1963. 518 p.

Includes biographies. Some volumes issued in a 2 ed.

412
Encyklopedie praktického lékaře; abecední slovník současného lékařského vědění [Encyclopedia for the general practitioner; alphabetical index of current medical knowledge] Ed. by Duchoslav Panýrek, et al. Praha, Borský a Šulc, etc., 1939– .

413
Medicinska enciklopedija [Medical encyclopedia] Ed. by Ante Šercer. Zagreb, Leksikografski zavod F.N.R.J., 1957– .

v. 8 (ending with Shistosomijaza) was published in 1963. Includes biographies.

HISTORY OF MEDICINE

BIBLIOGRAPHIES AND INDEXES

414

Bibliography of the history of medicine. Bethesda, 1, 1965– . U. S. National Library of Medicine.

About 2600 citations in first issue, covering material indexed in 1965. Arranged by persons as subjects, topics with chronological and geographical subdivisions, and authors. Includes monographs, analytics for congresses, etc., and journal articles. Annual, with five-year cumulation planned.

415

Choulant, Johann Ludwig. Bibliotheca medico-historica; sive, Catalogus librorum historicorum de re medica et scientia naturali systematicus. Lipsiae, Engelmann, 1842. 269 p. Additamenta. Julius Rosenbaum, ed. Halis Saxonum, Lippert, 1842–47. 2 v.

Classified bibliography with subject and author indexes. Reprinted Hildesheim, Olms, 1960 (omits *Additamenta*).

416

Choulant, Johann Ludwig. Handbuch der Bücherkunde für die ältere Medicin. 2 ed. Leipzig, Voss, 1841. 434 p.

Contains biographic and historical notes and lists editions of the works of early Greek, Latin, and Arabic writers. Reprinted Leipzig, W. Heims, 1911; München, Verlag d. Münchner Drucke, 1926; Graz, Akademische Druck und Verlagsanstalt, 1956.

417

Current work in the history of medicine. An international bibliography. 1, Jan./Mar. 1954– . Wellcome Historical Medical Library, London.

Quarterly subject index to periodical literature on medical history, with author index. Includes addresses of authors. Lists new books alphabetically by author. A recent number (44, Oct./Dec., 1964) contained 1320 subject entries (including duplicate entries for articles indexed under more than one subject). "Address Supplement" [no. 1, 1960] contains list of periodicals on the history of medicine and science.

418

Emmerson, Joan S. Translations of medical classics; a list. Newcastle upon Tyne, 1965. 82 p. (Newcastle upon Tyne. Unisity Library. Publications, no. 3)

Lists alphabetically by author translations of classic works originally published before 1900. Not comprehensive.

419

Garrison, Fielding H., and Morton, Leslie T. Garrison and Morton's medical bibliography, an annotated checklist of texts illustrating the history of medicine. 2 ed. London, Grafton; New York, Argosy, 1954. 655 p.

6808 entries, mostly annotated, arranged by broad subjects, with outstanding contributions listed chronologically, followed by histories. Includes list of periodicals devoted to the history of medicine, general histories of medicine, and histories by period and locality. Name and subject indexes. Supplemented by Lee Ash, *Serial publications containing medical classics. An index to citations contained in Garrison-Morton*, New Haven, The Antiquarium, 1961, 147 p.

Reprinted with minor revisions 1965.

419.1

Index zur Geschichte der Medizin und Biologie. München, Urban & Schwarzenberg, 1–2, 1945/48–1949/52. Im Auftrag der Deutschen Gesellschaft für Geschichte der Medizin, Naturwissenschaft und Technik.

Over 10,000 items in v. 1, over 7,000 in v. 2. Lists books and articles in classified arrangement. v. 2 has name index (authors and personal subjects), v. 1 does not.

v. 1 as *Index zur Geschichte der Medizin, Naturwissenschaft und Technik, im Auftrag der Deutschen Vereinigung für Geschichte der Medizin, Naturwissenschaft und Technik*. v. 1, 1953, ed. by Walter Artelt; v. 2, 1966, ed. by Johannes Steudel.

420

Mitteilungen zur Geschichte der Medizin

und der Naturwissenschaften. Leipzig, 1, 1902– . Deutsche Akademie der Naturforscher Leopoldina in cooperation with Deutsche Gesellschaft für Geschichte der Medizin, Naturwissenschaft und Technik.

Semiannual. Mainly devoted to current classified bibliography with signed descriptive and critical annotations. Nearly complete coverage of German books and articles, extensive coverage of other countries. Includes some original studies, bibliographies, and news items. Annual subject and name indexes.

v. 1–40 issued by the Gesellschaft (1902–31 under name Deutsche Gesellschaft für Geschichte der Medizin und der Naturwissenschaften). 1932–43 as *Mitteilungen zur Geschichte der Medizin, der Naturwissenschaften und der Technik*. Publication suspended 1943–60, resumed with v. 41, 1961. Founded by Karl Sudhoff, currently edited by Rudolph Zaunick.

421
Pagel, Julius L. Historisch-medicinische Bibliographie für die Jahre 1875–1896. Berlin, Karger, 1898. p. [585]–959 (His Geschichte der Medicin, 2. Th.)

Classified; no author index. Notable lists of local histories, individual biographies. Includes articles and monographs. Supplements Pauly (no. 422).

422
Pauly, Alphonse. Bibliographie des sciences médicales. Paris, Tross, 1874. 1758 columns.

Divided into sections on bibliography (general medical, by period, by country, by subject, manuscripts); biography, including individuals; history (general medical and by subject); schools, institutions, and societies; controversies and doctrines; hospitals; epidemics; medical geography. Cites both articles and books. Notable for local listings under general and special subjects. Author index. Supplemented in part by Pagel (no. 421).

423
Thornton, John L. Medical books, libraries and collectors; a study of bibliography and the book trade in relation to the medical sciences. 2 ed. London, Deutsch, 1966. 445 p.

Narrative chronological biobibliography of important contributions to medical knowledge, with chapters on medical societies, periodicals, bibliographies, and libraries. Author bibliography: p. 355–405. 1 ed. 1949.

424
Vierordt, Hermann. Medizin-geschichtliches Hilfsbuch, mit besonderer Berücksichtigung der Entdeckungsgeschichte und der Biographie. Tübingen, Laupp, 1916. 469 p.

Selective author bibliography, with some notes on important contributions of particular authors, eponyms, etc. Brief biographical data, references to critical studies in separate section. Subject index.

Manuscripts

Only general works on medical or scientific manuscripts are included. Catalogs of individual library collections have been omitted: most listings of medical manuscripts will be found in comprehensive catalogs; to list all these would be inappropriate, to list the few special catalogs of medical manuscripts misleading. For a guide to such catalogs, see Paul O. Kristeller, *Latin manuscript books before 1600; a list of the printed catalogues and unpublished inventories of extant collections*, New York, 1960, 234 p. For holdings of U. S. libraries, see Seymour De Ricci and William J. Wilson, *Census of medieval and renaissance manuscripts in the United States and Canada*, New York, Wilson, 1935–40, 3 v., and its *Supplement*, New York, Bibliographical Society of America, 1962, 626 p., edited by C. V. Faye and W. H. Bond.

425
Beccaria, Augusto. I codici di medicina del periodo presalernitano (secoli IX, X, e XI). Roma, Edizioni di Storia e letteratura, 1956. 500 p. (Storia e letteratura, 53)

Descriptive catalog of 145 medical manuscripts, arranged by country, city, and collection, with analyses of contents and bibliographies of published editions and studies. Introduction on nature of texts and problems of identification, dating, and localization. Indexes, bibliographies.

426
Devreesse, Robert. Introduction à l'étude des manuscrits grecs. Paris, Impr. nationale, Librairie C. Klincksieck, 1954. 347 p.

Ch. XVIII, "La médecine," p. 259–272, lists

more than 200 medical authors and their principal works. Supplements Diels (no. 427).

427
Diels, Hermann, ed. Die Handschriften der antiken Ärzte. Berlin, Akademie der Wissenschaften, 1905–06. 2 pts. Nachtrag, Berlin, 1908, p. 23–72.

Catalog of manuscripts of texts and translations of classical Greek physicians in European and Near Eastern libraries. Gives Greek and Latin title, incipit and explicit of each work, lists critical editions, and locates manuscripts, with dates. Pt. 1: Hippocrates and Galen; pt. 2: other Greek physicians. List of printed catalogs and studies, by country, city and library: pt. 2, p. xi–xxiii.

Reprinted from *Abhandlungen* of the Akademie der Wissenschaften, Berlin, 1905–07.

428
Thorndike, Lynn, and Kibre, Pearl. A catalogue of incipits of mediaeval scientific writings in Latin. Rev. ed. Cambridge, Mass., 1963. 1938 p. (Mediaeval Academy of America. Publication no. 29)

Fundamental source for identifying texts from their incipits.

Incunabula

Only specialized medical and scientific bibliographies have been included. Holdings of U. S. libraries are listed in Frederick Goff, ed., *Incunabula in American libraries; a third census*, New York, Bibliographical Society of America, 1964, which also serves as a guide to published catalogs of collections.

429
Choulant, Johann Ludwig. Graphische Incunabeln für Naturgeschichte und Medicin. Enthaltend Geschichte und Bibliographie der ersten naturhistorischen und medicinischen Drucke des XV. und XVI. Jahrhunderts, welche mit illustrirenden Abbildungen versehen sind. Leipzig, Weigel, 1858. 168 p.

Detailed bibliographical descriptions and analyses of contents of three anonymous works and works of eight authors. Originally printed in *Archiv für die zeichnenden Künste*, 3. Jahrg., 1857. Reprinted München, Verlag der Münchener Drucke, 1924; Hildesheim, Olms, 1963.

430
Klebs, Arnold C. Incunabula scientifica et medica. Bruges, St. Catherine Press, 1938. 359 p. (New York Academy of Medicine. Library. History of medicine series, no. 1)

Checklist with references to bibliographic descriptions of each edition. Reprinted from *Osiris*, 4: pt. 1, 1937. Reprinted Hildesheim, Olms, 1963.

431
Osler, Sir William. Incunabula medica; a study of the earliest printed medical books, 1467–1480. Oxford, Bibliographical Society, 1923. 140 p. (Bibliographical Society. Illustrated monographs, no. 19)

List of 217 editions, edited by Victor Scholderer, with a long introduction.

432
Sarton, George. The scientific literature transmitted through the incunabula. In Osiris, 5:41–245, 1938.

Appendixes contain the most popular authors of scientific incunabula; the best sellers; anonymous scientific incunabula; chronologic list of authors whose scientific works were printed before 1501.

433
Sudhoff, Karl. Deutsche medizinische Inkunabeln; bibliographisch-literarische Untersuchungen. Leipzig, Barth, 1908. 278 p. (Studien zur Geschichte der Medizin, v. 2/3)

Annotated, arranged by subject. Includes some editions after 1500.

History of Bibliography

434
Brodman, Estelle. The development of medical bibliography. Baltimore, Medical Library Association, 1954. 226 p. (Medical Library Association. Publication no. 1)

Historical study of general medical bibliographies, with a list of 255 appearing since 1500.

435
Fulton, John F. The great medical bibliographers; a study in humanism. Philadelphia, Univ. of Pennsylvania Press, 1951. 107 p. (Yale University, School of Medicine Library. Historical Library. Publication no. 26 [i.e., 28])

Brief essays.

436
Viets, Henry R. The bibliography of medicine. In Bulletin of the Medical Library Association, 27:105–17, 1938.

Descriptive accounts of medical bibliographies from the 15th century to the *Index-catalogue*. Checklist of 34 items, some not included here.

HISTORIOGRAPHY

437
Artelt, Walter. Einführung in die Medizinhistorik, ihr Wesen, ihre Arbeitsweise und ihre Hilfsmittel. Stuttgart, Enke, 1949. 240 p.

Manual, covering research methods (location, establishment, criticism, and interpretation of texts and other sources), and composition and style in writing, editing, and printing. Extensive lists of reference works, standard treatises, and bibliographies, often with annotations. "Anhang: Die Geschichte der Medizingeschichtschreibung," by Edith Heischkel: p. 202–237. Subject index only.

438
Galdston, Iago, ed. On the utility of medical history. New York, International Universities Press, 1957. 73 p. (New York Academy of Medicine. Institute on Social and Historical Medicine. Monograph I)

Essays by six different authorities. Subjects include medical historiography and teaching of medical history. References cited include several key articles.

439
Granjel, Luis Sánchez. Estudio histórico de la medicina; lecciones de metodología aplicadas a la historia de la medicina española. Salamanca, Librería Cervantes, 1961. 177 p.

Classified bibliography (p. 95–177) includes general histories of medicine, special periods, areas, and topics; emphasizes Spanish and Spanish American medicine (p. 115–171). No index.

440
Pazzini, Adalberto. Elementi propedeutici di storia della medicina. Roma, Società Editrice "Humanitas," 1944. 280 p.

Emphasis on Italian history and scholarship. Includes the history of medical historiography; the study and teaching of medical history (with accounts of study centers, societies, museums, etc.); historical methods; classified listing of reference works, bibliographies, and serial publications; synoptic tables and chronology; biobibliography of medical historians.

SOURCE COLLECTIONS

441
Camac, Charles N. B., ed. Epoch-making contributions to medicine, surgery, and the allied sciences; being reprints of those communications which first conveyed epoch-making observations to the scientific world, together with biographical sketches of the observers. Philadelphia, Saunders, 1909. 435 p.

Contains texts in English of twelve papers, by Lister, Harvey, Auenbrugger, Laennec, Jenner, Morton, Warren, Simpson, and Holmes. Reprinted New York, Dover, 1959, under title: *Classics of medicine and surgery*.

442
Clendening, Logan. Source book of medical history. New York, Hoeber, 1942. 685 p.

Translated excerpts from some 120 authors, from the Egyptian papyri to Roentgen, with brief historical and biographic notes, references to the original publications and to recent histories and commentaries. Reprinted New York, Dover, 1960.

443
Sudhoffs Klassiker der Medizin und der Naturwissenschaften. Leipzig, Barth, 1, 1910– .

A monographic series of German editions or translations of works by authors of various nationalities, mainly 16th–19th century. Each volume has introduction and notes; v. 33– have full bibliographies of editions and critical studies.

v. 1–33, 1910–42, as *Klassiker der Medizin*; v. 34–37, 1960–61, as *Sudhoffs Klassiker der Medizin*. General eds.: v. 1–32, Karl Sudhoff; v. 34– Johannes Steudel and Rudolph Zaunik for the Deutsche Akademie der Naturforscher Leopoldina.

BIOGRAPHIES

Bibliographies

444
Garrison, Fielding H. Available sources

and future prospects of medical biography. In Bulletin of the New York Academy of Medicine, ser. 2, 4:586–607, 1928.

Lists works which include biographic material, arranged by countries; also general medical biographic collections, biographies of individual men, and dictionaries of anonymous and pseudonymous works. Reprinted in his *Contributions to the history of medicine . . . 1925–1935*, New York, Hafner, 1966, p. 697–718.

445
New York Academy of Medicine. Library. Catalog of biographies. Boston, Hall, 1960. 165 p.

Photocopy of shelflist cards for single biographies, chiefly books, arranged by subject.

Biographical Dictionaries

446
Biographisches Lexikon der hervorragenden Ärzte aller Zeiten und Völker . . . unter Spezial-Redaktion von E. Gurlt und A. Wernich hrsg. von August Hirsch. 2 ed. By W. Haberling, F. Hübotter and H. Vierordt. Berlin, Urban & Schwarzenberg, 1929–34. 5 v. Ergänzungsband: Nachträge zu den Bänden I-V. By W. Haberling and H. Vierordt. Berlin, 1935. 426 p.

Biographical sketches, listing principal publications, of some 17,000 physicians who had arrived at maturity before 1880. References at end of each article.

Mainly a reprint, with entries intercalated, of the 1884–88 Leipzig edition by August Hirsch and of Julius L. Pagel's *Biographisches Lexikon hervorragender Ärzte des neunzehnten Jahrhunderts*, Berlin, 1901, with some new biographies. Additions, corrections, and new biographies mostly in *Ergänzungsband*. Indispensable, but because of duplicate entries, editorial defects, errors, and misprints, must be used with caution and does not entirely supersede original works on which it was based.

Reprinted Munich and New York, 1962. Continued by no. 447.

447
Biographisches Lexikon der hervorragenden Ärzte der letzten fünfzig Jahre. Ed. by I. Fischer. Berlin, Urban & Schwarzenberg, 1932–33. 2 v.

Continuation of Hirsch's *Biographisches Lexikon* (no. 446), similar in scope and arrangement. Covers the period 1880–1930. Reprinted München, Urban & Schwarzenberg, 1962.

448
Dechambre, Amédée, ed. Dictionnaire encyclopédique des sciences médicales. Paris, P. Asselin, V. Masson, 1864–89. 100 v.

Includes many brief biographies of major and minor medical figures of all centuries. Bibliographies vary in completeness, include books and articles. Also useful for subject bibliographies.

449
Dezeimeris, Jean E., Ollivier, Charles P., and Raige-Delorme, Jacques. Dictionnaire historique de la médecine ancienne et moderne. Paris, Béchet jeune, 1828–39. 4 v.

Dezeimeris, Jourdan (no. 450), and Eloy (no. 451) are especially useful for bibliographies of authors cited; the sketches are generally longer than those in Hirsch (no. 446).

450
Dictionaire des sciences médicales. Biographie médicale. Paris, Panckoucke, 1820–25. 7 v. Ed. by A. J. L. Jourdan. (Supplement to Dictionaire des sciences médicales, par une société de médecins et de chirurgiens. Paris, Panckoucke, 1812–22. 60 v.)

See no. 449.

451
Eloy, Nicolas F. J. Dictionnaire historique de la médecine ancienne et moderne; ou Mémoires disposés en ordre alphabétique pour servir à l'histoire de cette science, et à celle des médecins, anatomistes, botanistes, chirurgiens et chymistes de toutes nations. Mons, Hoyois, 1778. 4 v.

A pioneer biobibliography with over 5000 entries, especially good for France, Belgium, and Italy. Used extensively by later compilers. Biographies include full listing of works and editions, often with annotations. Contains some articles under subjects, places, etc. 1 ed. 1755. The Italian translation (*Dizionario storico della medicina*, Napoli, Gessari, 1761-65, 7 v.) adds some notes, corrections, and new articles.

452
Kestner, Christian W. Medicinisches Gelehrten-Lexicon, darinnen die Leben der berühmtesten Aerzte, samt deren wichtigsten Schrifften, sonderbaresten Entdeckungen und merckwürdigsten Streitig-

keiten. Aus den besten Scribenten in möglichster Kürze nach alphabetischer Ordnung beschrieben. Jena, Bey J. Meyers seel. Erben, 1740. 940, [4] p.

Biographical sketches include titles of works, with brief imprint data. References to sources in notes. Based on general reference as well as medical works. Sources described in preface and listed by author, p. [1–4] at end.

Collected Biographies

453
Gibson, William C. Young endeavor. Contributions to science by medical students of the past four centuries. Springfield, Ill., Thomas, 1958. 292 p.

Brief biographical studies, arranged by subject or specialty. Classified bibliography: p. 273–283.

454
Monro, Thomas K. The physician as man of letters, science, and action. 2 ed. Edinburgh, Livingstone, 1951. 245 p.

Short sketches of about 550 physicians, mainly British, who achieved distinction in other fields. Chapters on various fields. Indexes of names and topics. Sketches include important works. Chief sources used mentioned in preface and introduction. 1 ed. 1933.

455
Rosen, George, and Caspari-Rosen, Beate, ed. 400 years of a doctor's life. New York, Schuman, 1947. 429 p.

Autobiographical excerpts in English from writings of physicians, from Paracelsus to Seagrave, arranged in 10 sections representing phases of the medical life. Brief biographical introductions. Bibliography (sources used): p. 426–429.

456
Sourkes, Theodore L. Nobel prize winners in medicine and physiology, 1901–1965. New York, Abelard-Schuman, [c. 1966] 464 p. (The life of science library, 45)

For each gives biographical sketch, description of work, and its consequences in theory and practice. Revision of an earlier edition (1953) by Lloyd G. Stevenson.

DICTIONARIES AND CHRONOLOGIES

457
Aschoff, Ludwig. Kurze Übersichtstabelle zur Geschichte der Medizin. 7 ed. by Paul Diepgen and Heinz Goerke. Berlin, Springer, 1960. 85 p.

Chronological tables with brief historical introductions. Name and subject indexes. No bibliography. First published 1898.

458
Clark, Paul F., and Clark, Alice S. Memorable days in medicine; a calendar of biology and medicine. Madison, Univ. of Wisconsin Press, 1942. 305 p.

Entries for each day of the year cite birth and death dates of significant contributors to medicine from early days to the present. Other dates celebrate outstanding events. Bibliography: p. 293–294.

459
Kelly, Emerson C. Encyclopedia of medical sources. Baltimore, Williams & Wilkins, 1948. 476 p.

Lists by author's name medical syndromes, signs, test methods, and discoveries, with citations of key works. Subject index.

460
Pagel, Julius L. Zeittafeln zur Geschichte der Medizin. Berlin, Hirschwald, 1908. 16 p. 26 tables.

Tables show contemporaneous medical, cultural, and scientific developments, including historical, biographical, and bibliographic data.

COMPREHENSIVE HISTORIES

461
Baas, Johann H. Outlines of the history of medicine and the medical profession. Tr. and rev. by H. E. Handerson. New York, Vail, 1889. 1173 p.

Includes biobibliographical notices of important physicians of each period and specialty, arranged by nationality. No bibliography. Translation of *Grundriss der Geschichte der Medizin und des heilenden Standes*, Stuttgart, 1876.

462
Bariéty, Maurice J. C., and Coury, Charles R. Histoire de la médecine. Paris, Fayard, 1963. 1217 p.

General history, undocumented, with appendix on special topics (p. 827–928), synoptic chronology of general and medical history (p. 929–1049), biographic index with identifying data (p. 1051–1155), brief bibliography (p. 1201–1206). Detailed table of contents, but no subject index.

463
Castiglioni, Arturo. A history of medicine. Tr. and ed. by E. B. Krumbhaar. 2 ed. New York, Knopf, 1947. 1192, lxi p.

General survey, by periods. Includes annotated classified subject bibliography of secondary works, by chapters and general, p. 1147–1192. Additional references to sources in text. 1st Italian ed. 1927.

464
Diepgen, Paul. Geschichte der Medizin; die historische Entwicklung der Heilkunde und des ärztlichen Lebens. Berlin, Gruyter, 1949–55. 2 v. in 3.

General survey; emphasizes German contributions. Classified bibliography in each volume. 2 ed. of v. 2, pt. 1–2, appeared in 1959–65.

465
Garrison, Fielding H. An introduction to the history of medicine, with medical chronology, suggestions for study and bibliographic data. 4 ed. Philadelphia, Saunders, 1929. 996 p.

Still the standard English-language reference history. Classified bibliography: p. 884–922; footnote references throughout. Reprinted Philadelphia, Saunders, 1960. 1 ed. 1914.

466
Haeser, Heinrich. Lehrbuch der Geschichte der Medicin und der epidemischen Krankheiten. 3 ed. Jena, Dufft, 1875–82. 3 v.

Detailed history, with extensive bibliographical references in each section. v. 1–2, chronological history through the early 19th century; v. 3, history of epidemic diseases. No subject index, but detailed table of contents. Reprint Hildesheim, Olms, 1963.

467
Major, Ralph H. A history of medicine. Springfield, Ill., Thomas, 1954. 2 v. (1155 p.)

Most recent comprehensive text in English. Includes biographical sketches at end of each section. Bibliography: p. 1057–1081.

468
Mettler, Cecilia C. History of medicine, a correlative text, arranged according to subjects. Ed. by Fred A. Mettler. Philadelphia, Blakiston, 1947. 1215 p.

Arranged by broad subject sections. Includes excerpts from original writings. General references: p. xv. Extensive bibliographical footnotes.

469
Neuburger, Max. Geschichte der Medizin. v. 1–v. 2, pt. 1. Stuttgart, Enke, 1906–11.

Left incomplete. Comprehensive history through Middle Ages, including Oriental medicine. Extensive bibliographical data. English translation by Ernest Playfair, London, 1910–25, omits or abridges some passages, including bibliographic data.

470
Puschmann, Theodor. Handbuch der Geschichte der Medizin, begründet von Th. Puschmann; bearb. von Dr. [Rudolf] Arndt [et al.] Hrsg. von Max Neuberger und Julius Pagel. Jena, Fischer, 1902–05. 3 v.

Monographs by various authors, with bibliographies. v. 1, general history of medicine through the Middle Ages; v. 2 and 3, histories of special subjects in medicine.

471
Sprengel, Kurt P. J. Versuch einer pragmatischen Geschichte der Arzneykunde. 3 ed. Halle, Gebauer; Wien, Gerold, 1821–40. 6 v.

Examines contributions of important authors, with extensive bibliographical references. v. 1–5, originally published 1801–03, cover earliest times through 1800; v. 6, in 2 parts, 1837–40, is a continuation by Burkard Eble, covering 1800–1825. Chronological tables at end of v. 1–5; name index only in each volume.

The French translation by Antoine J. L. Jourdan (*Histoire de la médecine*, Paris, Deterville, 1815–20, 9 v.), based on 2 ed., revised by Édouard F. M. Bosquillon, includes translation of Kurt Sprengel and Wilhelm Sprengel's *Geschichte der Chirurgie* (Halle, 1805–19) and a general subject index in v. 9.

Shorter Histories

472
Ackerknecht, Erwin H. A short history of

medicine. New York, Ronald Press, 1955. 258 p.

Brief but well balanced. Suggestions for further reading.

473
Gotfredsen, Edvard. Medicinens historie. Kjøbenhavn, Busck, 1950. 513 p.

Largely biographical; useful for names and dates. Classified bibliography of sources and secondary works: p. 433–476.

474
King, Lester S. The growth of medical thought. Chicago, Univ. of Chicago Press, 1963. 254 p.

Chapters on successive periods, with emphasis in each on selected individuals representing trends in medical science and theories of disease.

475
Leibbrand, Werner. Heilkunde: eine Problemgeschichte der Medizin. Freiburg, Alber, 1953. 436 p. (Orbis Academicus, v. 2, pt. 4)

Interpretative study, with many quotations from the sources. Classified bibliography, partially annotated, p. 389–413.

476
Meyer-Steineg, Theodor, and Sudhoff, Karl. Illustrierte Geschichte der Medizin. 5 ed. Ed. by Robert Herrlinger and Fridolf Kudlien. Stuttgart, Fischer, 1965. 349 p.

Comprehensive survey through the 19th century, without scholarly apparatus. Emphasis on development of medical science rather than literature. 1–4 ed., 1920–1950, under title: *Geschichte der Medizin in Überblick, mit Abbildungen.*

477
Osler, Sir William. The evolution of modern medicine. New Haven, Yale Univ. Press, 1921. 243 p. (Silliman Memorial Lectures)

Interpretation of a great physician, notable for style. No bibliography.

478
Sigerist, Henry E. The great doctors; a biographical history of medicine. Tr. by Eden and Cedar Paul from the 2 German ed. New York, Norton, 1933. 436 p.

Outlines principal trends in medical history through biography. Bibliography (p. 405–415) includes standard editions of key works and biographical studies. Reprinted Garden City, N. Y., Doubleday, 1958. 1st German ed. 1932. 4th German edition, München, Lehmann, 1959, 495 p., includes 7 biographies not in English translation.

479
Singer, Charles J., and Underwood, Edgar A. A short history of medicine. 2 ed. Oxford, Clarendon, 1962. 854 p.

Brief survey through 18th century, extended view (p. 205–755) of 19th and 20th. Classified and selected list of reference material, p. 761–795.

480
Sudhoff, Karl. Kurzes Handbuch der Geschichte der Medizin. Berlin, Karger, 1922. 534 p.

Extensive bibliographical references and biobibliographical notices in the text. Chronological table, p. 505–511. Constitutes 3d and 4th ed. of J. L. Pagel, *Einführung in die Geschichte der Medizin*, 1898.

Pictorial Histories

481
Ackerknecht, Erwin H. Das Reich des Asklepios; eine Geschichte der Medizin in Gegenständen. The world of Asclepios; a history of medicine in objects. Bern, Huber [1963] 92 p.

70 illustrations, 7 in color, of selected objects and portraits from the medical historical collection, University of Zurich, with brief explanatory text in German and English. No index.

482
Bettmann, Otto L. A pictorial history of medicine; a brief, nontechnical survey of the healing arts from Aesculapius to Ehrlich. Springfield, Ill., Thomas, 1956. 318 p.

Illustrations copious but poorly reproduced and largely undocumented. Based mainly on author's Archive. Brief text.

483
Dumesnil, René. Histoire illustrée de la médecine. Paris, Plon, 1950. 195 p.

125 illustrations, documented. Name index only.

484
Hahn, André, Dumaître, Paule, and Sa-

mion-Contet, Janine. Histoire de la médecine et du livre médical à la lumière des collections de la Bibliothèque de la Faculté de médecine de Paris. Paris, Perrin, 1962. 430 p.

Mainly a survey of the illustrated medical book, 15th–19th centuries, with 274 annotated illustrations, including facsimiles and portraits. Emphasis on French contributions. Name index only. Bibliography: p. 377–394.

485
Laignel-Lavastine, Maxime, ed. Histoire générale de la médecine, de la pharmacie, de l'art dentaire et de l'art véterinaire. Paris, Michel, 1936–49. 3 v.

Articles by various authors. Valuable especially for illustrations.

486
Peters, Hermann. Der Arzt und die Heilkunst in der deutschen Vergangenheit. Mit 153 Abbildungen u. Beilagen nach den Originalen aus dem 15–18. Jahrhundert. Leipzig, Diederich, 1900. 136 p. (Monographien zur deutschen Kulturgeschichte, v. 3).

Reproductions of early illustrations, woodcuts, engravings, broadsides, etc., with sources indicated. No index. Reprinted Jena, 1924.

HISTORY BY PERIODS

Ancient

487
Allbutt, Sir Thomas C. Greek medicine in Rome . . . with other historical essays. London, Macmillan, 1921. 633 p. (Fitzpatrick lectures, 1909–10)

Interpretive essays of literary distinction. Occasional bibliographic footnotes.

488
Sigerist, Henry E. A history of medicine. New York, Oxford Univ. Press, 1951–61. 2 v.

v. 1: Primitive and archaic medicine; v. 2: Early Greek, Hindu, and Persian medicine. v. 1 includes introduction on historical approach to medicine (p. 3–37) and appendices (p. 499–541) listing histories of medicine, source books of medical history (periodicals; sets of classics), biographical and bibliographical reference works, museums of medical history, and bibliography of paleopathology since 1930. Intended as 8 v. work; no more published.

489
Steuer, Robert O., and Saunders, John B. de C. M. Ancient Egyptian & Cnidian medicine, the relationship of their aetiological concepts of disease. Berkeley, Univ. of California Press, 1959. 90 p.

Semantic analysis of etiological terms used in Egyptian papyri and Greek texts reflecting Cnidian doctrines, designed to illustrate the influence of Egyptian on early Greek medicine. Bibliography: p. 83–84.

490
Tabanelli, Mario. La medicina nel mondo degli etruschi. Firenze, Olschki, 1963. 123 p. (Biblioteca delle Rivista di storia delle scienze mediche e naturali, v. 11)

Study based on literary and archeological sources. Bibliographical footnotes. General bibliography: p. 119–120.

Babylonia

491
Contenau, Georges. La médecine en Assyrie et en Babylonie. Paris, Maloine, 1938. 230 p. (La Médecine à travers le temps et l'espace, 2)

Includes many extracts translated from the sources. Bibliography: p. 207–227.

Egypt

492
Ghalioungui, Paul. Magic and medical science in ancient Egypt. London, Hodder and Stoughton, 1963. 188 p.

Exposition of underlying concepts and clinical and surgical practices, based on medical papyri and other evidence. Relates Egyptian medicine to that of neighboring areas and considers its influence especially on Greek medicine. Bibliography and references: p. 173–182.

493
Goldstein, Miron. Internationale Bibliographie der altaegyptischen Medizin 1850–1930. Berlin, Aegyptologischer Verlag M. Goldstein, 1933. [48] p.

243 items arranged chronologically under subjects, with name index.

494
Grundriss der Medizin der alten Ägypter. Berlin, Akademie-Verlag, 1, 1954– .

Critical studies, texts and translations, and dictionaries. By Hermann Grapow and others. Includes bibliographical references. 8 v. in 10 published through 1962.

495
Leake, Chauncey D. The old Egyptian medical papyri. Lawrence, Univ. of Kansas Press, 1952. 108 p. (Logan Clendening lectures on the history and philosophy of medicine)

Chiefly about the Hearst medical papyrus, with a list of prescriptions in it and chapters on Egyptian weights and measures, drug measurements, and therapeutics. List of papyri, with locations and printed editions: p. 7. References: p. 98–103.

496
Lefebvre, Gustave. Essai sur la médecine égyptienne de l'époque pharaonique. Paris, Presses universitaires de France, 1956. 216 p.

Arranged topically; extensive quotations from sources. Bibliographic footnotes throughout.

Greece

497
Brock, Arthur J. Greek medicine; being extracts illustrative of medical writers from Hippocrates to Galen. London, Dent, 1929. 256 p. (Library of Greek thought)

In English, with annotations.

498
Schumacher, Joseph. Antike Medizin: die naturphilosophischen Grundlagen der Medizin in der griechischen Antike. 2 ed. Berlin, De Gruyter, 1963. 327 p.

Documented study based on original texts. Bibliography, arranged alphabetically by author, p. 251–298. 1 ed. 1940.

Medieval

The best general accounts of medieval medicine will be found in the larger comprehensive histories and in studies of special subjects.

499
MacKinney, Loren C. Early medieval medicine, with special reference to France and Chartres. Baltimore, Johns Hopkins Press, 1937. 247 p. (Johns Hopkins University, Institute of the History of Medicine. Publications, ser. 3, v. 3)

Lectures on "The dark age concept and early medieval medicine"; "Medicine in Merovingian and Carolingian France"; and "Medical progress at Chartres in the tenth and eleventh centuries." Notes (p. 153–211) include extracts from sources and bibliographical references.

500
Moulin, Daniël de. De heelkunde in de vroege middeleeuwen. Leiden, Brill, 1964. 166 p.

Survey of medical practice and education, followed by account of medical texts available in the period and detailed examination of selected texts. Account of surgical techniques and instruments. English summary: p. 155–159. Bibliography: p. 161–166. No index.

501
Riesman, David. The story of medicine in the Middle Ages. New York, Hoeber, 1935. 402 p.

An introduction to the subject intended for medical students and laymen. Occasional bibliographic references.

Arabic

502
Browne, Edward G. Arabian medicine. Cambridge, Univ. Press, 1921. 138 p. (Fitzpatrick lectures, 1919–20)

Account of contributions of Islamic physicians, Arabic and Persian, based on manuscript and printed sources. Bibliographical references in text and footnotes. Reprinted 1962.

503
Campbell, Donald. Arabian medicine and its influence on the Middle Ages. London, K. Paul, Trench, Trubner, 1926. 2 v.

General history, including transmission from Greek and into Latin, with extensive biobibliographic data, lists of translations and translators, etc.

504
Hamarneh, Sami. Bibliography on medicine and pharmacy in medieval Islam. Stuttgart, Wissenschaftliche Verlagsgesellschaft, 1964. 204 p. (Internationale Gesellschaft für Geschichte der Pharmazie. Veröffentlichungen, new ser., v. 25).

Guide to original texts and other sources and secondary works, including material on general historical background, pertaining to medicine and related sciences during 7th–14th centuries in the Islamic domain from Spain to Pakistan. Arabic and other non-Western titles transliterated. Annotated throughout.

505
Khairallah, Amin A. Outline of Arabic contributions to medicine and the allied

sciences. Beirut, American Press, 1946. 228 p.

Briefly describes writings of Arabic physicians. Arranged topically. Appendices include extensive lists of physicians and their works, translations from Greek and to Latin.

506
Leclerc, Lucien. Histoire de la médecine arabe. Exposé complet des traductions du grec: les sciences en Orient, leur transmission à l'Occident par les traductions Latins. Paris, Leroux, 1876. 2 v.

Exhaustive history, not yet superseded. Survey by periods and geographic areas, with sketches of authors and translators, lists of their works. Preface includes some account of the manuscript and printed sources used. No index. Reprint (New York, Franklin, 1960) includes reproduction of a manuscript index of names.

507
Wüstenfeld, Ferdinand. Geschichte der arabischen Aerzte und Naturforscher. Nach den Quellen bearbeitet. Göttingen, Vandenhoeck & Ruprecht, 1840. 167 p.

Brief biographies, with bibliographies, of men who lived before 1000 A. D. Useful chiefly for identifying obscure men. Reprinted 1963. 183 p.

Modern

508
Foucault, Michel. Naissance de la clinique; une archéologie du regard médical. Paris, Presses Universitaires de France, 1963. 212 p.

Interpretive study, based mainly on French sources, of changes in theories of disease and medical practice, ca. 1770–1830. Classified bibliography (sources): p. 203–212.

509
Galdston, Iago. Progress in medicine; a critical review of the last hundred years. New York, Knopf, 1940. 347 p.

Interpretive survey of main trends. No bibliography.

510
Haagensen, Cushman D., and Lloyd, Wyndham E. B. A hundred years of medicine. New York, Sheridan House, 1943. 443 p.

General historical review. Bibliography (by chapter, largely secondary): p. 413–430.

511
King, Lester S. The medical world of the eighteenth century. Chicago, Univ. of Chicago Press, 1958. 346 p.

Essays on various topics. Notes, by chapters, p. 327–340.

512
Shryock, Richard H. The development of modern medicine, an interpretation of the social and scientific factors involved. 2 ed. New York, Knopf, 1947. 457 p.

Outstanding contribution. Covers the period from the 17th century. Bibliographical footnotes. 1 ed. 1936.

NATIONAL HISTORIES AND SPECIAL GROUPS

American Indians

513
Corlett, William T. The medicine-man of the American Indian and his cultural background. Springfield, Ill., Thomas, 1935. 369 p.

Includes chiefly information about the Indians of recent past. Bibliography: p. 337–354.

514
Harcourt, Raoul d'. La médecine dans l'ancien Pérou. Paris, Maloine, 1939. 242 p. (La médecine à travers le temps et l'espace, 3).

Study based on archeological and anthropological sources. Bibliography (134 references, by author): p. 217–235.

515
Pardal, Ramón. Medicina aborigen Americana. Buenos Aires, Anesi, 1937. 377 p. (Humanior; biblioteca del Americanista moderno, sec. C, 3)

Survey of primitive medicine and magic, followed by accounts of medicine of the most important native cultural groups of Mexico, Central, and South America, and of trephining, archeological evidence of diseases, and materia medica. References at ends of chapters.

516
Rodríguez, Luis A. La ciencia médica de los Aztecas. México, Editorial Hispano Mexicana, 1944. 170, [5] p.

Chiefly about the medicinal plants used. Appendixes, p. 117–[171], contain La medicina de los Aztecas, and La medicina en el Perú de antaño by Hans Dietschy. Bibliography (18 items): p. [173]. No index.

517
Stone, Eric P. Medicine among the American Indians. New York, Hoeber, 1932. 139 p. (Clio medica, no. 7)

General account of Indian medical practices. Bibliography: p. 123–125. Reprinted New York, Hafner, 1962.

518
U. S. Bureau of American Ethnology. Bibliography on American Indian medicine and health. Comp. by William C. Sturtevant. Washington, 1962. 39 p. (Smithsonian Institution. Smithsonian information leaflet 99, rev.)

Approximately 400 references, arranged in broad subject categories.

Argentina

519
Aráoz Alfaro, Gregorio. Crónicas y estampas del pasado. Buenos Aires, El Ateneo, 1938. 363 p.

Biographies of some 30 notable 19th century Argentine doctors, with historical background and medical history of period. No bibliography or index.

520
Cantón, Eliseo. Historia de la medicina en el Río de la Plata desde su descubrimiento hasta nuestros días, 1512 a 1925. Madrid [Sociedad de Historia Hispano-Americana] 1928. 6 v.

Exhaustive medical history of Argentina with emphasis on the University of Buenos Aires, including also data on Uruguay and Paraguay. Contains extensive extracts from archival and other sources, with references. Bibliography (sources and general works): v. 6, p. 471–475. Detailed tables of contents, but no index.

521
Furlong Cardiff, Guillermo. Médicos argentinos durante la dominación hispánica. Buenos Aires, Editorial Huarpes, 1947. 311 p. (His Cultura colonial argentina, 6)

Survey of native and Spanish medicine of period, accounts of physicians, and reviews of special subjects. List of colonial medical works: p. 244–249; medical imprints to 1810 (14 books and broadsides, 132 articles in 4 journals): p. 264–276. Bibliographical references: p. 277–302.

Armenia

522
Oganesian, Leon A. Istoriia meditsiny v Armenii s drevneishikh vremen do nashikh dnei; vrachi, meditsinskaia literatura i lechenye uchrezhdenia u Armian v Armenii i za ee predelami [History of medicine in Armenia from ancient times to our days; physicians, medical literature and health institutions of Armenians in Armenia and beyond its borders] Erevan, Akademiia nauk Armianskoi SSR, 1946–47. 5 v.

From earliest times to 1947. References at ends of chapters, including works in Russian and other foreign languages as well as Armenian. No index. Supplemented by his *Illiustratsii k Istorii meditsiny v Armenii . . .* Erevan, Akademiia nauk Armianskoi SSR, 1958, 85 p. Text in Armenian, Russian, and French.

An epitome in French appeared in 1962: *Histoire de la médecine en Arménie des origines au debut du XIX siècle*, Erevan, Éditions de l'Académie des sciences de la RSS d'Arménie, 1962, 42 p.

Australia

523
Gandevia, Bryan. An annotated bibliography of the history of medicine in Australia. [Sydney, Australasian Medical Pub. Co., 1957] 139 p. (Federal Council of the British Medical Association in Australia. Monographs, no. 1)

About 680 items in a classified list, with descriptive and critical notes. Attempts comprehensive coverage. Name and subject indexes.

524
Tovell, Ann, and Gandevia, Bryan. References to Australia in British medical journals prior to 1880. [Melbourne] Museum of Medical History, Medical Society of Victoria, 1961. [52] l.

673 articles, mainly in 7 journals, 1799–1880, listed under the journals indexed, with a section of references in miscellaneous sources. Author and subject indexes.

Austria

525
Breitner, Burghard. Geschichte der Medi-

zin in Österreich. Wien, Rohrer, 1951. 270 p. (Österreichische Akademie der Wissenschaften. Philosophisch-historische Klasse, Sitzungsberichte, 226. Bd., 5. Abhandlung. Veröffentlichungen der Kommission für Geschichte der Erziehung und des Unterrichts, Heft 2)

Includes popular medicine, histories of medicine at Universities (Vienna, Graz, Innsbruck), local history. With bibliographic references. Name index only.

526

Puschmann, Theodor. Die Medicin in Wien während der letzten 100 Jahre. Wien, Perles, 1884. 327 p.

Medical education, hospitals, public health, societies. Includes lists of professors in the University from 1742 and in the Josefs-Akademie from 1781, and of the directors of the Allgemeine Krankenhaus from 1784. Name index only.

527

Schönbauer, Leopold. Das medizinische Wien; Geschichte, Werden, Würdigung. 2 ed. Wien, Urban & Schwarzenberg, 1947. 484 p.

Detailed account to 1938. Bibliography: p. 457–569. Name index only. 1 ed. 1944.

Belgium

528

Broeckx, Corneille. Essai sur l'histoire de la médecine belge, avant le XIXe siècle. Gand, Leroux, 1837. 322 p.

General survey, followed by accounts of specialties. Includes biographical notices. References at ends of chapters. "Bibliographie médicale belge" (original works to 1796, by author): p. 246–322.

529

Faidherbe, Alexandre J. Les médecins et les chirurgiens de Flandre avant 1789. Lille, Danel, 1892. 347 p.

Documented history, including biographical sketches. Covers medical education; professional organization; public health; and social, literary and scientific contributions. Bibliography of works by Flemish physicians or published in Flanders, with biographical data: p. 296–336. Index of sources: p. 337–347. No index.

Bolivia

530

Balcázar, Juan Manuel. Historia de la medicina en Bolivia. La Paz, Ediciones Juventud, 1956. 721 p.

Comprehensive history from the precolonial period to 1954. Text not documented, but includes extracts from sources. Brief biographies: p. 689–708. Bibliography (sources and secondary works, including periodicals): p. 709–721. No index.

Brazil

531

Guerra, Francisco. Bibliografia medica brasileira, periodo colonial, 1808–1821. New Haven, 1958. 54 p. (Yale University School of Medicine. Dept. of the History of medicine. Publication, no. 34)

Chronological list of 55 publications, with annotations and location of copies.

532

Santos, Lycurgo de Castro, filho. História da medicina no Brasil (do século XVI ao século XIX). São Paulo, Editora Brasiliense, 1947. 2 v.

Arranged by subject. Includes numerous extracts from sources. With lists of hospitals, medical societies, and journals, and short biographies. Bibliography (by author, including sources): v. 2, p. 413–429. Extensive lists of early works, theses, etc., in text. No index.

Bulgaria

533

Golemanov, Khristo. Vuzrozhdenskata meditsinska knizhnina [Medical literature of the national awakening] Sofiia, Meditsina i fizkultura, 1964. 139, [4] p.

Covers medical and public health literature in Bulgaria from 1806 to 1878. Classified list of 222 books and selected articles published in the period (p. 96–136) with chronological subarrangement. No indexes. References: p. 137–140.

Canada

534

Ahern, Michael J., and Ahern, George. Notes pour servir à l'histoire de la médecine dans le Bas-Canada depuis la fondation de Québec jusqu'au commencement du XIXe siècle. Québec, Imprimerie Laflamme, 1923. 563 p.

Documented biographical notes, in alphabetical order, with data and some quotations from contemporary sources. Name index only.

535

Canniff, William. The medical profession

in Upper Canada, 1783–1850: an historical narrative, with original documents relating to the profession. Toronto, Briggs, 1894. 688 p.

Biographical sketches: p. 217–677. No bibliography, but sources of data often given in text.

536
Heagerty, John J. Four centuries of medical history in Canada and a sketch of the medical history of Newfoundland. Toronto, Macmillan, 1928. 2 v.

Comprehensive survey. Bibliography (by topic, mainly sources): v. 2, p. 311–338.

537
Seaborn, Edwin. The march of medicine in western Ontario. Toronto, Ryerson Press, 1944. 386 p.

Brief sketches of Indian and French medicine. Chiefly on English medicine, with emphasis on cholera epidemics and hospitals. Includes numerous biographical sketches.

Chile

538
Laval Manríquez, Enrique. Noticias sobre los médicos en Chile en los siglos XVI, XVII, y XVIII. Santiago, Universidad de Chile. Centro de Investigación de Historia de la Medicina, 1958. 137 p. (Biblioteca de historia de la medicina en Chile, 3)

Includes chapter on regulation of practice, Spain and America, 16th–18th centuries, and survey of each century. With biographies. References: p. 125–134.

China

539
Huard, Pierre A., and Wong, Ming. La médecine chinoise au cours des siècles. Paris, Dacosta, 1959. 190 p.

Bibliography: p. 185–186.

540
Morse, William R. Chinese medicine. New York, Hoeber, 1934. 185 p. (Clio medica, no. 11)

References (in Western languages): p. 169–172. Account of Chinese sources: p. xiii–xv of preface.

541
Wang, Chi-min, and Wu, Lien-Teh. History of Chinese medicine. 2 ed. Shanghai, National Quarantine Service, 1936. 906 p.

Comprehensive and detailed study. Index of Chinese books: p. 241–246; bibliography: p. 247–254. 1 ed. 1932.

Colombia

542
Robledo, Emilio. Apuntaciones sobre la medicina en Colombia. Cali, Colombia, 1959. 112, 21 p. (Biblioteca de la Universidad del Valle, 7 [i.e. 5])

Five lectures on medicine of the 15th–17th centuries, native medicine, medical education and the establishment of scientific medicine, medical doctrines, and European and American influences. Bibliography: p. 1–2 at end.

Cuba

543
Martínez Fortún y Foyo, José A. Cronología médica cubana: contribución al estudio de la historia de la medicina en Cuba. La Habana, 1947–58. 16 fasc.

Chronology, 1492–1958, with occasional long notes. No index. Reproduced from typewritten copy.

544
——. Historia de la medicina en Cuba. La Habana, 1956– .

General survey. No index, no bibliography. Pt. 5, 1957, covers 1801–1825.

Czechoslovakia

545
Rippa, B. K. K histórii medicíny na Slovensku [Contributions to the history of medicine in Slovakia] Bratislava, Slovenská akadémia vied, 1956. 200 p.

Contains an outline history; collection of documents (p. 49–83); description of the more important Slovak publications, with extracts; and index of outstanding physicians, with biographical data (p. 119–192). List of basic literature (17 items): p. 195. Name index only.

546
Vinař, Josef. Obrazy z minulosti českého lékařství [Pictures from the history of Czech medicine] Praha, Státní zdravotnické nakladatelství, 1959. 240 p.

Brief but reliable general account covering Czech provinces (Bohemia, Moravia, and Silesia) from the oldest times to second half of the

18th century. Describes early manuscripts, bio-bibliographical data for outstanding physicians, etc. Bibliographical footnotes. Name index only.

Denmark

547
Carøe, Kristian. Den danske laegestand, 1479–1900. København, Gyldendal, 1904–22 (v. 1, 1909) 5 v.

A series of biographical dictionaries of physicians and surgeons who died before 1901, giving education, professional, and family data. v. 1–4 list those licensed or examined during the period covered; v. 5 supplements v. 1–4 and lists medical officials. v. 1, Doktorer og licentiater, 1479–1788; v. 2, Kirurger, 1738–1785; v. 3, Laeger. og kirurger, 1786–1838; v. 4, Laeger, 1838–1900 (issued as a supplement to *Den danske laegestand*, 7 ed.) Continued by no. 548.

548
Den danske laegestand. 7- ed. København, Lund [etc.] Almindelige danske laegeforening, 1901– .

A series of biographical dictionaries continuing no. 547. The 7th ed. includes physicians living on Jan. 1, 1901. Successive editions include licensed physicians living at the date of publication or who died after the previous edition. The 7th and 9th eds. include notices of Icelandic physicians. 1st–6th eds. largely superseded by no. 547.

549
Ingerslev, Vilhelm. Danmarks laeger og laegevaesen fra de aeldste tider indtil aar 1800. Kjøbenhavn, Jespersen, 1873. 2 v.

Scholarly history, with extensive footnote references. Includes many biographical sketches of physicians with lists of their works.

550
Møller-Christensen, Vilhelm. Middelalderens laegekunst i Danmark. With an English summary. København, Munksgaard, 1944. 247 p. (Acta historica scientiarum naturalium et medicinalium, v. 3)

Comprehensive study. Includes antiquities, magic and folk medicine, dissemination of classical and European medicine through the church, therapeutics, surgery, and special diseases. "Litteraturliste": p. 232–237. Survey of earlier works on Danish medical history and antiquities and paleopathology, p. 1–9.

551
Norrie, Gordon, Kirurger og doctores; et kritisk bidrag til laegeuddannelsens historie i Danmark før 1800. København, Levin & Munksgaard, 1929. 194 p.

Account of medical education and professional history, with extensive biographical data on leading professors. Name index only. Bibliographical references: p. 189–191.

Ecuador

552
Paredes Borja, Virgilio. Historia de la medicina en el Ecuador. Quito, Casa de la Cultura Ecuatoriana, 1963. 2 v.

Includes prehistoric and aboriginal medicine. No index or bibliography, but some chronological lists of publications in the text.

553
Samaniego, Juan J. Cronología médica ecuatoriana. Quito, Casa de la Cultura Ecuatoriana, 1957. 562 p.

Detailed chronology, 1500–1947, with appendix listing various officials, professors, congresses, periodicals, etc. Detailed index.

Estonia

554
Brennsohn, Isidorus. Die Aerzte Estlands vom Beginn der historischen Zeit bis zur Gegenwart; ein biographisches Lexikon, nebst einer historischen Einleitung über das Medizinalwesen Estlands. Riga, Neuner, 1922. 550 p. (His Biographien baltischer Aerzte, 3)

Introduction (p. 23–114) includes histories of hospitals and lists of medical officials. Biographical dictionary in two parts, the second including Estonian physicians of the areas united with Estonia in 1917 and 1920. Manuscript and and printed sources: p. 17–21.

555
——. Die Aerzte Livlands von den ältesten Zeiten bis zur Gegenwart; ein biographisches Lexikon nebst einer historischen Einleitung über das medizinalwesen Livlands. Riga, Bruhns, 1905. 481 p.

The historical introduction (p. 19–75) includes a list of medical officials. Manuscript and printed sources: p. 13–17.

France

556
Académie de Médecine, Paris. Index bio-

graphique des membres, des associés et des correspondants . . . de décembre 1820 à juillet 1939. Paris, Masson, 1939. 145 p.

Lists entire membership 1820–1939, giving full name, place and date of birth and death, date of election, and offices held in the Académie.

557
Delaunay, Paul. La vie médicale aux XVIe, XVIIe et XVIIIe siècles. Paris, Editions Hippocrate, 1935. 556 p. (Collection Hippocrate, no. 4)

Study of medical education and the profession, and of various aspects of the private, professional, and public life of the French physician. References in footnotes and at ends of chapters. Full index of names only.

558
Lévy-Valensi, Joseph. La médecine et les médecins français au XVIIe siècle. Paris, Baillière, 1933. 668 p.

Covers medical sciences, teaching, care of sick poor (mainly on hospitals), practitioners, and biographies (p. 439–661). Sources described in introduction; few bibliographical footnotes. No index, but detailed table of contents.

559
Wickersheimer, Ernest. Dictionnaire biographique des médecins en France au moyen âge. Paris, Droz, 1936. 2 v. (867 p.)

Scholarly biobibliography, giving biographical data, manuscript and printed works, and extensive references to secondary sources. Alphabetically by forename, with index of family and variant names.

560
——. La médecine et les médecins en France, à l'époque de la Renaissance. Paris, Maloine, 1906. 693 p. (Bibliothèque de curiosités et singularités médicales, v. 3)

Covers all phases of medical science and practice, with data on education, schools, hospitals, and professional history. Based largely on the sources, but with few references and no bibliography or index.

French Colonies

561
Brau, Paul. Trois siècles de médecine coloniale française. Paris, Vigot, 1931. 205 p.

Covers medical administration in the American, African, and Asian colonies, 17th–20th centuries. Includes many documents and extracts from contemporary sources. A few bibliographical footnotes. No index, but detailed table of contents.

Germany

562
Haberling, Wilhelm. German medicine. Tr. by Jules Freund. New York, Hoeber, 1934. 160 p. (Clio medica, no. 13)

Brief history, no bibliography.

563
Hirsch, August. Geschichte der medicinischen Wissenschaften in Deutschland. München, Oldenbourg, 1893. 739 p. (Geschichte der Wissenschaften in Deutschland. Neuere Zeit. v. 22).

Brief review (p. 1–162) through the 17th century, more detailed history of the 18th and 19th centuries. Extensive bibliographical footnotes referring to original sources and works. Name index only. Reprinted New York, Kraus, 1966.

Great Britain

564
Bonser, Wilfred. The medical background of Anglo-Saxon England; a study in history, psychology, and folklore. London, 1963. xxxv, 448 p. (Wellcome Historical Medical Library. Publications. New ser., v. 3)

Bibliography: p. xvii–xxxv.

565
Bloom, James H., and James, Robert R. Medical practitioners in the Diocese of London, licensed under the Act of 3 Henry VIII, c. 11. An annotated list, 1529–1725. Cambridge, Univ. Press, 1935. 97 p.

Alphabetical list with brief biographical sketches. Appendix of documents, p. 75–86. Name index.

566
Clark, Sir George N. A history of the Royal College of Physicians of London. Oxford, Clarendon Press for the Royal College of Physicians, 1964–66. 2 v.

To 1858. Explores broadly the social history of British medicine. Footnote references, no bibliography.

567
Comrie, John D. History of Scottish medicine. 2 ed. London, Wellcome Historical Medical Museum, 1932. 2 v.

Comprehensive history through the 19th century. Bibliographical footnotes.

568
Copeman, William S. C. Doctors and disease in Tudor times. London, Dawson, 1960. 186 p.

General survey. Select bibliography: p. 177–181.

569
Munk, William. The roll of the Royal College of Physicians of London; comprising biographical sketches of all the eminent physicians, whose names are recorded in the annals from the foundation of the College in 1518 to . . . 1825. 2 ed. London, The College, 1878. 3 v.

The sketches vary widely in length, with usually incomplete bibliographies. Arranged chronologically, with name and subject index. Contains a brief history of the College and its library with lists of lecturers, Harveian orators, and the College's pharmacopoeias. Supplemented by G. H. Brown, *Lives of the fellows of the Royal College of Physicians of London, 1826–1925*, London, The College, 1955, 637 p. (Half title: Munk's roll, v. IV).

570
Power, Sir D'Arcy, ed. British medical societies. London, Medical Press and Circular, 1939. 311 p.

Brief historical accounts of 34 societies, beginning 1617. Reprinted, with additions, from the *Medical Press and Circular*, 1936–38.

571
Poynter, F. N. L., ed. The evolution of medical practice in Britain. London, Pitman, 1961. 168 p.

From the time of Henry VIII. Eleven varied papers read at the first British Congress on the History of Medicine and Pharmacy, Sept. 1960. References at end of most papers. Index mainly of names.

572
Raach, John H. A directory of English country physicians, 1603–1643. London, Dawsons, 1962. 128 p.

Alphabetical list with brief data and references for each.

573
Russell, Kenneth F. Checklist of medical books published in English before 1600. In Bulletin of the history of medicine 21: 922–58, 1947.

574
Talbot, Charles H., and Hammond, E. A. The medical practitioners in medieval England. A biographical register. London, Wellcome Historical Medical Library, 1965. 503 p. (Wellcome Historical Medical Library. Publications. New ser., v 8.)

From the Anglo-Saxon period to the founding of the Royal College of Physicians in 1518, the starting point of Munk's *Roll* (no. 569). Brief biographical notes in alphabetical arrangement with references to archival, documentary, and secondary sources. "Books consulted": p. 427–449.

Guatemala

575
Martínez Durán, Carlos. Las ciencias médicas en Guatemala: origen y evolución. 3 ed. Guatemala, Editorial Universitaria, 1964– .

v. 1 covers pre-Columbian period through the 19th cent.; v. 2 to cover 1900–1950. Includes extensive extracts from original documents and bibliographies. Previous editions, 1941 and 1945, in 1 v., covered through ca. 1920.

Haiti

576
Parsons, Robert P. History of Haitian medicine. New York, Hoeber, 1930. 196 p.

Revised and elaborated text of article appearing in *Annals of medical history*, new ser. 1:291–324, 1929. References: p. 190–192.

Honduras

577
Reina Valenzuela, José. Bosquejo histórico de la farmacia y la medicina en Honduras. Tegucigalpa, "Ariston," 1947. 233 p.

General survey, pre-Columbian to 1936. Detailed table of contents; no index or bibliography.

Hungary

578
Gortvay, György. Az újabbkori magyar orvosi müvelödés és egészségügy története

[History of modern Hungarian medical culture and public health] Budapest, Akadémiai Kiadó, 1953– .

References: v. 1, p. 283–286. Chronology, 1526–1868: v. 1, p. 287–304.

579
Magyary-Kossa, Gyula. Magyar orvosi emlékek; értekezések a magyar orvostörténelem köréből [Hungarian medical reminiscences; essays on Hungarian medical history] Budapest, 1929–40. 4 v. (Magyar Orvosi Könyvkiadó Társulat. Könyvtára, v. 121, 122, 128, 168)

Documented studies. v. 3-4 present a chronology of medical history, 1000–1800, with notes and indication of sources, including manuscripts and archives. Extensive bibliographical footnotes in v. 1-2. References for the chronology: v. 3, p. ix–xviii; v. 4, p. vii–xii. Partial German translation: *Ungarische medizinische Erinnerungen*, Budapest, 1935, 368 p.

580
Weszprémi, István. Magyarország és Erdély orvosainak rövid életrajza. Fordította Kővári Aladár. Budapest, Medicina Könyvkiadó, 1960– .

Reprint of original Latin edition, *Succincta medicorum Hungariae et Transylvaniae biographia*, Lipsiae, Ex Officina Sommeria, 1774–88, 4 v., with added Hungarian text on facing pages. Contains some 320 biographies, with extensive bibliographies of manuscript and printed works.

India

581
Chakraberty, Chandra. An interpretation of ancient Hindu medicine. Calcutta, Ramchandra Chakraberty, 1923. 509 p.

Systematic summary of classical Hindu teachings in various fields of medicine. Includes extracts in Sanskrit. No index.

582
Filliozat, Jean. The classical doctrine of Indian medicine: its origins and Greek parallels. Delhi, Munshiram Manoharlal, 1964. 298 p.

Analysis of texts, with exposition of terminology. Bibliography (297 items referred to in text, classic and modern): p. 281–290. Translation by Dev Raj Chanana of *La doctrine classique de la médecine indienne*, Paris, 1949.

583
Jolly, Julius. Indian medicine. Translated from the German and supplemented with notes by C. G. Kashikar. Poona, C. G. Kashikar, 1951. 238 p.

Detailed analysis of ancient texts. Sources: p. 1–29. Additional references in Kashikar's supplementary notes: p. 185–208. Translation of the section "Medicin" in *Grundriss der indoarischen Philologie und Altertumskunde*, v. 3, pt. 10, Strassburg, 1901.

584
Khanolkar, Vasant R. Fifty years of science in India: progress of medical science. Calcutta, Indian Science Congress Association, 1963. 50 p.

Surveys of medical education and medical research in various areas and specialties during the past fifty years. Bibliography (19 items): p. 49–50.

585
Kutumbiah, P. Ancient Indian medicine. Bombay, Orient Longmans, 1962. xiv, liv, 225 p.

Well organized survey for the general reader. The introduction (p. i–liv) presents an account of origins, schools, and doctrines, a listing of the sources (p. xxvi–xxvii), and a study of relations to Greek medicine. Chapters on subject areas and specialties. Notes and references: p. 203–212.

586
Müller, Reinhold F. G. Grundsätze altindischer Medizin. København, Munksgaard, 1951. 163 p. (Acta historica scientiarum naturalium et medicinalium, v.8)

Based mainly on the Ayurvedic texts. Notes (including bibliographical references): p. 90–161.

587
Mukhopādhyāya, Girindranāth. History of Indian medicine. Calcutta, Univ. of Calcutta, 1923–26. 2 v.

Detailed study of the works of Ayurvedic physicians, with translated excerpts.

588
Zimmer, Heinrich R. Hindu medicine. Ed. by Ludwig Edelstein. Baltimore, Johns Hopkins Press, 1948. 203 p. (Johns Hopkins University. Institute of the History of Medicine. Publications, ser. 3, v. 6)

Vedic and classical Hindu views of the body, medicine, and the physician. Extracts from texts in English. References, p. 194–201.

Indonesia

589
Schoute, Dirk. De geneeskunde in den dienst der Oost-Indische Compagnie in Nederlandsh-Indië. Amsterdam, De Bussy, 1929. 347 p.

This work, covering 1602–1798, and the following one present a survey of medicine and public health, based largely on contemporary sources. Lists of sources at ends of chapters. A concise summary in English of the two works appeared in 1937 under title: *Occidental therapeutics in the Netherlands East Indies during three centuries of Netherlands settlement, 1600–1900*, Batavia, Netherlands Indies Public Health Service, 1937, 214 p.

590
——. De geneeskunde in Nederlansch-Indië gedurende de negentiende eeuw. Batavia, Kolff, 1936. 381 p.

See no. 589.

Iran

591
Elgood, Cyril L. The medical history of Persia and the Eastern caliphate from the earliest times until the year A.D. 1932. Cambridge, Univ. Press, 1951. 616 p.

Comprehensive survey, with emphasis on historical background, medical practice, and biography. Covers medicine in the Avesta and Persian authors who wrote in Pahlavi, Syriac, Arabic, and other languages as well as Persian; Arabian medicine in the Islamic period; the introduction of European medicine and developments in modern Iran. Occasional bibliographic footnotes, references in text, but no bibliography. Index mainly of names and titles.

592
Fonahn, Adolf M. Zur Quellenkunde der persischen Medizin. Leipzig, Barth, 1910. 152 p.

Lists 408 works in classified arrangement, with entries under Persian titles. Transliterated and translated titles, authors if known, description of contents, location of MSS., citation of printed editions. Bibliography of modern Persian medicine (151 items): p. 135–140.

Ireland

593
Cameron, Sir Charles A. History of the Royal College of Surgeons in Ireland and of the Irish schools of medicine, including a medical bibliography and a medical biography. 2 ed. Dublin, Fannin, 1916. 882 p.

Includes chapter on medical knowledge and literature to 1700, accounts of barber-surgeons and surgical education and examination prior to the foundation of the College (chartered 1784), and of the schools of surgery. Annotated bibliography of medical books published in Ireland during the 18th century, p. 17–59. Biographical sketches of presidents, professors, etc. 1 ed. 1886.

594
Fleetwood, John. History of medicine in Ireland. Dublin, Browne and Nolan, 1951. 420 p.

Chronologic account, with chapters on medical societies and schools, hospitals, and professional publications. Classified bibliography: p. 384–399.

595
Widdess, J. D. H. A history of the Royal College of Physicians of Ireland, 1654–1963. Edinburgh, Livingstone, 1963. 255 p.

Sponsored by the College and based on its archives and other sources. Includes the history of its predecessors. Valuable for the history of medical education and the profession. Bibliography: p. 245–247.

Italy

596
Castiglioni, Arturo. Italian medicine. Tr. by E. B. Krumbhaar. New York, Hoeber, 1932. 134 p. (Clio medica, no. 6)

Bibliography: p. 111–112.

597
De Renzi, Salvatore. Storia della medicina in Italia. Napoli, Filiatre-Sebezio, 1845–48. 5 v. 2 ed., v. 1, 1849; suppl. to v. 2, 1849. 136 p.

Scholarly history, based largely on sources, from classical times to ca. 1815, with surveys of special fields and accounts of authors and their works. Index of names only in v. 5 and in 2 ed., v. 1.

598
Pazzini, Adalberto. Bibliografia di storia della medicina italiana. Roma, Tosi, 1939. 455 p. (Encyclopedia biografica e bibliografia "Italiana," ser. 31, La medicina, v. 1)

Classified list of 7451 books and articles, some annotated, in Italian medical history and biography, planned as the first of 5 volumes. No more published. Lack of index makes the work difficult to use. Reprinted 1946.

Japan

599

Fujikawa, Yu. Japanese medicine. Tr. by John Ruhräh; with a chapter on the recent history of medicine in Japan by Kageyas W. Amano. New York, Hoeber, 1934. 114 p. (Clio medica, no. 12)

Surveys of successive periods, with analyses of important works and bibliographic lists of contributions of each period. Chronological table (414–1932): p. 75–92. Translation of *Geschichte der Medizin in Japan*, Tokyo, 1911.

600

——. Nippon igaku shi [History of Japanese medicine] Rev. ed. Tokyo. Nisshin shoin, 1941. 1 v.

From ancient times to the Meiji period. Includes a list of pre-Western medical bibliographies.

600.1

Nippon Ishi Gakkai. Shiryo de miru kindai Nippon igaku no akebono. Catalogue of the historical writings and materials in early stage of the development of modern medicine in Japan. Kyoto, Benrido, 1959. 52, 40 p.

108 illustrations and facsimiles from 17th–19th century works important for history of Western medicine in Japan, with bibliographical descriptions. List of illustrations (in English): p. 29–40, with data concerning authors and works.

601

Whitney, Willis N. Notes on the history of medical progress in Japan. Yokohama, Meiklejohn, 1885. 245–469 p.

The pioneer Western study, not yet superseded. Based mainly on studies by Japanese scholars, especially Kōchi Zensetsu. Includes translated extracts from the sources. Bibliography of Western works used: p. 395–399. Chinese and Japanese medical works (1594 items, by original title, with transliteration; author index): p. 405–467. Subject index. Issued separately from Asiatic Society of Japan, *Transactions*, v. 12. Reprinted Tokyo, 1905, in a reprint of the *Transactions*.

Korea

601.1

Kim, Tu-jong. Hanguk uihaksa [History of Korean medicine] Seoul, Chongumsa, 1955. 314 p.

Covers ancient and medieval Korean medicine, including veterinary medicine. Includes footnotes.

601.2

Miki, Sakae. Chosen igakushi oyobi shitsubyoshi. The history of Korean medicine and of disease in Korea. Sakai, Japan, 1955. various pagings.

Covers the earliest period to end of the Yi dynasty. 1 ed., limited to 100 copies. A later ed. has been printed.

Lapps

602

Qvigstad, Just K. Lappische Heilkunde; mit Beiträgen von K. B. Wiklund. Oslo, Aschehoug, 1932. 270 p. (Instituttet for samenlignende kulturforskning, Oslo. [Publikasjoner] Ser. B: Skrifter, 20)

Detailed survey of folk beliefs and practices relating to various diseases, with accounts of specific remedies and therapeutic procedures. Preliminary chapter on shamanism and magical cures. Glossary of Lapp terms. Early accounts of Lapp folk medicine: p. 2–4. Bibliography (including manuscript and archival material): p. 259–265.

Latin America

603

Guerra, Francisco. Historiografía de la medicina colonial hispanoamericana. México, Abastecedora de Impresos, 1953. 322 p.

Bibliography, regionally arranged, with historical introduction for each colony. No index.

604

Moll, Aristides A. Aesculapius in Latin America. Philadelphia, Saunders, 1944. 639 p.

General survey, poorly documented and unreliable. Bibliography (by country, and general): p. 582–594.

Latvia

605

Brennsohn, Isidorus. Die Ärzte Kurlands vom Beginn der herzoglichen Zeit [1562] bis zur Gegenwart: ein biographisches Lexikon nebst einer historischen Einleitung über das Medizinalwesen Kurlands. 2 ed. Riga, Plates, 1929. 492 p.

Historical introduction (p. 5–63) includes a list of public health officials by date and locality. Bibliography (sources): p. 1–4. A revision of Brennsohn's *Die Aerzte Kurlands von 1825–1900*, Mitau, 1902, combined with Gustav Otto's *Das Medicinalwesen Kurlands . . . bis zum Jahre 1825*, Mitau, 1898.

606
Vasil'ev, Konstantin G., Grigorash, Fedor F., and Krauss, A. A. Materialy po istorii meditsiny i zdravookhraneniia Latvii [Materials for the history of medicine and public health in Latvia] Riga, Latviiskoe gosud. izd-vo, 1959. 360 p.

Covers 12th century to 1950, with emphasis on period since the Revolution. Classified bibliography: p. 316–355. No index.

The first two authors published a revised abridged version in 1964, with new material on medical care in ancient Latvia and period since 1950: *Ocherki istorii meditsiny i zdravookhraneniia Latvii* [Essays on the history of medicine and public health in Latvia] Moskva, Izd-vo "Meditsina," 1964, 216 p.

Malta

607
Cassar, Paul. Medical history of Malta. London, Wellcome Historical Medical Library, 1964. 586 p. (Wellcome Historical Medical Library. Publications. New ser., v. 6).

From the paleolithic age through World War II. Includes folk and popular medicine, public health and welfare, nursing, midwifery, pharmacy, dentistry, hospitals, communicable diseases.

Mexico

608
Aguirre Beltrán, Gonzalo. Medicina y magia; el proceso de aculturación en el estructura colonial. [Mexico] Instituto Nacional Indigenista [1963] 443 p. (Colección de antropología social)

Based largely on documents in the national archives. References in notes: p. 279–356; bibliography: p. 359–427.

609
Chavez, Ignacio. México en la cultura médica. México, Colegio Nacional, 1947. 187 p.

Survey with bibliography (p. 171–173) and chronology. No index.

610
Flores, Francisco A. Historia de la medicina en México desde la época de los Indios hasta la presente. México, Officina Tip. de la Secretaría de Fomento, 1886–88. 3 v.

Exhaustive history, including numerous extracts. Prefaces describe sources used; v. 2–3 contain chapters on bibliography (p. 275–301; p. 373–424). v. 1 (389 p.) on Aztec and primitive medicine. Includes biological sciences, pharmacy, veterinary medicine, and public health. No index, but full tables of contents.

611
Guerra, Francisco. Iconografía médica mexicana: catálogo gráfico descriptivo de los impresos médicos mexicanos de 1552 a 1833, ordenados cronológicamente. México. Diario español, 1955. xvi, ccclxxviii p.

Lists about 852 titles, mostly with facsimile. References: p. xiii–xvi. Author index.

612
Somolinos d'Ardois, Germán. Historia y medicina: figuras y hechos de la historiografía médica mexicana. México, Imprenta Universitaria, 1957. 160 p. (Cultura mexicana, 18)

Account of historical and bibliographical works and sources, including nonmedical materials. Bibliographical references throughout. No index.

Netherlands

613
Banga, Jelle. Geschiedenis van de geneeskunde en van hare beoefenaren in Nederland, vóór en na de stichting der Hoogeschool te Leiden tot aan den dood van Boerhaave; uit de bronnen toegelicht. Leeuwarden, Eekhoff, 1868. 2 v.

Documented biographies of physicians of the Netherlands, from Frisius to Boerhaave, in chronologic order. Name and subject indexes.

614
Baumann, Evert D. Uit drie eeuwen Nederlandse geneeskunde. Amsterdam, Meulenhoff [1951] 320 p.

Mainly devoted to leading physicians and their contributions, 14th–19th centuries. Brief bibliography by author, largely secondary works, unannotated: p. 308–316.

615
Schulte, Benedictus P. M., ed. Viftig jaren der geneeskunde, wiskunde en natuurwetenschappen in Nederland, 1913–1963. Leiden, Genootschap voor Geschiedenis der Geneeskunde, Wiskunde en Natuurwetenschappen, 1963. 118 p.

Includes bibliographies of contributions in several fields (medicine: p. 19–23).

Norway

616
Norges laeger, 1800– Oslo, Aschehoug; [etc., etc.] 1888– .

A series of biographical dictionaries of Norwegian physicians, with full listing of their publications. Each issue contains entries for physicians holding licenses during the period covered, and usually additional data on physicians entered in previous issues. Most sketches include portraits. Current issues serve as directories. Original issue by Frantz C. Kiaer; publication continued 1915–46 by Isak Kobro, and 1956– by Bernhard Getz. Some issues under the auspices of the Norske medicinske selskab.

Comprises: (1) Norges laeger i det nittende aarhundrede (1800–1886), 2 ed., Christiania, Cammermeyer, 1888–90, 2 v. (2) Norges laeger, 1800–1908, 3 ed., Kristiania, Cammermeyer, 1915, 2 v., and Tillegg, Oslo. Aschehoug, 1944, 644 p. (This supplements rather than supersedes volumes for 1800–1886). (3) 1909–1925, Oslo, Aschehoug, 1927, 434 p. (4) 1926–1936, Oslo, Centraltr., 1938, 740 p. (5) 1937–1946, Oslo, Aschehoug, 1951, 446 p. (6) 1947–1951, Oslo, 1956, 417 p.

617
Reichborn-Kjennerud, Ingjald, Grøn, Fredrik, and Kobro, Isak. Medisinens historie i Norge. Oslo, Grøndal, 1936. 328 p.

Bibliographical references (by section): p. 295–323. Name indexes only.

Peru

618
Lastres, Juan B. Historia de la medicina peruana. Lima, Impr. Santa María, 1951. 3 v. (Eguiguren, Luis A., ed. Historia de la Universidad de San Marcos, v. 5)

v. 1 on Inca medicine; v. 2–3, from the Spanish conquest through the 19th century. Documented. Includes frequent extracts from the sources, facsimiles. Bibliography at end of each volume.

619
Valdizán, Hermilio. Apuntes para la bibliografía médica peruana. Lima, Impr. Americana, 1928. 390 p.

429 items (manuscripts, documents, printed books, articles, and extracts) from the 16th through the 18th centuries, with full descriptions and many quotations. Chronologically arranged, with index of names.

620
——. Diccionario de medicina peruana. Lima, 1923– .

Includes historical, biographical, and topical entries, often with bibliographies. v. 7, pt. 1, U-V, 1960. No more published?

Philippines

621
Bantug, José P. A short history of medicine in the Philippines during the Spanish regime, 1565–1898. Manila, Colegio Medico-Farmaceutico de Filipinas, 1953. 182 p.

Survey, based on general as well as medical sources. Includes account of primitive native medicine. References: p. 163–166. Translation of *Bosquejo histórico de la medicina hispanofilipina*, Madrid, 1952.

Poland

622
Gasiorowski, Ludwik. Zbiór wiadomości do historyi sztuki lekarskiéj w Polsce od czasów najdawniejszych, aż do najnowszych [Collection of information concerning the history of the art of medicine in Poland from the oldest times up to the present] W Poznaniu, 1839–55. 4 v.

Comprehensive treatise. v. 1–3 cover successive periods to 1854, each beginning with a general survey of developments but mainly devoted to detailed biographical and bibliographical data on physicians of Polish origin or foreign physicians working in Poland, grouped by specialties. v. 4 contains supplements to v. 3. Bibliographical footnotes. Index reliable only for names.

623
Skarzyński, Bołeslaw. Histoire de la médecine en Pologne: aperçu sur son évolution. Varsovie, Editions médicales d'état [1954?] 23 p.

Sketch of the historiography of Polish medicine, with accounts of important historians and their works, and of teaching centers, societies, and serial publications.

624
Sokół, Stanisław. Medicina w. Gdańsku w dobie odrodzenia [Medicine in Gdansk during the Renaissance] Wrocław, Zakład Norodowy im. Ossolińskich, 1960. 253 p. (Polska Akademia Nauk. Komitet Historii Nauki. Monografie z dziejów nauki i techniki, 14)

Summary in French and German. Bibliographical references in footnotes. Name index only.

Portugal

625
Mira, Matias B. Ferreira de. História da medicina portuguesa. Lisboa, Empresa Nacional de Publicidade, 1947. 558 p.

General history through early 20th century. Bibliographical references at ends of chapters.

Spain

626
Bibliografia española de historia de la medicina. Salamanca. 1, 1957– . (Salamanca. Universidad. Seminario de historia de la medicina. Publicaciones. Ser. B: Repertorios biobibliográficos. v. 1, no. 1)

Annotated author list of recent books and articles on general and Spanish medical history by Spanish authors. v. 1: 1521 items. Indexes of biographies, subjects, and "patobiografías." Compiled by Luis Sánchez Granjel and María T. Santander Rodríguez.

627
Chinchilla, Anastasio. Anales históricos de la medicina en general, y biográfico-bibliográficos de la española en particular. Valencia, Lopez, 1841–46. 8 v.

v. [3–6], *Historia de la medicina española*, form an exhaustive biobibliography of Spanish physicians, with synopses of and extracts from their works, arranged by period. For name index, see no. 629. v. 1–2 on general medicine, v. 7 on surgery, v. 8: *Vade mecum.* Reprint, New York, Johnson Reprint, 1964– (Sources of science, 8).

628
García del Real, Eduardo. Historia de la medicina en España. Madrid, Editorial Reus, 1921. 1148 p. (Biblioteca médica de autores españoles y extranjeros, v. 23.)

Comprehensive biographical survey through the 19th century, with bibliographical data and analysis of works. Extensive lists of references for some sections. Full table of contents but no index. For name index, see no. 629.

629
Granjel, Luis Sánchez, and Santander Rodríguez, María T. Indice de médicos españoles. Salamanca, 1962. 111 p. (Acta Salmanticensia. Medicina, v. 7, no. 1)

Analyzes 66 collective biographical works, including books and articles.

630
Hernández Morejón, Antonio. Historia bibliográfica de la medicina española. Madrid, 1842–52. 7 v.

Exhaustive history. Chronologic table of contents. For name index, see no. 629. Reprinted New York, Johnson Reprint, 1965 (Sources of science, 9)

631
Indice histórico médico español. In Cuadernos de historia de la medicina española 1: 113–8, 1962– .

Author list of recent publications on the history of Spanish medicine.

632
López Piñero, José M. Medicina y sociedad en la España del siglo XIX. Madrid, Sociedad de Estudios y Publicaciones, 1964. 485 p. (Estudios de humanidades, 3)

Studies of the medical profession and science in relation to society, industry, and government, and of the effect of the cholera epidemic of 1885 on social conditions. Bibliography: p. 403–420.

Sudan

633
Squires, Herbert C. The Sudan medical service: an experiment in social medicine. London, Heinemann, 1958. 138 p.

Covers 1904–54.

Sweden

634
Hjelt, Otto E. A. Svenska och Finska medicinalverkets historia, 1663–1812. Helsingfors, Helsingfors Central-Tryckeri, 1891–93. 3 v.

v. 1: medical education, societies and professional history; v. 2: public health; v. 3: hospitals, military medicine, legal medicine, pharmacy, etc., with a final section (p. 675–754) containing short biographic notes. Numerous texts and extracts from original documents. Bibliographical footnotes. Name index.

635
Sveriges läkarehistoria ifrån Konung Gustaf den I: s [1523–1560] till närvarande tid. [1.]–4. följden. Stockholm [etc], Norstedt, 1822–1935.

Basic biographical dictionary with new series covering physicians of later periods. Supplements include new entries and corrections and additional data on physicians previously entered. Biographies list publications and biographical and critical references.

[1.] följden, Nyköping, 1822–24, 2 v. in 3, ed. by Johan F. Sacklén. Supplement. 1835, 664 p., ed. by J. F. Saklén. Nytt supplementhäfte, Stockholm, 1853, 466 p., ed. by Alfred Hilarion Wistrand. Ny [2.] följden, 1873–76, 2 v. (926 p.) ed. by Wistrand, Anders J. Bruzelius, and Carl Edling. 3. följden, 1895–1901, 4 v., ed. by A. J. Bruzelius, also entitled *Svensk läkare-matrikel* (v. 3: Tillägg: v. 4. Supplement) Förteckning öfver svenska läkare intill år 1901. Tillika utgörande register [name index to 1.–3. följden] 1902. 107, xcviii p. 4. följden, 1930–35, 5 v., published under the auspices of the Svenska läkaresällskapet, ed. by Axel Widstrand (v. 4, p. 327–742: Supplement)

Switzerland

636
Olivier, Eugène. Médecine et santé dans le pays de Vaud. Lausanne, Payot, 1962–63. 2 pts. in 4 v. (Bibliothèque historique vaudoise, 29–32)

Detailed and comprehensive, through 18th century. Pt. 2 is reissue of 1939 edition.

Tibet

637
Illion, Theodor. Tibetische Heilkunde. Zürich, Origo, 1957. 170 p.

Mainly concerned with present-day popular and folkloristic medical concepts and practice, but refers to Chinese, Indian, and classic Tibetan influences. Includes (p. 47–66) description of works in Tibetan including versions of Indic and Chinese classical texts.

638
Krasinski, Cyrill von Corvin. Die tibetische Medizinphilosophie: der Mensch als Mikrokosmos. [2 ed.] Zürich, Origo, 1964. xlvii, 363 p. (Mainzer Studien zur Kultur- und Völkerkunde, 1)

Study of classical and folk medicine of Lamaism. Introduction by W. A. Unkrig includes an account of the Tibetan sources and a list of references in European languages (p. xxvi-xxxi). A reissue of the 1953 ed. with a new foreword containing additions and revisions.

639
Laufer, Heinrich. Beiträge zur Kenntnis der tibetischen Medizin. Berlin, Unger, 1900. 2 v. (90 p.)

Studies of special topics, based on analysis of the sources. Includes some translated excerpts. Bibliography (p. 11–17) describes classical works and versions in Tibetan and Mongolian. Extensive references in footnotes.

Tunisia

640
Société des sciences médicales de Tunisie. Médecine et médecins de Tunisie de 1902 à 1952. Tunis, 1952. 335 p.

Published under the direction of Raoul Dana, Maurice Uzan, and Raymond Didier. A history of the society, and essays on medicine in Tunisia. No bibliography or references, except works mentioned in text.

Union of South Africa

641
Burrows, Edmund H. A history of medicine in South Africa up to the end of the nineteenth century. Cape Town, Balkema, 1958. 389 p.

Includes biographical sketches. References: p. 370–377, and at ends of chapters. Published under the auspices of the Medical Association of South Africa.

U. S. S. R.

642
Bogoiavlenskii, Nikolai A. Drevnerusskoe vrachevanie v XI–XVII vv. Istochniki dlia izucheniia istorii russkoi meditsiny [Old Russian medicine from the 11th to the 17th century. Sources for the study of the history of Russian medicine] Moskva, Medgiz, 1960. 325 p.

Description of the sources in medical and nonmedical literature, and fine arts. List of manuscripts, with locations: p. 296–308. Bibliography: p. 309–324.

643
Gantt, William A. Horsley. Russian medicine. New York, Hoeber, 1937. 214 p. (Clio medica, no. 20)

Survey, from primitive medicine to ca. 1936. Bibliography (mainly secondary works in English): p. 199–201.

644
Grombakh, Sergei M. Russkaia meditsinskaia literatura XVIII veka [Russian medical literature of the 18th century] Moskva, Izd-vo Akademii meditsinskikh nauk SSSR, 1953. 281, [3] p.

Describes historical development of medical literature, including medical material in general literature and history of early journals. Bibliography (p. 273–[282]) of 18th century Russian language books in 2 parts: (1) medical books; (2) nonmedical books containing medical material.

645
Kanevskii, Lazar' O., Lotova, Elena I., and Idel'chik, Khasia I. Osnovnye cherty razvitiia meditsiny v Rossii v periode kapitalizma (1861–1917) [Basic features of the development of medicine in Russia during the period of capitalism (1861–1917)] Moskva, Medgiz, 1956. 192 p.

Describes developments in general medicine, including education, organizations, and publication, and the various specialties. Politically colored, but contains valuable information. Bibliography: p. 175–183. Index of names only.

646
Richter, Wilhelm M. von. Geschichte der Medicin in Russland. Moskwa, Wsewolojsky, 1813–17. 3 v.

Pioneer work largely based on original sources, many unpublished; still not superseded in a Western European language. Covers to 1761. General surveys by periods followed by biobibliographical notices. Each volume has appendix of texts, mainly in Russian and Latin. Bibliographical footnotes. Index (adequate for names only) in v. 3.

647
Rossiiskii, Dmitri M. Istoriia vseobshchei i otechestvennoi meditsiny i zdravookhraneniia: bibliografiia (996–1954 gg.) [History of world and national medicine and public health: bibliography (996–1954)] Pod red. B. D. Petrova. Moskva, Medgiz, 1956. 935 p.

8707 items (books, manuscripts, articles) in Russian and other Soviet languages, with introduction on Russian medical history. Classified arrangement, with subject and name indexes. General reference works and bibliographies and universal medical history: p. 93–235 (1608 items); Russian and Soviet medicine and public health: p. 236–779; supplements: p. 779–808. Some brief annotations.

648
Zabludovskii, Pavel E. Istoriia otechestvennoi meditsiny. Chast'I. Period do 1917 goda [History of national medicine. Part I. Up to 1917] Moskva, Tsentral'nyi institut usovershenstvovaniia vrachei, 1960. 399 p.

Brief but reliable history of medicine in Russia from the beginnings to 1917. Chronology of important events and list of references at end of each chapter. To be continued.

648.1
Zmeev, Lev Fedorovich. Russkie vrachi pisateli [Russian physician-writers] S. Peterburg', 1886–89. 5 pts.

Biobibliographical dictionary of Russian physicians. Pts. 1–2 physicians who published from about 1800 to 1863; pt. 3 additional bibliographic data to 1887; pts. 4–5 new names and publications 1863 to 1888.

United States

BIBLIOGRAPHIES

649
Gilbert, Judson B. A bibliography of articles on the history of American medicine compiled from "Writings on American history," 1902–1937. New York, 1951. 44 p. (New York Academy of Medicine. Library. History of medicine series, no. 9)

Approximately 650 references, mainly on the United States. Valuable for indexing of local history and other nonmedical journals. Excludes citations printed in the *Index-catalogue* (no. 29), *Index medicus* (no. 36), and *Quarterly cumulative index medicus* (no. 34).

650
Miller, Genevieve, ed. Bibliography of the history of medicine in the United States and Canada, 1939–1960. With a historical

introd. by W. B. McDaniel, 2d. Baltimore, Johns Hopkins Press, 1964. 428 p.

A reissue in consolidated form of an annual bibliography published in *Bulletin of the history of medicine* since 1940. Arranged by broad topics. Detailed table of contents, author index. Sponsored by American Association for the History of Medicine. Annual bibliographies continued in *Bulletin*, 1962–66.

BIOGRAPHICAL DICTIONARIES

651
Atkinson, William B. The physicians and surgeons of the United States. Philadelphia, Robson, 1878. 788 p.

Includes some less well known men. Especially good for the 19th century. Many portraits. Arrangement haphazard, but well indexed by name, locality, and subject. A 2d ed., entitled *A biographical dictionary of contemporary American physicians and surgeons*, Philadelphia, Brinton, 1880, 747 p., has some new biographies and revisions of others, but omits the portraits and subject index.

652
Kelly, Howard A. A cyclopedia of American medical biography, comprising the lives of eminent deceased physicians and surgeons from 1610 to 1910. Philadelphia, Saunders, 1912. 2 v.

See no. 654.

653
Kelly, Howard A., and Burrage, Walter L. American medical biographies. Baltimore, Norman, Remington, 1920. 1320 p.

See no. 654

654
Kelly, Howard A., and Burrage, Walter L. Dictionary of American medical biography; lives of eminent physicians of the United States and Canada, from the earliest times. New York, Appleton, 1928. 1364 p.

This constitutes in effect the third edition of no. 652 and 653. Some material is included here that was not in either of the other works and vice versa. Together they represent the best resource for American medical biography to 1927.

655
Stone, Richard F., ed. Biography of emient American physicians and surgeons. Indianapolis, Carlon & Hollenbeck, 1894. 729 p.

Especially good for last half of 19th century. Bibliographies and many portraits.

656
Thacher, James, American medical biography. Boston, Richardson, 1828. 2 v.

Fundamental resource for early biographies, much used by later compilers. Contains also brief history of medicine in United States, arranged by state.

657
Watson, Irving A., ed. Physicians and surgeons of America . . . a collection of biographical sketches of the regular medical profession. Concord, N. H., Republican Press Association, 1896. 843 p.

Almost wholly a record of men then living; hundreds of portraits. Locality index.

658
Williams, Stephen W. American medical biography; or, memoirs of eminent physicians, embracing principally those who have died since the publication of Dr. Thacher's work. Greenfield, Mass., Merriam, 1845. 664 p.

SOCIETIES

659
American Medical Association. Digest of official actions, 1846–1958. 1st ed. [Chicago, 1959] 779 p. Supplement, 1959–1963. [Chicago, 1966]

Compiled by Susan Crawford, Arranged alphabetically by broad subjects, with actions in chronological order, and with references to documents or publications. Subject index.

660
Bates, Ralph S. Scientific societies in the United States. 2 ed. New York, Columbia Univ. Press, 1958. 297 p.

History from 1683 to 1955, with accounts of organization, activities, and publications of individual societies. Extensive footnote references. Classified bibliography: p. 225–268.

661
Burrow, James G. AMA: voice of American medicine. Baltimore, Johns Hopkins Press, 1963. 430 p.

Historical survey, with special emphasis on economic and social affairs.

662
Fishbein, Morris. A history of the American Medical Association, 1847 to 1947; with biographies of the presidents . . . by Walter Bierring; and with the histories of the publications, councils, bureaus and other official bodies [by various authors] Philadelphia, Saunders, 1947. 1226 p.

Official history. Based largely on archival materials and official publications, with numerous extracts from the documents. "Publications" (histories of journals and collective works): p. 1109–1185.

HISTORIES

663
A century of American medicine. 1776–1876. Philadelphia, Lea, 1876. 366 p.

Contents: E. H. Clarke, Practical medicine; H. J. Bigelow, Discovery of modern anesthesia; S. D. Gross, Surgery; T. G. Thomas, Obstetrics and gynaecology; J. S. Billings, Literature and institutions. No index. First published in the *American journal of the medical sciences*, 1876. Reprinted Brinklow, Md., Old Hickory Bookshop [1962].

664
Flexner, James T. Doctors on horseback; pioneers of American medicine. New York, Viking, 1937. 370 p.

Biographies of John Morgan, Benjamin Rush, Ephraim McDowell, Daniel Drake, William Beaumont, and a sketch of the discovery of ether anesthesia. Reprinted New York, Macmillan, 1962.

665
Gross, Samuel D. History of American medical literature from 1776 to the present time. Philadelphia, Collins, 1875, 85 p.

Survey arranged under different subjects as well as under biography, translations and reprints, journals, theses, book publishers, etc.

666
——, ed. Lives of eminent American physicians and surgeons of the nineteenth century. Philadelphia, Lindsay & Blakiston, 1861. 836 p.

Articles on 32 important physicians of the late 18th and early 19th centuries.

667
Malloch, Archibald. Medical interchange between the British Isles and America before 1801. Based on the Fitzpatrick lectures of the Royal College of Physicians of London for 1939. [London, The College, 1946] 143 p.

Covers Mexico, West Indies, Canada, and United States. Arranged by state or region. Many bibliographical references in the text and in footnotes.

668
Martí-Ibañez, Felix, ed. History of American medicine. A symposium. New York, MD Publications, 1958. 181 p. (MD international symposia, no. 5)

Series of articles, with a bibliography following each one.

669
Packard, Francis R. History of medicine in the United States. 2 ed. New York, Hoeber, 1931. 2 v.

Comprehensive history, based largely on secondary sources. Reprinted New York, Hafner, 1963.

670
Pickard, Madge E., and Buley, Roscoe Carlyle. The midwest pioneer, his ills, cures, and doctors. Crawfordsville, Ind., Banta, 1945. 339 p.

Chiefly about first half of 19th century. Chapters on home remedies; doctors: bleed, blister and purge; the people's doctors; patent medicines. References: p. 291–306; bibliographical note: p. 307–324.

671
Postell, William D. The health of slaves on southern plantations. Baton Rouge, Louisiana State Univ. Press, 1951, 231 p. (Louisiana State University. Studies. Social science series, no. 1)

Chiefly from contemporary manuscript records. Bibliography: p. 214–226.

672
Rosen, George. Fees and fee bills: some economic aspects of medical practice in nineteenth century America. Baltimore, Johns Hopkins Press, 1946. 93 p. (Bulletin of the history of medicine. Suppl. no. 6)

673
Shafer, Henry B. The American medical profession, 1783 to 1850. New York,

Columbia Univ. Press, 1936. 271 p. (Columbia University. Faculty of Political Science. Studies in history, economics and public law, no. 417)

Study of medical practice of the period, with chapters on medical fees, medical education, and medical societies. Bibliography: p. 250–257.

674
Shryock, Richard H. Medicine and society in America, 1660–1860. New York, New York Univ. Press, 1960. 182 p.

Traces rise of medical profession, and changes in medical thought, practice, and public health.

674.1
——. Medicine in America: historical essays. Baltimore, Johns Hopkins Press, 1966. 332 p.

Brief general survey (p. 1–45), followed by 15 special studies reprinted from various journals, 1930–1962.

675
Sigerist, Henry E. American medicine. Tr. by Hildegard Nagel. New York, Norton, 1934. 316 p.

Interpretive survey. Classified bibliography: p. 289–304.

ARIZONA

676
Quebbeman, Frances E. Medicine in territorial Arizona. Phoenix, Arizona Historical Foundation, 1966. 424 p.

From earliest times to 1912. Documented. Biographical notes: p. 325–381; bibliography: p. 383–406.

CALIFORNIA

677
Harris, Henry. California's medical story. San Francisco, Stacey, 1932, 421 p.

Detailed history to 1900. References (by sections, including sources): p. 397–410.

COLORADO

678
Colorado State Medical Society. Medical Coloradoana; a jubilee volume in celebration of the semi-centennial anniversary, 1871–1921. Denver, The Society, 1922. 144 p.

"Historical notes": p. 1–18. "Medical periodicals published in Colorado": p. 19. "List of . . . books and papers published by the medical profession of Colorado" (with dates of authors if known): p. 22 142.

CONNECTICUT

679
Russell, Gordon W. Early medicine and early medical men in Connecticut. Connecticut Medical Society Proceedings, 100: 69–176, 177*–224*, 1892.

Short history to 1800, with brief biographies.

680
Thoms, Herbert K., ed. The heritage of Connecticut medicine. New Haven, 1942. 223 p.

Brief sketches by various authors on different phases of the history of medicine in Connecticut. Many reprinted from the *Connecticut state medical journal.* Some bibliographies. No index. dex.

DISTRICT OF COLUMBIA

681
Cobb, William M. The first Negro medical society: a history of the Medico-Chirurgical Society of the District of Columbia, 1884–1939. Washington, Associted Publishers, 1939. 159 p.

Publications of the Society and its members: p. 104–119; bibliography: p. 135.

682
Medical Society of the District of Columbia. History of the . . . 1817–1909. Washington, The Society, 1909. 501 p. Pt. 2, 1833–1944. 1947. 357 p.

Includes biographies, lists of members, and extensive data on other medical developments and institutions in the District. Compiled by committees under the chairmanship of Daniel S. Lamb and John B. Nichols. Includes many extracts from documents and records.

FLORIDA

683
Merritt, Webster. A century of medicine in Jacksonville and Duval County. Gainesville, Univ. of Florida Press, 1949. 201 p.

Covers 1798–1888. Includes biographical sketches and data on epidemics, hospitals, sanitation, education, etc. Notes and bibliography: p. 169–195.

HAWAII

684
Halford, Francis J. 9 Doctors and God. Honolulu, Univ. of Hawaii, 1954, 322 p.

Describes work of medical missionaries, 1819–98. Appendices include chronology of medical events, 1778–1899, and selected bibliography (p. 315–322). No index.

ILLINOIS

685
Bonner, Thomas N. Medicine in Chicago, 1850–1950; a chapter in the social and scientific development of a city. Madison, Wis., American History Research Center, 1957. 302 p.

Notes and references: p. 227–266; bibliography (sources and secondary works, no annotations): p. 267–288.

686
Chicago Medical Society. History of medicine and surgery and physicians and surgeons of Chicago. Chicago, Biographical Pub. Corp., 1922. 928 p.

Biographies of 172 physicians, 1803–1922: p. 9–186. Physicians and surgeons living in 1922: p. 373–912. Historical accounts of medical colleges, hospitals, medical societies, and the health department: p. 187–371. Indexes of personal and corporate names only.

687
Illinois State Medical Society. History of medical practice in Illinois. Chicago, 1927–1955. 2 v.

Documented, detailed history to 1900. v. 1 comp. by Lucius H. Zeuch, v. 2 ed. by David J. Davis.

INDIANA

688
Kemper, General W. H. A medical history of the State of Indiana. Chicago, American Medical Association Press, 1911. 393 p.

Includes historical sketches of counties and cities, with biographical data, accounts of public health and of medical organizations, and war medicine (with lists of surgeons). List of deceased physicians (with biographical data and works): p. 231–371. No bibliography.

689
Russo, Dorothy R., ed. One hundred years of Indiana medicine, 1849–1949. Published in connection with the centennial of the Indiana State Medical Association. [Indianapolis?] 1949. 195 p.

Fourteen studies on various aspects of Indiana medical history. Bibliographical footnotes; general bibliography: p. 173–180; Indiana medical periodicals: p. 180–184. Name index.

IOWA

690
Fairchild, David S. History of Medicine in Iowa. v. 1. Des Moines, Iowa State Medical Society, 1927. 356, 95 p.

Mainly on period to 1870. Biographies, historical sketches of medical journals, hospitals for the insane, societies, and Iowa medical profession in World War I. Disorganized, but has extensive data. Reprinted from material published in *Journal of the Iowa State Medical Society*.

691
Iowa State Medical Society. One hundred years of Iowa medicine; commemorating the centenary of the Iowa State Medical Society, 1850–1950. Iowa City, Athens Press, 1950. 483 p.

Includes a survey of Iowa medicine to 1850; biographies of presidents; directory of local associations; reviews of medical education, journalism, hospitals, and other topics. No index.

KANSAS

692
Bonner, Thomas N. The Kansas doctor; a century of pioneering. Lawrence, Univ. of Kansas Press, 1959. 334 p.

An excellent state history.

KENTUCKY

693
McCormack, Joseph N., ed. Some of the medical pioneers of Kentucky. Bowling Green, Kentucky State Medical Association, 1917. 173 p.

Biographical studies by various authors, with a history of the state medical society and essays on the medical history and literature of

Kentucky. Also published as a special issue of the *Kentucky medical journal*, v. 15, no. 11, 1917.

694
Medical Historical Research Project. (W. P. A.) Kentucky. Medicine and its development in Kentucky. Louisville, Standard Print. Co., 1940. 373 p.

General survey, emphasizing public health and social aspects. References by chapters.

LOUISIANA

695
Duffy, John. The Rudolph Matas history of medicine in Louisiana. Baton Rouge, Louisiana State Univ. Press, 1958–62. 2 v.

An outstanding state history.

MARYLAND

696
Cordell, Eugene F. The medical annals of Maryland, 1799–1899. Prepared for the centennial of the Medical and Chirurgical Faculty. Baltimore, 1903. 889 p.

In part a revision of Quinan (no. 697) but abridges data on publications. Includes history of the Faculty, chronology (1608–1902), about 2400 biographical sketches, and detailed memoirs of 12 founders and leaders.

697
Quinan, John R. Medical annals of Baltimore from 1608 to 1880, including events, men and literature. Baltimore, Friedenwald, 1884. 274 p.

Largely based on contemporary sources. Contains a chronology, 1608–1880; a record of public services of Baltimore physicians, 1730–1880; and a biobibliography of Baltimore physicians, 1730 to 1880, with a subject index (p. 54-235). Not entirely superseded by Cordell (no. 696).

MASSACHUSETTS

698
Burrage, Walter L. A history of the Massachusetts Medical Society, with brief biographies of the founders and chief officers, 1781–1922. Norwood, Mass., Priv. printed, 1923. 505 p.

Documented, comprehensive history.

699
Green, Samuel A. History of medicine in Massachusetts. Boston, Williams, 1881. 131 p.

Frequent quotations from sources. No index or bibliography.

700
Viets, Henry R. A brief history of medicine in Massachusetts. Boston, Houghton, 1930. 194 p.

Colonial period to 1930, with emphasis on biography. References: p. 185.

MICHIGAN

701
Anderson, Fanny J. Doctors under three flags. Detroit, Wayne Univ. Press, 1951. 185 p.

The history of medicine in Michigan (chiefly Detroit) through 1837. Bibliographic notes at end of each chapter, chiefly sources; bibliography (sources and secondary): p. 170–185.

702
Michigan State Medical Society. Medical history of Michigan. Comp. and ed. by a committee, C. B. Burr, chairman. Minneapolis, Bruce, 1930. 2 v.

A collection of studies by different authors, providing a detailed history. References at ends of the studies.

MISSISSIPPI

703
Underwood, Felix I., and Whitfield, Richard N. Public health and medical licensure in the State of Mississippi 1798–[1947] Jackson, Tucker Printing House, 1938–[51] 2 v.

Includes texts of legislation and extracts from other sources; biographies and lists of officials, and chronologies. v. [1], 1798–1937 (only 9 p. on 1798–1877); v. 2, 1938–1947. Index for v. 2 only.

MISSOURI

704
Goldstein, Max A. One hundred years of medicine and surgery in Missouri. St. Louis, St. Louis Star, 1900. 364 p.

Includes biographies (p. 208–360), histories of hospitals, medical schools, medical journals, etc. No subject index. No bibliography.

705
Goodwin, Edward J. A history of medi-

cine in Missouri. St. Louis, Smith, 1905. 284 p.

Institutions and biographies (p. 179–278). Name index. No documentation.

MONTANA

706
Phillips, Paul C. Medicine in the making of Montana. Missoula, Montana University Press, 1962. 564 p.

Documented history covering the period to 1890 only. Many biographical sketches in the text, with supplementary biographical notes by counties. Bibliography (by chapters, including sources): p. 467–525.

NEBRASKA

707
Tyler, Albert F., and Auerbach, Ella F. History of medicine in Nebraska. Omaha, Magic City Print. Co., 1928. 662 p.

A biographic history. Includes chapters on publications, organizations, colleges, hospitals, with a directory of living physicians (p. 549–662). No index.

NEVADA

708
Walker, Moses R. A life's review and notes on the development of medicine in Nevada from 1900 to 1944. Reno, The Author, 1944. 92 p.

An autobiography, but includes such subjects as legislation affecting medicine; hospitals; physicians; medical organizations; industrial medicine.

709
Walder, Moses R. Story of . . . Nevada State Medical Society and Nevada medicine. Reno, The Author, 1937. 45 p.

Covers from 1864 to 1937. Bibliography: p. 43–44.

NEW JERSEY

710
Cowen, David L. Medicine and health in New Jersey; a history. Princeton, Van Nostrand, 1964. 229 p. (New Jersey historical series, v. 16)

General survey. Sources (by chapter): p. 184–202. Bibliographical notes (significant works, classified and annotated): p. 203–212.

711
Wickes, Stephen. History of medicine in New Jersey, and of its medical men, from the settlement of the province to A. D. 1800. Newark, Dennis, 1879. 449 p.

Largely based on original sources. Pt. 1 is a brief history stressing the profession. Pt. 2, p. 123–438, is a comprehensive biographical dictionary.

NEW YORK

712
Van Ingen, Philip. The New York Academy of Medicine; its first hundred years. New York, Columbia Univ. Press, 1949. 573 p. (New York Academy of Medicine Library. History of medicine series, no. 8)

Chronologic account with brief biographies of the presidents. Useful for New York City, 1847–1946.

713
Walsh, James J. History of medicine in New York; three centuries of medical progress. New York, National Americana Society, 1919. 5 v.

Contains extensive data, but not well organized, incomplete in some areas, and very little documentation. v. 1, general survey, with accounts of specialities; v. 2 mainly on medical schools; v. 3 on societies and hospitals; v. 4–5, biographies (with lists of publications). Inadequate indexes in v. 3 and 5.

NORTH DAKOTA

714
Grassick, James. North Dakota medicine: sketches and abstracts. Grand Forks, North Dakota Medical Association, 1926. 378 p.

Early history, societies, biographies of presidents, public health, local history. Roster of registered physicians 1885–1925: p. 283–365.

OHIO

715
Dittrick, Howard, comp. Pioneer medicine in the Western Reserve. Cleveland, Academy of Medicine of Cleveland, 1932. 110 p.

Biographical sketches, reprinted from the *Bulletin* of the Academy.

716
[Ohio medical history] Ohio state archaeological and historical quarterly, v. 48, 1939–v. 54, 1945, *passim*.

Series of articles on various phases. Lack of overall index or table of contents limits usefulness for reference.

717
Ohio State University. College of Medicine. The Ohio State University College of Medicine: a collection of source material covering . . . medical progress, 1834–[1958] Blanchester, Ohio, Brown; Columbus, The University, 1934–61. 2 v.

v. 1, 1834–1934, includes histories of various medical schools, current biographies; v. 2 limited to University's College of Medicine.

718
Striker, Cecil, ed. Medical portraits. Cincinnati, Academy of Medicine of Cincinnati, 1963. 259 p.

Biographical sketches of 79 Ohio physicians, reprinted from the *Cincinnati journal of medicine*.

OREGON

719
Larsell, Olof. The doctor in Oregon; a medical history. Portland, Ore., Binfords & Mort for the Oregon Historical Society, 1947. 671 p.

Comprehensive, including Indian medicine, medical education, journals, societies, hospitals, and public health. Physicians to 1900 (biographies, by county): p. 161–342. Women physicians to 1900: p. 414–419. Bibliography and notes (including sources, by chapter): p. 623–650.

PENNSYLVANIA

720
Diller, Theodore. Pioneer medicine in western Pennsylvania. New York, Hoeber, 1927. 230 p.

Mainly biographical, with emphasis on period to 1850. Brief surveys of epidemics, institutions, and journals. Name index only.

721
Henry, Frederick P., ed. Standard history of the medical profession of Philadelphia. Chicago, Goodspeed, 1897. 544 p.

Includes many biographical sketches, data on institutions and literature, including accounts of works of important authors, annotated chronology of 45 journals. Detailed table of contents but no index.

722
Norris, George W. The early history of medicine in Philadelphia. Philadelphia, Collins Print Co., 1886. 232 p.

25 biographies, p. 9–100. Accounts of epidemics, institutions, etc. Mainly 17th–18th centuries. Written about 1845. A few footnote references; no index.

SOUTH CAROLINA

723
South Carolina Medical Association. A brief history of the South Carolina Medical Association, to which are added short historical sketches of various medical institutions and societies. Charleston, The Association, 1948. 197 p.

Prepared by a committee under the chairmanship of Joseph I. Waring. Includes data on general medical history, county and other societies, institutions. References (including sources): p. 81–82.

724
Waring, Joseph I. A history of medicine in South Carolina, 1670–1825. Charleston, South Carolina Medical Association, 1964. 407 p.

Narrative survey, with biographical section (p. 173–330), documents, lists, bibliographies, etc. To be continued.

TENNESSEE

725
Tennessee State Medical Association. The centennial history . . . 1830–1930. Ed. by P. M. Hamer. Nashville, The Association, 1930. 580 p.

History of the Association, biographies of officers, pioneer physicians, specialties, education, public health, periodicals, and organizations. Documents, lists of members, etc.

726 and 727 not used.

TEXAS

728
Nixon, Patrick I. A century of medicine in San Antonio, the story of medicine in Bexar County, Texas. San Antonio, The Author, 1936. 405 p.

Detailed history, including 20th century. Bibliography: p. 390–393.

729
——. A history of the Texas Medical Association, 1853–1953. Austin, University of Texas Press, 1953. 476 p.

Comprehensive survey.

730
——. The medical story of early Texas, 1528–1853. San Antonio, Mollie Bennett Lupe Memorial Fund, 1946. 507 p.

Includes Indian medicine, hospitals, diseases, physicians, etc. With a list of physicians from 1836 to 1853, and bibliography (p. 489–502).

731
Red, Mrs. George P. The medicine man in Texas. Houston, Standard Printing. 1930. 344 p.

Short history to mid-19th century, plus collection of biographies (p. 111-340). Bibliography (sources, by chapters): p. 343–344. No index.

UTAH

732
Richards, Ralph T. Of medicine, hospitals, and doctors. Salt Lake City, Univ. of Utah Press, 1953. 266 p.

Survey of Utah medical history from 1847, with emphasis on hospitals in Salt Lake City. Includes accounts of mining and medicine and of special diseases. Bibliography (sources and secondary works): p. 261–262.

VIRGINIA

733
Blanton, Wyndham B. Medicine in Virginia . . . [17th–19th centuries]. Richmond, W. Byrd, 1930; Garrett & Massie, 1931–33. 3 v.

Exhaustive history with a wealth of information, bibliographic references, and such helpful lists as those of Virginia surgeons in the Revolutionary and Civil Wars, medical fees, and acts of the Assembly concerning medicine.

734
Hughes, Thomas P. Medicine in Virginia, 1607–1699. Williamsburg, Virginia 350th Anniversary Celebration Corporation, 1957. 78 p. (Jamestown 350th anniversary historical booklet, no. 21)

Bibliographical note: p. 77–78.

WISCONSIN

735
Frank, Louis F. The medical history of Milwaukee, 1834–1914. Milwaukee, Germania Pub. Co., 1915. 272 p.

Includes biographies; a directory of physicians, 1834–1914; chronological accounts of institutions, etc. No index; no bibliography.

Uruguay

736
Schiaffino, Rafael. Historia de la medicina en el Uruguay. Montevideo, Imprenta Nacional, 1927–52. 3 v.

Exhaustive history through 1828. Extracts from sources. References in footnotes. Name index for v. 3 only. Full table of contents in each volume.

Venezuela

737
Archila, Ricardo. Historia de la medicina en Venezuela: época colonial. Caracas, Vargas, 1961. 617 p.

Documented, with extensive citations to original sources. Bibliographies at ends of chapters.

738
Perera, Ambrosio. Historia de la medicina en Venezuela. Obra editada por el Ministerio de Sanidad y Asistencia Social. Caracas, Imprenta Nacional, 1951. 278 p.

Comprehensive survey through the 19th century, with emphasis on medical education, professional history, and public health. Documents: p. 237–267. Bibliography (including sources): p. 269–270. No index.

Yugoslavia

739
Zbor liječnika Hrvatske, Zagreb. Iz hrvatske medicinske prošlosti [From the medical past of Croatia] Zagreb, 1954. 314 p.

Contributions by 24 authors on the history of medicine in Croatia, published on the 80th anniversary of the Medical Association of Croatia. Edited by Mirko D. Grmek and Stanko Dujmušić. Annotated table of contents in English (7 p.) inserted at end. Bibliographical notes at ends of essays. No index.

SPECIAL TOPICS IN HISTORY

Art and Medicine

Medical Illustration and Portraiture

740
Kisch, Bruno. Iconographies of medical portraits. In Journal of the history of medicine 12:366–87, 524, 1957.

Bibliography (p. 376–387) arranged chronologically includes over 160 items from 1570 to 1957.

741
MacKinney, Loren C. Medical illustrations in medieval manuscripts. Berkeley, Univ. of California Press, 1965. (London ed. published as Wellcome Historical Medical Library. Publications, New ser., v. 5)

Pt. I: Early medicine in extant manuscripts (survey by subjects with descriptions of the miniatures, including the reproductions). Pt. II: Medical miniatures in extant manuscripts: A checklist (by location) compiled with the assistance of Thomas E. Herndon: p. 103–185. Plates (96 illustrations, 20 in color): p. 193–253. The index provides a subject approach to the manuscripts in the checklist as well as to the text and plates.

742
New York Academy of Medicine. Library. Illustration catalog. Boston, Hall, 1960. 200 p.

Photographic reproduction of card file. Indexes under specific topics about 20,000 illustrations in early and rare books, histories, and journals.

743
— . —. Portrait catalog. Boston, Hall, 1960. 5 v. First supplement, 1959/65. Boston, Hall, 1965. 842 p.

Photographic reproduction of card catalog, listing alphabetically by subject 10,784 separate portraits and 151,792 portraits appearing in books and journals. Supplement adds 1,073 separate portraits and 35,976 in books and journals.

744
Royal College of Physicians, London. Catalogue of engraved portraits, by A. H. Driver. London, 1952. 219 p.

Lists 4500 prints of medical men and scientists, a large proportion British. Arranged alphabetically by subject, with identification and dates, giving provenance, type, painter, and engraver. Index of engravers.

745
——. Index of portraits in books: physicians, surgeons, and others, maintained in the Library of the Royal College of Physicians. London, Royal College of Physicians and Micro Methods, Ltd., 1964.

Microfilm: 2 reels. Copy of card file. Does not include portraits in serials, or in individual biographies of or works by an author.

746
——. Portraits. Ed. by Gordon Wolstenholme. The portraits described by David Piper. London, Churchill, 1964. 468 p.

Includes sculpture as well as original paintings, drawings, and pastels arranged alphabetically by subject. Mainly English physicians or foreign members of the College. Biographical notice of the subject, full description, artist, provenance, and references for each portrait. Index of artists. Illustrated.

747
Royal College of Surgeons of England. A catalogue of the portraits and other paintings, drawings, and sculpture; by William LeFanu. Edinburgh, Livingstone, 1960. 118 p.

Describes fully 240 portraits, 54 other paintings, 48 drawings, and 10 sculptures. 145 illustrations, including 100 portraits. Artist and subject indexes.

Medicine in Art

748
Behne, Adolf B. Läkaren i konsten; en medicinsk bildatlas med beledsagande konsthistorisk text. Oldenburg, Stalling, 1937. 233 p.

A collection of reproductions of medical illustrations, some in color.

749
Cabanès, Augustin. Esculape chez les artistes. Paris, Le François, 1928. 401 p.

Chapters on various deformities and infirmities, surgery, medicine, dentistry, etc., in art. With 196 illustrations, usually documented. Bibliographical footnotes. No index.

750
Holländer, Eugen. Die Medizin in der klassischen Malerei. 4 ed. Stuttgart, Enke, 1950. 488 p.

From the late Middle Ages through the 18th century. Includes anatomy, surgery, and dentistry. Topically arranged; no index. 308 illustrations, some colored, with sources given. 1 ed. 1903. 4 ed. is reimpression of 3 ed., 1923.

751
——. Plastik und Medizin. Stuttgart, Enke, 1912. 576 p.

Topically arranged; no index. 434 illustrations. "Literatur- und Quellenverzeichnis": p. 572–576.

752
Lemke, Rudolf. Psychiatrische Themen in Malerei und Graphik. Bearbeitet von Helmut Rennert. Jena, Fischer, 1958. 144 p.

Studies of 109 works, from the Renaissance to the present, with reproduction of each. Index of artists.

753
Mazzini, Giuseppe. Il bambino nell'arte, vista da un medico. Milano, Hoepli, 1933. 363 p.

With 30 plates and 267 illustrations, documented. Bibliography: p. 343–347. Name index.

754
Richer, Paul M. L. P. L'art et la médecine. Paris, Gaultier, Magnier, 1902. 562 p.

Studies of artistic representation of the possessed, the deformed, dwarfs, clowns, idiots, the handicapped, the sick, etc.; and of physicians, surgeons, and dentists, and of the dead, mainly in European art before 1750. Partly based on two earlier works by Jean M. Charcot and Richer: *Les démoniaques dans l'art*, 1887; and *Les difformes et les malades dans l'art*, 1889. 345 illustrations and plates, with sources given. Index of artists and anonymous works listed by type.

Caricatures

755
Hein, Wolfgang Hagen. Die Pharmazie in der Karikatur. Pharmacy in Caricature. Frankfurt a/M, Govi, 1964. 222 p.

Brief introductory discussions, 210 illustrations. Bibliography: p. 219–220; index of artists. Captions and text in German and English.

756
Holländer, Eugen. Die Karikatur und Satire in der Medizin; mediko-kunsthistorische Studie. 2 ed. Stuttgart, Enke, 1921. 404 p.

From ancient times to the beginning of the 20th century. Includes literary extracts. 262 illustrations, some in color, with sources given. 1 ed. 1905.

757
U. S. National Library of Medicine. Caricatures from the art collection. [Sheila M. (Parker) Durling, comp.] Washington, 1959. 24 p.

Lists 288 medical and dental caricatures by artist, giving title, date, and subject. Index of subjects, including persons.

758
Veth, Cornelis. Der Arzt in der Karikatur. Berlin, Stollberg, 1927. 153 p.

Historical survey: p. 1–38; illustrations: p. 39–153. No documentation, no index.

759
Vogt, Helmut. Medizinische Karikaturen von 1800 bis zur Gengenwart. München, Lehmann, 1960. 184 p.

Includes 315 illustrations, arranged by topic. Bibliography: p. 182–184. No index.

760
Weber, A. Tableau de la caricature médicale depuis les origines jusqu'à nos jours. Paris, Éditions Hippocrate, 1936. 143 p.

Chronological survey, with 125 illustrations, not documented. No bibliography; no index except "Table des gravures."

Bookplates

761
Radbill, Samuel X. Bibliography of medical ex libris literature. Los Angeles, Hilprand Press, 1951. 40 p.

Lists 141 books and articles, with annotations.

Famous Persons

762
Gilbert, Judson Bennett. Disease and destiny; a bibliography of medical references to the famous. With additions and introd. by Gordon E. Mestler. London, Dawsons, 1962. 535 p.

Arranged alphabetically by names of the famous. Publications cited from ca. 1600 to 1950, with selected additions to 1961. Earlier histories and bibliographies listed, p. 11–16.

763
Lange, Wilhelm. Genie, Irrsinn und Ruhm; eine Pathographie des Genies. Vollstandig neu bearb. und um über 1500 neue Quellen vermehrt von Wolfram Kurth. [5 ed.] München, Reinhardt, 1961. 628 p.

"Pathographien" (over 500 persons alphabetically by name): p. 264–450. Sources (2860 references, including 1650 on individuals alphabetically by name): p. 451–580. Unaltered reprint of 4 ed., 1956; 1 ed. 1927.

764
Marx, Rudolf. The health of the presidents. New York, Putnam, 1960, 376 p.

Popular, undocumented essays.

765
Roos, Charles A. Physicians to the presidents, and their patients: a biobibliography. Bulletin of the Medical Library Association, 49:291–360, 1961.

Chronological listing by presidents, with bibliographical references and list of physicians, giving brief identification. Name index of physicians.

766
Stevenson, Robert Scott. Famous illnesses in history. London, Eyre and Spottiswoode, 1962. 239 p.

Accounts of illnesses of 15 famous persons, the majority English and American. References at end of each chapter. No index.

767
Treue, Wilhelm. Mit den Augen ihrer Leibärzte. Von bedeutenden Medizinen und ihren grossen Patienten. Düsseldorf, Droste, 1955. 479 p.

Chapters on France, England, Russia, and Germany. Emphasis on kings, princes, and other rulers. Index of persons, with dates. Bibliography (by country): p. 459–474. English translation by Frances Fawcett (*A doctor at court*, London, 1958) omits bibliography and index.

768
Wold, Karl C. Mr. President, how is your health? St. Paul, Bruce, 1948. 214 p.

Medical history of each president, to F. D. Roosevelt. Brief bibliography for each.

Homeopathy

769
Bradford, Thomas L. Homoeopathic bibliography of the United States, from the year 1825 to the year 1891, inclusive. Philadelphia, Boericke & Tafel, 1892. 596 p.

Books and pamphlets (including many reprints), journals, directories, institutions, etc., in several lists alphabetically by author, with occasional annotations. Includes books attacking homeopathy.

770
Bradford, Thomas L. The pioneers of homoeopathy. Philadelphia, Boericke & Tafel, 1897. 677 p.

Biographical sketches of some 500 homeopathic physicians of all countries who were practitioners prior to 1835; intended to be complete. Sketches include lists of works and biographical references.

771
Cleave, Egbert. Biographical cyclopaedia of homoeopathic physicians and surgeons. Philadelphia, Galaxy Pub. Co., 1873. 512 p.

Covers United States only.

772
King, William H., ed. History of homoeopathy and its institutions in America, New York, Lewis, 1905. 4 v.

A compilation; includes state histories, biographies, and accounts of medical colleges, hospitals, societies, and periodicals. No bibliography.

773
Tischner, Rudolf. Geschichte der Homö-

opathie. Leipzig, Schwabe, 1932–39. 4 pts. in 2 v.

Exhaustive history with biographies.

Jews

774
Friedenwald, Harry. Jewish luminaries in medical history ... and a catalogue of works bearing on the subject of the Jews and medicine from the private library of Harry Friedenwald. Baltimore, Johns Hopkins Press, 1946. 199 p.

Includes author catalog (p. 25–199) of over 1700 items, with occasional brief notes on the authors or works. Pt. 1: writings of individual physicians and works about them. Pt. 2: works of general reference. No index.

775
——. The Jews and medicine; essays. Baltimore, Johns Hopkins Press, 1944. 2 v. (The Johns Hopkins University. Institute of the History of Medicine. Publications. Monographs, no. 2 and 3)

Biographical, bibliographical and historical studies mostly reprinted from journals. Includes: "The bibliography of ancient Hebrew medicine," v. 1, p. 99–145; "Use of the Hebrew language in medical literature" (with lists of writers and translators), v. 1, p. 146–180; "History of the Jewish physicians of Spain, Portugal and southern France" (with annotated alphabetical list; only introduction previously published), v. 2, p. 613–771. Many facsimiles. Bibliographical footnotes. "Works of reference": p. 773–787. Name index only.

776
Kagan, Solomon R. Jewish contributions to medicine in America from colonial times to the present. 2 ed. Boston, Boston Medical Pub. Co., 1939. 792 p.

Largely biographical, with chapter on Jewish medical institutions. Reprint of 1 ed., 1934, with supplement, p. 549–792.

777
——. Jewish medicine. Boston, Medico-Historical Press, 1952. 575 p.

Mainly biographical sketches, from ancient times to the present. Emphasis on 19th–20th centuries (p. 142–564). Name index.

778
Muntner, Süssmann. Contribution to the history of the Hebrew language in medical instruction. Jerusalem, Geniza, 1940. xv, 128 p. (Sources of reference of the history of Hebrew medicine, v. 1–2)

In Hebrew, with English summary (p. v–xv). Survey of medical literature in Hebrew, including translations, from Old Testament times, in manuscript and in print.

Literature and Medicine

For references to works on individual authors, see Gilbert, *Disease and Destiny* (no. 762), and Lange (no. 763).

779
Dana, Charles L. Poetry and the doctors: a catalogue of poetical works written by physicians, with biographical notes and an essay on the poetry of certain ancient practitioners of medicine. Woodstock, Vt., Elm Tree Press, 1916. xxiii, 83 p.

Alphabetical catalog of Dana's collection, with brief biographical notes on the authors and bibliographical descriptions. Appendix of works not in Dana's library: p. 81–83.

780
Davenport, James H. Literary doctors of medicine; a catalogue of the extra-professional writings of physicians and surgeons in the library of James Henry Davenport. Providence, Privately printed, 1926. 306 p.

Arranged by forms and topics; includes contributions to subject fields as well as *belles lettres.* Index of authors, with biographical notes. p. 207–306.

781
Oppenheimer, Heinrich. Medical and allied topics in Latin poetry. London, Bale and Danielsson, 1928. 445 p.

Chapters on various topics. Mainly quotations in Latin, with English translations and brief comments. Subject index.

782
Simpson, Robert R. Shakespeare and medicine. Edinburgh, Livingstone, 1959. 267 p.

Comprehensive account, with numerous extracts.

783
Witkowski, Gustave J. Les médecins au

théatre, de l'antiquité au dix-septième siècle. Paris, Maloine, 1905. 568 p.

Brief accounts of plays, arranged by period, with numerous quotations. No index. Table of contents lists plays by title.

784
Yearsley, Percival Macleod. Doctors in Elizabethan drama. London, J. Bale, Sons & Danielsson, 1933. 128 p.

Studies of medical education, practice, and practitioners. Frequent quotations.

Music and Medicine

785
Schullian, Dorothy M., and Schoen, Max, ed. Music and medicine. New York, Schuman. 1948. 499 p.

Studies by different authors on historical aspects and modern musical therapy. Includes chapters on primitive peoples, American Indians, classical antiquity, tarantism, the Renaissance through the 18th century, musical physicians, etc. Selected references: p. 407–471.

Numismatics

786
Holzmair, Eduard. Katalog der Sammlung Dr. Josef Brettauer Medicina in Nummis, Wien, 1937. 384 p.

5557 items: nos. 1–1347 medals honoring physicians and natural scientists, alphabetically by name; the rest classified by subject. 26 plates reproducing selected medals. References to works on numismatics and medical history: p. 371–377. Subject index.

787
Johns Hopkins University. John Work Garrett Library. Medals relating to medicine and allied sciences in the numismatic collection of the Johns Hopkins University. A catalogue by Sarah Elizabeth Freeman. Baltimore, 1964. xx, 430 p. (Evergreen House Foundation. Publication no. 2)

Describes 922 items. Sect. 1 by person, with biographical notes; sect. 2 by subject, including schools, societies, etc. 32 plates. Index of medallists. Bibliography: p. xiv–xx.

788
Storer, Horatio R. Medicina in nummis; a descriptive list of the coins, medals, jetons relating to medicine, surgery, and the allied sciences. Ed. by Malcolm Storer. Boston, Wright and Potter, 1931. 1146 p.

8343 entries, plus addenda, in 2 sections: personal names and subject. Reference list (396 items) p. 11–19; bibliography: p. 1135–1140. Subject index.

Paleopathology

789
Moodie, Roy L. Paleopathology; an introduction to the study of ancient evidences of disease. Urbana, Univ. of Illinois Press, 1923. 567 p.

Bibliography (p. 545–557) thoroughly covers literature to 1922. Repeated in Pales (no. 790).

790
Pales, Léon. Paléopathologie et pathologie comparative. Paris, Masson, 1930. 352 p.

Bibliography (p. 293–348) lists 660 titles, including those in Moodie (no. 789) and additional items published from 1923 to 1930. Supplemented by H. E. Sigerist's "Literature on paleopathology since 1930," in his *History of medicine*, New York, 1951–61, v. 1, p. 532–541 (no. 488).

791
Palla, Ákos, ed. Paläopathologie. Jena, Fischer, 1962– .

v. 1: Tasnádi-Kubacska, Andras, *Pathologie der vorzeitliche Tiere*, 1962, 269 p. Bibliography: p. 241–255. Translanted from Hungarian.

792
Wells, Calvin. Bones, bodies, and disease: evidence of disease and abnormality in early man. London, Thames and Hudson, 1964. 288 p. (Ancient peoples and places, v. 37)

Survey for the general reader. Text not documented, but references (p. 201–212) listed in order of text.

Philately

793
Bishop, William J., and Matheson, Norman M. Medicine and science in postage stamps. London, Harvey and Blythe, 1948. 82 p.

Biographical notes. Illustrations: p. 25–56. Bibliography: p. 57–59. Catalogue of portrait stamps: p. 60–82. No general index.

794
Gottfried, Oscar. Doctors philatelic. New York, The American Physician, 1954. 96 p. Supplements no. 1–2, 1958–62. 16 p.; 29 p.

Physicians depicted on postage stamps, with biographical sketches. One stamp under each entry is illustrated. Consolidated name index in Suppl. 2, April 1962.

795
Newerla, Gerhard J. Medical history in philately. Milwaukee, American Topical Assn., [1964]–

Contains sections on persons and topics, catalogue of stamps, list of charity seals of medical interest, bibliography (172 items) and indexes of names and issuing countries. Large sections of additions and corrections. Not illustrated. Mostly previously published in the *Weekly philatelic gossip.*

796
Stroppiana, Luigi. Catalogo dei francobolli a soggeto medico. Roma, Tipografia Guerra & Belli, 1956. 185 p.

Arranged by country, with indexes of medicinal plants and of persons. Many stamps illustrated.

Primitive Medicine, Magic & Folklore

797
Black, William G. Folk-medicine; a chapter in the history of culture. London, Stock, 1883. 227 p. (Folk-lore Society, London. Publications, 12)

Documented survey based on literary and miscellaneous sources, with many extracts, especially from British texts. "Books of reference": p. 221–222.

798
Budge, Ernest A. T. W. Amulets and superstitions; the original texts with translations and descriptions. London, Oxford Univ. Press, 1930. 543 p.

Study of ancient and medieval amulets, talismans, symbols, magic, divination, astrology, superstitions, etc. Reprinted New York, University Books, 1961, as *Amulets and talismans.*

799
Caillet, Albert L. Manuel bibliographique des sciences psychiques ou occultes. Paris, Dorbon, 1912. 3 v.

11,648 entries, frequently annotated, listing magic, hermetic, astrological, cabalistic, and similar works, many by medical men. Reprinted 1964.

800
Ferguson, John. Bibliographical notes on histories of inventions and books of secrets. London, Holland Press, 1959. 2 v.

Covers popular and pseudo-scientific works concerned with inventions and "secrets" (techniques, receipts, etc.) in medicine, pharmacy, and other arts and sciences, frequently anonymous, pseudonymous, or falsely ascribed. Describes editions, with account of contents and discussion of problems. Author and title indexes. Previously published in 6 parts and 7 supplements, Glasgow, 1894–1915.

801
Hovorka, Oskar, Edler von Zderas, and Kronfeld, Adolf, ed. Vergleichende Volksmedizin; eine Darstellung volksmedizinischer Sitten und Gebräuche, Anschauungen und Heilfaktoren, des Aberglaubens und Zaubermedizin. Stuttgart, Strecker & Schröder, 1908–09. 2 v.

Exhaustive. v. 1 contains accounts of special beliefs and practices, and descriptions and histories of the use in folk medicine of plants, chemical substances, animals, magic words, parts of the body, etc., with frequent quotations and references. v. 2 is devoted to diseases of different parts of the body, surgery, dentistry, etc. Bibliography: v. 2, p. 920–960.

802
Reichborn-Kjennerud, Ingjald. Vår gamle trolldomsmedisin. Oslo, Dybwad, 1928–47. 5 v. (Norske videnskaps-akademi i Oslo. Historisk-filosofisk klasse. Skrifter. 1928, no. 6; 1933, no. 2; 1940, no. 1; 1943, no. 2; 1947, no. 1)

Detailed history of Scandinavian folk medicine, with extensive references to sources and bibliography in each volume.

803
Thompson, Charles J. S. Magic and healing. London, Rider, 1947. 176 p.

Covers early periods and British Isles through 18th century. Includes such subjects as: healing by incantation; healing and astrology; by sympathy; by touch; herb lore; precious stones, etc. No bibliography or index.

804
Wilke, Georg. Die Heilkunde in der europäischen Vorzeit. Leipzig, Rabitzsch, 1936. 418 p.

Covers anatomy, concepts, diagnosis, and treatment of diseases, pregnancy and childbirth, surgery, dentistry, magical medicine, etc. Extensive bibliographical references. Place and subject indexes.

Quackery

805
Francesco, Grete de. The power of the charlatan. Tr. by Miriam Beard, New Haven, Yale Univ. Press, 1939. 288 p.

Includes chapters on alchemy, the medicine show, handbills, broadsides, etc., and mechanical devices. References: p. 279–283. Translation of *Die Macht des Charlatans*, Basel, 1937.

806
Holbrook, Stewart H. The golden age of quackery. New York, Macmillan, 1959. 302 p.

Popular account of patent medicines in America, Bibliography: p. 293–295.

807
Jameson, Eric. The natural history of quackery. London, Joseph, 1961. 224 p.

Discusses various types of quacks, chiefly English and American. Bibliography: p. 215–217.

808
Thompson, Charles J. S. The quacks of old London. London, Brentano, 1928. 356 p.

Popular account. No bibliography or notes.

809
Young, James Harvey. The toadstool millionaires; a social history of patent medicines in America before Federal regulation. Princeton, Princeton Univ. Press, 1961. 282 p.

Historical analysis. Bibliographic footnotes (chiefly sources); note on sources: p. 263–269.

Religion and Medicine

Religious and Mental Healing

810
Jayne, Walter A. The healing gods of ancient civilizations. New Haven, Yale Univ. Press, 1925. 569 p.

On Egyptian, Assyro-Babylonian, Indian, Iranian, Greek, Roman and Celtic deities. Classified bibliography: p. 523–542. Reprinted New Hyde Park, N.Y., University Books, 1962.

811
Podmore, Frank. From Mesmer to Christian science; a short history of mental healing. New Hyde Park, N. Y., University Books, 1964. 306 p.

Popular history of hypnotism, spiritualism, new thought, Christian Science, etc. Bibliographical footnotes throughout. Reprint of the 1909 London ed., entitled *Mesmerism and Christian Science*, with new introduction.

812
Weatherhead, Leslie D. Psychology, religion and healing. A critical study of all the non-physical methods of healing, with an examination of the principles underlying them and the techniques employed to express them, together with some conclusions regarding further investigation and action in this field. 2 ed. London, Hodder and Stoughton, 1963. 544 p.

Includes early methods of healing through religion and psychology. Bibliography: p. 525–532.

Bible, Talmud, and Koran

813
Brim, Charles J. Medicine in the Bible, the Pentateuch, Torah. New York, Froben Press, 1936. v. 1, The Pentateuch, Torah. 384 p.

Chapters on special subjects. Emphasis on terminology, the Hebrew terms transliterated. Biblical citations and references in footnotes.

814
Fenner, Friedrich. Die Krankheit im Neuen Testament; eine religions- und medizingeschichtliche Untersuchung. Leipzig, Hinrichs, 1930. 115 p.

Interpretative, historical, and semantic study of the texts. Includes psychotherapy. Bibliography: p. 111–115. Enlargement of a thesis, Jena, 1920.

815
Opitz, Karl. Die Medizin im Koran. Stuttgart, Enke, 1906. 92 p.

Studies of special topics in medicine, hygiene, and sanitary law. Bibliographical references in notes (p. 68–79). Sources: p. 80. Indexes of passages cited and of subjects and names.

816
Preuss, Julius. Biblisch-talmudische Medizin. Berlin, Karger, 1911. 735 p.

Detailed studies of special subjects. Indexes of passages cited and of topics. Classified bibliography of medicine in the Bible and Talmud: p. 688–704. Reprinted 1921, 1923.

817
Short, Arthur. The Bible and modern medicine: a survey of health and healing in the Old and New Testaments. London, Paternoster Press, 1953. 142 p.

Compact guide for the general reader in medical history or Biblical studies.

818
Snowman, Jacob. A short history of Talmudic medicine. London, J. Bale, Sons & Danielsson, 1935. 94 p. (Short history series)

Based chiefly on Preuss. No bibliography.

The Church

819
Delaunay, Paul. La médecine et l'église: contribution à l'histoire de l'exercice médicale [par les clercs] Paris, Editions Hippocrate, 1948. 135 p.

Documented. Chiefly on France. No index.

820
Pazzini, Adalberto. I santi nella storia della medicina. Roma, Casa editrice "Mediterranea", 1937. 605 p.

Detailed work. Includes extracts in Italian from the sources and plates reproducing artistic representations. Bibliography: p. 521–605.

Research

821
Bretschneider, Hubert. Der Streit um die Vivisektion im 19. Jahrhundert: Verlauf, Argumente, Ergebnisse. Stuttgart, Fischer, 1962. 158 p. (Medizin in Geschichte und Kultur, 2)

Chiefly on Germany. Bibliography (165 items): p. 144–150.

822
Shryock, Richard H. American medical research, past and present, New York, Commonwealth Fund, 1947. 350 p. (New York Academy of Medicine. Committee on Medicine and the Changing Order. Monograph studies)

Formative influences, economic and social background, research trends.

Symbolism, Medical

823
Bergman, Emanuel. Medicinska emblem och symboler. Karlshamn, Sweden, Sveriges Läkarforbunds Förlagsaktiebolag, 1941. 104 p.

Discussion of medical emblems and symbols, with 111 illustrations, described and documented. Bibliography (48 items): p. 102–104. No index.

824
Potter, Edwin S. Serpents in symbolism, art and medicine: the Babylonian caduceus and Aesculapius club. Santa Barbara, Calif., Privately printed, 1937. 85 p.

With 36 illustrations. Bibliography: p. 81–82.

825
Sozinskey, Thomas S. Medical symbolism in connection with historical studies in the arts of healing and hygiene. Philadelphia, Davis. 1891. 171 p. (Physicians' and students' ready reference series, no. 9)

Chapters on the serpentine god of medicine, Aesculapian staff and serpent, medical amulets, the pentacle, pharmacists' symbols, etc. Bibliographical footnotes. No index.

Women in Medicine

826
Bell, Enid H. C. M. Storming the citadel: the rise of the woman doctor. London, Constable, 1953. 200 p.

On British women physicians, including those practicing in British India. List of books consulted: p. 192.

827
Hughes, Muriel J. Women healers in medieval life and literature. New York, King's Crown Press, 1943. 180 p.

Documented study, mainly based on literary and historical sources. Women practitioners of the later Middle Ages (list by specialties, with bibliographical references): p. 139–147. Bibliography: p. 155–171.

828
Lipinska, Mélina. Les femmes et le progrès des sciences médicales. Paris, Masson, 1930. 235 p.

General historical survey. Bibliographical footnotes throughout; no bibliography or index.

829
Lovejoy, Esther P. Women doctors of the world. New York, Macmillan, 1957. 412 p.

Women physicians and their achievements since about 1850. A few bibliographical footnotes.

830
Mead, Kate C. H. A history of women in medicine from the earliest times to the beginning of the nineteenth century. Haddam, Conn., Haddam Press, 1938. 569 p.

Detailed survey. Weak in synthesis and sometimes inaccurate. Occasional footnote references.

831
——. Medical women of America; a short history of the pioneer medical women of America and a few of their colleagues in England. New York, Froben Press, 1933. 95 p. (Historia medicinae, v. 7)

Short bibliography included in preface.

832
Schönfeld, Walther. Frauen in der abendländischen Heilkunde vom klassischen Altertum bis zum Ausgang des 19. Jahrhunderts. Stuttgart, Enke, 1947. 176 p.

Survey, with biographic notes. Bibliography: p. 157–164. More reliable than Mead (no. 830).

SPECIAL SUBJECTS

AEROSPACE AND SUBMARINE MEDICINE

Indexes and Abstracts

Current

833
Abstracts of current literature. Aerospace medicine and biology. In Aerospace medicine, 29, 1958– .

931 numbered abstracts in 1966. Includes books, chapters in books. Minimum time lag 1966, 3 months.

834
U.S. National Aeronautics and Space Administration. Aerospace medicine, a continuing bibliography. Washington, July 1964– .

Abstracts. Includes reports, books. Minimum time lag 1966, 2 months. Supersedes no. 835.

Noncurrent

835
U.S. Library of Congress. Science and Technology Division. Aerospace medicine and biology; an annotated bibliography. Washington, 1–11, 1952–62/63.

15,236 entries. Includes reports, journal articles, and books. Occasional coverage of nonmedical journal titles. Superseded by no. 834.

Cumulative indexes v. 1–10 published as a separate.

Bibliographies

836
Hoff, Ebbe C. A bibliographical sourcebook of compressed air, diving and submarine medicine. Washington, Bureau of Medicine and Surgery, 1948–54. 2 v. (NAVMED 1191 and P-5033)

Selective review of references. Includes books, research reports. v. 1: 2958 items through 1945; v. 2: 3805 items, mainly 1946–51.

v. 2 by Ebbe C. Hoff and Leon J. Greenbaum; sponsored by the Office of Naval Research and Bureau of Medicine and Surgery.

837
Hoff, Ebbe C., and Fulton, John F. A bibliography of aviation medicine. Springfield, Ill., Thomas, 1942. 237 p. (Yale Medical Library. Historical Library. Publication no. 5).

5745 entries from 1660 through 1941. Includes books.

838
Hoff, Phebe M. [et al.] A bibliography of aviation medicine; supplement. Washington, 1944. 109 p. (Yale Medical Library. Historical Library. Publication no. 9)

2336 entries numbered consecutively with the original [no. 837]. Mainly 1942–44 references.

839
Monge, Carlos M. Aclimatación en los Andes; extractos de investigaciones sobre biologia de altitud. Lima, 1960. 165 p.

538 references, most with abstracts. Includes books, theses, reports.

840
National Research Council. Division of Medical Sciences. Committee on Aviation Medicine. Bibliography on aviation medicine. [Washington] 1946. 2 v. 802 p.

Largely U. S. and foreign government research reports.

841
Nelson, David R. [et al.] Electrical generation of oxygen; literature survey. 106 p. (WADC technical report 57–739, August 1958).

Lists in excess of 550 references and 691 patents.

842
Schmidt, Ingeborg. Bibliographie der Luftfahrtmedizin; eine Zusammenstellung von Arbeiten über Luftfahrtmedizin und Grenzgebiete bis Ende 1936. Berlin, Springer, 1938. 136 p.

843
——. ——. Zweite Folge. Eine Zusammenstellung von Arbeiten über Luftfahrtmed-

izin und Grenzgebiete 1937 bis ende 1940. 127 p.

Issued as v. 8 (1), 1943 of *Luftfahrtmedizin*.

844
Snyder, Richard G. et al. Biomedical research studies in acceleration, impact, weightlessness, vibration, and emergency escape, and restraint systems: a comprehensive bibliography. [n. p.] 3072 p. (U. S. Federal Aviation Agency, Civil Aeromedical Research Institute, CARI report 63–30, December 1963).

10,306 entries, most with abstracts. Includes reports, articles and books.

844.1
——. ——. Supplement one. By John Ice, Richard G. Snyder [et al.] 3010 p. (CARI Report 63–30, Supplement one, September 1966)

3872 entries, most with abstracts.

845
Space Technology Laboratories. Technical Library. Physiological and psychological effects of space flight: A bibliography. By J. F. Price. Redondo Beach, Calif., 1962–63. 2 v. (Research bibliography no. 43, October 1962; no. 44, January 1963)

v. 1, Acceleration, deceleration, and impact (1020 references); v. 2, Weightlessness and subgravity (385 references). Includes books, government and private research reports. Most references annotated.

846
U.S. Library of Congress. Aerospace Technology Division. Soviet biotechnology and bioastronautics, December 1964 to June 1965; compilation of abstracts. Washington, 1966. 228 p. (Surveys of Soviet Scientific and Technical Literature. Report no. 2)

132 abstracts. Includes reports of conferences and symposia and books.

847
U.S. National Aeronautics and Space Administration. Scientific and Technical Information Division. Bibliography related to human factors system program (July 1962–February 1964). By Richard J. Potocko. Washington, 1964. 237 p.

Includes articles, monographs, research reports, translations (mainly JPRS documents), congresses. Emphasis on the research report literature.

847.1
Waga kuni ni okeru koku igaku bunken mokuroku. Bibliography of aviation medicine in Japan. 1 [ed.] Tokyo, Aero-Medical Laboratory, JASDF, 1963. 303 p.

Covers 1903 to 1962.

Directories

848
Aerospace Medical Association. Directory of members. Washington [1] 1960?– .

Irregular. Alphabetical listing of members with addresses; also includes officers of the association, past presidents, constitution and bylaws, and awards. Published in 1960 and 1961 as a supplement to one issue of its *Journal*.

Histories

Official histories are listed under Military Medicine.

849
Benford, Robert J. Doctors in the sky; the story of the Aero Medical Association. Springfield, Ill., Thomas, 1955. 326 p.

Detailed account of aviation medicine in U. S. from 1929.

850
Fulton, John F. Aviation medicine in its preventive aspects, an historical survey. London, Oxford University Press, 1948. 174 p. (Univ. of London, Heath Clark lectures, 1947)

Includes altitude sickness and acclimatization, decompression sickness. References.

ALLERGY

Indexes and Abstracts

851
Allergy abstracts. Brooklyn, 1, 1936– Jewish Hospital of Brooklyn. Allergy Division.

Bimonthly. 1964 had 200 abstracts of primarily English language journals. Minimum time lag (1965) 4 months.

v. 1–8, 1936–43, mimeographed; v. 9, 1944– , published as a separately volumed and paged section of *Journal of allergy* (v. 15, 1944–).

v. 2, no. 1, as *Review of the current American and foreign literature of experimental and applied immunology*; v. 2, nos. 2–3, as *Quarterly review of American and foreign literature of experimental and applied immunology.*

852
Review of allergy; selected abstracts of allergology. St. Paul, etc., 1, 1947– .

Monthly. 1964 contained about 550 abstracts. Minimum time lag (1965) 2 months.

v. 1–10, 1947–56, as *Quarterly review . . .*; v. 11–19, 1957–65, as *Review of allergy and applied immunology; selected abstracts . . .*

853
A current bibliography on allergy and applied immunology. In Review of allergy, 4(3), Sept. 1950– .

Includes drug allergy, iatrogenic diseases, air pollution.

Monthly. "Supplement" to abstracts in *Review* (no. 852). References only. Abstracted articles not listed. No indexes.

References no. 1–8071 (ser. 1) in *Letters of the International Correspondence Society of Allergists* (not listed).

Reviews

854★
Progress in allergy. Fortschritte der Allergielehre. Basel, Karger, 1, 1939– .

v. 1, as *Fortschritte der Allergielehre.*

Dictionaries

854.1
Wilken-Jensen, Knud. Lexikon allergologicum. 2 ed. Leipzig, Barth, 1966. 119 p.

Equivalent words in German, English, French, Italian, Russian, and Spanish. Brief section defining some 70 terms, including syndromes, in the languages covered.

ANATOMY

Indexes and Abstracts

Current

855
Internationale Bibliographie der Anatomie des Menschen und Wirbeltiere. In Anatomischer Anzeiger, 1, 1896– .

Articles and books listed alphabetically by author under subject breakdowns. The *Bibliographie* is published as a separately and cumulatively paged section of the individual issues of the *Anzeiger.*

v. 12–67, 1896–1928, issued under the title *Literatur* (except for v. 13–14, 1897–98, when it was entitled *Bibliographia anatomica*) and separately paged. Prior to this most issues of the *Anzeiger* included within its regular pagination a section entitled "Literatur."

856
Referátovy výběr z patologické anatomie [Selected abstracts on pathological anatomy] Praha, 1, 1959– . Ústav pro zdravotnickou dokumentaci.

Abstracts in Czech or Slovak of selected articles, most from foreign periodicals.

Noncurrent

857
Anatomischer Bericht; referiendes Organ für das Gesamtgebiet der Anatomie. Jena, 1–45, no. 6–7, 1922–44. Im Auftrage der anatomischen Gesellschaft.

2–3 volumes a year, several issues a volume. Each volume contains about 1500 abstracts.

858
Bericht über die Fortschritte der Anatomie und Physiologie. Leipzig, 1856–71.

Annual literature review. Articles and books listed by author under subject and then reviewed in order of listing.

Title on spine: *Zeitschrift für rationelle Medicin*; 1856 has added t.p., *Zeitschrift für rationelle Medicin*; subtitle 1856–68, Als besondere Abtheilung der Zeitschrift für rationelle Medicin.

Ed. by J. Henle and G. Meissner. See also 2271.

858.1
Bibliographie anatomique; revue des travaux en langue française; anatomie-histologie-embryologie-anthropologie. Paris, 1–25, 1893–1918.

859
Jahresberichte über die Fortschritte der Anatomie und Entwicklungsgeschichte. Jena, n. s. 1–20, 1892–1914.

v. 1, 1892–95, references only; with v. 2, articles and books listed under subject and then summarized in order of listing. With v. 4, the three principal subject divisions, Allgemeine Anatomie, Entwicklungsgeschichte, Spezielle Anatomie und Entwicklungsgeschichte des Menschen und der Wirbeltiere, have separate title pages and paging.

Separately published author and subject index (Gesamtregister) to v. 1–7, 1892–1901.

Ed. by G. Schwalbe.

Continues Abt. 1 of no. 860.

860
Jahresbericht über die Fortschritte der Anatomie und Physiologie. Leipzig, 1–20, 1872–91.

Annual literature reviews. Articles and books listed under subject, then abstracted or reviewed in order of listing.

From v. 12, 1883, published in two separately paged parts: Erste Abt., Anatomie und Entwicklungsgeschichte; Zweite Abt., Physiologie. 1–12, 1872–83, as *Jahresberichte . . .*

Separately published author indexes (General-Register) to v. 1–10, 11–20.

Continued by nos. 859 and 2271.

861
Zentralblatt für normale Anatomie und Mikrotechnik. Berlin, 1–11, 1904–14.

v. 11 contained 1013 entries, most with abstracts.

v. 1 as *Zentralblatt für normale und pathologische Anatomie mit Einschluss der Mikrotechnik.*

Reviews

862
Advances in morphogenesis. New York, 1, 1961–

Annual reviews.

863
Ergebnisse der Anatomie und Entwicklungsgeschichte. Berlin, 1, 1891– .

Irregular. Suspended 1945–55. Some vols. issued in revised ed. Text in German or English, 1956– .

864 (Not used)

865
Recent advances in anatomy. 2 ser. Ed. by F. Goldby and R. J. Harrison. London, Churchill, 1961. 477 p.

1 ed., 1927. No author index.

Bibliographies

866
Haller, Albrecht von. Bibliotheca anatomica; qua scripta ad anatomen et physiologiam facientia a rerum initiis recensentur. Tiguri, Orell, Gessner, Fussli, 1774–77. 2 v.

Similar in arrangement and method to no. 970. 1796 chapters devoted to individual authors or groups of authors. v. 1, to 1700; v. 2, 1701–1776. Index of authors and of anonymous works by subject.

867
Isaev, Petr O. Bibliografiia otechestvennoi literatury po anatomii cheloveka [Bibliography of national literature on anatomy of man] Moskva, Gos. izd-vo medits. literatury, 1962. 451 p.

More than 10,000 titles of books and journal articles published over a period of some 200 years. The most recent entries are for 1959.

868
Krogman, Wilton M. A bibliography of human morphology, 1914–1939. Chicago, Univ. of Chicago Press, 1941. 385 p.

869
Russell, Kenneth F. British anatomy, 1525–1800; a bibliography. Melbourne, Melbourne Univ. Press, 1963. 254 p.

Lists 901 items by author with full descriptions. Includes works by British authors published outside Great Britain, and other European works translated into English or published in Great Britain. Locates copies examined.

Dictionaries

870
Abadir, Fahim M. Etymologica anatomica; comprising anatomical terms, their origin, derivation and meaning. Alexandria, Egypt, 1957. 150 p.

No eponyms.

871
Abd-El-Malek, Shafik. English-Arabic glossary of anatomical terms. [Cairo, 1940] 144 p.

872
Dobson, Jessie. Anatomical eponyms; being a biographical dictionary of those

anatomists whose names have become incorporated into anatomical nomenclature, with definitions of the structures to which their names have been attached and references to the works in which they are described. 2 ed. Edinburgh, Livingstone, 1962. 235 p.

873
Donáth, Tibor. Erläuterndes anatomisches Wörterbuch; vergleichende Übersicht der Baseler, Jenaer und Pariser Nomenklaturen, gruppiert nach Organen. Budapest, Verlag Medicina, 1960. 538 p.

Translated from Hungarian, *Anatómiai értelmezö szótár*, Budapest, 1959. Also translated into Russian, *Tolkovyi, anatomicheskii slovar'*, Budapest, 1964.

Contains comparative nomina anatomica and an "explanatory dictionary" which gives German equivalents of Latin terms and definition or description of the terms. Includes brief biographies of eponyms.

874★
Field, Ephraim J. and Harrison, R. J. Anatomical terms: their origin, and derivation. 2 ed. Cambridge, Eng., Heffer, 1957. 190 p.

Includes eponyms, with brief biographical notes; intended for the student.

875
Fonahn, Adolf M. Arabic and Latin anatomical terminology, chiefly from the Middle Ages. Kristiania, Dybwad, 1922. 174 p. (Videnskapsselskapet i Kristiania. Historisk-filosofisk Klasse. Skrifter. 1921, no. 7)

Arabic transliterations (followed by term in Arabic) and Latin in one alphabet. English equivalents.

876
Herber, Otto. Slovník anatomických jmen. 2 ed. Praha, Stát. zdrav. nakl., 1955. 207 p.

Pt. 1, Czech equivalents for Latin, Greek, or other term of origin; pt. 2, short biographical sketches of famous anatomists; pt. 3, *Nomina anatomica* (Basle, 1895, and Jena, 1935).

877
Krüger, Gerhard. Der anatomische Wortschatz, unter Mitberücksichtigung der Histologie und der Embryologie für Studierende, Ärzte und Tierärzte. 8 ed. Leipzig, Hirzel, 1964. 131 p.

Title varies slightly. 1 ed., 1950.

878
Lovasy, E. and Veillon, E. Dictionnaire des termes d'anatomie, d'embryologie, et d'histologie. Paris, Maloine, 1954. 624 p.

879
Mori, Masaru. Gakushū hikkei kaibōgaku yōran [Handbook of anatomical terminology, especially designed for students] Tokyo, Nanzando, 1960. 553 p.

880
Olivier, Georges. Les nouveaux termes anatomiques; lexique conforme à la nomenclature internationale (P.N.A.). Paris, Vigot, 1959. 146 p.

French term followed by the international term in Latin and a free translation in French.

881
Rodriguez Rivero, Placido Daniel. Eponimias anatomicas. [n.p.] Sociedad Venezolana de Historia de la Medicina [1939] 371 p.

882
Schaller, Anton [et al.] Lateinisch (deutsch)—arabisches Wörterbuch der Anatomie. Wien, Hammer-Purgstall-Gesellschaft [1965?] 240 p.

Latin and German in one alphabet followed by Arabic equivalent.

Added t.p. in Arabic.

883
Sørensen, Edward C., and Høeg, L. Terminologia anatomica; etymologien af de i den makroskopiske og den mikroskopiske anatomi samt i embryologien anvendte termini technici. København, Busck, 1958. 85 p.

Danish equivalents of Latin and Greek terms.

884
Triepel, Hermann. Die anatomischen Namen; ihre Ableitung und Aussprache. Mit einem Anhang; Eigennamen die früher in der Anatomie verwendet wurden. 27 ed. München, Bergmann, 1965. 99 p.

Includes eponyms and biographies. 1 ed., 1905.

Nomenclature

884.1
Barcia Goyanes, Juan J., Moncayo Marques, J. La Nomina anatomica de Paris (P.N.A.) y su concordancia con la Nomina anatomica de Jena (I.N.A.) y las denominaciones anatomicas usuales en español. 2 v. Valencia, Garcia Muñoz, 1960. 345 p.

885★★
Eycleshymer, Albert C., and Schoemaker, Daniel M. Anatomical names, especially the Basle Nomina Anatomica (BNA) . . . . with biographical sketches. By Roy Lee Moodie. New York, Wood, 1917. 744 p.

886
International Anatomical Nomenclature Committee. Nomina anatomica. 3 ed. Amsterdam, Excerpta Medica, 1966. 112 p.

Introduction provides detailed account of various congresses and the decisions made. Terminology arranged first by parts of body and then by systems.

887★
Leutert, Gerald. Die anatomischen Nomenklaturen von Basel, Jena, Paris in dreifacher Gegenüberstellung. Leipzig, Thieme, 1963. 378 p.

Three lists: comparison of Paris, Jena and Basel nomenclature; comparison of Basel and Paris nomenclature; comparison of Jena and Paris nomenclature. Terms are in alphabetical order side by side.

888
Woerdeman, M. W. Nomina anatomica Parisiensia (1955) et B.N.A. (1895). Utrecht, Oosthoek, 1957. 174 p.

Preface presents brief historical sketch of the systems of anatomical nomenclature. Terms arranged in alphabetical order.

Histories

889
Choulant, Johann Ludwig. History and bibliography of anatomic illustration; translated and annotated by Mortimer Frank. Further essays by Fielding S. Garrison, Mortimer Frank [and] Edward C. Streeter, with a new historical essay by Charles Singer. [Rev. ed.] New York, Schuman's, 1945. 435 (i. e. 453) p.

Standard reference. Describes illustrated works of anatomists from the 14th to the mid-19th century, with biographical and bibliographical data. List of works on artistic anatomy: p. 351–361. Appendix by F. H. Garrison on anatomical illustration since Choulant, with bibliography, p. 404–412. Many illustrations, with sources indicated. Name index only.

Translation (first published Chicago, 1920) of *Geschichte und Bibliographie der anatomischen Abbildung*, Leipzig, 1852, with corrections and additions by Choulant published in *Archiv für die zeichnenden Künste*, 3. Jahrg., 1857, and also in his *Graphische Incunabeln für Naturgeschichte und Medicin* (no. 429), p. 122–159. The sections on the pre-Vesalian periods include supplementary material from the works of Karl Sudhoff and an essay on manuscript anatomic illustration by Mortimer Frank.

890
Cole, Francis J. A history of comparative anatomy from Aristotle to the eighteenth century. London, Macmillan, 1944. 524 p.

Includes scientific contributions, biographical notes, institutions. Bibliography: p. 490–507.

891
Corner, George W. Anatomy. New York, Hoeber, 1930. 82 p. (Clio medica, no. 3.)

From the Greeks on. References: p. 69–74. Reprinted, London, Hafner, 1963.

892
Faller, Adolf. Die Entwicklung der makroskopisch-anatomischen Präparierkunst von Galen bis zur Neuzeit. Basel, Karger, 1948. 115 p. (Acta anatomica. Supplementum 7)

Scholarly study. 45 documented illustrations. References: p. 111–115.

893
Meyer, Arthur W. The rise of embryology. Stanford, Calif., Stanford University Press, 1939. 367 p.

Detailed studies of special subjects. Bibliography: p. 343–361.

894
Needham, Joseph. A history of embryology. 2 ed. New York, Abelard-Schuman, 1959. 303 p.

From ancient times to ca. 1900. Bibliography: p. 241–292. 1st separate ed. Cambridge, Eng., 1934.

895
Portal, Antoine. Histoire de l'anatomie et de la chirurgie. Paris, Didot, 1770–73. 6 v. in 7.

Biobibliographical survey of the development of anatomy, physiology, and surgery through 1755. Notices of individual authors list theses, books, and articles, frequently with annotations. v. 6 includes classified bibliographies and author indexes.

896
Premuda, Loris. Storia della iconografia anatomica. Con un' appendice di Gaetano Ottaviani. Milano, Martello, 1957. 235 p.

From prehistoric times through the 19th century, with a brief account of contemporary developments by Ottaviani. Mainly studies of particular works. References at ends of chapters. 120 documented plates. General bibliography by author: p. 209–217. Name index only.

897
Singer, Charles J. A short history of anatomy and physiology from the Greeks to Harvey. New York, Dover, 1957. 209 p.

Reprint of *The evolution of anatomy*, London, 1925, with minor changes.

898
Wegner, Richard N. Die Anatomenbildnis; seine Entwicklung im Zusammenhang mit der anatomischen Abbildung. Basel, Schwabe, 1939. 199 p.

Survey by periods, with emphasis on history of various types of prints. 105 documented illustrations (mainly portraits). List of anatomists, with biographies and portraits: p. 177–184; Bibliography: p. 185–190.

Cytology

Reviews

899★
International review of cytology. New York, 1, 1952– . International Society for Cell Biology.

Annual. Reviews with bibliographies.

Histories

900
Baker, John R. The cell-theory: a restatement, history, and critique. Pt. 1–5. In Quarterly journal of microscopical science 89:103–25, 1948; 90:87–108, 1949; 93: 157–90, 1952; 94:407–40, 1953; 96:449–81, 1955.

Review of origin and development of cell theory from 17th century. Extensive references.

901
Hughes, Arthur. A history of cytology. London, Abelard-Schuman, 1959. 158 p.

Traces development of scientific knowledge about structure and function of cells, from 17th century. List of references at end of each chapter.

902
Keilin, David. The history of cell respiration and cytochrome. Cambridge, Univ. Press, 1966. 416 p.

Survey to 1884, detailed account of scientific developments thereafter. Bibliography (references): p. 360–399.

Congenital Anomalies and other Abnormalities

Indexes and Abstracts

902.1
Birth defects; abstracts of selected articles. New York, 1, 1964– . National Foundation.

Monthly. 1966 contains 1020 abstracts selected from over 2600 journals. Random arrangement. No indexes.

Supersedes no. 902.

903
Current literature — congenital anomalies. New York, 1–3, 1960–62. National Foundation.

Monthly. About 1500 abstracts a year from approximately 2200 journals. Quarterly subject indexes. Superseded by no. 902.1.

Directories

903.1
Directory of birth defects centers. Clinical research centers supported by National Headquarters; treatment centers and evaluation centers supported by local chapters. 5 ed. New York, National Foundation, 1966. 1 v.

Arranged by state.

Histories

904
Caffaratto, Tirsi M. I mostri umani: fan-

tasie d'altri tempi e realtà attuali. Torino, Edizioni Vitalità, 1965. 232 p.

From antiquity to the present. 166 bibliographical citations in text, additional references, 16th–20th centuries, p. 217–232. Many illustrations. No index.

904.1
Holländer, Eugen. Wunder, Wundergeburt und Wundergestalt in Einblattdrucken des fünfzehnten bis achtzehnten Jahrhunderts. Kulturhistorische Studie. Stuttgart, Enke, 1921. 373 p.

Preliminary chapter on classical antecedents, followed by studies of special topics as presented in the broadsides. 202 illustrations and facsimiles. No index.

Histology

Indexes and Abstracts

904.2
Bibliographia histochemica. In Acta histochemica, Jena, 7(5/8) 1959– .

Irregular. 19,643 references through 1966.

905
Current tissue culture literature; a key to the world periodicals and abstract indexes. New York, 1965– .

3 times a year. Includes proceedings of societies, congresses, and theses.

By M. R. Murray and G. Kopech. Author and subject index in each issue.

905.1
Histochemical titles from current literature, 1952– . In Journal of histochemistry and cytochemistry, 1, 1953– .

Irregular. Approximately 500 entries in 1966. Arranged by author under journal title. No indexes.

906
Tissue culture bibliography. Bethesda, 1, 1960– . Microbiological Associates.

Bimonthly. About 1200 references a year. Author arrangement. No indexes.

Reviews

907
International review of connective tissue research. New York, 1, 1963– .

Annual. Critical appraisals with bibliographies.

Bibliographies

908
Murray, Margaret R., and Kopech, Gertrude. A bibliography of the research in tissue culture, 1884 to 1950; an index to the literature of the living cell cultivated in vitro. New York, Academic Press, 1953. 2 v. (1741 p.) Supplementary author list, 1950–[53] 11 p.

15,000 references to articles, books, and chapters in books arranged by author and subject in one alphabet. Articles selected from 1035 journals. Sponsored by the Tissue Culture Association.

908.1
Velez Boza, Fermin. Bibliografia venezolana de histologia, embriologia y genetica. Caracas, Universidad Central de Venezuela, 1961. 259 p.

Author arrangement under principal subjects.

Dictionaries

908.2
China (People's Republic) Wei shêng pu [Ministry of Health] Tsu chih hsüeh p'ei t'ai hsüeh ming tz'ŭ ho pien [Glossary of terms in histology and embryology] Shanghai, 1953. 65 p.

Chinese-English, English-Chinese.

ANTHROPOLOGY

Reviews

909
Biennial review of anthropology. Stanford, Calif., Stanford University Press, 1959– .

Bibliographies

910
Mandelbaum, David G. [et al.], ed. Resources for the teaching of anthropology, including basic list of books and periodicals for college libraries. Compiled by Rexford S. Beckham. Berkeley, University of California Press, 1963. 316 p.

Bibliography contains 1714 items.

911
Pearsall, Marion. Medical behavioral science; a selected bibliography of cultural

anthropology, social psychology, and sociology in medicine. Lexington, University of Kentucky, 1963. 134 p.

3064 references. Includes books, chapters in books, theses, reports. English language material, except for a few Spanish references.

BIOLOGY

Indexes and Abstracts

Current

Special attention is called to *Biological abstracts* (no. 916) one of the essential tools for comprehensive medical reference work.

912

Abstracts of Bulgarian Scientific Literature. Biology and Biochemistry. Sofia, 1, 1963– . Bulgarian Academy of Sciences. Centre of Scientific Information and Documentation.

Semiannual. About 500 abstracts a year from Bulgarian journals.

Supersedes in part *Abstracts of Bulgarian scientific literature. Biology and medicine.*

913 (not used)

914

Berichte über die wissenchaftliche Biologie. (Berichte über die gesamte Biologie. Abt. A) Berlin, 1, 1926– .

Currently more than 20 volumes a year, each volume in 3 issues. A separately published index covers several volumes. A recent volume listed in excess of 1300 references, most with abstracts. Includes books. Time lag (1964) rarely less than 8 months. Covers literature on human microbiology as well as plant and animal morphology, physiology, etc.

Subtitle: Referierendes Organ der deutschen botanischen Gesellschaft (from v. 70, 1950–51) und der deutschen zoologischen Gesellschaft (from v. 94, 1955). See also no. 921.

915

Bibliographia biotheoretica. Leiden, 1, 1925/29– . (Leiden. Universiteit. Jan van der Hoeven Stichting voor Theoretische Biologie van Dier en Mensch. Geschriften. Series C)

Irregular. Includes behavioral sciences. Lists books, chapters in books, congresses, etc. No annual indexes.

1925/29 published in 1938.

916

Biological abstracts. Philadelphia, 1, 1926/27– .

Currently semimonthly. 120,102 entries in 1966 most with abstracts. Covers basic biological sciences from agronomy to zoology, and medicine selectively, but frequently in depth. Coverage also includes the behavioral sciences. Minimum time lag for 1966, 3 months, but some entries as much as 2 years delayed.

Semimonthly keyword index entitled *B.A.S.I.C.*, v. 36 (20) Oct. 15, 1961– . Published as a separate v. 45, 1964– . Currently each issue of *B.A.* has Author, Biosystematic, and CROSS index, the latter corresponding to titles of sections and subsections. All indexes cumulated annually.

v. 1–3, 1926/27–29 irregular; 4–12, 1930–38, 9–11 issues a year including indexes; 13–23 monthly, except bimonthly June-Sept.; v. 24–33 (2) 1950–1959 (Feb) monthly; 33(3) – 34(5) Feb. 12–Dec. 3, 1959, tri-weekly; v. 35, 1960– semimonthly.

Subtitles: v. 1–28, 1926/27–1954, A comprehensive abstracting and indexing journal of the world's literature in theoretical and applied biology, exclusive of clinical medicine; v. 1–3, 1926/27–1929, In its departments dealing with theoretical and applied bacteriology and botany the journal represents a continuation of Abstracts of bacteriology [no. 1541] and Botanical abstracts [no. 966]

Published under the auspices of, or sponsored by, the Union of American Biological Societies. v. 1–22, 1926/27–1948.

Absorbed no. 966 and no. 1541.

For list of periodicals indexed see no. 944.

A condensed history of Biological abstracts B. A. 30(7): 1805–21, 1956.

917 (not used)

918

International abstracts of biological sciences; a comprehensive survey of the world literature. London, 1, 1954– . Physiological Society, the Biochemical Society, etc.

Monthly. 4 volumes a year. v. 41 (1966) listed in excess of 8000 entries, most with abstracts. Abstracts more than 83 journals fully and about 400 selectively. Of the total number of journals abstracted about 275 are *Index medicus* titles. Each issue includes a list of titles from reviews, symposia, and society proceedings. Quarterly subject and author indexes.

Attempts to cover the more important papers in experimental biology, with emphasis on preclinical sciences, including pharmacology, animal behavior, and odontology. Applications of biology to clinical medicine included insofar as they underlie the development of fundamental research.

v. 1–3, 1954–56, as *British abstracts of medical sciences*. Continues no. 27.

919
Japan science review: Biological sciences. Tokyo, 1, 1952– . Zoological Society of Japan, etc.

Annual. In 2 [parts] Title list of papers on biological sciences; Abstracts of papers in biological sciences (selective abstracts of the title list) v. 9, 1958 listed 2422 papers and contained 388 abstracts in English from the Japanese literature.

Includes list of leading biological societies in Japan.

919.1
Science abstracts of China. Biological sciences. Chung kuo k'o hsuch wen chai. Sheng wu k'o hsueh. Peking, 1, 1958– . Institute of Scientific and Technical Information of China.

Bimonthly. 500 English abstracts from the Chinese literature through v. 2, no. 4, 1964. No indexes.

Noncurrent

920
Bibliografia italiana. Biologia. Roma, 1928–43. Consiglio Nazionale delle Ricerche.

1941 contained 4031 entries, most with abstracts. Includes books.

1928 as *Bibliografia scientifico-tecnica italiana. Gruppo 7. Biologia-medicina*; 1929–31, *Gruppo A. Scienze matematiche, fisiche e biologiche, geografia*; 1932–40, *Gruppo A bis. Biologia.*

920.1
Bioresearch titles, reporting the world's research literature in the life sciences. Philadelphia, BioSciences Information Service of Biological Abstracts, 1965–66.

Monthly. Approximately 5000 references each issue. Indexes articles not abstracted in no. 916, with the same subject coverage. Minimum time lag 2 months, but many entries 2–3 years old.

In 3 sections: Subject index (keyword), Bibliography (references arranged alphabetically by journal title) and Author index. No annual indexes. No abstracts.

920.2
Current titles from biological journals; a monthly register of selected tables of contents. Chicago, v. 1, no. 1–3, 1937.

Monthly. No. 3 listed 134 journals.

921
Jahresbericht über die wissenschaftliche Biologie, zugleich bibliographisches Jahresregister der Berichte über die wissenschaftliche Biologie. Berlin, 1–6, 1926–31.

In 1928, 1640 periodicals indexed (200 American).

Cumulates references of no. 914.

921.1
Zentralblatt für allgemeine und experimentelle Biologie. Leipzig, 1–2, 1910/11–11/12.

v. 2, 1787 entries, most with abstracts. Indexes books, theses, reports, proceedings of societies. Includes material on clinical medicine. Abstracts in German, English or French.

Reviews

922
Advances in marine biology. New York, Academic Press, 1, 1963– .

922.1
Année biologique. Comptes rendus annuels des travaux de biologie générale. Paris, 1, 1895– . Fédération Française des Sociétés de Sciences Naturelles.

Bimonthly. Since May 1952 review articles only. Includes book reviews.

923
Biological reviews of the Cambridge Philosophical Society. Cambridge, Eng., 1, 1923– .

Quarterly. Through 1964, 570 reviews from 27 countries.

v. 1 as *Proceedings of the Cambridge Philosophical Society biological sciences*; v. 2–9 as *Biological reviews and biological proceedings of the Cambridge Philosophical Society*. Cumulative index for every ten volumes.

924
Ergebnisse der Biologie. Berlin, 1, 1926– .

Annual. Review articles in English, French, and German with bibliographies. Suspended 1944–57.

925
Quarterly review of biology. Stony Brook, New York, etc., 1, 1926– . Stony Brook Foundation, Inc.

Each issue contains extensive book review section covering the basic sciences.

1957–65 published by the American Institute of Biological Sciences.

926
Seibutsu kagaku saikin no shinpo [Recent advances in biology] Tokyo, 1, 1956– .

927
Survey of biological progress. New York, Academic Press, 1, 1949– .

4 v. since 1949. Reviews with bibliographies.

928
Viewpoints in biology. London, 1, 1962– .

Reviews with bibliographies.

Bibliographies

929
Nikitin, Vladimir N. Otechestvennye raboty po vozrastnoĭ fiziologiĭ, biokhimii i morfologii; istoricheskiĭ ocherk i bibliografiia [National works on physiology of growth, biochemistry and morphology; a historical essay and bibliography] Khar'kov, Izd-vo Khar'kovskogo universiteta, 1958. 200 p.

Bibliography: p. 41–200. Over 3000 references. Includes books. Covers period 1761–1956. Author arrangement. No subject index.

Manuals

930
Levin, V. L. Spravochnoe posobie po bibliografii dlia biologov [A reference book of bibliography for biologists] Moskva-Leningrad, Izd-vo Akademii nauk SSSR, 1960. 406 p.

Description of selected domestic and foreign bibliographic tools, giving scope and evaluation. Foreign titles are listed in the original language. Emphasis is given to the organization of Soviet bibliographic services and to Soviet publications.

Monographs

Nos. 931, 932, and 934 contain quantitative data on all aspects of biology. Data is comparative, giving, for example, weights of organs in man and a number of animals, enzymes in urine, etc.

931★★
Federation of American Societies for Experimental Biology. Committee on Biological Handbooks. Biology data book. Washington, 1964. 633 p.

General data derived in part from the other *Handbooks*. Supplements and supersedes in part no. 934.

931.1
——. ——. Environmental biology. Comp. and ed. by Philip L. Altman and Dorothy S. Dittmer. Bethesda, 1966. 694 p.

Includes tolerance data (temperature extremes, acceleration, etc.), physiological responses to atmospheric pressure, air pollutants, etc.

932
——. ——. Growth, including reproduction and morphological development. Comp. and ed. by Philip L. Altman and Dorothy S. Dittmer. Washington, 1962. 608 p.

Contains verifiable data collected from the world literature, together with references, on various aspects of normal growth.

933
Gray, Peter, ed. The encyclopedia of the biological sciences. London, Reinhold, 1961. 1119 p.

Intended to provide succinct information for biologists in those fields in which they are not themselves experts. Each article has list of references. Contains personal names.

934
National Research Council. Handbook of

biological data. Ed. by William S. Spector. Philadelphia, Saunders, 1956.

Tables of quantitative data with references given at end of each table.

935
Tabulae biologicae. The Hague, 1, 1925– .

Biological and physiological data similar to no. 931 and 934. Some volumes constitute monographs in a special field.

Cumulative indexes for v. 1–10, 11–20.

Dictionaries

936
Abercrombie, Michael, et al. A dictionary of biology. 5 ed. Baltimore, Penguin, 1966. 283 p. (Penguin reference books)

2000 terms. No biographies. [1 ed.] 1951.

937
Artschwager, Ernst. Dictionary of biological equivalents; German-English. Baltimore, Williams and Wilkins, 1932. 239 p.

937.1
Genzel, Peter. Die Lebensfunktionen der Menschen und Säugetiere im Spiegel der englischen Sprache. Halle, Niemeyer, 1959. 351 p.

Comparative terms for human and animal bodily structure and function. Examples from N.E.D. and literature. Includes slang.

938★★
Henderson, Isabella F., and Henderson, W. D. A dictionary of biological terms; pronunciations, derivation, and definition of terms in biology, botany, zoology, anatomy, cytology, genetics, embryology, physiology. 8 ed. By John H. Kenneth. Edinburgh, Oliver and Boyd, 1963. 640 p.

939
Husson, Roger. Glossaire de biologie animale. Paris, Gauthier-Villars, 1964. 280 p.

940
Jaeger, Edmund C. A source-book of biological names and terms. 3 ed. Springfield, Ill., Thomas, 1962. 360 p.

About 15,000 elements with origins and meanings. Brief biographies of persons commemorated in botanical and zoological generic names.

941
——. The biologist's handbook of pronunciations. Springfield, Ill., Thomas, 1960. 317 p.

Some 9,000 scientific terms.

942
Russian-English biological dictionary. Comp. by C. Dumbleton. Edinburgh, Oliver & Boyd, 1964. 512 p.

Directories

943
Hirsch, Gottwalt C., ed. Index biologorum; investigatores, laboratoria, periodica. Berlin, Springer, 1928. 545 p.

Pt. 1, lists biologists with brief professional notes. Pt. 2, lists laboratories and biologic institutions by subject, then by city. Includes a list of biologic journals.

Periodicals

944★
Biological abstracts. List of serials with word abbreviations. In Biological abstracts 12(7), Oct. 1938–

1966 lists 6,876 serials published in 91 countries and territories. Includes institutional annual reports, review annuals, reports of periodically scheduled conferences, congresses and symposia, and numbered unclassified reports of research supported or conducted by various U. S. government agencies.

Irregular through 1944; 1945–58, complete lists or supplements published annually in the May issue; 1960 in Oct. 15 issue; 1962, May 1 issue; 1963 and 1964 in July 1 issue; 1965-in November 1, issue.

Title varies.

Some complete lists, or supplements published as separates.

See also no. 944.1

944.1
U.S. Library of Congress. Science Division. Biological sciences serial publications, a world list, 1950–1954. Philadelphia, Biological Abstracts, 1955. 269 p.

Includes annual and other reports of governmental and private institutes. Geographic index.

Titles abstracted in *Biological abstracts* indicated.

Histories

945
Bodenheimer, Friedrich S. The history of biology; an introduction. London, Dawson, 1958. 465 p.

Pt. 1, methodology and relationships to general culture; pt. 2, a short factual history; pt. 3 (p. 147–457), extracts from sources, in English translation, with brief notes on the authors and bibliographical references. Intended as an aid to teaching the history of science.

946
Dawes, Ben. A hundred years of biology. London, Duckworth, 1952. 429 p.

Covers 1850–1950. Chapters on protoplasm and cell, reproduction, development, growth, heredity, taxonomy, functional problems, receptors and effectors, nervous system and coordination, behavior, evolution, parasites and parasitic diseases, antibiotics, research institutes. Bibliography (by chapter): p. 385–418.

947
Callot, Émile. La renaissance des sciences de la vie au XVIe siècle. Paris, Presses universitaires de France, 1951. 204 p.

Sections on methodology, morphology, anatomy, physiology, taxonomy. Bibliography: p. 197–201. No index.

948
Greene, John C. The death of Adam; evolution and its impact on western thought. Ames, Iowa State University Press, 1959. 388 p.

Traces the rise of evolutionary concepts and the decline of traditional views of nature as shown in all the sciences from Newton to Darwin, from the viewpoint of an intellectual historian. References: p. 341–377.

949
Guyénot, Émile. L'évolution de la pensée scientifique: les sciences de la vie aux XVIIe et XVIIIe siècles; l'idée d'évolution. Paris, Michel, 1941. 462 p. (L'Evolution de l'humanité, synthèse collective, 3. sect., 68)

Sections cover classification, anatomy and physiology, generation, evolution. Footnotes references and brief bibliography. Reprinted 1957.

950
Nordenskiöld, Erik. The history of biology: a survey. Tr. by Leonard B. Eyre. New York, Knopf, 1928. 629 p.

Comprehensive, detailed. Emphasis on 19th and 20th centuries (p. 299–616).

Bibliography (by chapter): p. 617–629. Reprinted New York, Tudor, 1935 and 1960; Swedish original, *Biologins historia*, 3 v., 1920–24.

951
Rádl, Emanuel. The history of biological theories. Tr. by E. J. Hatfield. London, Milford, 1930. 408 p.

Covers 19th century, primarily on development and implications of Darwinism. Abridged from pt. 2 of *Geschichte der biologischen Theorien seit dem Ende des siebzehnten Jahrhunderts*, Leipzig, 1902–09, 2 v. Rev. ed. of pt. 1, *Geschichte der biologischen Theorien in der Neuzeit*, Leipzig, 1913, covers Renaissance also.

952
Ritterbush, Philip C. Overtures to biology: the speculations of eighteenth-century naturalists. New Haven, Yale University Press, 1964. 287 p.

Interpretive study of development of speculative concepts, especially of the significance of electricity in nature and of botanical and zoological analogy. Bibliography: p. 211–273.

953
Roger, Jacques. Les sciences de la vie dans la pensée française du XVIIIe siècle. La génération des animaux de Descartes à l'Encyclopédie. Paris, Colin, 1963. 842 p.

First 160 p. cover 1600–1670. Bibliography (877 items): p. 781–814. Name index only.

954
Singer, Charles J. A history of biology to about the year 1900; a general introduction to the study of living things. 3 ed. London, Abelard-Schuman, 1959. 580 p. (The Life of science library, 38)

For student and general reader; not documented. 1 ed., Oxford, 1931, had title *A short history of biology* (American ed.: *The story of living things*).

955
Sirks, Marius J. and Zirkle, Conway. The evolution of biology. New York, Ronald, 1964. 376 p.

Survey from prehistory to present, including early Oriental and Arabic contributions, with especially full treatment of the period prior to the Renaissance. Bibliography: p. 350–365.

956
Zimmermann, Walter. Evolution. Die Geschichte ihrer Probleme und Erkenntnisse. Freiburg, Alber, 1953. 623 p.

Discusses works of leading authors in relation to central problems of biological evolution, primarily before Darwin. References: p. 557–579; bibliography: p. 580–606.

957
Zuckerman, Sir Solly, ed. Classics in biology. A course of selected reading by authorities. Introductory reading guide. New York, Philosophical Library, 1960. 351 p.

Includes bibliography.

BIOPHYSICS

Indexes and Abstracts

958
Medical electronics and communications abstracts. Brentwood, Essex, Eng., Multiscience Publishing Co., 1, 1966– .

Quarterly. Abstracts. Covers all aspects of instrumentation in biomedical research, diagnosis and practice. Includes some reports. Indexes a number of nonmedical journals.

Reviews

959
Advances in biological and medical physics. New York, Academic Press, 1, 1948– .

Irregular.

960
Biomedical sciences instrumentation. Pittsburgh, 1, 1963– . Instrument Society of America.

Proceedings of the National Biomedical Sciences Instrumentation Symposium.

961
Progress in biophysics and molecular biology. New York, Pergamon, 1, 1950– .

Annual. v. 1–12, 1950–62, as *Progress in biophysics and biophysical chemistry.*

Bibliographies

962
Rockefeller Institute for Medical Research. Medical Electronics Center. Bibliography of medical electronics. New York, Professional Group on Medical Electronics, 1958. 91 p. Supplement 1, 1959– .

Through Supplement 2 (1960) 7599 references. Includes books. Covers some nonmedical sources.

Directories

963
Bioelectronics directory. Fort Worth, 1, 1961– . Institute of Behavioral Research, Texas Christian University.

2 ed., 1963, lists 1280 names from the United States and 25 other countries. Data include name, title, affiliation, location, and current research interests. Geographic index.

1. ed. issued as *Survey of bioelectronic approaches to the study of behavior*, report no. 1; 2 ed. as *Bioelectronics report*, no. 3.

BOTANY AND AGRICULTURE

Indexes and Abstracts

Current

964
Bibliography of agriculture. Washington, 1, 1942– . National Agricultural Library.

Monthly. "Index to the literature of agriculture and the allied sciences received in the National Agricultural Library. Publications from any country are indexed, provided they are in one of the languages of western Europe or in Russian or have summaries or abstracts in one of those languages." Approximately 100,000 entries in 1966. Last issue of each volume is subject and cumulative author index. Each issue includes listings of translations, new periodicals and serials, and checklists of publications of the U. S. Department of Agriculture, State Agricultural Experiment Stations, and State Agricultural Extension Services. The 1964 annual list of serials indexed includes 8254 titles.

For list of periodicals indexed see no. 983.

965
Biological and agricultural index. New York, 1, 1916– .

Monthly except September. About 40,000 references a year from English language literature. Indexes 146 periodicals, 30 of which are *Index Medicus* titles. v. 1–49, 1916–63, as *Agricultural index.* Cumulated annually without volume number and biennially with different voluming.

Noncurrent

966
Botanical abstracts. Baltimore, 1–15, 1918–26.

The series contains 60,071 abstracts.
United with no. 1541 to form no. 916.

Reviews

967
Advances in botanical research. London, Academic Press, 1, 1963– .

968 (Not used)

Bibliographies

969
Carnegie Institute of Technology, Pittsburgh. Rachel McMasters Miller Hunt Botanical Library. Catalog of botanical books in the collection. Comp. by Jane Quinby. Pittsburgh, Hunt Botanical Library, 1958–61. 2 v. in 3.

Extensive collection, described in detail. Covers printed books 1477–1800 and some earlier manuscripts. v. 2 comp. by Allan Stevenson.

970
Haller, Albrecht von. Bibliotheca botanica, qua scripta ad rem herbariam facientia a rerum initiis recensentur. Tiguri, Orell, Gessner, Fuessli, 1771–72. 2 v. (His Bibliothecae medicae, pars I) Index emendatus; perfecit J. Christian Bay. Bernae, Benteli, 1908. 57 p.

Arrangement by periods and by countries or schools; 1921 chapters devoted to individual authors or groups of authors. Lists works, editions (indicating special features), and translations, some with summaries and evaluations. Original indexes authors (about 6000 entries) and anonymous works (by subject, including academy publications, manuscripts, dictionaries, pharmacopeias, etc.). Bay's revised author index adds some 900 names, corrects 1200 errors, and improves entry for 200 names.

971
Jackson, Benjamin D. Guide to the literature of botany; being a classified selection of botanical works, including nearly 6000 titles not given in Pritzel's 'Thesaurus.' London, Longmans, Green, 1881. 626 p. (Index Society. Publications, no. 8)

In 123 classes, with large section of local floras and sections on botanical gardens and serial publications. Chronological subarrangement. Index of authors and of headings used. Reprinted New York, Hafner, 1964.

971.1
Merrill, Elmer D. and Walker, Egbert H. A bibliography of Eastern Asiatic botany . . . Sponsored by the Smithsonian Institution, Arnold Arboretum of Harvard University . . . [etc.] Jamaica Plain, Mass., Arnold Arboretum of Harvard University, 1938. 719 p.

Through 1936–37. Includes books. Mainly an author list, with works listed chronologically under author. Appendices include: Older Oriental works; Reference list of Oriental serials; Reference list of Oriental authors. Subject, systemic and geographic indexes.

972
Pritzel, Georg A. Thesaurus literaturae botanicae omnium gentium, inde a rerum botanicarum initiis ad nostra usque tempora, quindecim millia operum recensens. Rev. ed. Lipsiae, Brockhaus, 1872–[77] 576 p.

Pt. 1, author bibliography of 10,871 numbered works with brief biographical data; pt. 2, classified subject list, with chronological subarrangement. Indexes of variant names of authors and of editors, translators, etc., and of anonymous titles. Reprinted Milan, Görlich, 1950. 1 ed. Leipzig, 1847–51.

973
Utkin, L. A. [et al.] Bibliografiia po lekarstvennym rasteniiam; ukazatel' otechestvennoĭ literatury: Rukopisi XVII–XIX vv., pechatnye izdaniia 1732–1954 gg[Bibliography of medicinal plants; index of national literature: Manuscripts from 17th–20th century, printed works from 1732–1954] Moscow, Izd-vo Akademii nauk SSSR, 1957. 724 p.

Pt. 1, manuscripts, lists 431 items, giving location of each. Pt. 2, printed works, contains books and articles by about 5,000 authors in Russia (Soviet Union) from 1732 through 1954. Chronological arrangement with alphabetical subarrangement. Includes an index of Latin names for *genera* and a Russian-Latin index of names of plants and plant products.

Monographs

974
U. S. National Agricultural Library. Report of Task Force ABLE: Agricultural biological literature exploitation; a systems study of the National Agricultural Library and its users. Washington, 1965. 477 p.

Dictionaries

975
Berger, Franz. Synonyma-Lexikon der Heil- und Nutzpflanzen. Wien, Österreichische Apotheker-Verlags Ges., 1955. 1221 p.

976
Chopra, Ram N. [et al.]. Glossary of Indian medicinal plants. New Delhi, Council of Scientific and Industrial Research, 1956. 328 p.

Alphabetically arranged by scientific name, with some vernacular names given; information includes medicinal uses, references to the literature and goographical distribution of plants.

977
Davydov, N. N. Botanicheskiĭ slovar' russko-angliĭsko-nemetsko-frantsuzsko-latinskiĭ [Botanical dictionary. Russian-English-German-French-Latin] Moskva, Fizmatgiz, 1960. 335 p.

Contains about 6000 terms. Title page in Russian, English, German, French and Latin; preface in Russian, English, German and French.

978
Héraud, Auguste. Nouveau dictionnaire des plantes médicinales; description, habitat et culture, récolte, conservation, partie usitée, composition chimique, formes pharmaceutiques et doses, action physiologique, usages dans le traitement des maladies, memorial thérapeutique. 7 ed. Paris, Baillière, 1949. 657 p.

The "memorial thérapeutique" consists of an alphabetical list of diseases with designation of plants appropriate for treatment.

979
Schoen, Ernest. Nomina popularia plantarum medicinalium. Berne, Galenca, 1963. 202 p.

Latin, French, and German terms in parallel columns. Substantial index arranged alphabetically.

980
Strugger, Siegfried. Biologie I (Botanik). Frankfurt a. M., Fischer, 1965. 349 p. (Das Fischer Lexikon, 27).

First published 1962.

981
Wren, R. C. Potter's New cyclopaedia of botanical drugs and preparations. Re-ed. and enl. by R. W. Wren. London, Isaac Pitman & Sons for Potter & Clarke, 1956. 400 p.

Both scientific and vernacular names given; data include description, medicinal use and preparations. Illustrated.

Nomenclature

982
Lanjouw, Joseph [et al.] International Code of Botanical Nomenclature. Utrecht, International Bureau for Plant Taxonomy and Nomenclature, 1956. 338 p. (Regnum vegetabile; a series of handbooks for the use of plant taxonomists and plant geographers. v. 8)

Provides rules and regulations for the nomenclature of plants including fungi adopted by the Eighth International Botanical Congress, Paris, July 1954. Supersedes the rules of earlier congresses, 1867–1952. Title pages and text in English, French, German, and Spanish.

Referred to as the "Paris Code".

Directories

982.1
International Association of Agricultural Librarians and Documentalists. World directory of agricultural libraries and documentation centers. Ed. by D. H. Boalch. Harpenden, Herts, 1960. 280 p.

Geographical arrangement. Includes veterinary medicine, food and nutrition. Gives date founded, number of volumes, number of current periodicals received, publications, staff, specialization, when known. Data from 1956–58 or earlier. Polyglot subject index.

Periodicals

983
U. S. National Agricultural Library. Serial publications indexed in Bibliography of Agriculture. Washington, 1963. 163 p. (Library list no. 75).

Alphabetical list of 7,186 serials.

Histories

984
Arber, Agnes R. Herbals; their origin and evolution. A chapter in the history of botany, 1470–1670. 2 ed. Cambridge, University Press, 1938. 325 p.

Includes chronologic list of principal herbals, 1470–1670, p. 271–285; "works consulted": p. 286–303.

985
Blunt, Wilfrid. The art of botanical illustration. 3 ed. London, Collins, 1955. 304 p.

General survey of the development from antiquity. Bibliography (secondary works): p. 287–294.

986
Davy de Virville, Adrien [et al.] Histoire de la botanique en France. Paris, Société d'édition d'enseignement supérieur, 1954. 392 p.

Includes concise sketches of leading authors with bibliographical accounts of their works. Name index only.

987
Fischer, Hermann. Mittelalterliche Pflanzenkunde. München, Verlag der Münchner Drucke, 1929. 326 p.

Particularly useful for its table of synonyms and indexes of plant names.

988
Humphrey, Harry B. Makers of North American botany. New York, Ronald, 1961. 265 p. (Chronica botanica, 21)

Sketches of 121 botanists of the United States and Canada. Biographical references for each. No subject index.

989
Langkavel, Bernhard A. Botanik der spaeteren Griechen vom dritten bis dreizehnten Jahrhundert. Berlin, Berggold, 1866. xxiv, 207 p.

Systematically arranged, with index of Latin and Greek names. Citations under each species to original sources and secondary works and to variant names. Sources listed, p. xii–xxiv. Reprinted Amsterdam, Hakkert, 1964.

990
New York. Botanical Garden. Library. Biographical notes upon botanists. Comp. by John Hendley Barnhart. Boston, Hall, 1965. 3 v.

Reproduction of card file on some 45,000 botanists, past and present, maintained in New York Botanical Garden Library, with brief biographical data and references.

991
Nissen, Claus, Die botanische Buchillustration; ihre Geschichte und Bibliographie. Stuttgart, Hiersemann, 1951. 2 v.

v. 1, history, from antiquity; extensive footnote references; general bibliography: p. 255–264; v. 2, 2387 author or title entries, with biographic references, other notes; indexes of titles, artists, plants, countries, authors.

992
Reed, Howard S. A short history of the plant sciences. Waltham, Mass., Chronica Botanica, 1942. 320 p. (A new series of plant science books, v. 7)

Chronological survey through the 18th century, followed by chapters on selected, highly specialized areas during 19th and 20th centuries. Fields which the author considered adequately treated elsewhere are omitted. References, mainly secondary, at ends of chapters.

993
Rohde, Eleanour S. The old English herbals. London, Longmans, Green, 1922. 243 p.

Detailed descriptions of early herbals; also discusses manuscript recipe books. Chronological bibliographies (manuscript and printed English herbals, chief foreign printed herbals): p. 189–235.

CHEMISTRY AND BIOCHEMISTRY

Indexes and Abstracts

Current

Of the items listed below, no. 996 is of special importance; one of the most comprehensive specialized indexes published, it will be the tool of choice for literature searches in this field.

994
Analytical abstracts. Cambridge, Eng., 1, 1954– . Society of Analytical Chemistry.

Monthly. 5835 abstracts in 1964 covering all branches of analytical chemistry.

995
Bibliography of reviews in chemistry. Washington, 1–5, 1958–63. American Chemical Society.

Annual. Compilation of abstracts of review articles appearing in *Chemical abstracts*.

v. 1–4 as *Bibliography of chemical reviews*.

996★
Chemical abstracts; key to the world's chemical literature. Easton, Pa., 1, 1907– . American Chemical Society.

Biweekly. About 165,000 abstracts in 1964. Minimum time lag (1965) 2 months. Each issue has keyword, author, and numerical patent indexes. Cumulative indexes every five years now instead of the former ten-year cumulations.

Annual author, numerical patent, formula and subject indexes.

Collective formula index 1920–1946; Collective patent number index 1907–1936.

For list of periodicals abstracted see no. 1080.

Supersedes no. 1010.

997
Chemical-biological activities; an index to current literature on the biological activity of organic compounds. Easton, Pa., 1, 1965– . American Chemical Society.

Biweekly. In four sections: digest section (journals listed alphabetically by title, with title and author of pertinent articles and digest of important research results following under journal title); keywork-in-context index; molecular formula index; author index. Approximately 300 journals covered.

"Biological" is exclusive of botanical kingdom.

998
Chemical titles; current author and keyword indexes from selected journals. Washington, 1, 1961– . American Chemical Society.

Biweekly. About 75,000 references a year from approximately 650 world journals. Each issue contains three parts: keyword index; bibliography, which is a listing of journal contents arranged alphabetically by journal title; and author index.

999
Chemisches Zentralblatt. Berlin, etc., 1, 1830– . Im Auftrage der Deutschen Akademie der Wissenschaften zu Berlin, der Chemischen Gesellschaft in der DDR, etc.

Weekly. Currently in excess of 100,000 abstracts a year. Each issue has author and patent indexes. Annual author, subject, patent and formula indexes. Also quinquennial indexes (since 1925). Said to give more complete coverage of the pre-1930 literature than 996. Minimum time lag (1963) about 6 months, though many entries are considerably older.

v. 1–20, 1830–49, as *Pharmaceutisches Central-Blatt*; v. 21–26, 1850–55, as *Chemisch-Pharmaceutisches Central-Blatt*.

1856–86 had subtitle: Repertorium für reine, pharmaceutische, physiologische und technische Chemie; 1887–1963: Vollständiges Repertorium für alle Zweige der reinen und angewandten Chemie.

1000
Current chemical papers. London, 1954– . Chemical Society.

Monthly. Lists references from a maximum of 262 periodical titles. Minimum time lag (1966) zero months.

1001
Gas chromatography abstracts. London, Butterworths, 1958– .

1963 contains 1051 abstracts. Includes books, pamphlets.

1002
Howell, M. Gertrude, ed. Formula index to NMR literature data. New York, Plenum Press, 1–2, 1965–66.

v. 1, references through 1960; v. 2, references for 1961–62.

1003
Index chemicus. Philadelphia, 1, 1960– .

Semimonthly. Contains some 100,000 abstracts a year in graphic form of newly synthesized chemical compounds. Each issue has author, molecular formula, and journal indexes. Indexes cumulated three times a year.

1004
Science abstracts of China. Chemistry and chemical technology. Chung kuo k'o hsueh wen chai. Hua hsueh yu hua kung. Peking, 1, 1963– Institute of Scientific and Technical Information of China.

Semi-annually. 235 English abstracts from the Chinese literature through v. 2, no. 2, 1964. No author index.

Noncurrent

1005
Abstracts of chemical papers issued by the Bureau of Chemical Abstracts. A. Pure chemistry. In Journal of the Chemical Society, London, 24–128, 1871–1925.

Later volumes include some patents and an occasional thesis.

v. 24–32, 1871–77, as *Journal of the Chemical Society containing papers read before the Society and abstracts of chemical papers published in other journals*; v. 34–62, 1878–92, *Journal of the Chemical Society . . . Abstracts*; v. 64–104, 1893–1913, pt. 1 as *Abstract of papers on organic chemistry*, pt. 2 as *Abstract of papers on physical, inorganic, mineralogical, physiological, agricultural and analytical chemistry*; v. 106–124, 1914–23, pt. 1 as *Abstracts of papers on organic, physiological and agricultural chemistry*, pt. 2 as *Abstracts of paper on physical, inorganic, mineralogical and analytical chemistry*; v. 126–128, 1924–25, pt. 1 as *Organic chemistry and biochemistry*, pt. 2 as *Physical, inorganic, mineralogical, and analytical chemistry.*

With v. 34, 1878, *Abstracts* published as separate volumes. With v. 34 two consecutive and continuing volume numbers assigned each year, one for the *Transactions* and a second for the *Abstracts*. With the exception of v. 37, 1880, the *Abstracts* bear even numbers.

Continued by no. 1007.

1006
Biophysikalisches Centralblatt (Centralblatt für gesamte Biologie, Abt. 2) Leipzig, 1–4, 1905–10.

Review articles and 1500 to 1800 abstracts per volume. Includes books.

Merged with *Biochemisches Zentralblatt* to form no. 1011.

1007
British chemical abstracts. A. Pure chemistry. London, 1926–37.

Monthly. Includes biochemistry. Author indexes. No annual indexes.

Issued by the Bureau of Chemical Abstracts representing the Chemical Society and the Society of Chemical Industry.

Continues 1005.

Continued as no. 27.

1008
Jahresbericht über die Fortschritte der Tier-Chemie oder der physiologischen, pathologischen und Immuno-Chemie und der Pharmakologie. Wien, 1–49, 1871–1919.

Abstracts, arranged by subject with a brief review.

v. 1–10, 1871, without *oder . . .*; v. 11–37, 1881–1907, *. . . oder physiologischen und pathologischen Chemie.*

v. 1–13, ed. by R. Maly; v. 14–15, R. Maly and R. Andreasch; v. 16–20, R. Andreasch; v. 21–30, M. V. Nencki and R. Andreasch; v. 31–43, R. Andreasch and K. Spiro.

General register for Jahrg. 1–10, 11–20, 21–30, 31–40.

Continued in nos. 2269 and 2270.

1009
Kharasch, Norman [et al.] Index to reviews, symposia volumes and monographs in organic chemistry for the period 1940–1960. New York, Pergamon Press, 1962. 345 p.

Pt. 1, reviews in journals and periodic publications; pt. 2, reviews in symposia, collective volumes and nonperiodical publications; pt. 3, monographs on organic chemistry, 1940–1960. Limited to French, German, and English language literature. Pt. 1, arranged alphabetically by journal title. Except for monographs, subarrangement of sections is by date.

1010
Review of American chemical research. Easton, Pa., 1–12, 1895–1906.

Abstracts, rather than review articles. Includes federal and state documents as well as journals.

v. 1–7, 1895–1901, in *Technology quarterly*, v. 8–14; v. 1–2 also issued separately; v. 3–12, 1897–1906, in *Journal of the American Chemical Society*, v. 19–28. v. 1–7 contributed by the Massachusetts Institute of Technology instructing staff. Superseded by no. 996.

1011
Zentralblatt für Biochemie und Biophysik. Berlin, etc., 1–23, 1902–21.

Abstracts of articles and books. v. 1–9 had occasional literature reviews.

v. 1–9, 1902–10, had subtitle: Vollständiges Sammelorgan für die Grenzgebiete der Medizin und Chemie; v. 10–23, 1910–21: mit Einschluss der theoretischen Immunitätsforschung.

Generalregisterband for v. 1–9 and v. 1–4 of no. 1006.

Continued by no. 2269.

Reviews

1012
Advances in analytical chemistry and instrumentation. New York, 1, 1960– .

1013
Advances in carbohydrate chemistry. New York, 1, 1945– .

Annual reviews with extensive bibliographies. Each volume has cumulative author and subject index for previous volumes.

1014
Advances in catalysis and related subjects. New York, Academic Press, 1, 1948– .

1015
Advances in chemical physics. New York, Interscience, 1, 1958– .

1016
Advances in clinical chemistry. New York, Academic Press, 1, 1958– .

1017
Advances in colloid sciences. New York, Interscience, 1–3, 1942–50.

1018
Advances in heterocyclic chemistry. New York, Academic Press, 1, 1963– .

2 volumes a year.

1019
Advances in inorganic chemistry and radiochemistry. New York, Academic Press, 1, 1959– .

1020
Advances in lipid research. New York, Academic Press, 1, 1963– .

1021
Advances in organic chemistry; methods and results. New York, Interscience, 1, 1960– .

Irregular.

1022
Advances in organometallic chemistry. New York, Academic Press, 1, 1964– .

1023
Advances in protein chemistry. New York, Academic Press, 1, 1944– .

Annual reviews with bibliographies.

1024 (Not used)

1025
Annual reports on the progress of chemistry. London, Chemical Society, 1, 1904– .

Reviews with bibliographies.

1026
Annual review of biochemical and allied research in India. Bangalore, Society of Biological Chemists, 1, 1930– .

v. 1–6, 1930–35, as *Biochemical and allied research in India.*

1027★★
Annual review of biochemistry. Palo Alto, 1, 1952– .

Annual reviews with bibliographies. Quinquennial cumulative indexes, both subject and author, in each volume. Decennial index last appeared in 1960.

1028
Chemical reviews. Baltimore, American Chemical Society, 1, 1924– .

Reviews with bibliographies.

1029
Chromatographic reviews; progress in chromatography, electrophoresis and related methods. Amsterdam, 1, 1959– .

Annual. Review articles with bibliographies. v. 1–5 contain reviews previously published in *Journal of Chromatography*; beginning with v. 6, the reviews consist entirely of previously unpublished material.

1030
Exposés annuels de biochimie médicale. Paris, 1, 1938– .

Review articles with bibliographies. Each volume contains cumulative author (with title) index of previous volumes.

1031
Fortschritte der Chemie organischer Naturstoffe. Progress in the chemistry of

organic natural products. Progrès dans la chimie des substances organiques naturelles. Wien, 1, 1938– .

Annual. Reviews in German, English, and French, with bibliographies.

1032
Methods of biochemical analysis. New York, Interscience, 1, 1954– .

Annual reviews with bibliographies. Cumulative indexes in each volume.

1033
Progress in inorganic chemistry. New York, Interscience, 1, 1959– .

1034
Progress in nucleic acid research. New York, Academic Press, 1, 1963– .

Irregular.

1035
Progress in organic chemistry. New York, Academic Press, 1, 1952– .

Irregular.

1036
Progress in physical organic chemistry. New York, Interscience, 1, 1963– .

1037
Progress in stereochemistry. Washington, Butterworths, 1, 1954– .

1038
Progress in the chemistry of fats and other lipids. New York, Academic Press, 1, 1952– .

Annual reviews. v. 5 devoted to advances in technology.

1039
Review of physical chemistry of Japan. Kyoto, 1, 1926– . Physico-Chemical Society of Japan.

Semiannual. Issued also in Japanese, 1926–45, with title *Butsuri kagaku no shinpo.*

Bibliographies

1040
Bolton, Henry C. A select bibliography of chemistry, 1492–1892. Washington, Smithsonian Institution, 1893. 1212 p. Suppl. 1, 1492–1897. 1899. 489 p. Suppl. 1, Sect. VIII, Academic dissertations, 1492–1898. 1901. 534 p. Suppl. 2, 1492–1902. 1904. 462 p.

A comprehensive checklist of books published in Europe and America. Sections on: bibliography; dictionaries; history and biography; chemistry, pure and applied; alchemy; periodicals; dissertations.

1041
Cincinnati. University. College of Medicine. Kettering Laboratory of Applied Physiology. Annotated bibliography: the occurrence and biological effects of fluorine compounds. v. 1. The inorganic compounds. Books 1–2. By Irene R. Campbell, Evelyn M. Widner, and Irene P. Kukainis. Cincinnati, 1958– . 1955 p.

8600 abstracts, 1798–1957, chronologically arranged within 16 major subject headings.

Earlier edition (1950–53) has title: *Classified bibliography of publications concerning fluorine and its compounds in relation to man, animals, and their environment including effects on plants.* Pt. 1, inorganic compounds; pt. 2, organic fluorine compounds.

1042
Henley, Alfred, ed. Electrophoresis bibliography. Comp. by Charles L. Schuettler. [2 ed.] Silver Spring, Md., Biochemical Instruments Division, American Instrument Co. [1955] 290 p.

1043
Kiev. Respublikanskaia nauchnaia meditsinskaia biblioteka. Komponenty krovi i krovozameniteli; bibliograficheskiĭ ukazatel' otechestvennoĭ literatury, 1948–1958 [Components of the blood and blood plasma substitutes; bibliographical index of national literature, 1948–1958] Kiev, 1961. 145 p.

Covers all medical literature except books. Contains 1296 references.

1044
Macek, Karel [et al.] Bibliography of paper chromatography 1957–1960 and survey of applications. Prague, Publishing House of the Czechoslovak Academy of Sciences, 1962. 706 p.

8292 references.

1044.1
Nakazawa, Ryōji. Bibliography of fermentation and biological chemistry. 11 v.

[Tokyo] Nippon Gakujutsu Shinkōkai, 1950–64.

From 1800 to 1940. Subject arrangement. Title also in Japanese.

1045
The nucleic acids: an annotated bibliography. Washington, etc., 1, 1962– . U. S. National Library of Medicine.

v. 2, 1963 contained 3451 numbered entries, arranged by author.

v. 1–v. 2, pt. 1, 1962–Jan–June 1963, published by Special Bibliographies. Loma Linda. Ed. R. S. Scharffenberg and R. E. Beltz.

v. 2, pt. 2, July-Dec. 1963, issued in 1966, published by the National Library of Medicine. Ed. R. E. Beltz.

v. 1–v. 2, pt. 1 as ... *an annotated bibliography of current literature.*

1046
Pierce, Charles M., comp. The detailed composition of feces, sweat, and urine: An annotated bibliography. Sunnyvale, Calif., Lockheed Missiles and Space Co., 1962. 210 p. ([Lockheed] Special bibliography, SB–62–56, March 1962)

598 selected references. Includes books and chapters in books.

1047
Signeur, Austin V. Guide to gas chromatography literature. New York, Plenum Press, 1964. 351 p.

7577 references. Includes titles of unpublished papers presented at various scientific meetings. Alphabetical author arrangement.

1048
U.S. Library of Congress. Aerospace Technology Division. CBE factors; an annotated bibliography. Washington, 1, 1962– . (Surveys of Soviet-Bloc scientific and technical literature. ATD report B–65–43)

Title: *Chemical-biological-environmental factors.*

Nos. 1–2 consisted of 301 partly annotated references covering aerosols, biological pathogens, chemical substances, etc. Coverage begins 1959.

1049
West, Clarence J., and Berolzheimer, D. D., comp. Bibliography of bibliographies on chemistry and chemical technology, 1900–24. Washington, 1925. 308 p. (National Research Council. Bulletin no. 50)

Includes biochemistry and some pharmacology.

Personal bibliographies: p. 304–08.

1050
——. ——. First supplement, 1924–28. Washington, 1929. 161 p. (National Research Council. Bulletin no. 71)

Personal bibliographies: p. 161.

1051
——. ——. Second supplement, 1929–31. Washington, 1932. 150 p. (National Research Council. Bulletin no. 86)

Personal bibliographies: p. 149–50.

Catalogs

1052
Duveen, Denis I. Bibliotheca alchemica et chemica; an annotated catalogue of printed books on alchemy, chemistry, and cognate subjects in the library of Denis I. Duveen. London, Weil, 1949. 669 p.

Lists by author some 2000 items, mainly 17th–19th centuries, with annotations and references. Reprinted London, Dawson's, 1965.

1053
——. The Duveen collection of alchemy & chemistry, supplementing the Bibliotheca alchemica et chemica. New York, Kraus, 1953. 98 p.

654 items. Includes section on balneology.

1054
Ferguson, John. Bibliotheca chemica. A catalogue of the alchemical, chemical and pharmaceutical books in the collection of the late James Young of Keely and Durris. Glasgow, Maclehose, 1906. 2 v.

Careful bibliographical descriptions with extensive contents notes, annotations, and copious references. Reprinted London, Holland Press, 1954.

1055
Glasgow. University. Library. Catalogue of Ferguson collection of books, mainly relating to alchemy, chemistry, witchcraft and gypsies. Glasgow, Maclehose, 1943. 2 v. (820 p.)

About 4900 items. Brief author entries, including many rare works.

1056
Pennsylvania. University. Edgar Fahs Smith Memorial Library. Catalog of the Edgar Fahs Smith memorial collection in the history of chemistry, University of Pennsylvania Library. Boston, Hall, 1960. 524 p.

Photographic reproduction of author and added entry catalog cards. No subject entries.

1057
Wisconsin. University. Library. Chemical, medical and pharmaceutical books printed before 1800 in the collections of the University . . . Libraries. Ed. by John Neu. Madison, University of Wisconsin Press, 1965. 280 p.

Author catalog of 4402 items, about 3000 of which are from the Duveen collection (no. 1052). Includes some author and title added entries, but no index.

Manuals

1058
American Chemical Society. Division of Chemical Literature. Searching the chemical literature. Based on papers presented by the Division of Chemical Literature and the Division of Chemical Education of the American Chemical Society at national meetings from 1947 to 1956. 2 ed. Washington, 1961. 326 p. (Advances in Chemistry Series, no. 30)

Extensive bibliographies.

1059
Bottle, R. T. Use of the chemical literature. London, Butterworths, 1962. 231 p.

Chapters on chemical periodicals, Beilstein etc.

1060
Crane, Evan J. [et al.]. A guide to the literature of chemistry. 2 ed. New York, Wiley, 1957. 397 p.

Sections on current journals classified according to subjects and under subjects by country; classified and annotated list of abstract journals; list of journals discontinued before 1910; American and Canadian libraries of interest to chemists, etc.

1061★
Dyson, G. Malcolm. A short guide to chemical literature. London, Longmans, Green, 1958. 157 p.

Essentially an annotated bibliography of the literature of chemistry.

1062★
Mellon, M. G. Chemical publications; their nature and use. 4 ed. New York, McGraw-Hill, 1965. 324 p.

1063
Van Luik, James [et al.] Searching the chemical and chemical engineering literature, with an analysis of 229 journals and handbooks. 2 ed. Lafayette, Ind., Purdue University, 1957. Various pagings.

A discussion of literature searching with detailed analysis of periodicals.

Dictionaries

1064
Bennett, Harry. Concise chemical and technical dictionary. 2 ed. New York, Chemical Publishing Company, 1962. 1039 p.

Some 5500 definitions covering new trademark products (including manufacturer), chemicals, and drugs.

1065
Callaham, Ludmilla I. Russian-English chemical and polytechnical dictionary. 2 ed. prepared with the assistance of E. B. Uvarov. New York, Wiley, 1962. 892 p.

Emphasis is on Soviet terminology, although little-used Russian words are frequently included for translation value; includes abbreviations.

1066
The condensed chemical dictionary. 6 ed. by Arthur and Elizabeth Rose. New York, Reinhold, 1961. 1256 p.

Concise encyclopedia of information on chemicals, drugs, raw materials, and brand or trade name products. Includes specifications for commercial products, fire and poison hazards, and shipping regulations.

1067
Granderye, Leon M. Dictionnaire de chimie. Paris, Dunod, 1962. 655 p.

Describes chemical products; includes formulas and tables. Selective.

1068★
Grant, J. Hackh's chemical dictionary. 4 ed. London, McGraw-Hill, 1964.

About 80,000 words are defined including most new words created during the last 18 years.

1069
Honig, J. M. [et al.] ed. The Van Nostrand chemist's dictionary. Princeton, Van Nostrand, 1962. 761 p.

More than 11,000 commonly used chemical terms defined.

1070
Hoseh, Mordecai, and Hoseh, Melanie L. Russian-English dictionary of chemistry and chemical technology. New York, Reinhold, 1964. 522 p.

1071
Hsu, Shan-hsiang, comp. Ying han hua hsueh hsin tzu tien. A modern English-Chinese chemical lexicon. Shanghai, Chung-Kuo-K'o-hsuĕh tu-shu, 1951. [China Science Corporation]. xiv. 1265 p.

Title page has: Compiled by Zai-Ziang Zee and Lan Hua Cheng (an alternative transliteration)

1072
Karpovich, Eugene A. Russian-English chemical dictionary: chemistry, physical chemistry, chemical engineering, materials, minerals, fuels, petroleum, food industry, pharmacology. 1 ed. New York, Technical Dictionaries Co., 1961. 352 p.

About 29,000 Russian entries.

1073
Neville, H. H. [et al.] A new German-English dictionary for chemists. London, Blackie, 1964. 330 p.

Contains about 40,500 terms.

1074
Patai, Saul. Glossary of organic chemistry, including physical organic chemistry. New York, Interscience, 1962. 227 p.

Written for nonspecialists in organic chemistry. Terms illustrated by equations and documented with references to literature.

1075
Snell, Foster D., and Snell, Cornelia T. Dictionary of commercial chemicals. 3 ed. Princeton, N. J., Van Nostrand, 1962. 714 p.

Information on the composition of commercial products. Appendix contains information about the U. S. Caustic Poison Act, the Food, Drug and Cosmetic Act, Federal Insecticide, Fungicide, and Rodenticide Act.

1076
Sobecka, Z. [et al.] ed. Dictionary of chemistry and chemical technology in four languages: English, German, Polish, Russian. Oxford, Pergamon Press, 1962. 724 p.

Nomenclature

1077
Cahn, Robert S. An introduction to chemical nomenclature. London, Butterworths, 1959. 96 p.

Uses the nomenclature accepted by the Chemical Society. Indicates main differences from American practice.

1078
International Union of Pure and Applied Chemistry. Nomenclature of applied chemistry. Definitive rules for Section A. Hydrocarbons; Section B. Fundamental heterocyclic systems . . . Definitive rules for nomenclature of steroids . . . Tentative rules for nomenclature in the Vitamin B12 field . . . London, Butterworths, 1958. 92 p.

1079
International Union of Pure and Applied Chemistry. Commission on Codification. Ciphering and punched card techniques. Rules for I. U. P. A. C. notation for organic compounds. London, Longmans, Green, 1961. 107 p.

1080
International Union of Pure and Applied Chemistry. Inorganic Chemistry Section. Nomenclature of inorganic chemistry; definitive rules . . . 1957 report of the Commission on the Nomenclature of Inorganic Chemistry. London, Butterworths, 1959. 93 p.

T. p. and text also in French.

1081
National Research Council. Chemical-

Biological Coordination Center. Key to the biology code; a manual for the use of the symbols of the code, for coding results, procedures, and conditions of tests for biological responses to chemicals. Ed. by Philip G. Seitner, George A. Livingston, and Ann S. Williams. Washington, 1960. 210 p. (NAS-NRC Publication 790K)

1082
Synthetic Organic Chemical Manufacturers Association. SOCMA handbook, commercial organic chemical names. Washington, American Chemical Society, 1965. Various pagings.

Directories

For Current listing of chemists in the United States see no. 2499.

1083
American Chemical Society. Committee on Professional Training. Directory of graduate research 1963; faculties, publications and doctoral theses in departments or divisions of chemistry, biochemistry and chemical engineering at United States universities. Washington, 1963. 655 p.

Lists university and department with members and full citation to publications. Includes brief biographical information.

1083.1
Adressbuch deutscher Chemiker. Weinheim, 1950/51– Gesellschaft Deutscher Chemiker.

Brief professional information. 1965/66 listed more than 15,000 chemists under name and place.

1084
Chemical who's who, 1956; biography in dictionary form of the leaders in chemical industry, research and education. 4 ed. Ed. by Winfield S. Downs. New York, Lewis Historical Publishing Company, 1956. 1267 p.

Biographies alphabetically arranged with geographic index. Mainly U. S.

1085
Laboratories in the chemical bio-sciences. 6 ed., 1957/58. Beloit, Wisc., Burns Compiling & Research Organization, 1957. 80 p.

Geographical arrangement; gives address, name of president or director, brief summary of activities.

1 ed., 1941. 1–5 ed. as *Directory of biological laboratories.*

Periodicals

1086★
American Chemical Society. Chemical abstracts list of periodicals, with key to library files, 1961. Washington, 1962. 397 p.

Alphabetical listing of over 7,000 journals scanned by the staff of *Chemical abstracts.* Gives frequency, volume number, publisher, and libraries subscribing.

Annual supplements 1962 (38 p.), 1963 (48 p.).

1087
Periodica chimica. Verzeichnis der im Chemischen Zentralblatt referierten Zeitschriften mit den entsprechenden genormten Titelabkürzungen. 2 ed. by Maxmilian Pflücke und Alice Hawelek. Berlin, Akademie Verlag, 1952. 411 p. Nachtrag, 1962. 245 p.

List of periodicals abstracted in *Chemisches Zentralblatt.* Many medical and biological science journals included. Information includes titles, abbreviations, title changes, mergers, suspensions, publishers and addresses. Transliterations given for non-Roman alphabet languages.

Histories

For guides to the extensive literature on the history of chemistry, see the recent surveys by Frick (no. 1090) and Ihde (no. 1091).

1088
Crosland, Maurice P. Historical studies in the language of chemistry. London, Heinemann, 1962. 406 p.

From alchemy through the 19th century, with emphasis on symbols and nomenclature. Bibliography (sources): p. 355–379.

1089
Farber, Eduard, ed. Great chemists. New York, Interscience, 1961. 1642 p.

Biographical sketches of about 115 chemists from ancient times to the present century, by 94 authors.

1090
Frick, Karl. Einführung in die alchimiegeschichtliche Literatur. In Sudhoffs Archiv für Geschichte der Medizin und der Naturwissenschaften 45:147–163, 1961.

Critical review of recent and older publications, with a classified bibliography of books, articles, and manuscript catalogs. Includes works on ancient Egyptian, Greek, and oriental alchemy.

1091
Ihde, Aaron J. The development of modern chemistry. New York, Harper & Row, 1964. 851 p.

Critical bibliography: p. 759–823.

1092
Partington, James R. A history of chemistry. London, Macmillan, 1961– .

Comprehensive history with extensive bibliographical data in text and footnotes. Organization mainly biographical within each period, with critical account of contributions of each author. To be in 4 v.

Enzymes

Reviews

1093
Advances in enzyme regulation. Oxford, Pergamon, 1, 1963– .

v. 1, Proceedings of a symposium on regulation of enzyme activity . . . held at Indiana University School of Medicine, Oct. 1–2, 1962.

1094★★
Advances in enzymology and related subjects of biochemistry. New York, 1, 1941– .

1095
De Long, Chester W. Enzymology in the USSR; a review of the literature. Washington, National Institutes of Health, 1960. 189 p. (Public Health Service. Publication no. 782).

References, 1935–1959. Includes list of institutes at which enzymological research is conducted with names of some associated personnel.

1096
Ergebnisse der Enzymforschung. Leipzig, 1, 1932–54.

Bibliographies

1097
Novokreshchenov, B. V. Sistema gialuronovaia kislota—gialuronidaza v biologii i meditsine; annotirovannyĭ bibliograficheskiĭ ukazatel' [System of hyaluronic acid—hyaluronidase in biology and medicine; annotated bibliographic index] Pod red. S. M. Rassudova. Vyp. 1. Chita, Chitinskiĭ institut epidemiologii, mikrobiologii i gigieny, 1961. 218 p.

Contains about 1300 alphabetically arranged entries, 1940–61, most with annotations or abstracts, covering the literature in Russian or in other languages of the Soviet Union.

Nomenclature

1098
Florkin, Marcel, and Stotz, Elmer H., ed. Comprehensive biochemistry. v. 13. 2 ed. Enzyme nomenclature. Amsterdam, Elsevier, 1965. 219 p.

Recommendations (1964) of the International Union of Biochemistry on the nomenclature and classification of enzymes, together with their units and the symbols of enzyme kinetics.

CIRCULATORY SYSTEM

Indexes and Abstracts

1099
Cardiovascular abstracts; selected from world literature. New York, 1, 1960– . American Heart Association.

Annual. About 500 abstracts a year from 88 journals; originally published in *Circulation*.

1100
Cardiovascular compendium. Philadelphia, 1, 1965– .

Abstracts arranged under alphabetically listed journal titles. In 1966 indexed 44 serials. No indexes.

1101
Cerebrovascular bibliography. Bethesda, Md., 1961– . Joint Council Subcommittee on Cerebrovascular Disease, National

Institute of Neurological Diseases and Blindness.

Quarterly. Consists of cerebrovascular and related listings in the *Index medicus*. Subject headings more detailed than in *Index medicus*. Keyword and author indexes in each issue.

1102
Documenta cardioangiologica. Darmstadt, 1, 1965– .

1965 indexed 215 serials under a rather minute subject breakdown. No annual subject indexes.

1103
Referátový výběr z kardiologie; fysiologie a patologie oběhového ústrojí [Selected abstracts on cardiology; physiology and pathology of the circulation system] Praha, 1, 1960– . Ústav pro zdravotnickou dokumentaci.

4 issues a year. Abstracts in Czech or Slovak of selected articles chiefly from foreign periodicals.

Reviews

1104★
Advances in cardiopulmonary diseases. Chicago, Year Book Medical Publishers, 1, 1963– .

Selected lectures from the series of postgraduate courses presented by the Council on Postgraduate Medical Education of the American College of Chest Physicians.

1105
Fortschritte der Kardiologie. Advances in cardiology. Progrès en cardiologie. Basel, 1, 1956– . (Bibliotheca Cardiologica, Suppl. to Cardiologia, Fasc. 6–).

Triennial. Articles in English, German, or French.

1106
Modern trends in cardiology. New York, 1961– . (Hoeber's Modern trends series)

1107
Progress in cardiovascular diseases. New York, Grune and Stratton, 1, 1958– .

1108
Progress in hematology. New York, Grune and Stratton, 1, 1956– .

Irregular.

1109
Recent advances in cardiology. 5 ed. by Terence East and Curtis Bain. London, Churchill, 1959. 421 p.

Chapter bibliographies (omitting titles of articles). No overall author index. 1 ed., 1929; 4 ed., 1948.

1110★
Year book of cardiovascular and renal diseases. Chicago, Year Book Medical Publishers, 1961/62– . (The practical medicine year books)

Bibliographies

1111
Československá kardiologická společnost. Československá kardiologická literatura, 1861–1946. Seznam prací o ústrojí krevního oběhu v československé literatuře [Czechoslovak literature on cardiology, 1861–1946. Index to works on the system of circulation of blood in Czechoslovak periodical literature] Praha, 1948. 184, 43 p.

Lists over 2,000 references, chiefly journal articles but including some monographs by Czech or Slovak authors. In 3 parts covering different time spans, separate author entries for each part. Pt. 4, Subject indexes, in Czech and English by author.

1112
Dávid, József. Magyar haematologiai és transfúziós bibliográfia (1945–1960) [Hungarian bibliography on hematology and blood transfusion (1945–1960)] Budapest, Országos Orvostudományi Könyvtár és Dokumentációs Kózpont, 1964. 472 p.

Lists 3328 references, including books. Covers the literature published in Hungary or by Hungarian authors abroad. Into two parts, hematology and blood transfusion, with chronological subarrangement. Includes a list of periodicals indexed with abbreviations.

1113
Etingen, L. E., and Kraev, A. V. Bibliografiia otechestvennykh rabot po limfaticheskoĭ sisteme [Bibliography of national works on the lymphatic system] Red. Ia. A. Rakhimov. Stalinabad, Gosudarstvennaia nauchnaia meditsinskaia biblioteka, 1958. 218 p.

Indexes 2082 books, articles, dissertations, etc. in Russian and other languages. Covers the period from the end of the 18th century.

1114
Gergeley, János. Az atherosclerosis pathomechanizmusának válogatott bibliográfiája [Selected bibliography on pathological mechanism of atherosclerosis] Budapest, Országos Orvostudományi Könyvtár és Dokumentácios Központ, 1961. 144 p.

Lists 690 articles selected from non-Hungarian journals for the period 1944 to 1960, chiefly from Western countries.

1115
Kiev. Respublikanskaia nauchnaia meditsinskaia biblioteka. Ateroskleroz; bibliograficheskiĭ ukazatel' otechestvennoĭ literatury (1947–1957) [Atherosclerosis; bibliographic index of national literature (1947–1957)] Sost. F. S. Aronova-Zlatopol'skaia. Kiev, 1958. 81 p.

725 references, including monographs, textbooks, collections of works, serials, and journal articles. Entries are in Russian. Includes some 1958 publications.

1116
—. —. Profilaktika serdechnososudistykh zabolevaniĭ; bibliograficheskiĭ ukazatel' otechestvennoĭ literatury 1947–1957 [Prevention of cardiovascular diseases; bibliographical index to national literature, 1947–1957] Kiev, 1959. 40 p.

400 references listed. Includes books.

1117
Massachusetts. Recess Commission on Hypertension. A bibliography of the world literature on blood pressure, 1920–1950. Ed. by Ernest K. Koller and Jacob Katz. [Boston] 1952. 3 v.

v. 1, alphabetical author listing of 16,460 references, including journal articles, symposia reports, textbooks, monographs, etc.; v. 2, subject and co-author indexes; v. 3, approximately 15,000 abstracts of items listed in v. 1.

1118
Moscow. Gosudarstvennaia tsentral'naia nauchnaia meditsinskaia biblioteka. Zabolevaniia serdechno-sosudistoĭ sistemy; bibliografiia otechestvennoi literatury za 1950–1957 gg. [Diseases of cardiovascular system; bibliography of national literature, 1950–1957] Sost. M. L. Vil'shanskaia i dr. Pod red. E. I. Sokolova. Moskva, 1962. 964 p.

About 12,000 entries. Includes books and dissertations.

1119
——. ——. ——, 1917–1949 gg. Sost. M. A. Nazarova. Moskva, Medgiz, 1953. 518 p.

Contains about 8000 references, chiefly in Russian, but also in other Slavic languages of the USSR. Titles of indexed sources p. 5–70.

1120★
National Research Council. Division of Medical Sciences. Index-handbook of cardiovascular agents. v. 1. New York, McGraw-Hill, 1963. 2067 p. v. 2. Washington, National Research Council, 1960. 2 pts.

Based on examination of some 400 medical and scientific periodicals for data concerning the effects of chemical agents upon the anatomy, physiology and pathology of the cardiovascular system.

v. 1 covers literature 1931–1950; v. 2, 1951–1955.

1121
Selye, Hans. Thrombohemorrhagic phenomena. Springfield, Thomas, 1966. 337 p.

Essentially abstracts, with commentary, of references listed by author, p. 267–319.

1122
U.S. National Aeronautics and Space Administration. Scientific and Technical Information Division. Ballistocardiography; a bibliography. Washington, 1965. 46 p. (NASA SP-7021) (FAA AM 65–15)

Covers the period 1877–1964. Includes books. Author arrangement. No subject index.

Published under the joint auspices of NASA and the Federal Aviation Agency.

1123
U. S. National Heart Institute. Committee on Thrombolytic Agents. Fibrinolysis, thrombolysis, and bloodclotting; a bibliography. Bethesda, 1, 1965– .

Monthly. MEDLARS print-out. Published with the cooperation of the National Library of Medicine.

1124
U.S. Public Health Service. Division of Chronic Diseases. Endocarditis; bibliography compiled from the English language, 1957–1962. Washington, 1963. 22 p. (Public Health Service. Publication no. 1064).

335 references. "Covers all articles written in English on endocarditis and related subjects included in *Index Medicus* during the period January 1, 1957, through December 31, 1962."

1125
—. —. —, 1963–64. Washington, 1966. 8 p. (Public Health Service. Publication no. 1064 (Supplement 1. October 1965))

132 references.

Monographs

1126
Federation of American Societies for Experimental Biology. Committee on Biological Handbooks. Blood and other body fluids. Comp. by Philip L. Altman and Dorothy S. Dittmer. Washington, 1961. 540 p. (Biological Handbooks).

Comparative data arranged in the form of 166 tables, graphs, diagrams, nomograms, and line charts.

1127
National Research Council. Committee on the Handbook of Biological Data. Handbook of circulation. Philadelphia, Saunders, 1959. 393 p.

Comparative data, physiologic, anatomic, pharmacologic, etc. Includes effect of pathologic conditions.

Dictionaries

1128
Romei Braconi, L. Hematology; a glossary of terms in English-American, French, Spanish, Italian, German, Russian. New York, Elsevier, 1964. 306 p. (Glossaria interpretum)

2210 words or terms.

Nomenclature

1129★
New York Heart Association. Diseases of the heart and blood vessels; nomenclature and criteria for diagnosis. Boston, Little, 1, 1928– .

Gives full definitions and frequently lists signs; subject matter divided into 5 parts; cardiac, vascular, pathologic, roentgenologic, and electrocardiographic diagnosis.

Early editions have title, *Criteria for the classification and diagnosis of heart disease*; 4–5 ed. *Nomenclature and criteria for diagnosis of diseases of the heart and blood vessels.*

4 ed. translated into Spanish; 5 ed. translated into Italian and Spanish.

Directories

1130
American College of Cardiology. Directory, October 1, 1964. [New York] 1964. 111 p.

Alphabetical list of members, followed by a geographical listing, giving name, degrees, type of membership, and address. Includes officers and past presidents.

Histories

1131
Burch, George E., and De Pasquale, Nicholas P. A history of electrocardiography. Chicago, Year Book Medical Publishers, 1964. 309 p.

Thorough survey, with brief biographies of important figures. Bibliography (by date of publication, 1791–1960): p. 268–296.

1132
East, Charles F. Terence. The story of heart disease. London, Dawson, 1958. 148 p. (Fitzpatrick lectures, 1956–57)

Lectures on diagnosis, morbid anatomy, coronary circulation, and therapeutics. References at end of each lecture. No index.

1133
Fishman, Alfred P., and Richards, Dickinson W., ed. Circulation of the blood: men and ideas. New York, Oxford University Press, 1964. 859 p.

Twelve historical surveys on special topics from antiquity to the present by different authors. Includes analyses of and translated excerpts from key works. Extensive lists of references to original and secondary works.

1134
Graubard, Mark, ed. Circulation and respiration: the evolution of an idea. New York, Harcourt, Brace & World, 1964. 278 p.

Excerpts from 17 authors from Aristotle to Borelli, with commentaries.

1135
Ruskin, Arthur, ed. Classics in arterial hypertension. Springfield, Ill., Thomas, 1956. 358 p. (American lecture series, no. 290. American lecture series classics in science and medicine, v. 1)

Papers and excerpts, in English, A. D. 400–1934, with brief introductions. Bibliography: p. 353–358.

1136
Willius, Frederick A., and Dry, Thomas J. A history of the heart and the circulation. Philadelphia, Saunders, 1948. 456 p.

In three parts: chronologic sketch 500 B. C.–1925 A. D.; special biographies of 20 important figures; chronologic presentation under 18 subjects. Extensive bibliographical reference lists.

1137
——, and Keys, Thomas E. Cardiac classics. A collection of classic works on the heart and circulation with comprehensive biographic accounts of the authors. Fifty-two contributions by fifty-one authors. St. Louis, Mosby, 1941. 858 p.

Papers in English (some abridged) from Harvey to Herrick. Sources given in footnotes. References (for each author): p. 840–846. Reprinted New York, Dover, 1961, as *Classics of cardiology*.

COMMUNICABLE DISEASES

General

Indexes and Abstracts

1138
Referátový výběr z chorob infekčních [Selected abstracts on infectious diseases] Praha, 1, 1960– . Státní ústav pro zdravotnickou dokumentačni a knihovnickou službu.

Quarterly.

1138.1
References to literature of interest to mosquito workers and malariologists. In Mosquito news, 2, 1942–

Quarterly. Includes monographs, annual and special reports and unpublished papers of WHO.

v. 2(2)-v. 3(1), June 1942–Mar. 1943 as *References to literature on mosquitoes and their control;* v. 3(2)-7, 1943(June)–1947 as *References to literature of interest to mosquito control workers*; v. 8–16, 1948–56 as *References . . . to mosquito control workers and malariologists.*

1139★
Tropical diseases bulletin. London, 1912– . Bureau of Hygiene and Tropical Diseases.

1964 listed 2174 references, most with abstracts. Includes reports and surveys, proceedings of congresses, book reviews.

Since 1939 each issue (Dec. excepted) contains a section "Summary of recent abstracts" covering a selected disease. The abstracts summarized are those which appeared in the *Bulletin* for the previous year. The diseases summarized are cholera (Jan.), yellow fever (Feb.), malaria (Mar., April), trypanosomiasis (May), leishmaniasis (June), plague (July), helminthiasis (Aug.-Sept.), rickettsial diseases (Oct.), leprosy (Nov.)

Annual index includes geographic index. Index for 1962 published in 1965.

Reviews

1140
International review of tropical medicine. London, Academic Press, 1, 1961– .

1140.1
Recent advances in tropical medicine. 3 ed., by N. H. Fairley, et al. London, Churchill, 1961. 480 p.

1 ed., 1928; 2 ed., 1929.

Bibliographies

1141
Bloomfield, Arthur L. A bibliography of internal medicine; communicable diseases. Chicago, University of Chicago Press, 1958. 560 p.

Lists references of "fundamental importance" in the history of 31 diseases, with annotations.

1142
Farmhouse, João C. R. Bibliografia portuguesa de medicina tropical e ciencias

afins. Lisboa, Instituto de Medicina Tropical, 1958. Unpaged.

2355 entries; includes books. Breakdown by Portuguese colonies.

At head of title: VI congressos internacionais de medicina tropical e paludismo, Lisboa, 5–13 de setembro de 1958.

Revision of 1952 ed., by the author and Manuel Farmhouse.

1143
Haeser, Heinrich. Bibliotheca epidemiographia; sive Catalogus librorum de historia morborum epidemicorum cum generali tum speciali conscriptorum. 2 ed. Gryphiswaldiae, Ex Libraria Academica, 1862. 230 p.

Lists collections, histories (general, by region, by disease), special epidemics arranged chronologically from antiquity to 1860.

1144
Norman-Taylor, W. Annotated bibliography on medical research in the South Pacific. Nouméa, New Caledonia, 1963. 371 p.

Includes books and reports.

Histories

1145
Corradi, Alfonso. Annali delle epidemie occorse in Italia dalle prime memorie fino al 1850. Bologna, Gamberini e Parmeggiani, 1865–94. 8 v.

Monumental compilation of historical data from archival and printed sources, with extensive bibliographical citations in text and footnotes. Indexes in v. 8 include authors and anonymous works; epidemics by place and date and by disease; cattle epidemics; meteorological and astronomical events and disasters; military, naval, and prison epidemics.

1146
Creighton, Charles. A history of epidemics in Britain. With additional material by D. E. C. Eversley, E. Ashworth Underwood and Lynda Ovenall. 2 ed. New York, Barnes and Noble, 1965. 2 v.

Classic study, comprehensive and detailed, based on contemporary works and other sources, with references in footnotes. Reprint of the original edition, Cambridge, Eng., 1891–94, with 177 p. of new material, including a select classified bibliography of epidemiological literature relating to Great Britain since 1894, by Lynda Ovenall, v. 1, p. 137–166.

1147
Duffy, John. Epidemics in colonial America. Baton Rouge, Louisiana State University Press, 1953. 274 p.

Studies of the various epidemic diseases and their effect on social and economic life, based on a variety of original and secondary sources, with extensive footnote references. Classified bibliography: p. 249–265.

1148
Greenwood, Major. Epidemics and crowd diseases; an introduction to the history of epidemiology. London, Williams & Norgate, 1935. 409 p.

A review of principles and methods from Hippocrates and Galen to the present with emphasis on the modern period, followed by studies of 13 special diseases. References for further study at ends of chapters.

1149
Hare, Ronald. Pomp and pestilence: infectious disease, its origins and conquest. London, Gollancz, 1954. 224 p.

Aspects of epidemiology in historical perspective. References (by chapters): p. 203–217.

1150
Olpp, Gottlieb. Hervorragende Tropenärzte in Wort und Bild. München, Gmelin, 1932. 446 p.

Nearly 300 biographical sketches, each with references and lists of publications, alphabetically arranged.

1151
Parish, Henry J. A history of immunization. Edinburgh, Livingstone, 1965. 368 p.

Review of the main contributions made by immunology to the control of infections. Chap. 1, Historical introduction (1683–1949) has list of general historical references (p. 15–16). Remaining chapters on special diseases, usually brought down to present, with references for each.

1152
Scott, H. Harold. A history of tropical medicine. London, Arnold, 1939. 2 v. (1219 p.)

Detailed history, chiefly by diseases, infectious and deficiency. Additional chapters on military and maritime aspects, slave trade, biographical sketches of 15 leading figures. Selective author bibliography: p. 1091–1099.

1153
Sticker, Georg. Abhandlungen aus der Seuchengeschichte und Seuchenlehre. Giessen, Töpelmann, 1908–12. 2 v.

v. 1: Die Pest (in 2 pts.); v. 2: Die Cholera. Detailed and comprehensive. Bibliographies: v. 1, pt. 1, p. 423–478; pt. 2, p. 491–538; v. 2, p. 523–586. Full tables of contents; no index.

1154
Top, Franklin H., ed. The history of American epidemiology. Sponsored by the Epidemiology Section, American Public Health Association. St. Louis, Mosby, 1952. 190 p.

Four studies, by C. E. A. Winslow, W. G. Smillie, J. A. Doull, and J. E. Gordon, on successive periods from 1607 to the present. Extensive lists of references for each study.

1155
Winslow, Charles E. A. The conquest of epidemic disease; a chapter in the history of ideas. Princeton, N.J., Princeton University Press, 1943. 411 p.

Epidemiologic theory from primitive times to early 20th century, with critical evaluations of significant works. References: p. 384–397.

Anthrax

Bibliographies

1155.1
U.S. Army Chemical Corps. Technical Library, Fort Detrick, Md. Bibliography of anthrax and *Bacillus anthracis*. Rev. ed. Fort Detrick, 1956. 100 p.

From 1930. Includes books, chapters in books, theses.

Bilharziasis

Bibliographies

1156
Bouillon, Albert. Bibliographie des schistosomes et des schistosomiases (bilharzioses) humaines et animales de 1931 à 1948. Bruxelles, 1950. 141 p. (Institut Royal Colonial Belge. Section des Sciences Naturelles et Médicales. Mémoires. v. 18, fasc. 5)

2078 entries. Includes monographs. Continues and supplements no. 1158.

1157
Brazil. Instituto Brasileiro de Bibliografia e Documentaçâo. Esquistossomose; bibliografia brasileira. Rio de Janeiro, 1, 1958– .

Arranged chronologically. [v. 1] 1958, 742 references, 1908–57; v. 2, 1963, 362 references, 1958–62. Brazilian and international literature relating to Brazil. Includes theses, monographs.

v. 2 has series note: Bibliografias brasileiras sôbre doenças tropicais, no. 3.

1158
Khalil, M. The bibliography of schistosomiasis (bilharziasis), zoological, clinical and prophylactic. Cairo, Egyptian University, 1931. 503 p. (The Faculty of Medicine. Publication no. 1)

1159
University of Puerto Rico. School of Medicine. School of Tropical Medicine. Library. Bilharzia (Schistosomiasis Mansoni) in Puerto Rico; a bibliography, 1904–1962. San Juan, 1963. 18 p.

271 English, French and Spanish references, nearly all journal articles.

1160
World Health Organization. Bibliography of bilharziasis, 1949–1958. Genève, 1960. 158 p.

2781 entries, alphabetically arranged. Includes monographs.

Combined subject and geographical index.

Title also in French.

Updates nos. 1156 and 1158.

Botulism

Bibliographies

1160.1
U.S. Army Chemical Corps. Technical Library. Camp Detrick, Md. Bibliography on botulism and *Clostridium botulinum*. Camp Detrick, 1952. 69 p.

From 1930. Includes books, chapters in books, theses.

Brucellosis

Bibliographies

1161
Beklemishev, N. D., and Karakulov, I. K. Brutsellez; annotirovannyĭ ukazatel' literatury (do 1951 g.) [Brucellosis; annotated index to literature (up to 1951)] Alma-Ata, Izd-vo Akademii nauk Kazakhskoĭ SSR, 1955. 508 p.

1850 annotated references to works in the Russian language by Soviet authors, chiefly since 1920. Includes books and dissertations. Alphabetical author arrangement.

1162
Hoptman, Julian. Brucellosis in the USSR; a review of the literature. Washington, National Institutes of Health, 1959. 77 p.

1163
Khrushchev, N. F. [et al.] Ukazatel' literatury po brutsellezu (s 1952 po 1956 god vkliuchitel'no) [Index to literature on brucellosis (from 1952 to 1956 incl.)] In Akademiia nauk Kazakhskoĭ SSR. Institut kraevoĭ patologii. Trudy. Tom 6 (14). Sbornik rabot po brutsellezu. Alma-Ata, 1958. p. 146–223.

1377 titles of books, articles, dissertations in Russian and other languages of the Soviet Union. Author arrangement.

Cholera

Bibliographies

1164
Pollitzer, Robert. List of publications on cholera appearing during the period from 1 January 1959 to mid-March 1963. Geneva, World Health Organization, 1963. 30 p.

432 references, listed alphabetically by author. Does not include historical papers.

History

1165
Rosenberg, Charles E. The cholera years: the United States in 1832, 1849, and 1866. Chicago, Univ. of Chicago Press, 1962. 257 p.

Detailed and documented, concentrating on New York City. Annotated bibliography; p. 235–252.

Coccidioidomycosis

Bibliographies

1166
Cheu, Stephen H. Coccidioidomycosis bibliography. 1965 ed. Fresno, [1965] 77, 10 p.

Consists of articles 1891–1964 chronologically arranged.

1166.1
U.S. Army Chemical Corps. Fort Detrick, Frederick, Md. Bibliography on coccidioidomycosis. 2 ed. Frederick, 1959. 77 p.

1892–1959. Includes books, theses, reports.

Dengue

Bibliographies

1166.2
U.S. Army Chemical Corps. Technical Library. Fort Detrick, Frederick, Md. Bibliography on dengue and yellow fever. Part A. Dengue fever; part B. Yellow fever. Frederick, 1956. 104 p.

Mainly from 1928 to 1956. Includes books. Pt. B has geographic breakdown under *Epidemic countries.*

Filariasis

Bibliographies

1167
South Pacific Commission. Annotated bibliography of filariasis and elephantiasis. Pt. 1–[5] Nouméa, New Caledonia, 1954–[60] (Its Technical paper, nos. 65, 88, 109, 124, 129)

The 5 parts collectively contain in excess of 2000 abstracts. Includes books and reports. All parts arranged chronologically, the earliest reference being for the year 1716.

Pt. 2–5 by M. O. T. Iyengar. Each part on a different aspect of the subject.

Pt. 2 entitled *Annotated bibliography on filariasis.*

1168
——. A review of the literature on the distribution and epidemiology of filariasis in the South Pacific region. By M. O. T. Iyengar. Nouméa, New Caledonia, 1959. 172 p. (Its Technical paper, no. 126)

311 annotated references arranged chronologically. Includes books. Earliest reference 1785.

Foot-and-Mouth Disease

Bibliographies

1168.1
Bibliography of foot-and-mouth disease in man, 1695–1965. Comp. by B. Balassa. Greenport. Long Is., U.S. Dept. of Agriculture, Animal Disease and Parasite Research Division [1965?] 29 p.

310 references.

Hepatitis, Infectious

Bibliographies

1169
Kiev. Respublikanskaia nauchnaia meditsinskaia biblioteka. Infektsionnyĭ gepatit (bolezn' Botkina); bibliograficheskiĭ ukazatel' otechestvennoĭ literatury (1919–1959) [Infectious hepatitis (Botkin's disease); bibliographic index to national literature (1919–1959)] Kiev, Medgiz USSR, 1962. 266 p.

2292 entries. Includes books, lectures, annotations and abstracts. Lists separately: textbooks and handbooks; instructional materials; proceedings of congresses, conferences and meetings; symposia; collected works; and popular science and health education publications.

Histoplasmosis

Bibliographies

1170
U.S. Army Biological Laboratories. Technical library. Fort Detrick, Md. Bibliography on histoplasmosis. 1955. 84 p.

1171
——. Supplement, 1955–60. 1961. [47 p.]

511 entries.

No. 1170 published by U.S. Chemical Corps.

Influenza

Indexes and Abstracts

1172
Annotated bibliography of influenza. Washington, 1, 1960– .American Institute of Biological Sciences.

Quarterly. 1963 had 641 numbered annotations from approximately 2600 international journals. Supplement (no. 1173) covers the literature, January 1, 1957–May 31, 1960.

Bibliographies

1173
American Institute of Biological Sciences. An annotated bibliography of influenza, January 1, 1957, to May 31, 1960. Washington [1962] 225 p.

2339 numbered references, most with annotations. Includes monographs, editorials, reports.

Supplements, retrospectively, no. 1172.

1174
Vil'shanskaia, M. L. [et al.] Gripp; bibliografiia otechestvennoĭ literatury za 1939–1957 gg. [Influenza; bibliography of the national literature, 1939–1957] Pod red. N. D. Abramovoĭ. Moskva, Gos. tsentr. nauch. medits. biblioteka, 1961. 150 p.

Lists approximately 2100 references. Includes monographs and theses.

Leishmaniasis

Indexes and Abstracts

1175
Kala azar bulletin. London, 1, no. 1–3, 1911–12. Tropical Disease Bureau.

Literature reviews.

v. 1, no. 1–2, 1911–12 issued by the Sleeping Sickness Bureau.

Bibliographies

1176
Brazil. Instituto Brasileiro de Bibliografia e Documentaçâo. Leishmanioses; bibliografia brasileira. Rio de Janeiro, 1958. 57 p. (Bibliografias brasileiras sôbre doenças tropicais, no. 5)

Chronological arrangement. 499 selected references for the period 1909–57. Includes books. Not limited to Brazilian literature.

1177
Kala azar bulletin. List of references. London, Sleeping Sickness Bureau, 1911. 63 p.

Around 900 entries on affections known to be caused by *Leishmania*, 1787–1911. Author arrangement. Includes theses.

1178
Rodiakin, N. F., and Dvurechenskaia, N. V. Kozhnyĭ leishmanioz (bolezn' Borovskogo); bibliograficheskiĭ ukazatel' literatury (1862–1960) [Cutaneous leishmaniasis (Borovskii's disease); bibliographic index to literature (1862–1960)] Ashkhabad, Respublikanskaia nauchnaia meditsinskaia biblioteka, 1962. 134 p.

994 references including books, articles, and collected works in the Russian language. Brief historical review of the national literature.

Leprosy

Bibliographies

1179
São Paulo (State) Departamento de Profilaxia de Lepra. Biblioteca. Indice bibliográfico de lepra, 1500–1943. Organizado por Luiza Keffer. São Paulo, 1944–48. 3 v.

Authors and subjects in one alphabet.

v. 2 (I-P) has title *1500–1944*; v. 3 (Q-Z) 1500–1945.

1180
——. ——. Suplemento 1–[5] São Paulo, 1952–[62]

Supplements are on special subjects (Reação de Mitsuda, B.C.G., Profilaxia da Lepra) and cover different time periods. Most have abstracts.

1181
——. Sumário bibliográfia. São Paulo, no. 1-313, [19? –59]

Monthly or semimonthly. Superseded by no. 1182.

1182
——. Biblioteca e Documentacão. Indice bibliográfico de lepra. São Paulo, 1, 1960– .

Monthly. A sample issue listed 65 references, most with abstracts, generally in language of original publication. Issues occasionally on a special subject.

Has subtitle: suplemento mensal. Continues no. 1181.

1183
Torsuev, N. A. Bibliograficheskiĭ ukazatel' rabot otechestvennykh avtorov po lepre [Bibliographical index of works of national authors on leprosy] Rostov na Donu, 1959. 223 p.

2636 references to works published through 1957 by "national" authors in Russian and foreign languages. Includes monographs, collected works, serials, popular literature, unpublished dissertations, and journal articles.

Histories

1184
Fay, Henri M. Histoire de la lèpre en France; lépreux et cagots du Sud-Ouest. Notes historiques, médicales, philologiques, suivie de documents. Paris, Champion, 1910. 784 p.

Detailed study, with texts of documents (p. 337–534), local history (p. 535–702) and bibliography (p. 703–715).

1185
Feeny, Patrick. The fight against leprosy. London, Elek, 1964. 191 p.

Brief account of ancient and medieval history of the disease, followed by a fuller survey of scientific advances in the 19th and 20th centuries. Bibliography (mainly works used, by chapters): p. 181–191. No index.

1186
Frohn, Wilhelm. Lepradarstellungen in der Kunst des Rheinlandes. Berlin, Junker & Dünnhaupt, 1936. 105 p. (Neue deutsche Forschungen, v. 66; Abteilung Geschichte der Medizin und Naturwissenschaften, v. 1)

Includes medieval and renaissance literature, pictorial art, sculpture. Footnote citations. Bibliography: p. 104–105.

1187
Souza-Araujo, Heraclídes C. Historia da lepra no Brasil. Rio de Janeiro, Imprensa Nacional, 1946–56. 3 v.

Exhaustive history from 1500 through 1952, with extensive quotations from original documents. v. 2 is an album of plates. Bibliography for v. 1: p. 534–536. "Bibliografia leprológica brazileira de 1931 a 1952": v. 3, p. 599–657.

Leptospirosis

Bibliographies

1188
Blagodarnyĭ, Ia. A., and Medvedva, S. G. Leptospiroz; annotirovannyĭ ukazatel'

literatury (1948–1958) [Leptospirosis; annotated index to literature (1948–1958)] Alma-Ata, Izd-vo Akademii nauk Kazakhskoĭ SSR, 1961. 251 p.

840 books and articles by Soviet authors, 1948–58. Arranged by author. Includes a geographic index.

1189
U.S. Army Biological Laboratories. Technical Library. Fort Detrick, Md. Bibliography on leptospirosis. Frederick, Md., 1957. 117 p.

1190
——. ——. Supplement, 1957–1962. Frederick, Md., 1963. 91 p.

963 entries. No. 1189 published by the U.S. Army Chemical Corps.

1191
U.S. National Library of Medicine. Leptospirosis; a bibliography of literature 1957–1959. Comp. by Dorothy Bocker. Washington, 1959. 39 p.

319 entries arranged by continent.

Malaria

Bibliographies

1192
Brazil. Instituto Brasileiro de Bibliografia e Documentacão. Malaria; bibliografia brasileira. Rio de Janeiro, 1958. 129 p. (Bibliografias brasileiras sôbre doenças tropicais).

Lists 1,151 references selected from 169 journals (chiefly Brazilian) for the period 1884–1957. Chronological arrangement.

Dictionaries

1193
World Health Organization. Expert Committee on Malaria. Drafting Committee on Revision of Malaria Terminology. Terminology of malaria and of malaria eradication; report of a drafting committee. Geneva, World Health Organization, 1963. 127 p.

Text, p. 1–89; glossary, p. 91–124.

Histories

1194
Ackerknecht, Erwin H. Malaria in the upper Mississippi Valley, 1760–1900. Baltimore, Johns Hopkins Press, 1945. 142 p. (Bulletin of the History of Medicine. Supplements, no. 4.)

Documented history, emphasizing epidemiology. References: p. 134–142.

1195
Celli, Angelo. The history of malaria in the Roman Campagna from ancient times. Ed. by Anna Celli-Fraentzel. London, J. Bale, Sons & Danielsson, 1933. 226 p.

Documented study from pre-Roman times through the 19th century, with brief notes on the 20th. References: p. 176–214.

1196
Jaramillo-Arango, Jaime. The conquest of malaria. London, Heinemann, 1950. 125 p.

Valuable for history of mosquito-malaria theory and especially of cinchona.

1197
Jones, William H. S. Malaria and Greek history. Manchester, University Press, 1909. 175 p. (Manchester University Publications, no. 43; Historical series, no. 8)

Examination of references to malaria in non-medical and medical Greek texts, with studies on prevalence and effects. Footnote references; bibliography: p. 135–136.

1198
Russell, Paul F. Man's mastery of malaria. London, Oxford University Press, 1955. 308 p. (University of London, Heath Clark lectures, 1953)

Brief data on early periods, with full account of modern developments.References, by author, including sources and historical studies: p. 259–285.

Plague

Bibliographies

1199
U.S. Army Chemical Corps. Biological Laboratories. Technical Library. Camp Detrick. Bibliography on plague and *pasteurella pestis*. Frederick, Md., 1954. 182 p.

Selected journal references covering 1900–1954. Issued as ASTIA document.

Histories

1200
Campbell, Anna M. The black death and men of learning. New York, Columbia University Press, 1931. 210 p. (History of Science Society. Publications, no.1)

Documented history of the plague in the 14th century. Bibliography (sources and secondary works): p. 181–195; footnote references throughout.

1201
Crawfurd, Sir Raymond H. P. Plague and pestilence in literature and art. Oxford, Clarendon Press, 1914. 222 p. (Fitzpatrick lectures, 1912)

To the end of the 18th century. No index.

1202
Frari, Angelo A. Delle peste e della pubblica amministrazione sanitaria. v. 1. Venezia, Andreola, 1840. cxlix, xvii, 964 p.

No more published. Bibliography of works on plague (by language and author): p. 1–202.

1203
Hirst, Leonard Fabian. The conquest of plague; a study of the evolution of epidemiology. Oxford, Clarendon Press, 1953. 478 p.

From primitive man to the present, but valuable chiefly for discoveries since 1894. Bibliographical references at end of each of the 4 parts.

1204
Klebs, Arnold C., and Sudhoff, Karl. Die ersten gedruckten Pestschriften. Arnold C. Klebs: Geschichtliche und bibliographische Untersuchungen. Karl Sudhoff: Der Ulmer Stadtarzt und Schriftsteller Heinrich Steinhöwel. München, Verlag der Münchner Drucke, 1926. 222 p.

Lists 130 incunabula on the plague, with brief descriptions, references, locations of copies, and indexes by date and by place of printing (p. 14–82) followed by a historical and bibliographical study. 24 facsimiles from various tracts, and complete facsimile of the 1473 ed. of Steinhöwel's tract.

1205
Mullett, Charles F. The bubonic plague and England: an essay in the history of preventive medicine. Lexington, University of Kentucky Press, 1956. 401 p.

Study covering 14th through early 19th century. Valuable especially to the student of history and literature. Footnote references.

Poliomyelitis

Indexes and Abstracts

1206
Current literature, poliomyelitis and related diseases. New York, 1–16, 1946–62. National Foundation.

v. 1–12, 1946–58, as *Poliomyelitis current literature.*

Bibliographies

1207
Lega Italiana per la Lotta Contro la Poliomielite. Bibliografia italiana sulla poliomielite. . . A cura di S. Siggia. Roma, 1957. 630 p.

892 references, 1829–1956, arranged chronologically by author. Most entries have abstracts. Title and abstracts also in French, English and German.

1208★
National Foundation for Infantile Paralysis. A bibliography of infantile paralysis, 1789–1949, with selected abstracts and annotations. Prepared under the direction of the National Foundation for Infantile Paralysis, Inc. Ed. by Morris Fishbein and Ella M. Salmonsen, with Ludwig Hektoen. 2 ed. Philadelphia, Lippincott, 1951. 899 p.

10,367 entries from the international literature. Includes monographs. Chronological arrangement. 1 ed., 1946.

1209
Raettig, Hansjürgen. Poliomyelitis Immunität. Stuttgart, Fischer, 1963. Pts. 1–2. 301, 362 p. (Literatur-Dokumentation. Reihe 2)

5500 references, 1908–61. Pt. 1: Sachregister; pt. 2: Bibliographie. Title page, introduction, and subject headings in English and German. Bibliography arranged by author at random.

Psittacosis

Bibliographies

1209.1
U.S. Army Biological Laboratories. Tech-

nical Library Branch. Fort Detrick, Md. Bibliography on psittacosis. Supplement, 1950–1962. Fort Detrick, 1962. 63 p.

Includes books. Has section *Epidemic countries*, with listing by country. Supplements 1209.2

1209.2
[U.S. Army Chemical Corps. Technical Library. Camp Detrick, Md.] Bibliography on psittacosis. [Camp Detrick, 1950] [33 p.]

From 1883–1949.

Rickettsial Diseases

Bibliographies

1210
U.S. Army Chemical Corps. Camp Detrick. Technical Library. Bibliography on Q fever. Camp Detrick, Md., 1950. 30 p. [Supplement] 1954. 77p.

The original covers the literature from 1936 to about May 1950. The supplement lists additional references for the same period and updates.

1211
U.S. Army Chemical Corps. Technical Library, Fort Detrick, Md. Bibliography [on] the Rocky Mountain spotted fever group of Rickettsioses. [Fort Detrick, 1954] 34 p. Supplement. Fort Detrick, 1956. 46 p.

References from 1899 to 1956.

1211.1
U.S. Army Chemical Corps. Technical Library. Camp Detrick, Frederick, Md. Bibliography on epidemic, endemic, and scrub tryphus fevers. Part 1. Epidemic (human, louse borne) typhus. Frederick, 1952. 93 p.

Covers from about 1940 through 1951, with a few selected earlier articles. Books, theses, etc. p. 76–8.

1211.2
U.S. Army Chemical Corps. Technical Library. Camp Detrick, Frederick, Md. Bibliography of epidemic, endemic, and scrub typhus fevers. Part 2. Endemic (murine, flea borne) typhus. Part 3. Scrub typhus (Tsutsugamushi disease) Frederick, 1952. 63 p.

Covers from about 1940 through 1951, with a few selected earlier articles. Books, theses, etc. p. 51a.

Histories

1212
Aikawa, Jerry K. Rocky Mountain spotted fever. Springfield, Ill., Thomas, 1966. 140 p.

History of knowledge of the disease, its treatment and control. 168 references.

1213
Zinsser, Hans. Rats, lice and history; being a study in biography, which . . . deals with the life history of typhus fever. Boston, Atlantic Monthly, 1935. 301 p.

Relies heavily on secondary works; no bibliography, few footnotes. But author's knowledge of subject and literary skill make it a classic of epidemiology.

Salmonellosis

Bibliographies

1214
U.S. National Library of Medicine. Salmonella, salmonella infections; bibliography of literature, 1955–April 1960. Comp. by Dorothy Bocker. Washington, 1960. 40 p. (Public Health Service. Publication, no. 803).

755 references from English, French, German, Italian, and Spanish literature.

1215
Wisconsin. University. Bibliography on Salmonella, exclusive of *Salmonella typhi*, covering the years 1945 to 1954. [Madison, 1955?] 191 p.

1216
——. ——. Supplements 1–5, 1955/56–1960. [Madison, n.d.]

Original bibliography contains 3697 citations to periodical articles, books, theses, conferences, and patents. Most citations include reference to an abstract. All volumes issued as ASTIA documents.

Smallpox

Histories

1217
Crookshank, Edgar M. History and pa-

thology of vaccination. London, Lewis, 1889. 2 v.

Exhaustive history by an anti-vaccinationist. v. 2 is a collection of original essays on vaccination by various authors from Jenner to 1887, the foreign works in translation. No index.

1218
Gins, Heinrich A. Krankheit wider den Tod; Schicksal der Pockenschutzimpfung. Stuttgart, Fischer, 1963. 368 p.

Mainly based on a collection of documents and letters dated 1801–1858 in the Berlin Impfanstalt. Name index only.

1219
Miller, Genevieve. The adoption of inoculation for smallpox in England and France. Philadelphia, University of Pennsylvania Press, 1957. 355 p.

Detailed study, largely based on contemporary sources. Bibliography (classified, including primary and secondary sources): p. 294–339. Extensive footnote references throughout.

1220
Stearn, Esther A. W., and Stearn, Allen E. The effect of smallpox on the destiny of the Amerindian. Boston, Humphries, 1945. 153 p.

Factual survey, covering 16th–20th centuries. Bibliography: p. 140–149.

Staphylococcal Infections

Bibliographies

1221
National Research Council of Canada. Associate Committee on the Control of Hospital Infections. Bibliography on the control of staphylococcal and of other hospital infections. Ottawa, 1960. 148 p.

1154 numbered references, 1914–59.

1222
U.S. National Library of Medicine. Staphylococcal infection; a bibliography covering the literature of 1952 through May 1958. [By Dorothy Bocker] Washington, 1958. 43 p.

506 entries.

1223
——. ——. Supplement. A bibliography covering the literature of June 1958 through July 1959. [By Dorothy Bocker] Washington, 1959. 29 p.

285 entries.

Toxoplasmosis

Bibliographies

1224
Galuzo, I. G., and Zasukhina, D. N., ed. Toksoplazmoz cheloveka i zhivotnykh; ukazatel' otechestvennoĭ i inostrannoĭ literatury, 1908–1962 [Toxoplasmosis of man and animals; index to national and foreign literature, 1908–1962] Alma-Ata, Izd-vo Akademii nauk Kazakhskoĭ SSR, 1963. 412 p.

Includes monographs and sections of monographs, collected works, dissertations, proceedings of congresses, etc. In two sections: 691 Russian references; 3015 foreign references. Author arrangement.

1225
U.S. National Library of Medicine. Toxoplasmosis; a bibliography of literature 1956–September, 1960. Comp. by Dorothy Bocker. Washington, 1960. 15 p.

Trypanosomiasis

Indexes and Abstracts

1226
Sleeping sickness bulletin. London, 1–4, 1908–12. Tropical Disease Bureau.

Abstracts. Includes reports, theses, bibliographies on special subjects, and with v. 1, n. 7, *Monthly list of references.* Occasional review articles.

v. 1–3 issued by the Sleeping Sickness Bureau as its *Bulletin.*

Bibliographies

1227
Brazil. Instituto Brasileiro de Bibliografia e Documentação. Doença de Chagas; bibliografia brasileira. Rio de Janeiro, [1] 1958– . (Bibliografias brasileiras sôbre doencas tropicales, no. 2)

Chronological arrangement. v. 1–2 and supplement to v. 1 contain 2659 references 1909–1962. Includes books, theses. v. 1–2 list the international literature relating to Brazil. Supplement to v. 1 (1959) covers the literature relating to Chagas' disease outside of Brazil.

v. 1 without series note; *Supplement*, as 2-A.

Supplement as *Doença de Chagas; bibliografia.*

1228
Bureau Permanent Interafricain de la Tsé-Tsé et de la Trypanosomiase. Bulletin bibliographique et signaletique. Leopoldville, Congo, [1] 1949/50– .

Abstracts in French or English. Annual author index only.

No. 1-9, Nov. 1949-Jan./Feb. 1951, issued without volume number. Numbering commenced as v. 2, no. 1, Mar./Jul. 1951.

1229
Great Britain. Sleeping Sickness Bureau. Bibliography of trypanosomiasis; embracing original papers published prior to April 1909, and references to works and papers on tsetse-flies, especially *glossina palpalis*, Rob.-Desv. Comp. by C. A. Thimm. London, 1909. 229 p.

Tuberculosis

Indexes and Abstracts

CURRENT

1230
Kekkaku bunken no Shoroku sokuho [Abstracts of the current literature of tuberculosis] Tokyo, 1, 1950– .

Monthly. Abstracts 230 Japanese and 92 non-Japanese journals.

1231
Referátový výběr z tuberkulosy a pneumologie [Selected abstracts on tuberculosis and pneumology] Praha, 1, 1956– . Ústav pro zdravotnickou dokumentaci.

Eight issues a year. 1000–1500 abstracts a year from 110 to 170 journals, principally Czech, English, German, and some Russian.

1232
Zentralblatt für die gesamte Tuberkuloseforschung. Berlin, 1, 1906– . Organ der Deutschen Gesellschaft für Tuberkulose und Lungenkrankheiten.

Currently 3–4 volumes a year, several issues a volume. A recent volume had in excess of 1500 entries, most with abstracts. Pre-World War II volumes included literature reviews, reports of proceedings of societies, obituaries.

v. 1, 1906/07, as *Internationales Centralblatt für die gesamte Tuberkulose-Literatur;* v. 2–14, 1907–21, *Internationales Centralblatt für Tuberkulose-Forschung.*

Sponsoring bodies and their names vary. See also no. 1234.

NONCURRENT

1233
Chest disease index and abstracts including tuberculosis. London, 1–20, no. 2, 1946–65. Chest and Heart Association.

Quarterly. About 3000 abstracts a year from 365 journals, 307 of which are *Index medicus* titles. Includes mongraphs and reports.

[v. 1, no. 1] as *Tuberculosis index and digest of current literature;* [v. 1, no. 2]–v. 11, no. 2, as *Tuberculosis index and abstracts of current literature;* v. 11, no. 3–v. 14, no. 1, as *Tuberculosis index including chest diseases.* v. 1–13 issued by the National Association for the Prevention of Tuberculosis.

1234
Jahresbericht Tuberkuloseforschung. Berlin, 1–18, 1921–37.

Cumulation of references of no. 1232. v. 1–2, 4, 6, 8, 1921–22, 1924, 1926, 1928 also contained literature reviews.

v. 1–6, 1921–26, as *Jahresbericht über die gesamte Tuberkuloseforschung und ihre Grenzgebiete.*

Subtitle: Zugleich bibliographisches Jahresregister des Zentralblattes für die gesamte Tuberkuloseforschung; v. 7, 1927: without Zugleich.

Reviews

1235
Advances in tuberculosis research. Fortschritte der Tuberculoseforschung. Progrès de l'exploration de la tuberculose. Basel, 1, 1948– . (Bibliotheca tuberculosea, Fasc. 1, etc.)

Annual. Critical reviews in English, German, or French with bibliographies. v. 1–7 as *Fortschritte der Tuberkuloseforschung . . .*

1236
Ergebnisse der gesamten Tuberkulose- und Lungenforschung. Stuttgart, 1, 1930– .

Irregular. Suspended 1942–52. Title varies: 1930–56 as *Ergebnisse der gesamten Tuberkuloseforschung.*

1237
Kekkaku kenkyu no shinpo [Recent advances in tuberculosis research] Tokyo, 1, 1953– .

Irregular.

Bibliographies

1238
U.S. Veterans Administration. Medical and General Reference Library. Tuberculosis and mental illness; a selected bibliography, 1803–1952. Washington, 1953. 27 p.

Dictionaries

1239
Roloff, W. Tuberkulose-Lexikon für Ärzte und Behörden. 2 ed. Stuttgart, Georg Thieme, 1949. 372 p.

Defines terms and types of therapy, etc. Cites references. Includes biographies.

1 ed., 1943, by the Reichs-Tuberkulose-Ausschuss.

Directories

1240
American College of Chest Physicians. Membership roster. Silver anniversary ed. [9 ed.] Chicago, 1959. 964 p.

Arranged geographically by country (U.S. and foreign). Gives professional information.

1241
American Trudeau Society. Medical Section of the National Tuberculosis Association. Membership roster, 1959. New York, 1959. 88 p.

Geographic (U.S. and foreign) and alphabetic lists. Addresses only. Older lists give professional information.

1242
National Association for the Prevention of Tuberculosis and Diseases of the Chest and Heart. Handbook of tuberculosis activities. A complete directory of hospitals, sanatoria and clinics, regional hospital boards, hospital management committees and local health authorities, in the United Kingdom, the Irish Republic, and the British Commonwealth. Ed. by Harley Williams and Elizabeth Harrison. 15 ed. London, 1957, 365 p.

Histories

1243
Brown, Lawrason. The story of clinical pulmonary tuberculosis. Baltimore, Williams & Wilkins, 1941. 411 p.

Historical survey, mainly on the 18th–20th centuries, with accounts of important contributions. Bibliography, p. 382–391.

1244
Bochalli, Richard. Die Entwicklung der Tuberkuloseforschung in der Zeit von 1878 bis 1958; Rückblick eines deutschen Tuberkulosearztes. Stuttgart, Thieme, 1958. 122 p.

Review and evaluation of important contributions with emphasis on German research. Extensive references in text, but no bibliography. Lack of index hampers reference value.

1245
Burke, Richard M. An historical chronology of tuberculosis. 2 ed. Springfield, Ill., Thomas, 1955. 125 p.

From 5000 B.C. to 1953. Bibliography (general works including histories of tuberculosis and 476 reference citations): p. 81–112.

1246
Dubos, René, and Dubos, Jean. The white plague; tuberculosis, man and society. Boston, Little, Brown, 1953. 277 p.

Concerned with the incidence, and the human, social, and literary aspects of the disease, as well as the scientific. Mainly on the 19th century. General references: p. 241–242. Notes, including some references: p. 242–269.

1247
Flick, Lawrence F. Development of our knowledge of tuberculosis. Philadelphia, Wickersham Print. Co., 1925. 783 p.

Exhaustive history from the earliest times, presenting extensive summaries of and extracts from the works of important authors. Footnote references to sources; no bibliography.

1248
Piéry, Marius, and Roshem, Julien. Histoire de la tuberculose. Paris, Doin, 1931. 479 p.

Comprehensive history, from antiquity to 20th century, including the Orient. Classified bibliography of 729 items, p. 417–456.

1249
Predöhl, August. Die Geschichte der Tuberkulose. Hamburg, Voss, 1888. 502 p.

Detailed review, mainly of 19th century contributions. References to original publications throughout.

1250
Waksman, Selman A. The conquest of tuberculosis. Berkeley, University of California Press, 1964. 241 p.

Brief topical accounts of early history of the disease and its diagnosis and treatment, with about half of the book on chemotherapy, control, and conquest from 1943, based on the author's own experience. Bibliography (mainly works in English): p. 219–232.

Tularemia

Bibliographies

1251
U.S. Army Chemical Corps. Technical Library. Bibliography on tularemia. 4 ed. Fort Detrick, Md., 1958. 144 p.

Covers 1919–58.

Venereal Diseases

Indexes and Abstracts

CURRENT

1252★
Abstracts of current literature on venereal disease; an annotated bibliography. Atlanta, etc., 1952– . U.S. Public Health Service. Communicable Disease Center. Venereal Disease Branch.

Currently 3–4 times a year. Minimum time lag about 6 months.

1952–61 as *Current literature on venereal disease.*

With 1955 [no. 2] "an annotated bibliography" added to title.

1952–53 published by U.S. Public Health Service, Division of Special Health Services; 1955 [no. 2]–1956 by U.S. Public Health Service. Division of Special Health Services. Venereal Disease Program.

1956 [no. 1] Special issue. 1st International symposium on venereal diseases and the treponematoses. Washington, D.C., May 28–June 1, 1956. 164 p. Abstracts.

1253
Zentralblatt für Haut- und Geschlechtskrankheiten, sowie deren Grenzgebiete. Berlin, 1, 1921– . Kongressorgan der Deutschen dermatologischen Gesellschaft.

Currently 3–4 volumes a year in several issues a volume, including a separate index issue. A recent volume had about 1400 entries, most with abstracts. Includes books and proceedings of societies.

Subtitle: Zugleich Referatenteil des Archivs für Dermatologie und Syphilis; later, Archivs für klinische und experimentelle Dermatologie.

Continues no. 1349.

NONCURRENT

1254
Jahresbericht Haut- und Geschlechtskrankheiten. Berlin, 1–11, 1921–31.

Annual cumulation of references of no. 1253.

v. 1, 1921, as *Bibliographie der . . .*; v. 2–6, 1922–26, *Jahresbericht über . . .*

Subtitle: v. 2–6, 1922–26, Zugleich bibliographisches Jahresregister des Zentralblattes für Haut- und Geschlechtskrankheiten, sowie deren Grenzgebiete; v. 7–11, 1927–31, without "Zugleich".

Reviews

1255
Recent advances in venereology. By Ambrose King. London, Churchill, 1964. 496 p.

Chapter bibliographies (omitting titles of articles). No overall author index.

Bibliographies

1256
Alkiewicz, Jan. Materiały do polskiej bibliografii dermatologii i wenerologii; oraz ich progranicza od XVI wieku do 1951 roku [Materials of the Polish bibliography on dermatology and venerology and related fields from the 16th century up to 1951] Poznań, Państwowe wydawnictwo naukowe. 1957. 315 p.

Lists 7042 selected books and articles. Includes some entries in French, German, Russian, etc.

1257
Proksch, Johann K. Die Litteratur über die venerischen Krankheiten von den ersten Schriften über Syphilis aus dem Ende des fünfzehnten Jahrhunderts bis zum Jahre 1889 systematisch zusammengestellt. Bonn, Hanstein, 1889–91. 3 v.

Form (books, theses, bibliographies, etc.) and subject arrangement. Author index published separately.

v. 2, as . . . *bis Mitte 1889;* v. 3 . . . *bis Ende 1889.*

1258
——. ——. Supplementband I. Enthält die Litteratur von 1889–99 und Nachträge aus früherer Zeit. Bonn, Hanstein, 1900. 835 p.

Supplement, . . . *bis zum Beginn des Jahres 1899.*

1259
World Health Organization. Bibliography on yaws, 1905–1962. Bibliographie du pian, 1905–1962. Genève, 1963. 106 p.

1726 items arranged by author. Includes books and theses.

Directories

1260
World health organization. World directory of venereal-disease treatment centres at ports. Application of the International Agreement of Brussels, 1924, respecting facilities to be given to merchant seamen for the treatment of venereal disease. 2 ed. Geneva, 1961. 164 p.

Listing by country and city. Gives name of institution, address, and hours. In English and French.

Histories

1261
Bloch, Iwan. Der Ursprung der Syphilis; eine medizinische und kulturgeschichtliche Untersuchung. Jena, Fischer, 1901–11. 2 v.

Detailed study of the early history based on examination of the sources, with extensive bibliographic references in footnotes. No index.

1262
Jeanselme, Edouard. Histoire de la syphilis; son origine, son expansion. In his Traité de la syphilis, Paris, v. 1, 1931, p. 1–432.

Survey through 1930, with extensive bibliographical references to original and secondary sources in the text and in footnotes.

1263
Proksch, Johann K. Die Geschichte der venerischen Krankheiten. Bonn, Hanstein, 1895. 2 v.

Exhaustive history, from prehistoric times, with notices of authors and analyses of works, references to which are given in no. 1257. Name index only in each volume.

1264
Pusey, William A. The history and epidemiology of syphilis. Springfield, Ill., Thomas, 1933. 113 p.

Short sketch. No bibliography.

1265
Sticker, Georg. Entwurf einer Geschichte der ansteckenden Geschlechtskrankheiten. In Jadassohn, Josef, ed. Handbuch der Haut- und Geschlechtskrankheiten. Berlin, v. 23, 1931, p. 264–603; 606–616; 632–642.

Scholarly survey, arranged by special diseases and topics, including accounts of diseases historically confused with venereal diseases, paleopathology, and relations to the arts, mythology, and history. References for each section.

Yellow Fever

Bibliographies

1266
Brazil. Conselho Nacional de Pesquisas. Instituto Brasileiro de Bibliografia e Documentacão. Febre amarela; bibliografia brasileira. Rio de Janeiro, 1958. 88 p.

787 references, 1851–1957; includes monographs. Chronological arrangement.

See also no 1166.2.

History

1267
Carter, Henry R. Yellow fever; an epidemiological and historical study of its place of origin. Ed. by Laura A. Carter and Wade H. Frost. Baltimore, Williams & Wilkins, 1931. 308 p.

Detailed and comprehensive study, based on sources, illuminated by author's knowledge of the disease. Bibliography: p. 272–289.

DENTISTRY

Indexes and Abstracts

Current

1268★
Dental abstracts; a selection of world den-

tal literature. Chicago, 1, 1936– . American Dental Association

Monthly. Approximately 1000 abstracts a year. Has section: Important new books. Minimum time lag 6 months (1963).

1269★★
Index to dental literature. Chicago, etc., 1839/75– . American Dental Association and National Library of Medicine.

1950– published in four cumulations with the fourth cumulation appearing as a bound volume. Includes author listing of new books and of books reviewed. From 1961– contains a listing of dissertations and theses. Through 1927/29 contains occasional special bibliographies and historical literature surveys. Includes only material in the English language through 1961.

1839–1938 arranged by subject with author index; 1939–64 author-subject arrangement; 1965– subject with author index.

Commenced publication in 1921, with 1911/15 volume; volumes covering earlier and later years through 1949 published at irregular intervals. Literature for 1839/75, 1876/85, in two volumes; from 1886–1920 each volume covers 5 years; 1921–47, three years; 1948–49 two years. Literature for 1921 published in 1922 as a separate volume, with references later incorporated in 1921–23 volume.

1839/75–1936/38 had title *Index of the periodical dental literature*, which was also the cover title 1839/75–1948/49. 1839/75–1936/38 had subtitle: published in the English language; 1939/41–61: in the English language.

From 1965 published in cooperation with the National Library of Medicine.

1270
Indice de la literatura dental periódica en castellano y portugués. Buenos Aires, 1952– . Asociación Odontológica Argentina.

Annual. 3630 references in 1962 from 54 journals (44 Spanish, 10 Portuguese). Includes books, congresses, editorials, biographies, obituaries. Author-subject arrangements in one alphabet.

1271
Oral research abstracts. Chicago, 1, 1966– . American Dental Association.

Monthly. Includes nondental journals. First issue contains 613 abstracts.

1272
Periodontal abstracts; the journal of the Western Society of Periodontology. Los Angeles, 1, 1953– .

Quarterly. v. 12, 1964, contains 272 abstracts. v. 1–12, 1953–64, as *Journal of the Western Society of Periodontology.*

1273
Stomatology references; current medical literature; annotated title review. New York, 1, 1963– . Columbia University, School of Dental and Oral Surgery, William Jarvie Society.

1273.1
Zentralblatt für die gesamte Zahn- Mund- und Kieferheilkunde. Leipzig, 1, 1936– . In Deutsche Zahn- Mund- und Kieferheilkunde; mit Zentralblatt für die gesamte Zahn- Mund- und Kieferheilkunde. Leipzig, 11, 1948– . Deutsche Gesellschaft für Zahn- Mund- und Kieferheilkunde.

A sample volume listed approximately 1000 references, most with abstracts.

v. 1–9, 1936–44, issued separately. Suspended 1945–47. Assumed volume number (11) of *Deutsche Zahn-* . . . in 1948.

Continues no. 1277.

Noncurrent

1274
D.D.S. Digest of dental science. New York, 1–2, Oct. 1952–June 1953.

About 30 articles abstracted per issue.

1275
Dental abstracts. New York [ser. 1] 1941–44; [ser. 2] 1–6, 1945–50.

Ser. 1 and ser. 2, v. 1–2, sponsored by the Dental Abstracts Society of the Columbia University School of Dental and Oral Surgery. Beginning Feb. 1947, became official publication of the Columbia University School of Dental and Oral Surgery.

1276
Eichler, Max. Index der deutschen und wichtigsten ausländischen zahnärztlichen Literatur. Bonn, Georgi, 1904. 177 p.

6000 items.

1277
Index der deutschen und ausländischen zahnärztlichen Literatur und zahnärztlichen Bibliographie. Müchen, etc., 1902–

1934. Im Auftrage des Zentral-Vereins deutscher Zahnärzte.

Consists of approximately 100,000 numbered references to the German literature and the foreign literature principally as abstracted in German sources. Includes monographs, biographies, and obituaries.

1902 has title: *Index der deutschen zahnärztlichen Literatur und zahnärztlichen Bibliographie; umfassend die Literatur bis zum Jahre 1902*. Originally published as Lieferung 1–9, 1909–10. Covers the literature from 1847–1902.

1903–14 and 1930 has title: *Index der deutschen zahnärztlichen Literatur und zahnärztlichen Bibliographie*; 1915/18, *Index der deutschen und ausländischen zahnärztlichen Literatur.*

1278
Literaturarchiv der gesamte Zahnheilkunde. Leipzig, 1–9, 1925–33.

1929 volume had in excess of 1900 abstracts. Includes monographs and theses; covers general medicine. v. 5 has subject index to v. 1–5.

Forms second part of *Die Fortschritte der Zahnheilkunde nebst Literaturarchiv*. . .(not listed).

1279 (not used)

Reviews

1280
Advances in fluorine research and dental caries prevention. New York. [1] 1962– .

Comprises proceedings of the Congress of the European Organization for Research on Fluorine and Dental Caries Prevention, 9th, 1962– .

1281
Advances in oral biology. New York, Academic Press, 1, 1964– .

1282
Modern trends in dental surgery. Washington, 1, 1963– .

Each chapter reviews a field of dentistry in which there has been significant progress in fundamental concepts or method of treatment. Some with bibliographies.

1283
Progresos en la practica odontologica. Buenos Aires, 1, 1944– .

Irregular. 1944–47, as *Progresos anuales en la practica odontologica.*

1284
Shika kokugeka saikin no shinpo [Recent advances in dentistry and oral surgery] Tokyo, 1, 1956– .

Irregular.

1285★
Year book of dentistry. Chicago, Year Book Medical Publishers, 1936– . (The practical medicine year books)

Abstracts, with editorial comment.

Bibliographies

1286
Afonsky, D., comp. Saliva and its relation to oral health; a survey of the world literature. University, Ala., University of Alabama Press, 1961. 785 p.

1287
Bagnall, J. Stanley. Bibliography on caries research. Ottawa, National Research Council of Canada, 1950. 557 p.

Review of the literature, p. 1–448; references (2274) p. 449–557. Covers the period 1883–1948.

1288
Bernadskiĭ, Iuriĭ I. Sovetskaia stomatologicheskaia literatura [Soviet stomatological literature] Moskva, Medgiz, 1951–65. 2 v. 672, 696 p.

v. 1, 1951, covers the literature from 1917–45; v. 2, 1965, with 8207 entries, covers 1946–58.

1289
Brislin, Jane F., and Cox, Gerald J. Survey of the literature of dental caries, 1948–1960. Pittsburgh, University of Pittsburgh Press, 1964. 762 p.

3755 references, most with abstracts. Intended as the successor to no. 1287. Chronological arrangement, references cited alphabetically by author under year. Author and subject indexes.

1290
Campbell, J. Menzies. A dental bibliography: British and American, 1682–1880. London, David Low, 1949. 63 p.

Lists 723 books and pamphlets chronologically. Omits paging and publisher. No annotations.

1291
Crowley, C. George. Dental bibliogra-

phy: a standard reference list of books on dentistry published throughout the world from 1536 to 1885. Philadelphia, White, 1885. 180 p.

2047 items in chronological arrangement, with index of authors. Limited to Western Europe and America. The proposed classified list was never published.

1292
Fastlicht, Samuel. Bibliografía odontológica mexicana. México, La Prensa Médica mexicana, 1954. 220 p.

Describes 46 monographs, 37 periodicals, and lists 1635 theses from 1552 to 1950.

1293
David, Théophile. Bibliographie française de l'art dentaire. Paris, Alcan, 1889. 307 p.

3000 items. Includes books, theses. From about A.D. 1595.

1294
International Dental Federation. Special Commission on Oral and Dental Statistics. Epidemiology of selected dental conditions, 1950–1963. Ed. by Maynard K. Hine; comp. by L. Robert Newburn. [Indianapolis, 1964?] 124 p.

1500 citations to the monographic and periodical literature on dental caries, periodontal disease, malocclusion, and cleft lip and cleft palate. Country arrangement under each subject. No author or subject index.

1295
Martínez Sánchez, José. Bibliografía de la odontología española. Índice para formar un catálogo razanado, de las obras impresas en castellano que tratan sobre el arte del dentista. Madrid, Imprenta de La Odontología, 1911. 63 p.

Lists monographs by author, periodicals, congresses, society publications, etc., with appendix of reference works, bibliographies, etc. relating to dentistry; and a chronology of the publications, 1557–1911.

1296
National Research Council. A survey of the literature of dental caries. Prepared for the Food and Nutrition Board, National Research Council, under the supervision of the Committee on Dental Health . . . by Guttorm Toverud, et al. Washington, National Academy of Sciences—National Research Council, 1952. 567 p. (National Research Council. Publication 225).

Comprehensive review articles. Bibliography.

1297
Poletti, Gian B. De re dentaria apud veteres, sive Repertorium bibliographicum . . . 2 ed. Ed. by Lamberto Diotallevi. Mediolani, Görlich, 1951. 213 p.

Through 1900. Arranged by author, with occasional extensive notes. Includes some general works on medicine and surgery which have chapters on dentistry. Bibliography of dental bibliographies: p. 209–[214].

1298
Sternfeld, Alfred, and Kellner, Karl. Zahnärztliche Bücherkunde; bibliographisches Verzeichniss von Büchern, akademischen und sonstigen Abhandlungen, sowie der in medizinischen und naturwissenschafflichen Zeitschriften veröffentlichten Aufsatze. Karlsruhe, 1891. 211 p.

1299
Strömgren, Hedvig L. Index of dental and adjacent topics in medical and surgical works before 1800. Copenhagen, Munksgaard, 1955. 255 p. (Copenhagen. University Library. Scientific and Medical Department. Library Research monographs, v. 4)

Author list, subject index. Contains a few items published after 1800. Cites page references to dental material in nondental monographs.

1300
Taft, Jonathan. Index to the periodical literature of dental science and art, as presented in the English language. Philadelphia, Blakiston, 1886. 212 p.

Contains a chronologic bibliography of dental periodicals; a subject index to the periodical literature but without author and title of article; and an author index. Covers the period from 1839 to 1885, and includes some journals not in no. 1269.

1301
U.S. Library of Congress. Science and Technology Division. Bibliography Section. Bibliography on saliva. Washington, Office of Naval Research, 1960. 447 p.

(U.S. Office of Naval Research. ONR report, ACR-48)

1302
Vályi, Edit. Magyar stomatológiai bibliográfia (1945–1960) [Bibliography of Hungarian stomatology (1945–1960)] Budapest, Országos Orvostudományi Könyvtár és Dokumentációs Központ, 1961. 568 p.

4459 references, including books. Chronological subarrangement.

1303
U.S. Public Health Service. Division of Dental Public Health and Resources. Psychology in dentistry; selected references and abstracts. [Prepared by L. R. Borland et al.] Washington, 1962. 202 p. (Public Health Service. Publication no. 929. Bibliography series no. 35)

661 articles listed, most with abstracts. A few books and theses listed separately. Includes psychology of dentist and patient, education in psychology and psychiatry for the dentist, hypnosis, habits in relationship to dental conditions (thumb-sucking, etc.) Most of the references are from the late 1940's through 1961.

1304
Weber, Andrés G. Bibliographiae stomatologicae. Buffalo, 1922. 41 p.

A chronological list of dental bibliographies, 1530–1921. Most entries have annotations, some extensive.

Reprinted from no. 1269, 1916/20, p. xiv–liii.

1305
Weinberger, Bernhard W. Dental bibliography; a reference index to the literature of dental science and art as found in the libraries of the New York Academy of Medicine and Bernhard Wolf Weinberger. Pt. [1]–2. New York, First District Dental Society, State of New York, 1929–32. 183, 262 p.

Pt. 1, an author list, includes books, theses and periodical titles, but not periodical articles. Also contains Dental periodicals on file in the Academy of Medicine (p. 148–78) and Medical classics containing dental citations (p. 178–82). Pt. 2 consists of additional literature of dental science and an updated list of periodicals, Earliest dental books published 1530–1810 (chronological arrangement), and the subject index.

Pt. 1 is 2 ed. Pt. 2 as *Dental bibliography; a subject index . . .*

Dictionaries

1306
Academy of Denture Prosthetics. Nomenclature Committee. Glossary of prosthodontic terms. 1 ed. St. Louis, Journal of Prosthetic Dentistry, 1956. 34 p.

Terms with their special connotations in prosthodontics; choice of term is based on majority opinion.

1307★
Boucher, Carl O., ed. Current clinical dental terminology; a glossary of accepted terms in all disciplines of dentistry. St. Louis, Mosby, 1963. 501 p.

10,000 terms; contains further listing by subject and discipline.

1307.1
China (People's Republic) Wei shêng pu [Ministry of Health] K'ou ch'iang i hsüeh ming tz'ŭ [Glossary of terms in dentistry] Peking, 1955. 74 p.

Chinese-English, English-Chinese.

1308
Denton, George B. The vocabulary of dentistry and oral science, a manual for the study of dental nomenclature. Chicago, American Dental Association, 1958. 207 p.

Pts. 1–3 discuss foundations of scientific language (including list of combining forms) and nomenclature problems; pt. 4, selected dental vocabulary with critical notes.

1309
Durante Avellanal, Ciro, and Durante, M. I. Diccionario odontológico. Buenos Aires, Ediar, 1955. 739 p.

Comprehensive; includes some medical and pharmaceutical terms; contains abbreviations, biographical sketches, some portraits.

1310
Harris, Chapin A. A dictionary of dental science and such words and phrases of the collateral sciences as pertain to the art and practice of dentistry. [1]–6 ed. Philadelphia, Blakiston, 1849–98.

Comprehensive. Abbreviations. Biographies

are primarily of American dentists and include bibliographies.

1 ed. has title, *A dictionary of dental science, biography, bibliography, and medical terminology*; 2–4 ed., *A dictionary of medical terminology, dental surgery and the collateral sciences.* 3–6 ed. rev. by Ferdinand J. S. Gorgas.

1311
Heinemann modern dictionary for dental students. Comp. by Jenifer E. H. Fowler. London, Heinemann, 1952. 364 p.

1312
Hoffman-Axthelm, Walter, ed. Zahnärztliches Lexikon. Leipzig, 1962. 552 p.

Includes some medical terms; biographical sketches.

1312.1
Lexicon of English dental terms; with their equivalents in español, deutsch, français, italiano. Comp. by the Fédération Dentaire Internationale. The Hague, A. Sijthoff, 1966. 424 p.

7122 terms including some medical and technological words.

1313
Marie, Joseph S. F. English-Spanish, Spanish-English dental vocabulary; including many medical terms. Lancaster, Pa., Cattell, 1943. 159 p.

Equivalent terms.

1313.1
Moortgat, Paul. Odonto-stomatologie. Syndromes à noms propres. Paris, Prélat, 1966. 46 p.

No references.

1314
Scartezzini, Carmelino. Diccionário odontológico (contendo têrmos de medecina, farmácia, diagnósticos, fórmulas, produtos químicos e farmacêuticos, etc.) 2 ed. Rio de Janeiro, Editôra Cientifica, 1955. 471 p.

Portuguese dictionary of approximately 15,000 terms.

1315
Terra, Paul de. Manual of conversation for the dental profession: collection of professional terms and phrases in German, English, French and Italian. 2 ed. Stuttgart, Enke, 1922. 274 p.

Parallel columns of the four languages; pt. 1, terms commonly used; pt. 2, expressions and conversation. Index for each language.

Directories

Practicing dentists are usually listed in the medical directory of each country.

1316
Admission requirements of American dental schools. Chicago, 1, 1964/65– . American Association of Dental Schools.

Arranged by state; data include address, name of dean, entrance and acceptance requirements, fees, housing and financial aid. Information for Canadian schools given. 2 ed., 1965/66.

1317
American College of Dentists. Register of membership, as of January 1, 1963. St. Louis, Mo., 1963. 91 p.

Alphabetical and geographical listings with addresses.

1318★★
American dental directory. Chicago, 1947– . American Dental Association.

Annual. Arranged by state and city with name and address; professional data given in code. Lists dental schools, dental hygiene schools, officials of the American Dental Association, state dental organizations, examining boards in dental specialties, licensure requirements for dentists and dental hygienists, dental internships and residencies, national dental organizations, dental specialists. Includes name index. Triennial through 1953.

1319
Annuaire dentaire. Paris, [1] 1936– .

Alphabetical listing of practicing dentists with brief professional information. Lists officials, associations, schools. Includes overseas territories. 26 ed., 1965. 1017 p.

1320
Canadian Dental Association. Directory. Liste de membres. Toronto, 1, 1950?–

Frequency varies. Names and addresses of members, arranged by province. Includes list of dental schools, members of special dental societies, and list of dental hygienists. Continues the association's *List of members.*

1321
The Dentists register. London, 1879– . General Dental Council.

Annual. Alphabetical listing of dental practitioners registered in the United Kingdom, the Commonwealth, and those holding a foreign diploma. Gives brief professional data.

Issued 1879–1922 by the General Council of Medical Education and Registration; 1923–56, by the Dental Board of the United Kingdom.

1322
Deutsches zahnärztliches Adressbuch. [1 ed.] Dortmund-Mengede, 195?– . Bundesverband der deutschen Zahnärzte.

Geographical arrangement; gives very brief professional information.

1323
Indian dentists register. New Delhi, Dental Council of India, 1952?– .

Alphabetical listings of dentists registered under the Dentists Act of 1948, with brief professional information.

1961 ed., 241 p.; suppl. 1, 1961; suppl. 2, 1963.

1324
Oral surgery directory of the world. W. Harry Archer, ed.-in-chief. Pittsburgh, Pa., 1957. 298 p.

Professional data for oral surgeons in the United States: names and addresses for foreign surgeons; includes listing of members of American Society of Oral Surgeons, dental schools and professors of oral surgery, hospital dental internships and residencies.

1325
Orthodontic directory of the world. Nashville, 1, 1920– .

United States listing arranged by state and city, followed by Canada and other countries. Name index. Includes short lists of schools and societies. Other countries p. 199–254. World coverage, but limited to 1 or 2 names for countries such as Iran, Iraq, Korea, Morocco, etc.

22 ed., 1964, ed. by William H. Oliver. 1–2 ed. as *Orthodontic directory of America.*

1326
Polk's Dental register and directory of the United States and Dominion of Canada. Chicago, 1–14, 1893–1928.

Arranged by state; includes state laws and a list of dental colleges and societies.

1326.1
Svenska tandläkare. Stockholm, P. A. Norstedt, 1963. 515 p.

Brief professional data. Includes photographs.

1326.2
Svenska tandläkare i ord och bild. Stockholm, Biografiskt Galleri, 1939. 583 p. Supplements, 1948–54.

Brief professional data. Includes photographs.

1327
Who's who in American dentistry. Ed. by Alvin J. Debré. Los Angeles, Dale Dental Publishing Company, 1963. 198 p.

Alphabetical listing of 6000 dentists, gives personal and professional data.

1328
Who's who in dentistry; biographical sketches of prominent dentists in the United States and Canada. Ed. by Samuel Greif, New York, Who's who Dental Publishing Co., 1916–25. 2 v.

Personal and professional data, including bibliographies. v. 2 is enlarged ed. of v. 1.

1329★
World directory of dental schools. Geneva, World Health Organization, 1, 1961– .

Arranged alphabetically by country. Gives number of dentists, general information on enrollment, admission, curriculum, examinations, and licensure. Lists institutions with addresses, year founded, teaching staff, enrollment, annual admissions, graduates and tuition fees.

Periodicals

1330
Schmidt, H. J. Index der zahnärztlichen Zeitschriften der Welt. Stuttgart, Deutsche Dokumentenstelle für zahnärztliches Schrifttum, 1962. 126 p.

Arranged by country. Includes address of publisher, beginning date, and frequency.

Histories

1331
American Academy of Dental Science, Boston. A history of dental and oral science in America. Philadelphia, White, 1876. 271 p.

Pioneer study, ed. by James E. Dexter. Includes progress of practical and scientific dentistry, societies, and education. Annotated lists of standard works and periodicals: p. 215–235. No index.

1332
Colyer, Sir James Frank. Old instruments used for extracting teeth. London, Staples Press, 1952. 245 p.

Careful, detailed study. Bibliography (works consulted): p. 224–235.

1333
Guerini, Vincenzo. A history of dentistry from the most ancient times until the end of the eighteenth century. Philadelphia, Lea & Febiger, 1909. 355 p.

Bibliographical footnotes. Includes detailed analyses of key works.

1334
Koch, Charles R. E. History of dental surgery. Fort Wayne, National Art Pub. Co., 1910. 3 v.

The most detailed and comprehensive history. Includes chapters on dental specialties, literature, education, legislation, societies, and jurisprudence. v. 3: Biographies of pioneer American dentists and their successors, by B. L. Thorpe. The sketches of the earliest men are superseded by Weinberger (no. 1345).

1335
Lufkin, Arthur W. A history of dentistry. 2 ed. Philadelphia, Lea & Febiger, 1948. 367 p.

Brief survey by periods and countries, followed by chapters on dental caries, the specialties in dentistry, and mechanical progress, with a historical sketch of anesthesia by W. Harry Archer. References at ends of chapters.

1336
McCluggage, Robert W. A history of the American Dental Association; a century of health service. Chicago, American Dental Association, 1959. 520 p.

Study of development of organized dentistry, placing the Association in its historical context. References, p. 442–507.

1337
McNeil, Donald R. The fight for fluoridation. New York, Oxford University Press, 1957. 241 p.

References and bibliography: p. 199–236.

1338
Pindborg, Jens J., and Marvitz, Leif. The dentist in art. Chicago, Quadrangle Books, 1960. 144 p.

Includes 60 illustrations. Index of illustrations by artist only. Translation of *Tandlaegen i kunsten*, København, 1959.

1339
Prinz, Hermann. Dental chronology; a record of the more important events in the evolution of dentistry. Philadelphia, Lea & Febiger, 1945. 189 p.

1340
Proskauer, Curt. Iconographia odontologica. Berlin, Meusser, 1926. 231 p. (Kulturgeschichte der Zahnheilkunde in Einzeldarstellungen, 4)

Chiefly illustrations.

1341
——, and Witt, Fritz H. Bildgeschichte der Zahnheilkunde; Zeugnisse aus 5 Jahrtausenden . . . Köln, DuMont Schauberg, 1962. 220 p.

With 196 illustrations. Brief text in German, English, French, Italian, and Spanish. English title: *Pictorial history of dentistry.* Bibliography: p. 219–220.

1342
Strömgren, Hedvig L. Die Zahnheilkunde im achtzehnten Jahrhundert; ein Stück Kulturgeschichte. Kopenhagen, Levin & Munksgaard, 1935. 232 p.

Biographical notes: p. 219–227. Bibliography: p. 228–230.

1343
——. Die Zahnheilkunde im neunzehnten Jahrhundert. Kopenhagen, Munksgaard, 1945. 274 p.

Accounts of special topics and specialties, with a chapter on teaching, organizations, and periodicals. Bibliography: p. 267–269.

1344
Sudhoff, Karl F. J. Geschichte der Zahnheilkunde. 2 ed. Leipzig, Barth, 1926. 222 p.

Includes ancient and primitive dentistry. Emphasis on period to 1600, with brief treatment of 17th–19th centuries. Short bibliographies by chapter. Reprinted Hildesheim, 1963.

1345
Weinberger, Bernhard W. An introduction to the history of dentistry with medical and dental chronology and bibliographic data. St. Louis, Mosby, 1948. 2 v.

Survey to early 19th century. v. 2 covers U.S., with special section on George Washington. References at ends of chapters. Bibliographies (sources and secondary works): v. 1, p. 408–473; v. 2, p. 366–379.

1346
——. Orthodontics: an historical review of its origin and evolution, including an extensive bibliography of orthodontic literature up to the time of specialization. St. Louis, Mosby, 1926. 2 v.

Comprehensive history, from prehistoric times to 1900. Detailed accounts of key contributions, often with extensive quotations. References at ends of chapters. Author bibliography of orthodontic literature, 1728–1900: v. 2, p. 909–983.

DERMATOLOGY

Indexes and Abstracts

Current

1347
Bibliograficheskiĭ ukazatel' sovetskoĭ dermatologii i venerologii [Bibliographic index to Soviet dermatology and venerology] Moskva, [1] 1900/31– .

Includes books, proceedings of societies. v. 2, 1951, covers the period 1932–38; v. 3, 1958, covers 1939–50. v. 4, 1964, covering 1951–61, consists of 863 pages. v. 1, published in 1935, has title: *Bibliograficheskii ukazatel' russkoi dermatologii i venerologii.*

1348
Referátový výběr z dermatovenerologie a příbuzných oborů [Selected abstracts on dermatology and venerology and related fields] Praha, 1, 1959– . Ústav pro zdravotnickou dokumentaci.

Quarterly. Covers the foreign literature. Title in Czech or Slovak and in the original language; abstracts in Czech or Slovak. Includes a geographical list of newly published books.

Noncurrent

1348.1
Dermatologischer Jahresbericht. Wiesbaden, 1–4, 1905–8.

References with selective reviews following. v. 4 listed approximately 8550 references.

1349
Dermatologisches Centralblatt. Internationale Rundschau auf dem Gebiete der Haut- und Geschlechtskrankheiten. Leipzig, 1–23, 1897–1920.

Abstracts. Includes books, literature reviews, and brief reports of papers of dermatological interest presented at meetings of societies. Continued as no. 1253.

1350
Quarterly review of dermatology and syphilology. Washington, 1–3, 1946–48. Washington Institute of Medicine.

Abstracts. Does not include gonorrhea.
Merged into no. 35 in 1950.

Reviews

1351
Hifuka saikin no shinpo. [Recent advances in dermatology] Tokyo, 1, 1955– .

Irregular.

1351.1
Modern trends in dermatology. 3 [ed.] Ed. by R. M. B. MacKenna. Washington, Butterworths, 1966. 338 p.

Reviews with bibliographies (omitting titles of journal articles).
1 [ed.] 1948, 2 [ed.] 1954.

1352
Recent advances in dermatology. 2 ed. By W. Noel Goldsmith and Francis F. Hellier. London, Churchill, 1954. 461 p.

Chapter bibliographies (omitting titles of articles). No overall author index.
1 ed., 1936.

1353★
Year book of dermatology. Chicago, 1902– . (The practical medicine year books)

Abstracts, with editorial comment.
1902–06 as *Skin and venereal diseases. Nervous and mental diseases*; 1907–21 as *Skin and*

venereal diseases; 1922 as *Dermatology and syphilis . . . genito-urinary diseases*; 1923?–31 as *Dermatology and syphilis . . . urology*; 1932 as *Dermatology and syphilology*; 1933–59 as *Year book of dermatology and syphilology*.

1902–05, 1932 as Practical medicine series of year books; 1906–31 Practical medicine series.

Bibliographies

1354
Faragó, László, and Nékám, Lajos. Magyar börgyógyászati és venerológiai bibliográfia (1945–1960) [Bibliography of Hungarian dermatology and venerology (1945–1960)] Budapest, Országos Orvostudományi Könyvtár és Dokumentációs Központ, 1962. 668 p.

5113 references, including books. Chronological subarrangement.

Dictionaries

1355
Butterworth, Thomas, and Strean, Lyon P. Manual of dermatologic syndromes. New York, McGraw-Hill, 1964. 76 p.

Approximately 200 syndromes with synonyms.

Directories

1356
Löhe, Heinrich, and Langer, Erich. Die Dermatologen deutscher Sprache. Bio-bibliographisches Verzeichnis. Berlin, Berliner Medizinische Verlagsanstalt GMBH, 1955. 391 p.

Brief professional data. Extensive coverage of publications since 1929, including periodical articles. Alphabetical city index and list of dermatological clinics in Germany.

1356.1
Riecke, Erhard. Deutsches Dermatologen-Verzeichnis; Lebens- und Leistungsschau. 2 ed. Leipzig, Barth, 1939. 314 p.

Same content and arrangement as 1356. Includes earlier publications.

1 ed., 1929, as *Deutscher Dermatologenkalender; biographisch-bibliographisches Dermatologen-Verzeichnis*.

Histories

1357
Bechet, Paul E. History of the American Dermatological Association in commemoration of its seventy-fifth anniversary, 1876–1951. New York, Froben Press, 1952. 392 p.

History, lists of officers and meetings, and brief biographies (p. 53–358) of some 300 dermatologists, chronologically arranged. No index.

1358
Pusey, William A. The history of dermatology. Springfield, Ill., Thomas, 1933. 223 p.

Survey from ancient times to the present. "Historical index of dermatology" (with bibliographical references): p. 176–211.

1359
Richter, Paul. Geschichte der Dermatologie. In Jadassohn, Josef, ed. Handbuch der Haut- und Geschlechtskrankheiten, Berlin, v. 14, pt. 2, 1928, p. 1–252.

Detailed history, with analyses of contributions of important authors. Bibliography: p. 248–252. Indexed with the name and subject indexes for v. 14.

1360
Shelley, Walter B., and Crissey, John T., ed. Classics in clinical dermatology, with biographical sketches. Springfield, Ill., Thomas, 1953. 467 p.

Translated excerpts of writings from Robert Willan to 1944, with brief notices of authors and their publications.

DIAGNOSIS

Indexes and Abstracts

1361
Jahresbericht über die Fortschritte der Diagnostik. Leipzig, 1–10, 1894–1903.

Abstracts.

Bibliographies

1362
Graziano, Eugene E. Medical diagnosis with electronic computers; an annotated bibliography. Sunnyvale, Calif., Lockheed Missiles and Space Co., 1963. (Its Special bibliography, SB-63-8, April 1963)

125 references, listed by author. Covers 1953–

62. Issued by the Defense Documentation Center.

Dictionaries

1362.1
China (People's Republic) Wei shêng pu [Ministry of Health] Chên tuan hsüeh ming tz'ŭ [Glossary of diagnostic terms] Peking, 1954. 53 p.

Chinese-English, English-Chinese.

1363
Robertson, Harold F., and Gabriel, H. W. Clinical diagnosary. Philadelphia, Hercules Publishing Co., 1964. 476 p.

Pt. 1: Diseases and conditions alphabetically listed with description and identification; pt. 2: Irregularities and abnormalities, alphabetically listed followed by identification of the disease it signifies; pt. 3: Signs, reflexes, phenomena, complexes, and syndromes, alphabetically listed with description and identification of the disease. Contains almost 8,000 entries.

1364
Watanabe, Yoshitaka. Shokomei jiten [Dictionary of terms in symptomatology] Urawa, Chugai Isho, 1955. 577 p.

English terms followed by Japanese definitions (in Japanese characters). Contains primarily terms used in diagnosis, eponyms, syndromes, and tests. Extensive Japanese-English index.

EDUCATION, MEDICAL

Indexes and Abstracts

1365
Bibliography on medical education, [1964]- . In Journal of medical education, v. 41, 1966- .

Monthly with annual cumulations. Consists of citations derived from the National Library of Medicine's MEDLARS program.

Bibliographies

1365.1
U.S. National Library of Medicine. Bibliography on medical education for 1964 and 1965; an index to the world literature related to education for medicine. Bethesda, 1966. 249 p.

Issued as J. Med. Educ. v. 41(11, pt. 2) Nov. 1966.

Includes references for late 1963.

1366
World Health Organization. Medical education; annotated bibliography, 1946–1955. Geneva, 1958. 391 p.

2571 items listed.

Manuals

1366.1
Educational Council for Foreign Medical Graduates. Handbook for foreign medical graduates. Evanston, Ill., 1965. 132 p.

Sections on eligibility, examinations, residency, hospital practices, etc.

Directories

1367★★
Association of American Medical Colleges. Medical school admission requirements, U.S.A. and Canada. Evanston, Ill., 1951- .

Annual listing of United States and Canadian colleges arranged by state or province. Gives address, name of dean, general information, entrance requirements, application procedure, expenses, financial aid. Includes chapters on planning for medical careers, the medical specialties, and the medical school admission process; lists recommended reading for students. 17 ed., 1966/67.

1951–1964/65 as *Admission requirements of American medical colleges, including Canada.*

1367.1
——. Division of Business Affairs. Financial assistance available for graduate study in medicine. 7. ed. Evanston, 1963. 666 p.

Mainly Canada and U.S. Includes awards for writing, research, etc.

1368
CME Continuing medical education: medical symposia. Los Angeles, 1, 1963- . Current Medical Information, Inc.

Quarterly. Contents based upon official programs and announcements furnished by medical schools, universities, hospitals, and pharmaceutical houses. Arranged chronologically with subject and geographic index.

1369
Directory of administrative staff, depart-

ment chairmen and individual members in medical schools of the United States and Canada. Evanston, Ill., 1964– . Association of American Medical Colleges.

Arranged alphabetically by school; address, enrollment and clinical facilities given.

1370★★
Directory of approved internships and residencies. Chicago, 1947– . American Medical Association. Council on Medical Education and Hospitals.

Includes information on the National Intern Matching Program, essentials of approved internship and residencies, requirements for licensure and for certification by American specialty boards, and list of corresponding officers of boards of medical examiners in the United States. In lists of internships and residencies hospitals are arranged geographically by state and city and include number of positions offered and yearly salary.

Published separately since 1961; formerly given in condensed form in the internship and residency number of the *Journal of the American Medical Association.*

Title varies.

1371
Directory of medical colleges in India, 1964 [3 ed.] New Delhi, 1965. 380 p. Central Bureau of Health Intelligence.

Lists medical, nursing, and dental schools and colleges. Arranged by province. Gives history, attached hospitals, rules for admission, scholarships, prizes, number of graduates in recent years, library facilities (including number of books and journals), etc.

Continues in part no. 1371.2.

1371.1
The hospital atlas; announcements of . . . internships and residencies. Columbus, 1, 1953– .

1–12 ed., 1953–64, as *Major hospital atlas.* 14 ed., 1966.

1371.2
Medical colleges and training institutions in India. [1960] 2 ed. New Delhi, 1961. 381 p. Directorate General of Health Services, Ministry of Health.

Gives approximately the same information for schools as no. 1371. Lists Government and private research institutions. Chronological list of schools and research institutions, 1824–1960, p. 1–4.

1 ed. 1958. Continued in part by no. 1371.

1372★★
World directory of medical schools. Geneva, World Health Organization, 1, 1953–

3 ed., 1963, lists institutions in 87 countries. General information on number of physicians, administration of the schools, conditions of admission, curriculum, examinations, qualification, and licensure, followed by a list of institutions with addresses, year founded, teaching staff, enrollment, admissions, graduates, and tuition fees.

2 ed., 1957.

Histories

1373
Bonner, Thomas N. American doctors and German universities; a chapter in international intellectual relations, 1870–1914. Lincoln, Univ. of Nebraska Press, 1963. 210 p.

Thorough, balanced, documented. References and bibliography.

1374
Bowers, John Z. Medical education in Japan, from Chinese medicine to Western medicine. New York, Harper & Row, 1965. 174 p.

Includes review of history of medicine and medical education (p. 1–45). Bibliography includes history (p. 163–165).

1375
Lesky, Erna. Die Wiener medizinische Schule im 19. Jahrhundert. Graz-Köln, Böhlaus, 1965, 660 p. (Studien zur Geschichte der Universität Wien, v. 6)

The central role of Vienna makes this valuable for much of 19th century medicine. Lists of sources and references at ends of sections.

1376
Newman, Charles. The evolution of medical education in the nineteenth century. London, Oxford University Press, 1957. 340 p.

Covers Great Britain. Includes much information on professional history. References and notes: p. 311–327.

1377
Norwood, William F. Medical education in the United States before the Civil War. Philadelphia, University of Pennsylvania Press, 1944. 487 p.

Detailed, documented study, including broad trends and data on virtually every school. Bibliography (mostly sources): p. 435–462.

1378
Puschmann, Theodor. A history of medical education from the most remote to the most recent times. Tr. and ed. by E. H. Hare. London, Lewis, 1891. 650 p.

Comprehensive study, including the Orient and North America. Includes surveys of the teaching of special subjects and of education in various countries. Bibliographical footnotes; index of personal names only. Translation of *Geschichte der medicinischen Unterrichts von den ältesten Zeiten bis zur Gegenwart*, Leipzig, 1889, with some additional material on the United Kingdom. Reprinted New York, Hafner, 1966.

ENDOCRINOLOGY

Indexes and Abstracts

1379
Bibliographia neuroendocrinologica. Philadelphia, 1, 1964– . Albert Einstein College of Medicine. Dept of Anatomy.

Irregular. 631 abstracts thru v. 1, no. 3. Author listing; keyword index.

1380
Referátový výběr z endokrinologie [Selected abstracts on endocrinology] Praha, 1, 1957(?)– . Ústav pro zdravotnickou dokumentaci.

4 issues a year. Abstracts in Czech or Slovak. Frequently includes bibliographies and general reviews of the field. Issues for 1960 contain approximately 400 abstracts.

Reviews

1381
Advances in thryoid research. New York, Pergamon [1] 1961– .

Transactions of the International Goiter Conference, 4th, 1960– .

1382
Année endocrinologique. Paris, Libraires de l'Academie de Médecine, 1, 1949– .

Annual.

1383
Modern trends in endocrinology. New York, 1, 1958– . (Hoeber's Modern trends series)

Irregular. Ser. 2 published 1961. Reviews with bibliographies.

1384
Recent progress in hormone research. New York, Academic Press, 1, 1947– .

Annual. Proceedings of the Laurentian Hormone Conference.

1385★
Year book of endocrinology. Chicago, Year Book Medical Publishers, 1934– . (The practical medicine year books)

Abstracts with editorial comment.

1934–45 as *Year book of neurology, psychiatry and endocrinology*; 1946–49 *Year book of endocrinology, metabolism and nutrition*.

Bibliographies

1386
Airapetian, T. Ia., and Kagramanian, K. A. Zob; bibliograficheskiĭ ukazatel' za 1954–1958 gg. [Goiter; bibliographic index to literature from 1954 to 1958] Erivan, Resp. nauchno-meditsinskaia biblioteka, 1960. 41 p.

374 books, collected works, their chapters or parts, abstracts of dissertations, and journal articles in the Russian language. Summaries in non-Russian languages are indicated for each entry.

1386.1
Bernstein, Seymour, et al. Steroid conjugates; a bibliography. [Columbus, Ohio] Chemical Abstracts Service, 1966. 336 p.

2404 abstracts confined primarily to sulfate and glucuronide conjugates, covering chemical and detoxication and transport mechanisms, intermediate metabolism, biological activity *per se*, and diagnosis, etiology, and treatment of pathological disorders. Earliest references noted 1907.

1386.2
Chilean Iodine Educational Bureau. Endemic goitre; world distribution and incidence, select bibliography. London, 1958. 104 p.

1014 entries. Geographic arrangement.

1387
Ganis, Frank M. et al., comp. A selective

bibliography on the endocrine response to ionizing radiation. Rochester, University of Rochester Atomic Energy Project [1963] 361 p. (AEC Research and Development Report UR610)

References listed by author under organ. Current through January 1962. No author or subject index.

1388
Kitay, Julian I., and Altschule, Mark D. The pineal gland; a review of the physiologic literature. Cambridge, Harvard University Press, 1954. 280 p.

Review section and bibliography of 1762 items. Includes books, chapters in books, and theses.
Published for the Commonwealth Fund.

1389
Köves, Péter. Az endokrinológia és az anyagcserebetegségek magyar bibliográfiája (1945–1960) [Hungarian bibliography on endocrinology and metabolic diseases (1945–1960)] Budapest, Országos Orvostudományi Könyvtár és Dokumentácios Központ, 1965. 506 p.

3241 entries published in Hungary or by Hungarians abroad in any language. Includes books.

1390
Mikyška, J., and Blehová, E. Endokrinologická: literatura; bibliografický soupis článků ze zahraničnich časopisů za rok 1955 [Literature on endocrinology; a bibliographic index of foreign journal articles from the year 1955] Praha, Stát. lékařská knihovna, 1957. 3 pts.

3473 entries. Includes a selective list of 162 books on endocrinology in the National Medical Library.

Histories

1391
Iason, Alfred H. The thyroid gland in medical history. New York, Froben Press, 1946. 130 p.

Brief sketches of leading contributions, from antiquity. No bibliography.

Diabetes

Indexes and Abstracts

1392
Diabetes literature index. Washington, 1, 1966– . National Institute of Arthritis and Metabolic Diseases.

Monthly. Prepared from MEDLARS tapes of the National Library of Medicine. Minimum time lag 3 months.
Continues no. 1393.

1393
Diabetes-related literature index, by authors and by key words in the title. New York, 1960–64?

Annual. 1963 listed approximately 2800 articles selected from *Cumulated index medicus.* Subject headings more detailed than in *CIM*; some are geographic. Complete bibliographic citations listed under each key word and author.
Published as a supplement to *Diabetes*, v. 12– , 1963– .

1394
Diabetes research; an international review. Amsterdam, 1, 1963– . Excerpta Medica.

Bi-monthly. 1966 contains 86 abstracts. Excludes articles on clinical management of diabetes. No indexes.

Bibliographies

1395
Schumacher, Joseph. Index zum Diabetes melitus; eine internationale Bibliographie. München, Urban & Schwarzenberg, 1961. 877 p.

Earliest references through 1954.

Directories

1396
American Diabetes Association. Membership directory. [New York] 1961. 93 p.

Alphabetical and geographical listings.

Histories

1397
Papaspyros, Nikos S. The history of diabetes mellitus. 2 ed. Stuttgart, Thieme, 1964. 104 p.

Bibliography: p. 81–97.

FILMS

Only general compilations are listed below. Compilations of films on special subjects are listed under the subjects.

1398
AMA medical-health film library. Chi-

cago, American Medical Association, 1964. 57 p.

1399
American Medical Association. Medical and surgical motion pictures; a catalog of selected films. Rev. ed. Chicago, 1966. 485 p.

More than 4430 titles in basic science, clinical medicine, surgery, and the paramedical sciences, with abstracts and occasional evaluations by the AMA or other medical organizations.

1400★★
Film reference guide for medicine and allied sciences. Atlanta, etc., 1956– . U.S. Public Health Service. Communicable Disease Center for the Federal Advisory Council on Medical Training Aids.

Annual. Each film selected can be used in the medical program of at least one of the member agencies of the FACMTA and is currently available for borrowing or rental.

1401
Ruhe, David S., ed. Selected films for medical teaching; a suggested basic motion picture library. In Journal of medical education 40(4, pt. 2): 1–76, 1965.

Lists 154 motion pictures in the basic and clinical sciences, giving for each a description of the content, appraisal of content and presentation, and suggestions for instructional uses of the film. Includes a list of distributors.

GASTROENTEROLOGY

Indexes and Abstracts

1402
Bibliographie et listes courantes de gastro-entérologie. In Acta gastro-entérologica belgica, 10, 1947– .

Monthly. The 1965 *Bibliographie* consists of 955 numbered abstracts (includes books); the *Listes courantes* consists of selected periodical titles with relevant articles listed under issue number. Author and subject indexes to abstracts only.

With v. 11, 1948 *Acta gastro-entérologica belgica* issued in 2 [pts.] and since 1952 in 2 v., of which the *Bibliographie* . . . is v. 2.

1947 lacks the combined title, added annually since 1948.

1403
Gastroenterology abstracts and citations. Bethesda, 1, 1966– . National Institute of Arthritis and Metabolic Diseases.

Monthly. 11,961 entries in 1966, approximately one third with abstracts.

1404
Cystic fibrosis; quarterly annotated references. New York, National Cystic Fibrosis Research Foundation, 1, 1962– .

190 abstracts in 1966.

1404.1
Ulcerative colitis abstracts. Washington, 1, 1960– . Prepared for the National Foundation for Research in Ulcerative Colitis by Scientific Literature, Inc.

Reviews

1405
Modern trends in gastro-enterology. Washington, 1, 1952– .

Irregular. Ser. 2, 1958; ser. 3, 1961. Includes review with bibliographies.

1406
Progress in liver diseases. New York, Grune & Stratton, 1, 1961– .

Bibliographies

1406.1
Dvinianinov, L. I. Fiziologiia i patologiia zheludochno-kishechnogo trakta. Referaty dissertatsii otechestvennykh avtorov s 1765 po 1917 g. i bibliograficheskiĭ ukazatel' dissertatsii s 1918 po 1964 g. [Physiology and pathology of the gastro-intestinal tract. Abstracts of dissertations by national authors from 1765 to 1917 and a bibliographic index of dissertations from 1918 to 1964] Moskva, Akademiia nauk SSSR, Institut fiziologii im. I. P. Pavlova, 1966. 267 p.

Part 1, 277 dissertations; pt. 2, 1,379 dissertations. Dissertations prepared in the I. P. Pavlov Laboratory not listed.

1407
Khar'kovskaia gosudarstvennaia nauchno-meditsinskaia biblioteka. Fiziologiia i patologiia pishchevareniia; kratkiĭ bibliograficheskiĭ ukazatel' otechestvennoĭ literatury za 1953–1955 gg. [Physiology and pathology of digestion; a brief biblio-

graphic index of national literature from 1953–1955] Khar'kov, 1956. 84 p.

Over 800 entries including monographs, dissertations, and collected works. Clinical materials and works on pathological anatomy are excluded. Entries are in Russian with original language indicated. No indexes.

History

1408
Cope, Sir Zachary. A history of the acute abdomen. London, Oxford University Press, 1965. 123 p.

Brief review of antiquity, followed by chapters on knowledge and treatment of specific conditions. Occasional references in text.

GENETICS

Indexes and Abstracts

1409
Resumptio genetica. s'Gravenhage, 1–19, 1924–53.

References listed under subjects by author and selectively annotated in a separate section. Annotations in French, English, or German.

Reviews

1410
Advances in genetics. New York, 1, 1947– .

Irregular. Reviews with bibliographies.

1411
Bibliographia genetica. s'Gravenhage, 1, 1925– .

Irregular. Each issue on separate subject.

1412
McKusick, Victor A., comp. Medical genetics, 1958–1960, an annotated review. St. Louis, Mosby, 1961. 534 p.

950 entries. Arranged by year. First published in *Journal of chronic diseases* (v. 10(4) Oct. 1959; 12(1) July 1960; 14(1) July 1961). Reviews for 1961–63 (1131 entries) in the *Journal*, v. 15, May 1962; v. 16, June 1963; and v. 17, Dec. 1964.

1413
Progress in medical genetics. New York, 1, 1961– .

Reviews. Published every 1–2 years.

1414
Recent advances in human genetics. Ed. by L. S. Penrose. London, Churchill, 1961. 194 p.

Bibliographies

1415
Angúlo Carpio, María D. Agentes químicos en citogenética; notas bibliográficas. Madrid, Instituto José Celestino Mutis, 1956. 321 p. (Monografías de Ciencia Moderna, no. 53–54).

Over 1000 references under cytogenetic action of alkaloids, action of substances derived from alkaloids, specifically mutagenic chemical agents.

1416
——. Notas bibliográficas sobre agentes fisicos en citogenética. Madrid, Instituto José Celestino Mutis, 1955. 134 p. (Monografías de Ciencia Moderna, no. 45).

420 references under such subjects as x-rays, other types of radiation, mechanical agents, ultrasonics, and physical and chemical agents. English language references predominate.

1417
Bibliography of the genetics of Drosophila. Edinburgh, Oliver and Boyd, etc., 1939–63. 4 pts.

Four pts. cover 1900–62. Arranged alphabetically by author. Pts. 1 and 2 lack subject indexes.

Pt. 1, comp. by Henry J. Muller; pts. 2–4 comp. by Irwin H. Herskowitz.

Pt. 2, Farnham Royal, Bucks, Commonwealth Agricultural Bureaux, 1952; pt. 3, Bloomington, Indiana University Press, 1958; pt. 4, New York, McGraw-Hill, 1963.

1417.1
McKusick, Victor A. Mendelian inheritance in man; catalogs of autosomal dominant, autosomal recession, and X-linked phenotypes. Baltimore, Johns Hopkins Press, 1966. 344 p.

1487 references on genetic disorders and traits in man which show simple Mendelian inheritance. Categories generally preceded by brief literature reviews. Earlier reference noted 1886.

Dictionaries

1418
Clapper, Russell B. Glossary of genetics and other biological terms. New York, Vantage Press, 1960. 200 p.

1419
Knight, Robert L. Dictionary of genetics including terms used in cytology, animal breeding and evolution. Waltham, Mass., Chronica Botanica, 1948. 183 p. (Lotsya; a biological miscellany, no. 2).

1419.1
Rieger, Rigomar, and Michaelis, A. Genetisches und cytogenetisches Wörterbuch. 2 ed. Berlin, 1958. 648 p.

Author arranged bibliography p. 597–648. Includes books.

1419.2
Sánchez-Monge y Parellada, Enrique. Diccionario de genética. Madrid, Instituto Nacional de Investigaciones Agronómicas, 1962. 152 p.

Spanish-Spanish, giving derivations and definitions, followed by polyglot sections of equivalent terms for English, French, German, Italian, and Portuguese.

Histories

1420
Darlington, Cyril D. Genetics and man. London, Allen & Unwin, 1964. 382 p.

Interpretive history of man's knowledge and understanding of genetics. References: p. 361–369.

1421
Dunn, Leslie C., ed. Genetics in the 20th century; essays on the progress of genetics during its first 50 years. New York, Macmillan, 1951. 634 p.

Papers by different authors on the knowledge of heredity before 1900, genetics and immunology, genetic studies in bacteria, genetics and disease resistance, and genetics and the cancer problem. References at ends of papers.

1422
Peters, James A., ed. Classic papers in genetics. Englewood Cliffs, N.J., Prentice-Hall, 1959. 282 p.

29 papers in English from Mendel (1865) to Benzer (1955), with a brief note on each paper and citation to source.

1423
Stubbe, Hans. Kurze Geschichte der Genetik bis zur Wiederentdeckung der Vererbungsregeln Gregor Mendels. Jena, Fischer, 1963. 232 p. (Genetik; Grundlagen, Ergebnisse und Probleme in Einzeldarstellungen. Beitrag 1)

To 1900. Bibliography: p. 207–221.

GERONTOLOGY

Indexes and Abstracts

1424
Bibliography of gerontology and geriatrics. Tokyo, 1, 1961– .

Annual. Title also in Japanese.

1424.1
Current publications in gerontology and geriatrics. In Journal of gerontology (St. Louis) 1, 1946– .

Quarterly. Up-dates no. 1429. Since 1950 by Nathan W. Shock.
Title varies.

Reviews

1425★
Advances in geronotological research. New York, 1, 1964– .

Bibliographies

1426
Nazarevskiĭ, N. A. Kratkiĭ bibliograficheskiĭ ukazatel' otechestvennoĭ literatury po gerontologii i geriatrii, 1958–1962 [A brief bibliographic index to the national literature on gerontology and geriatrics, 1958–1962] Kiev, Institut gerontologii i eksperimental'noĭ patologii Akademii meditsinskikh nauk SSSR, 1962. 90 p.

631 entries in Russian and Ukrainian. Includes books, newspaper articles.

1426.1
Nitkin, V. N. Russian studies on age-associated physiology, biochemistry and morphology. Historic description with extensive bibliography. Bethesda, 1961

[1962] 203 p. (U.S. Public Health Service. Publication no. 857)

2953 author entries covering 1769–1958. Bibliography preceded by a historical review. A translation.

1427★
Shock, Nathan W. A classified bibliography of gerontology and geriatrics. Stanford, Calif., Stanford University Press, 1951. 599 p.

18,036 references through 1948. Includes books, parts of books, pamphlets, etc. Frequently cites abstract of original.

1428★
——. ——. Supplement one, 1949–55. Stanford, 1957. 525 p.

15,983 references.

1429★
——. ——. Supplement two, 1956–61. Stanford, 1963. 624 p.

18,121 references.

Directories

1430
American Association of Homes for the Aging. Directory of non-profit homes for the aged. New York, 1, 1962– .

Geographical by state and city. Gives name of institution, address, and name of administrative officer.

Histories

1431
Grmek, Mirko D. On ageing and old age. Basic problems and historic aspects of gerontology and geriatrics. Den Haag, Junk, 1958. 106 p. (Monographiae biologicae, v. 5, no. 2)

Discusses theories of cause and nature of aging from Aristotle to present, with historical background. Bibliographical references: p. 91–104.

1432
Lüth, Paul. Geschichte der Geriatrie: dreitausend Jahre Physiologie, Pathologie und Therapie des alten Menschen. Stuttgart, Enke, 1965. 271 p.

Includes many extracts from the texts, usually in German translation, with sources indicated. Selective bibliography (50 items): p. 253–255.

HOSPITALS

Of the items listed below, no. 1435 is of especial value. It is minutely classified and it may be regarded as the tool of choice for questions on hospital literature. It is also of primary value for related fields.

Indexes and Abstracts

1433
Abstracts of hospital management studies. Ann Arbor, 1, 1964– . University of Michigan. Cooperative Information Center for Hospital Management Studies.

Quarterly.

1434
Hospital abstracts; a monthly survey of world literature. London, 1, 1961– . Ministry of Health.

Monthly. Covers the field of hospitals and hospital administration with the exception of strictly medical matters. Volume for 1964 contained 1848 abstracts. Abstracts selectively some nonmedical titles. Approximately 54 percent of the journals abstracted are not *Index medicus* titles. Minimum time lag two months.

1435★★
Hospital literature index. Chicago, 1, 1945– . American Hospital Association.

Quarterly. Cumulated annually under the same title and quinquenially as *Cumulative index of hospital literature.* Covers all aspects of the literature including administration, architecture, housekeeping, personnel, health insurance, etc. Indexes approximately 578 English language journals of which 158 are *Index medicus* titles. Includes a number of popular nonmedical journals.

v. 1–10, 1945–54, as *Index of current hospital literature*; v. 11–13(1), 1955–June 1957, *Hospital periodical literature index.*

Bibliographies

1436
Stageman, Anne, and Baney, Anna Mae. Hospital utilization studies; selected references annotated. Washington, U.S.

Public Health Service, Division of Hospital and Medical Facilities, 1962. 29 p.

29 references, 1954 to April 1962, arranged by author or title. Supplement contains 25 unannotated references.

Directories

Canada

1437★
Canadian hospital directory. Toronto, [1] 1953– . Canadian Hospital Association.

Annual listing of hospitals by province, giving statistics on admissions, births, budget, personnel, and names of chief administrative personnel; lists hospital and related associations, information on education programs for personnel, hospital buyers' catalogue.

Denmark

1438
Det danske sygehus vaesen. København, Dyva, 1962. 1201 p.

Descriptive account of individual hospitals. Includes history, special services, statistics.

France

1439
Guide de la santé et de l'aide sociale. Paris, [1] 195?– .

Arranged by locality. Includes hospitals, nursing homes, clinics, mental homes, and rest homes, both public and private. Divided into categories: general, establishments for children, for tuberculosis, special treatment, and social welfare.

Germany

1440
Adressen- und Auskunftsbuch über die Kranken-, Heil-, Pflege-, Erziehungs- und Wohlfahrts-Anstalten Deutschlands. 5 ed. Leipzig, Leineweber, 1929. 744 p.

Arranged by city. Name of hospital, type, and capacity.

1441
Germany. Statistisches Bundesamt. Verzeichnis der Krankenanstalten in den Ländern der Bundesrepublik Deutschland und West-Berlin. Stand: 1952. Stuttgart, W. Kohlhammer, 1952. 157 p.

Gives name of hospital, type, bed capacity.

1442
Krankenhaus-Lexikon für das Deutsche Reich. By A. Guttstadt. Berlin, Reimer, 1900. 939 p.

Arranged by province and city. Gives brief history of hospitals.

Great Britain

1443
The hospital gazetteer. London, British Medical Association, 1960– .

Hospitals are listed under hospital management group. Gives number of beds, specialties, number of staff by grade in each specialty, library, approval for higher qualifications, and the various diplomas. Index to hospitals. Also a special section on examination requirements and regulations under college, university, and institute.

1444
The hospitals year book, an annual record of the hospitals of Great Britain and Northern Ireland, incorporating "Burdett's Hospitals and Charities", founded 1889. London, [1] 1931– . Institute of Hospital Administrators.

Listing of hospitals arranged geographically by type of hospital; includes directory of government departments, local health authorities, hospital and health organizations; gives hospital statistics, and guide to purchasing. Published 1931–49 by Central Bureau of Hospital Information.

India

1445
India. Directorate General of Health Services. Ministry of Health. The directory of hospitals in India [for 1957] New Delhi, 1960. 778 p.

Name, type, bed capacity. Arranged by province with subarrangement by districts, etc.

1446
——. ——. Specialized treatment centers in India, 1958. New Delhi, 1959. 141 p.

Arranged by disease. Lists hospitals, clinics, dispensaries, sanatoria.

Japan

1447
Byoin Yoran. Japanese hospital directory. Tokyo, [1] 1952– .

Geographic arrangement. Name, bed capacity, patient load, etc.

1958/59– compiled by Japan, Ministry of Health and Welfare, Medical Affairs Bureau. 1952 and 1955 ed. compiled by Igaku Shoin. 1958/59– have added t.p. in English. 5 ed. 1964.

United States

PERSONNEL

1448★★
American College of Hospital Administrators. Directory. Chicago, [1] 1938– .

4 ed. includes list of officials, brief history, and code of ethics. Alphabetical listing of honorary fellows, fellows, members, and nominees. Personal and professional data, followed by regionally classified listing.

Biennial since 1960.

1449
——. Roster of membership. Chicago, [1] 1938– .

Alphabetical listing of active members and their addresses.

Issued in those years when the Association's *Directory* is not published. 1938–53, as *Roster of membership* [and] *geographical index*.

INSTITUTIONS

1450
American and Canadian hospitals. 2 ed. Chicago, Physicians Record Company, 1937. 1464 p.

Subtitle (varies): A reference book of historical, statistical and other information regarding the hospitals and related institutions of the United States and possessions and the Dominion of Canada.

1451
Clark's Directory of southern hospitals. Charlotte, N.C., Clark-Smith Pub. Co., 1962.

1452
Hospital progress; directory issue. St. Louis, 1937– .

1937–48 as *Catholic hospitals and schools of nursing*; 1949–54, *Catholic hospital directory*; 1955, *Directory of Catholic hospitals and allied agencies in the United States and Canada*; 1956–57, *Directory*.

1453★★
Hospitals; guide issue. Chicago, [1] 1946– . American Hospital Association.

Lists hospitals by state and city. Other sections list inpatient care institutions, members of the American Hospital Association, health organizations and agencies (medical societies, medical care groups, health departments, etc.), medical and paramedical schools (medical technology, dietetics, etc.), hospital statistics, and guide for hospital buyers.

1945–48 as *American hospital directory*; 1949–50, *Hospitals*: *statistics and directory section*; 1951–55, *Hospitals*: *administrators guide issue*. 1945–54, pt. 2 of the June issue; 1955– , pt. 2 of the August 1 issue.

Histories

1454
Abel-Smith, Brian. The hospitals, 1800–1948. A study in social administration in England and Wales. London, Heinemann, 1964. 514 p.

Carefully documented study of administrative, economic, and professional aspects. Bibliography (sources used): p. 503–506.

1455
Candille, Marcel, and Lévy, Françoise. Bibliographie d'histoire des hôpitaux. Pt. 1–10 in Revue de l'assistance publique à Paris (Nov.–Dec. 1957)– ; Pt. 11– in L'hopital et l'aide sociale à Paris 1:97–101, 1960– .

Retrospective bibliography, including journal articles, and including local history, in France and elsewhere. Entries numbered sequentially, reaching 2295 in pt. 28 (v. 6, 1965, p. 341–346).

1456
Correia, Fernando da Silva. Origens e formação das misericórdias portuguesas. Lisboa, Torres, 1944. 661 p. (His Estudos sôbre a história da assistência)

Preliminary survey of ancient and medieval hospitals and charity in the Orient and Europe (p. 7–209) with full account of Portuguese history through the 15th century. List of Portuguese hospitals, almshouses, etc., with historical data and references: p. 405–447. Bibliographical footnotes.

1457
Dainton, Courtney. The story of England's hospitals. London, Museum Press, 1961. 184 p.

From the Middle Ages to the National Health Service. Includes brief histories of important hospitals. Bibliography (chiefly secondary): p. 176–180.

1458
Eaton, Leonard K. New England hospitals, 1790–1833. Ann Arbor, University of Michigan Press, 1957. 282 p.

Covers architecture, finance and administration, medicine, surgery, teaching, and research in the hospital, with special chapters on the Massachusetts General Hospital and the Hartford Retreat. References (mainly sources, by chapters): p. 247–274. "Bibliographical essay": p. 239–246.

1459
Imbert, Jean. Histoire des hôpitaux français; contribution à l'étude des rapports de l'église et de l'état dans le domaine de l'assistance publique: les hôpitaux en droit canonique. Paris, Vrin, 1947. 334 p. (L'Eglise et l'état au moyen âge, no. 8.)

Documented study to 1505, with extensive extracts from the sources. Bibliography (classified, chiefly sources): p. 311–334. No index.

1460
Meffert, Franz. Caritas und Krankenwesen bis zum Ausgang des Mittelalters. Freiburg i. Br., Caritasverlag, 1927. xvii, 443 p. (Schriften zur Caritaswissenschaft, im Auftrage des Deutschen Caritasverbands, v. 2)

History of the care of the sick and of hospitals in early and medieval Christianity, with accounts of the work of religious orders and of the relations of the church to the medical profession. Based mainly on historical and ecclesiastical sources, cited in footnotes. References: p. xi-xvii.

1461
Muriel de la Torre, Josefina. Hospitales de la Nueva España. México, 1956–60. 2 v. ([Mexico. Universidad Nacional] Instituto de Historia. Publicaciones. ser. 1, no. 35, 62)

Documented history through 18th century, with general surveys and detailed accounts of special hospitals. Appendix of documents in v. 2. Bibliography: v. 1, p. 291–297; v. 2, p. 360–369. Index of personal and hospital names.

1462
Poynter, F. N. L. The evolution of hospitals in Britain. London, Pitman, 1964. 294 p.

15 papers delivered at the 3d British Congress on the History of Medicine and Pharmacy, London, 1962. From medieval monastic infirmaries to the present, with papers on special types of institutions, teaching, design and planning, administration, and nursing. References at ends of papers. Classified bibliography of British hospital history by Eric Gaskell, p. 255–279.

1463
Reicke, Siegfried. Das deutsche Spital und sein Recht im Mittelalter. Stuttgart, Enke, 1932. 2 v.

Documented study on hospitals, related religious orders, civil and canon law. Extensive bibliographical footnotes; author index to secondary works, v. 2, p. 291–297. Reprinted Amsterdam, 1961.

LEGAL MEDICINE

Indexes and Abstracts

1464
Medicolegal cases; abstracts of court decisions of medico-legal interest. Chicago, 1932– . American Medical Association. Bureau of Legal Medicine and Legislation.

Federal and State coverage.

Previously published in *JAMA*. v. 1 (1932) covers the decisions of 1926–30; v. 2 (1936), 1931–35; v. 3 (1942), 1936–40; v. 4 (1950), 1941–46; and v. 5 (1955), 1947–52.

1465
The Citation. Chicago, 1, 1958– . American Medical Association, Law Department.

12 issues per volume. Information on medical jurisprudence and medical legislation. Cumulative subject and case indexes for v. 1–5 (May 1958–Sept. 1962).

1466
Deutsche Zeitschrift für die gesamte gerichtliche Medizin. [Referate] Berlin, 1, 1922– . Organ der deutschen Gesell-

schaft für gerichtliche und soziale Medizin.

1964 contained about 800 entries, most with abstracts. Includes clinical medicine and material in the behavioral sciences related to legal medicine.

1467
International digest of health legislation. Geneva, 1, 1948– . World Health Organization.

Quarterly. Selection of reprints, translations or extracts from the text of the most important laws and regulations dealing with public health. Arranged alphabetically by country. Time lag 2 to 4 years.

Cumulated subject index, v. 1–5, 1948–54; v. 11–15, 1960–64.

Continues section 1 of the *Bulletin mensuel de l'Office International d'Hygiène Publique* (not listed).

1468
Personal injury annual. Albany, N.Y., Bender, 1, 1961– .

Abstracts and selected articles from legal and medical periodicals, also abstracts of selected case reports.

1965 contains 5 year cumulative index.

Reviews

1469
Methods in forensic science. New York, 1, 1962– .

Annual. Reviews with bibliographies.

Bibliographies

1470
Brittain, Robert P. Bibliography of medico-legal works in English. London, Sweet & Maxwell, 1962. 252 p.

1651 references, including books, pamphlets, theses, and a few articles. Includes translations from foreign languages. Does not cover criminology. Alphabetical author arrangement. Issued under the auspices of the British Academy of Forensic Sciences.

1470.1
Kornblitt, Herbert, ed. Medico-legal reports. Miami, Current Medicine for Attorneys, 1956. 175 p.

Compilation of the opinions of 300 medical authorities on personal injury collected from both medical and legal literature. Includes also over 500 brief abstracts of related federal or state law cases. Covers 1954–55 and part of 1956. No indexes or lists of journals indexed or cases cited.

Cumulation of 23 issues of *Medico-legal reporter.*

1470.2
Krügelstein, Franz C. C. Promptuarium medicinae forensis; oder: Realregister über die in die gerichtliche Arzney-Wissenschaft einschlagenden Beobachtungen, Entscheidungen und Vorfälle. Erfurth und Gotha, 1822–41. 4 pts.

A collection of abstracts and citations. Includes books and dissertations. Only last name of author is given; no titles are given for journal articles. No author index.

1471
Smedt, Marc de. Essai de bibliographie médico-légale et criminologique. Contribution to a bibliography of legal medicine and criminology. Liège, Vaillant-Carmanne, 1953. 124 p.

Over 1500 references. Includes monographs and serials in Dutch, English, French, German, Italian, Portuguese, and Spanish. Excludes journal articles except for a few important items which appeared in other than medico-legal or criminological journals. Covers from the second half of the 19th century to 1953.

1472
Wildberg, Christianus F. L. Bibliotheca medicinae publicae, in qua scripta ad medicinam et forensem et politicam facientia ab illarum scientiarum initiis ad nostra usque tempora digesta sunt. Berolini, Flittner, 1819. 2 v. in 1.

Includes books, dissertations and journals; no journal articles. v. 1, forensic medicine, contains 2980 references; v. 2, medicina politica, which covers public hygiene, public care of the sick, health personnel, and the administration of medicine, contains 2013 references. Entries are in Latin, German, and French. Chronological subarrangement.

Supersedes C. F. Daniel's *Entwurf einer Bibliothek der Staatsarzneykunde,* Halle, 1784 (not listed).

Manuals

1473
Pittsburgh. University. Graduate School

of Public Health. Health Law Center. Hospital law manual. Pittsburgh, 1959– 2 v. (looseleaf)

Record of state legislation concerning hospitals in the United States. v. 1, Administrator's volume; v. 2, Attorney's volume. Kept up to date by *Newsletter and Quarterly Supplement.*

Dictionaries

1474
Elsevier's Fachwörterbuch der Kriminalwissenschaft in acht Sprachen. Von Johann Anton Adler. München, Oldenbourg, 1960. 1460 p.

Lists 10,930 terms with their equivalents in English/American, French, Italian, Spanish, Portuguese, Dutch, Swedish, and German. No definitions.

1475
Madia, Ernesto. Dizionario di medicina legale con l'etimologia di tutte le parole derivanti dal greco e dal latino. Napoli, Michele d'Auria, 1901–1904. 3 v.

Includes terms from related fields such as botany, chemistry, pharmacy, psychiatry. Contains some case reports and frequently provides legal commentary.

1476
Maloy, Bernard S. The simplified medical dictionary for lawyers. 1 ed. Mundelein, Ill., Callaghan, 1, 1941– .

Medical terms defined in language understandable by the layman. Gives etymology or history of Greek terms.

3 ed., 1960, 724 p.

1477 (not used)

1478
Neureiter, Ferdinand von, ed. Handwörterbuch der gerichtlichen Medizin und naturwissenschaftlichen Kriminalistik. Berlin, Springer, 1940. 969 p.

Encyclopedic coverage of subjects including legal and medical views, casuistics, German legislation, and occasionally historical development. Each article contains a bibliography.

1479
Schmidt, J. E. Attorneys' dictionary of medicine. Albany, Bender, 1962. 885 p.

Encyclopedic dictionary with definitions in layman's language; gives pronunciation. Includes abbreviations.

1479.1
Stedman, Thomas L. Medical dictionary, unabridged lawyers' edition based upon the twentieth edition of Stedman's. A vocabulary of medicine and its allied sciences, with pronunciation and derivations... Lawyers' section edited by William J. Curran. Cincinnati, Anderson; Washington, Jefferson Law Book, 1961. 1680 p.

Same as no. 238 except contains a section giving information on how to use a medical library, lists of medical and medicolegal libraries in the United States, abbreviations used in medical records, description of American specialty boards and medicolegal centers and institutes.

Directories

1480
Forensic Science Society, London. World list of forensic science laboratories. London, 1963. 30 p.

Information from 42 countries. Alphabetical arrangement by country, giving name and address of laboratory, name of director.

LIBRARIES, MEDICAL

Manuals

1481★
Guidelines for medical school libraries. Prepared by a Joint Committee of the Association of American Medical Colleges and the Medical Library Association. Journal of medical education 40(1, pt. 1):5–64, 1965.

Outlines the major considerations in developing, maintaining and assessing library services.

1482
Inke, Gabor. Quellen medizinischer Literaturangaben und Methodik ihrer Bearbeitung. Jena, Fischer, 1960. 165 p.

Lists 568 indexes, abstracts, bibliographies, and reviews. Discusses library use and techniques.

1483
Keys, Thomas E. Applied medical li-

brary practice . . . With chapters by Catherine Kennedy [and] Ruth M. Tews. Springfield, Ill., Thomas, 1958. 495 p.

1484
Kricker, Gottfried. Medizinische Bücherkunde und Bibliotheksbenutzung; ein Grundriss für Studierende und Ärzte. 3 ed. Leipzig, Barth, 1954. 68 p.

Includes historical section.

1485★★
Medical Library Association. Handbook of medical library practice; with a bibliography of the reference works and histories in medicine and the allied sciences. 2 ed. Janet Doe and Mary L. Marshall, ed. Chicago, American Library Association, 1956. 601 p.

The volume in hand constitutes a revision of the bibliography section of the *Handbook.*

1486
Morton, Leslie T. How to use a medical library; a guide for practitioners, research workers and students. 4 ed. London, Heinemann, 1964. 66 p.

Broad treatment. 1 ed., 1934.

1487
Postell, William D. Applied medical bibliography for students. Springfield, Thomas, 1955. 142 p.

Includes discussions of more general library problems.

1488
Zamkova, Zinaida N. Osnovnye printsipy meditsinskoĭ bibliografii [Basic principles of medical bibliography] Moskva, Medgiz, 1958. 102 p.

A handbook for physicians on Soviet medical libraries and their use.

Collections—Catalogs

1489
American College of Surgeons. Library. A catalogue of the H. Winnett Orr Collection and other rare books in the Library. By H. Winnett Orr. Chicago, 1960. 198 p.

2289 items in broadly classified arrangement, with index of names and selected titles. Includes early imprints and classics (468 items); important 19th–20th century medical works, especially in surgery, orthopedics, and military medicine; and medical history and biography.

1490
France. Bibliothèque Nationale. Département des Imprimés. Catalogue des sciences médicales. Paris, Didot, 1859–89. 3 v.

Classified catalog with entries arranged chronologically and sometimes geographically in each section. Detailed table of contents; no index. (Author approach through the Library's *Catalogue général: auteurs*, 1900– .) Includes lists of institutions, societies, periodicals.

1491
Glasgow. University. Hunterian Museum. The printed books in the library . . . A catalogue prepared by Mungo Ferguson, with a topographical index by David B. Smith. Glasgow, Jackson, Wylie, 1930. 396 p.

Valuable collection including many rare works (534 incunabula) in medicine and science. Topographical index of books printed before 1600 by place of printing and printer. Lacks cross references. No subject index.

1492
Nederlandsche Maatschappij tot Bevordering der Geneeskunst. Bibliotheek. Catalogus. Amsterdam, Internationaal Antiquariaat [etc., 1930–49] 2 v. Bibliotheca medica Neerlandica. Aanwinsten van de Bibliotheek . . . Juni 1949–Juni 1954. Amsterdam, Campen, 1954. 88 p.

Classified catalog of the Society's library, on deposit in the Amsterdam University Library. Contains works by Dutch authors on medicine and allied sciences, medical works of foreign authors printed in the Netherlands or in the colonies, and works of medical interest concerning Netherlands or the colonies. Special sections of periodicals, proceedings, reports, etc.; manuscripts; and letters. Index of names and selective titles. v. 2 is a combined ed. of the 2 supplements issued in 1935 and 1940. A new supplement is announced covering acquisitions 1955–1960.

1493
Osler, Sir William. Bibliotheca Osleriana: a catalogue of books illustrating the history of medicine and science. Collected, arranged, and annotated by Sir William

Osler, Bt., and bequeathed to McGill University. Oxford, Clarendon Press, 1929. 785 p.

7787 (i.e. 7965) items, with extensive annotations, including references, by Osler and the editors (William W. Francis and others). Arranged in groups as Bibliotheca prima; Bibliotheca secunda; Bibliothecae litteraria, historica, biographica, and bibliographica; Incunabula and manuscripts; and Oriental books donated by Dr. Casey A. Wood (181 items, numbered as 3). Author, subject, and selective title index.

1494
Putti, Vittorio. La raccolta Vittorio Putti: antiche opere di medicina, manoscritte, e stampate, lasciate all' Istituto Rizzoli di Bologna. Milano, Istituto grafico Bertieri, 1943. 107 p.

Includes descriptions of 17 manuscripts, catalog of 1141 printed books, and list of autographs of physicians and scientists (p. 95–107). Comp. by Tammaro de Marinis. No subject index. Reprinted Bologna, Forni, 1963, as *Catalogo della raccolta Vittorio Putti.*

1495
Royal College of Physicians, London. Library. Catalogue. London, Spottiswoode, 1912. 1354 p.

Author checklist of 20,000 items. Omits periodicals, reports, and transactions of societies, but contains lists such as Harveian orations, Goulstonian lectures, and pharmacopoeias. Occasionally cites biographic references.

1496
Royal College of Physicians of Edinburgh. Library. Catalogue. Edinburgh, Clark, 1863. 764 p. Supplements: 1863/70 (1870), 279 p.; 1871/79 (1879), 162 p.

Author checklists of about 23,000 volumes of printed books. Supplementary lists of engraved medical portraits.

1497
Royal Medical and Chirurgical Society of London. Library. Catalogue. London, The Society, 1879. 3 v. Suppl. 1–7. 1880–93.

Checklist of a collection of about 45,000 books, now in the Library of the Royal Society of Medicine. v. 1–2, author catalog, including form entries for catalogs, dispensatories, Harveian orations, and the like; and entries for biographical and critical works under persons as subjects; with a section of transactions, journals, reports, etc. (v. 2, p. 583–731). v. 3, index of subjects.

1498★
U.S. National Library of Medicine. Catalog. A list of works represented by National Library of Medicine cards. Washington, 1950–65. 18 v.

Two quinquennial and one sexennial cumulated editions: 1950–54. 6 v. (as U.S. Armed Forces Medical Library, *Catalog*); 1955–59, 6 v.; and 1960–65, 6 v. Cumulations supersede annual volumes. Published in 2 pts.: 1, Authors; 2, Subjects.

Cards printed Oct. 1946–Mar. 1948 were included in U.S. Library of Congress, *A catalog of books represented by Library of Congress printed cards. Supplement . . . 1942– . . . 1947*, and in its *Cumulative catalog . . . of printed cards*, 1948; Apr.–Dec. 1948, published as U.S. Army Medical Library, *Catalog cards, April–December 1948* (issued as a supplement to the L.C. *Cumulative catalog*, 1948); 1949, as U.S. Army Medical Library, *Author catalog* (issued as a supplement to the L.C. *Author catalog*).

Continued by no. 1499.

1499★★
U.S. National Library of Medicine. Current catalog. Washington, 1966– .

Biweekly, with quarterly and annual cumulations. Biweekly issues include citations for recent publications catalogued during period covered. Contains as many as 3 appendices: (1) directory of publishers of monographs published in the last year, (2) added volumes to sets, and (3) list of reprints of publications already in the collection. In 1966, biweekly has author and title section only; 1967– , has subject section also.

Cumulations include all publications cataloged during period except monographs published before 1801, an author and title section, and a subject section. Continues no. 1498.

For a list of subject headings used see no. 1531.

1500
Uppsala. Universitet. Bibliotek. Bibliotheca Walleriana. The books illustrating the history of medicine and science collected by Dr. Erik Waller and bequeathed to the Library of the Royal University of Uppsala; a catalogue compiled by Hans Sallander. Stockholm. Almqvist & Wik-

sell, 1955. 2 v. (Acta Bibliothecae R. Universitatis Upsaliensis, v. 8–9)

20,428 items. Broadly classified, with index of authors, subjects, and titles of anonymous works.

1501
Wellcome Historical Medical Library, London. A catalogue of printed books in the . . . Library. London, 1962– (Its Publications. Catalogue series, PB1–2)

1. Books printed before 1641. 1962. 407 p. 6959 items. Indexes of places of publication and of printers and publishers.

2. Books printed from 1641 to 1850. 1966– v. 1, A–E, 540 p. (items not numbered)

Alphabetically arranged by author or anonymous title. General editor, F. N. L. Poynter. No subject index.

1502
Yale University. Yale Medical Library. Historical Library. The Harvey Cushing collection of books and manuscripts. New York, Schuman, 1943. 207 p. (Yale University. School of Medicine. Library. Historical Library. Publication no. 1)

Short-title author catalog of 7959 manuscripts, Orientalia, incunabula, general works, and Cushing memorabilia, now in Yale Medical Library. Includes added entries, references under names used as subjects.

1503 (not used)

Collections—Periodicals

1504
Ch'uan kuo chung wen ch'i k'an lien ho mu lu 1833–1949 [Union list of Chinese serials 1833–1949] Peking, China, Peking National Library, 1961. 1252 p.

Holdings of 19,115 Chinese serials, 1833–1949, in the 50 leading libraries in Mainland China as of 1959. Some 500 are medical.

Serials are arranged by the stroke bases of Chinese character.

1505
Clermont-Ferrand, France. Université. Faculté mixte de médecine et de pharmacie. Bibliothèque. Catalogue des periodiques. Établi par Jacques Archimbaud. Clermont-Ferrand, 1962. 156 p.

Current and noncurrent periodicals listed, with holdings.

1506 (not used)

1507
Cuboni, E., and Roversi, A. S. Catalogo dei periodici medici raccolti nelle Biblioteche Lombarde. Milano, Istituto Sieroterapico Milanese "S. Belfanti," 1959. 326 p.

1508
India. Directorate-General of Health Services. Union Catalogue of medical periodicals in Indian libraries. Corrected up to January 1962. 5 ed. New Delhi, 1962. 386 p.

Holdings of 84 institutions indicated. 2282 titles listed. Titles include indexes and abstracts.

4 ed. 1956.

1508.1
Isché, John, P. ed. Checklist of periodical titles currently received in medical libraries in the Southern region. 2 ed. New Orleans, 1964. 178 p.

1509
Kondo, Jion, ed. Nippon-i-shi-yakugaku zasshi soran [Union catalogue of medical, dental and pharmaceutical periodicals in Japan, 1958]. Tokyo, Daigaku Shobo, 1958. 1 v. (various pagings)

Covers 1864 to 1958. 3240 Japanese journal titles in alphabetical arrangement giving beginning and ending date.

1510
List of periodicals in the World Health Organization Library. Jan. 1, 1963. Library news; Nouvelles de la bibliothèque, 16 (suppl. 1), 1963.

Revised periodically. Addenda and corrigenda published quarterly in *Library news*. Data given include full title, place of publication, and holdings in the WHO and UN Libraries in Geneva.

1511 (not used)

1512
Paris. Université. Faculté de médecine. Bibliothèque. Catalogue des principaux périodiques. 2 ed. . . . Publiée par les soins du . . . André Hahn avec le concours de . . . [Janine] Samion-Contet. Paris, 1958. 567 p.

1 ed., 1952, as *Catalogue des principaux périodiques et congrès.*

1513 (not used)

1514
Seppala, Arvo. Medical periodicals and serials in the libraries of Finland. Helsinki, University of Helsinki, 1960. 355 p.

1515★
U.S. National Library of Medicine. Biomedical serials, 1950–1960; a selective list of serials in the National Library of Medicine. Comp. by Lela M. Spanier. Washington, 1962. 503 p. (Public Health Service. Publication no. 910)

8939 substantive serials arranged alphabetically by title. Information given includes publishing body, place, covering date, and frequency. Proceedings of congresses not included.

1515.1
U.S. National Library of Medicine. Current holdings of mainland Chinese journals, October 1965. [By Stephen Kim] [Bethesda, 1965] 26 p.

Lists holdings largely from the 1950's for 92 journals. Includes list of publishers and variant title index.

1516
U.S. Veterans Administration. Library Division. Special Service Department of Medicine and Surgery. Union list of periodicals in medical libraries of the Veterans Administration. 3 ed. Washington, 1965. 138 p.

1517
Warsaw. Glowna Biblioteka Lekarska. Spis czasopism Głównej Biblioteki Lekarskiej otrzymywanych v roku . . . [A list of periodicals received in the Central Medical Library in the year . . .] Warszawa, 1960(?)- .

Covers the fields of medicine, dentistry, midwifery, nursing, pharmacy, veterinary medicine, applied science, chemistry, and psychology. Any serial received since 1900 is included. In English.

1964 volume lists 2114 titles, arranged alphabetically. For each entry gives the original title, place of publication, and frequency.

Title varies slightly. With 1963 issue the title expanded to: *Spis czasopism i wydawnictw ciaglych* . . . [A list of periodicals and serials . . .].

Selection Tools

1518★
Brandon, Alfred N. Selected list of books and journals for the small medical library. In Bulletin of the Medical Library Association 53:329–64, 1965.

Lists 358 books and 123 journals.

1519
Library Association. Medical Section. Books and periodicals for medical libraries in hospitals. London, [1] 1952– .

Books and journals arranged by subject; gives bibliographic citation and price. 3 ed., 1966, 31 p.

1520
Medical books in print, a select list. Palo Alto, Stacey, [1] 1955/56– .

Annual listing of books by medical publishers in the United States; includes number of pages and price. Also cites forthcoming books. 1967/68 (published 1966) listed about 4000 titles. No author index.

1520.1
[Nicole, Geneviève] Choix d'ouvrages et de périodiques proposé pour l'épuipement des bibliothèques médicales. Paris, 1966. 269 p.

At head of title: Ministère de l'Education Nationale. Direction des Bibliothèques et de la Lecture Publique.

1521
Referáty, kritiky, diskuse o nových lékařských knihách ve státních vědeckých knihovnách [Reviews, critiques and discussions concerning new medical books received in the national scientific libraries] Praha, Státní lékařská knihovna, 1, 1955– .

8 issues a year. Annually reviews between 250 and 300 books published chiefly in the Western languages. Entries are in the original language with reviews in Czech or Slovak. No indexes.

1522
Science books; a quarterly review. Washington, 1, 1965– . American Association for the Advancement of Science.

1523★
U.S. National Library of Medicine. Basic reference aids for small medical libraries. Washington, 1, 1959– .

Annotated list of selected reference books and serials most likely to be useful in the small library; arranged by subject, including book and periodical lists, indexes, abstract journals, dictionaries, directories, reviews, etc.

First published as *Check list of basic reference aids for small medical libraries.* Revised 1962, 1963, 1967.

1524
U.S. National Library of Medicine. Reference Services Division. Selected basic science books in the reference collection of the National Library of Medicine. Comp. by Marjory H. Wright. Washington, 1964. 30 p.

118 references.

1525
U.S. Veterans Administration. Dept. of Medicine and Surgery. Medical and General Reference Library. Basic list of books and journals for Veterans Administration medical libraries. Washington, [1] 1946– .

Lists latest recommended texts and journals in medicine and related fields, with publisher and price.

First issued under title *Minimum medical library requirements for Veterans Administration hospitals and centers;* in 1950, became *Basic list of medical books and journals for V.A. hospitals, centers and domiciliaries;* in 1956, issued under present title as its *Program guide, G-8.* Usually revised at 2-year intervals; 1964 had series designation G-14, 2d rev., M-2, pt. 13.

Classification Schemes

1526
Barnard, Cyril C. A classification for medical and veterinary libraries. 2 ed. London, Lewis, 1955. 278 p.

1 ed. as *A classification for medical libraries* . . . .

1527
Cunningham, Eileen. Classification for medical literature. 4 ed. Nashville, Vanderbilt University Press, 1955. 164 p.

1528
Kiev. Respublikanskaia nauchnaia meditsinskaia biblioteka. Skhema indeksov sistematicheskogo kataloga meditsinskoi literatury [Scheme of indexes for a systematic catalog of medical literature] Kiev, 1960. 200 p.

Based on the decimal classification originally prepared by N. V. Rusinov and expanded in accordance with the experience of the V.I. Lenin Library (Leningrad) and that of the compilers. Medicine comprises a part of class 6.

1528.1
Louisiana State Department of Hospitals. Classification for medical literature. By William D. Postell. Baton Rouge, 1966. 18 p.

Decimal system intended for hospital libraries.

1529
Moscow. Gosudarstvennaia nauchnaia meditsinskaia biblioteka. Spisok rubrik predmetnogo kataloga GTsNMB [A list of subject headings of the National Central Scientific Medical Library's subject catalog] Moskva, Izd-vo Vsesoiuznoĭ knizhnoĭ palaty, 1958. 336 p.

Alphabetical index of subject headings used in the classification of medical and related literature. Also includes a list of standard subheadings and "sub-subheadings."

1530
Quarterly cumulative index medicus. Subject headings and cross references; a guide to the classification of medical periodical literature. 2 ed. Chicago, American Medical Association, 1940. 431 p.

1 ed., 1931, has subtitle: a guide to medical classification.

1531★★
U.S. National Library of Medicine. Medical subject headings; main headings and cross references used in Index medicus and National Library of Medicine catalog. Washington, 1960– .

2 ed., 1963– , as pt. 2 of the January issue of *Index medicus.*

1532★★
U.S. National Library of Medicine. National Library of Medicine classification;

a scheme for the shelf arrangement of books in the field of medicine and its related sciences. 3 ed. Bethesda, 1964. 286 p.

1 ed. 1951.

Directories

1533
Directory of medical libraries in the British Isles. Comp. by the Medical Section of the Library Association. 2 ed. London, Library Association, 1965. 113 p.

1534
Germany (Democratic Republic). Ministerium für Gesundheitswesen. Abteilung Wissenschaft. Medizinische Bibliotheken in der Deutschen Demokratischen Republik; Verzeichnis medizinischer Fachbibliotheken und Literaturstellen sowie wissenschaftlicher Allgemeinbibliotheken mit reichen Beständen an medizinischer Literatur. Zusammengestellt von Edith Krauss. Berlin, 1962. 63 p.

294 libraries arranged by city. Gives number of monographs, bound periodicals, current periodicals, subject specialization.

1535★★
Medical Library Association. Directory. Chicago [1] 1950– .

Geographical listing of institutional members; data includes address, founding date, name of librarian, number of personnel, number of volumes, loan policy, and classification scheme. Alphabetical listing of individual members. 1 ed. lists institutional members only.

2 ed., 1959. Membership lists published irregularly in its *Bulletin* through July 1962. Latest separate listing, 1966. Lists of new members published irregularly in its *Bulletin* through January 1965; in the *MLA News*, May 1965– .

1536
Nippon igaku toshokanin meibo, Showa 37 nen 10 gatsu genzai [Directory of staff members in Japanese medical libraries, as of October 1962]. Kashihara, Fuzoku Toshokan, Nara Kenritsu Ika Daigaku, 1962.

Listed under the names of 44 medical libraries.

1537★
U.S. National Library of Medicine. Directory of medical libraries outside the United States and Canada. Preliminary ed., comp. by Edith D. Blair. Washington, U.S. Public Health Service, 1963. 77 p.

Arranged by continent, city and institution. Gives name and address, and if available, name of librarian and size of collection.

MICROBIOLOGY

Indexes and Abstracts

Current

1538
Bulletin de l'Institut Pasteur. Paris, 1, 1903– .

Monthly. Covers theoretical microbiology and immunology and related sciences as well as their medical, veterinary, agricultural and industrial applications. In 1964 listed 13,404 references, selectively abstracted. Includes books. Currently each issue devoted to a particular subject complex. Minimum time lag (1964) 6 months.

1538.1
Industrial microbiology abstracts. London, Information Retrieval, Ltd., 1, 1965– .

Monthly.

1538.2
Synthesis microbiologica; rassegna bibliografica bimestrale. Parma, 1, 1964– . Istituto di Microbiologia, Ospedale Maggiore.

Bimonthly. English abstracts. Author index in each issue. Minimum time lag 2 months. Supplement to *L'Igiene moderna.*

Subtitle: Microbiological current literature.

1539
Zentralblatt für Bakteriologie, Parasitenkunde, Infektionskrankheiten und Hygiene. Erste Abteilung. Medizinisch-hygienische Bakteriologie, Virusforschung und Parasitologie. Referate. Stuttgart, etc. 1, 1887– .

Currently four volumes a year in six issues each and a separately published seventh index issue. A recent volume listed in excess of 1500 references, most with abstracts. Includes book reviews and, on occasion, abstracts of proceedings of societies, and literature surveys. Indexes a few journals (mainly veterinary and sanitary engineering) not indexed by *Index medicus.*

v. 1–17, 1887–95, as *Centralblatt für Bakteriologie und Parasitenkunde;* v. 18–30, 1895–1901,

Centralblatt für Bakteriologie und Parasitenkunde. Erste Abteilung. Medizinisch-hygienische Bakteriologie und tierische Parasitenkunde; v. 31–125, 1902–37, *Centralblatt für Bakteriologie, Parasitenkunde und Infektionskrankheiten. Erste Abteilung . . . Referate.* With v. 125, 1937, . . . *Virusforschung und tierische Parasitologie;* with v. 146, 1947, *und Hygiene* added to title, *tierische* dropped.

With v. 17, 1895, divided into 2 parts, pt. 2 becoming no. 1540. The earlier volumes and v. 17–30 of Abt. 1 contained both original articles and abstracts. With v. 31, 1902, Abt. 1 divided into two separately published sections: Referate and Originale.

1540
Zentralblatt für Bakteriologie, Parasitenkunde und Infektionskrankheiten. Zweite-naturwissenschaftliche-Abteilung. Allgemeine, landwirtschaftliche und technische Mikrobiologie. Jena, 1, 1895– .

One volume or more a year in several issues. Recent volumes had in excess of 550 abstracts a volume. Includes books. Covers anatomy and physiology of microorganisms, microbiology of food, plant pathology, etc. Offshoot from 1539.

Noncurrent

1541
Abstracts of bacteriology. Baltimore, 1–9, 1917–25. American Society of Microbiologists.

Includes proceedings of the Society. Continued in 916.

1542
Jahresbericht über die Fortschritte in der Lehre von den pathogenen Mikroorganismen umfassend Bacterien, Pilze und Protozoen. Leipzig, etc., 1–27, 1885–1911.

Articles, books, theses listed under subject, then briefly characterized or selectively abstracted following lisitng. 1700–3700 items abstracted per volume.

Added title page: *Baumgarten's Jahresbericht* . . .

Separate index to v. 1–5, 1885–89.

1543
Jahresbericht über die Fortschritte in der Lehre von den Garungs-Organismen und Enzymen. Braunschweig, 1–22, 1890–1911.

Reviews

1544
Advances in applied microbiology. New York, 1, 1959– .

Annual. Reviews with bibliographies.

1545★★
Advances in virus research. New York, 1, 1953– .

Annual. Reviews with bibliographies.

1546★★
Annual review of microbiology. Palo Alto, Calif., Annual Reviews, Inc., 1, 1947– .

Reviews with bibliographies.

1547★★
Bacteriological reviews. Baltimore, American Society of Microbiologists, 1, 1937– .

Monthly. Critical surveys of current status of various areas of microbiology, immunology, genetics.

1548
Ergebnisse der Mikrobiologie, Immunitätsforschung und experimentellen Therapie. Berlin, 1, 1914– .

Annual reviews with bibliographies. Currently, articles in German, French, or English.

v. 1, 1914, as *Ergebnisse der Immunitätsforschung, experimentellen Therapie, Bakteriologie und Hygiene*; v. 2–29, 1917–55, *Ergebnisse der Hygiene, Bakteriologie, Immunitätsforschung und experimentellen Therapie.* Suspended 1944–48.

v. 1–29, 1914–55 had subtitle: Fortsetzung des Jahresberichts über die Ergebnisse der Immunitätsforschung und experimentellen Therapie; v. 33, 1960– , Fortsetzung . . . begründet von Wolfgang Weichardt.

Supersedes no. 1549.

1549
Jahresbericht über die Ergebnisse der Immunitätsforschung. Stuttgart, 1–8, 1905–12.

v. 1–4, 1905–08, references with abstracts. Arranged alphabetically by author.

With v. 5, 1909, issued in 2 parts: pt. 1, original reveiw articles; pt. 2, abstracts alphabetically by author.

v. 7–8?, 1911–12, had subtitle: und deren Grenzwissenschaften, der Chemotherapie, Zoonosologie, Hygiene u.s.f.

Superseded by no. 1548.

1550
Progress in industrial microbiology. London, Heywood, 1, 1959– .

Annual reviews with bibliographies. Includes more general aspects of microorganisms than title indicates.

1551
Progress in medical virology. Fortschritte der medizinischen Virusforschung. Progrès en virologie medicale. New York, 1, 1958– .

Annual reviews with bibliographies.

Bibliographies

1551.1
McCoy, Elizabeth, and McClung, Leland S. The anaerobic bacteria and their activities in nature and disease; a subject bibliography. Berkeley, University of California Press, 1939. 2 v. 295, 602 p.

v. 1. *Chronological author index.* Covers 1816–1938; v. 2. *Subject index.* Includes books, reports, theses, patents. Includes a number of nonmedical sources.

1551.2
——. Supplement one. Literature for 1938 and 1939. By Leland S. McClung and Elizabeth McCoy. Berkeley, University of California Press, 1941. 244 p.

Includes some literature for 1940.

1552
Raettig, Hansjurgen. Bakteriophagie, 1917 bis 1956. Zugleich ein Vorschlag Dokumentation wissenschaftlicher Literatur. Teil 1. Einführung, Sachregister, Stichwortverzeichnis. [Teil 2. Autorenregister]. Stuttgart, Fischer, 1958. 215, 344 p.

5655 references. Includes books, chapters in books, proceedings of conferences.

1553
Teah, B. A. Bibliography of germ free research, 1885–1963. South Bend, Ind., 1964. 43 p.

804 entries. Author arrangement.

1554
——. ——. 1964 suppl. [South Bend, Ind.] 1964. 19 p.

304 entries. Author arrangement. Includes references as early as 1901.

Dictionaries

1554.1
China (People's Republic) Wei shêng pu [Ministry of Health] Wei sheng wu hsüeh ming tz'ŭ [Glossary of microbiological terms] Peking, 1954. 37 p.

Chinese-English, English-Chinese.

1555
Hauduroy, Paul [et al.] Dictionnaire des bactéries pathogènes pour l'homme, les animaux et les plantes; suivi de la liste des êtres microscopiques conservés dans les collections de cultures types. 2 ed. Paris, Masson, 1953. 692, 64 p.

Bacteria are listed alphabetically with synonyms, brief morphologic descriptions, culture methods, biochemical and biologic properties, and references to the original descriptions.

1556
Jacobs, Morris B. [et al.] Dictionary of microbiology. Princeton, N. J., Van Nostrand, 1957. 276 p.

Includes bacteriology, mycology, virology, cytology, immunology, immunochemistry, serology, and microscopy.

1557
Partridge, William. Dictionary of bacteriological equivalents; French-English, German-English, Italian-English, Spanish-English. London, Bailliere, Tindall and Cox, 1927. 140 p.

In four sections by language.

Nomenclature

1558★★
Breed, R. S. [et al.] Bergey's Manual of determinative bacteriology. 7 ed. Baltimore, Williams and Wilkins, 1957.

1559★★
Buchanan, Robert E. [et al.] Index Bergeyana; an annotated alphabetic listing of names of the taxa of the bacteria. Baltimore, Williams and Wilkins, 1966. 1472 p.

". . . primarily an attempt to locate and annotate from the literature of bacteriology and related sciences all the 'scientific' (nonvernacular) names that have been proposed for the bacteria."

A companion volume to no. 1558.

1560
Mráz, Oldřich [et al.] Nomina und synonyma der pathogenen und saprophytären Mikroben, isoliert aus den wirtschaftlich oder epidemiologisch bedeutenden Wirbeltieren und Lebensmitteln tierischer Herkunft. Jena, Fischer, 1963. 488 p.

List of microorganisms which had occurred in the medical, veterinary, and nutrition literature of past three years. Written primarily for veterinary microbiologists. Three major parts: viruses and rickettsia, schizomycetes, and fungi. Each part in three sections: alphabetical index of accepted name, names plus synonyms with references to first time each used in literature, and alphabetical listings of synonyms. Schizomycetes has additional section on common names in German, English, French, and Russian literature. Appendix contains outlines of ten most important systems of nomenclature.

Directories

1561
American Society for Microbiology. Directory and constitution. Ann Arbor, Mich. [etc.] 196 – .

Continues same title issued by the Society of American Bacteriologists. Alphabetical list of names and addresses followed by geographical listing.

Histories

1562
Brock, Thomas D., ed. Milestones in microbiology. Englewood Cliffs, N.J., Prentice-Hall, 1961. 275 p.

From 16th to 20th century, mainly 19th. Source readings in English, in part abridged, with biographical notes and explanatory comments. No index.

1563
Bulloch, William. The history of bacteriology, London, Oxford University Press, 1938. 422 p. (Univ. of London, Heath Clark lectures, 1936)

Comprehensive history. Bibliography: p. 285–348. Reprinted 1960.

1564
Clark, Paul F. Pioneer microbiologists of America. Madison, University of Wisconsin Press, 1961. 369 p.

General survey, followed by chapters on local history. References: p. 333–355.

1565
Doetsch, Raymond N., ed. Microbiology, historical contributions from 1776 to 1908. New Brunswick, N.J., Rutgers University Press, 1960. 233 p.

Selections in English from the writings of 15 authors, with biobibliographical introduction and further readings for each.

1566
Grainger, Thomas H. A guide to the history of bacteriology. New York, Ronald Press, 1958. 210 p. (Chronica botanica, no. 18)

An annotated selective bibliography for students of the history of bacteriology. 2802 items, mostly in English. Includes many general reference works.

1567
Hahon, Nicholas, ed. Selected papers on virology. Englewood Cliffs, N.J., Prentice-Hall, 1964. 363 p.

39 papers from 1884 to 1962, in English or translated, plus Jenner's *Inquiry* (1798). References at end of each selection.

1568
Lechevalier, Hubert A., and Solotorovsky, M. Three centuries of microbiology. New York, McGraw-Hill, 1965. 536 p.

Review of the development of microbiology with biographical and interpretive data on leading figures and extensive quotations. Chapters on Fracastoro to Pasteur; Pasteur; Koch; special subjects. References at ends of chapters; general references: p. 529.

Immunology

Reviews

1569★
Advances in immunology. New York, Academic Press, 1, 1961– .

Annual reviews with bibliographies.

1570
Modern trends in immunology. Washington, 1, 1963– .

Irregular. Reviews with bibliographies.

Bibliographies

1571
U.S. Army Biological Laboratories. Fort Detrick, Md. Immunofluorescence; an annotated bibliography . . . [by] Warren R. Sanborn. 6 v. (Miscellaneous publication no. 3, 1965)

v. 1. Bacterial studies; v. 2. Viral studies; v. 3. Studies of fungi, metazoa, protozoa, and rickettsiae; v. 4. Studies of animal physiology; v. 5. Diagnostic applications and review articles; v. 6, Technical procedures.

Covers 1905–62. Separately issued author and brief subject index.

1572
U.S. Army Chemical Corps. Technical Library, Fort Detrick. Bibliography on vaccinia, variola, and animal pox. Fredrick, Md., 1956. 153 p. Supplement, 1956/60. 1961. [38] p.

Covers the world literature from 1798.

Mycology

Indexes and Abstracts

1573
Bibliography of systematic mycology. Kew, England, 1943/46– . Commonwealth Mycological Institute.

Semiannual.

Lists publications on all aspects of the taxonomy of fungi (including lichen fungi and fungal parasites of lichens but excluding lichens). Names of fungi are arranged systematically by Divisions, Classes, Orders, and Families. Regional and ecological lists arranged geographically. Author index in each issue.

Issues for 1943/46-1956 published as the Insitute's Mimeographed publication, no. 1–14.

1574
Index of fungi; published since the beginning of 1940. Oxford, University Press, 1, 1940– . Commonwealth Mycological Institute, Kew.

Semiannual with 10 year cumulative indexes.

Lists, with full bibliographical citations, the names of new genera, species and varieties of fungi, new combinations and new names, compiled from the world literature. The names are arranged alphabetically under genera and a host index is provided for each part.

v. 1, pt. 1–15, 1940–47, issued as Supplements to the *Review of applied mycology.*

1575
Review of applied mycology. Kew, Eng., 1, 1922– .

Monthly. About 3000 abstracts a year. Covers plant pathology as well as applied mycology.

1576
Review of medical and veterinary mycology. Kew, Eng., [1] 1943– . Commonwealth Mycological Institute.

Currently quarterly, each volume in 12 parts covering 3 years. v. 4, 1961–63, lists more than 2200 references, most with abstracts. Includes books, congresses, reports.

1943–50 issued annually as *An annotated bibliography of medical mycology*, without volume numbers. Voluming begins with v. 1, pt. 9, 1951.

Through 1946 sponsoring body called Imperial Mycological Institute.

Bibliographies

1577
Bachmann, Barbara J., and Strickland, Walter N. Neurospora bibliography and index. New Haven, Yale Univ. Press, 1965. 225 p.

Lists more than 2300 papers beginning with earliest.

1578
Ciferri, Rafaele, and Redaelli, Piero. Bibliographia mycopathologica, 1800–1940. Firenze, Sansoni, 1958. 2 v. (Contributi alla bibliografica Italica diretta da Marino Parenti, 18, 20).

14,506 numbered references to mycotic diseases in men and animals. Includes books, chapters in books, theses. Arranged alphabetically by author. No subject index.

1579
U.S. National Library of Medicine. Reference Division. Fungus infections; a bibliography covering literature of 1952 through September 1958. Comp. by Dorothy Bocker. Washington, 1959. 90 p.

943 selected and occasionally annotated references from the English, French, German, Italian, and Spanish literature.

1580
——. ——. Pulmonary mycotic infections; a

bibliography of literature 1957-April 1961. Comp. by Dorothy Bocker. Washington, 1961. 28 p.

347 selected references in English, French, German, Italian, and Spanish. Supplements no. 1579.

Dictionaries

1581
Ainsworth, Geoffrey C. Ainworth's and Bisby's Dictionary of the fungi. 5 ed. Kew, Eng., Commonwealth Mycological Institute, 1961. 547 p.

Listing of all generic names of fungi (Eumycetes and Myxothallophyta but not bacteria and lichens). Contains systematic arrangement of the genera of fungi and key to families. Includes terms used in the field and other information relating to mycology, e.g. list of societies and their publications and brief biographies of outstanding mycologists.

1 ed., 1943.

1582
Snell, Walter H., and Dick, Esther A. A glossary of mycology. Cambridge, Mass., Harvard Univ. Press, 1957. 171 p.

MICROSCOPY

Bibliographies

1583
Cosslett, V. E., ed. Bibliography of electron microscopy. London, Arnold, 1950. 350 p. Institute of Physics.

Over 2,500 references covering 1928–48, arranged alphabetically by author. Abstracts given for about half the references; titles in English only. No subject index.

1583.1
New York Society of Electron Microscopy. The International bibliography of electron microscopy. 2 v. New York, 1959–62. 166, 482 p.

v. 1, 1950–55; v. 2, 1956–61 and papers not reported in v. 1. Includes books, chapters in books, dissertations. Author arrangement. Includes co-author index.

Histories

1584
Clay, Reginald S., and Court, Thomas H. The history of the microscope compiled from the original instruments and documents, up to the introduction of the achromatic microscope. London, Griffin, 1932. 266 p.

Detailed history through early 19th century, with list of instrument makers. References in text.

1585
Conn, Harold J. The history of staining; with contributions from Lloyd Arnold [et al.] Geneva, N.Y., Biological Stain Commission, 1933. 141 p.

On men who have made contributions, and on dyes and staining methods in bacteriology, histology, and vital staining. References at ends of chapters. Articles originally published in *Stain technology*, 1928–33.

1586
Freund, Hugo, and Berg, Alexander, ed. Geschichte der Mikroskopie: Leben und Werk grosser Forscher. Frankfurt am Main, Umschau Verlag, 1963– .

To be in 3 v.: v. 1, Biologie, 1963; v. 2, Medizin, 1964 (506 p.; 46 biographies); v. 3 to be on other sciences. Each volume has general introduction and biographical sketches by various authors, arranged alphabetically, with bibliographies of contributions and of biographical and critical studies. Name index only in v. 1–2.

1587
Nachet, Albert. Collection Nachet. Instruments scientifiques et livres anciens. Notice sur l'invention du microscope et son évolution . . . Liste de savants, constructeurs & amateurs du XVIe au milieu du XIXe siècle. Paris, Petit, 1929. 145 p.

Illustrated catalog. Items 1–89: microscopes; 90–148: other instruments. List of early works on microscopes and mathematical instruments: p. 49–145.

1588
Rooseboom, Maria. Microscopium. Leiden, 1956. 59 p. (Leyden. Rijksmuseum voor de Geschiedenis der Natuurwetenschappen. Communication no. 95)

History of microscope. English text. 115 illustrations, many in color.

1589
Royal Microscopical Society. Origin and development of the microscope, as illustrated by catalogues of the instruments

and accessories, in the collections of the . . . Society, together with bibliographies of original authorities . . . Ed. by Alfred N. Disney . . . with Cyril F. Hill and Wilfred E. Watson Baker. Preceded by an historical survey on the early progress of optical science. London, The Society, 1928. 303 p.

Pt. 1, Historical survey from Euclid through the 17th century; pt. 2, descriptive catalogues of instruments to date of publication, with illustrations. Annotated bibliographies: p. 116–152; 284–297.

MILITARY MEDICINE

Indexes and Abstracts

Current

1590
Revue international des services de santé des armées de terre, de mer et de l'air. Bruxelles, 1, 1928– . Organe de l'Office International de Documentation de Médecine Militaire.

Currently contains: Revue-Reviews: abstracts of articles related to or of interest to military medicine arranged by country; Fiches bibliographiques des revues du mois: references listed under broad subjects, including history; Bibliographie; Book reviews.

1964 contained in excess of 600 abstracts.

Title also in English: *International review of the army, navy and air force medical service.* At head of title: Revue mensuelle; monthly review. But some issues bimonthly. v. 1–30, 1928–57 as *Bulletin international . . .*

Noncurrent

1591
Index medicus. War supplement. A classified record of literature on military medicine and surgery, 1914–1917. Washington, Carnegie Institution of Washington, 1918. 260 p.

1592
Jahrescherícht über die Leistungen in der Kriegesheilkunde. Würzburg, 1860–65?

Review of articles in medicine and surgery applicable to military medicine. Scant reference to military medical literature as such. No author or subject indexes.

1593
W. Roths Jahresbericht über die Leistungen und Fortschritte auf dem Gebiete des Militär-Sanitätswesens. Berlin, 1–39, 1873–1913.

Review of official reports and journal articles specifically relating to military and naval medicine. Country breakdowns. Breakdowns by wars in progress. Includes obituaries. Covers some nonmedical military publications.

v. 1–17, 1873–91, as *Jahresbericht . . .*

Bibliographies

1594
Fränkel, G.H.F. Bibliotheca medicinae militaris et navalis. Beiträge zur Literature der Militair- und Schiffsheilkunde. I. Inaugural-Abhandlungen. Thesen. Programme. Glogau, Mosche, 1876. 66 p.

Author listing. No more published.

1595
Human engineering bibliography. Washington, 1956/57–1961/62. U.S. Office of Naval Research.

Through 1961/62, 21,429 references, most with abstracts. Includes book. Emphasis on government and private research reports. Superseded and continued by no. 1597.1.

1596
Shellhase, Leslie J., ed. The bibliography of Army social work: The first twenty years, 1941–1962. Washington, Walter Reed Army Institute of Research, 1962. 55 p.

Chronological arrangement. Selectively annotated.

1597
Stich, Virginia, and Minton, Richard. A bibliography covering medical activity on the Canal Zone 1904–1954. [n.p., n.d.] 85 p.

Chronological subarrangement. At head of title: Gorgas Hospital, Medical Library.

1597.1
U.S. Army. Human Engineering Laboratories. Aberdeen Proving Ground, Md. Human factors engineering bibliographic series. 1, 1940/59– .

Abstracts. Includes books, research reports. 1960/64 published in 1966. Includes abstracts published in no. 1595.

1598
U.S. National Library of Medicine. Reference Division. A bibliography of military medicine relating to the Korean War, 1950–1956. Comp. by Charles Roos. Washington, 1957. 56 p.

505 entries, partially annotated.

1599
U.S. Veterans Administration. Medical and General Reference Library. Medical care of the veterans in the U.S., 1870–1960: a bibliography. Washington, 1963. 106 p.

Chronological arrangement of 1872 items.

Dictionaries

1599.1
Schmid-Daberkow, Gertrud. Wörterbuch der Militärmedizin. Teil 1. Russisch-Deutsch. Leipzig, VEB Verlag, 1963. 275 p.

Brief definitions. Largely general medical terms.

Encyclopedias

1600
Entsiklopedicheskiĭ slovar' voennoĭ meditsiny. [Encyclopedic dictionary of military medicine] Moskva, Medgiz, 1946–50. 6 v.

Chiefly concerned with current problems, but also includes history of military medicine and military medical institutions, biographies of military physicians, etc.

Histories

General

1601
Garrison, Fielding H. Notes on the history of military medicine. Washington, Association of Military Surgeons, 1922. 206 p.

1602
Germany (Territory under Allied Occupations, 1945– U.S. Zone) Military Tribunals. Trials of war criminals before the Nuremberg Military Tribunals under Control Council law No. 10. Nuremberg, October 1946-April 1949. v. 1–2. Washington, U.S. Government Printing Office [1949].

Cover title: The Medical Case. Title on Spine: U.S. vs. Brandt.

1603
Müller, S. Die Entwicklung und Stellung des militärärztlichen Standes in ausserdeutschen Heeren. p. 5–256 (Germany. Reichskriegsministerium. Heeres-Sanitätsinspektion. Veröffentlichungen aus dem Gebiete des Heeres-Sanitätswesens. Heft 102, 1937)

Includes most European countries, the Americas, Turkey, and Japan.

Australia

WORLD WAR I

1604
Butler, Authur G., ed. The Australian Army medical services in the war of 1914–1918. Melbourne, etc., Australian War Memorial, 1930–43, 3 v.

Half-title: *Official history . . .*

WORLD WAR II

1605
Australia in the war of 1939–1945. Ser. 5. Medical. Canberra, Australian War Memorial, 1952–61. 4 v.

v. 1–4 by Allen S. Walker; v. 5 by Allen S. Walker and others.

Canada

WORLD WAR I

1606
MacPhail, Andrew. Official history of the Canadian forces in the Great War 1914–19. The medical services. Ottawa, Acland, 1925. 428 p.

WORLD WAR II

1607
Feasby, William R., ed. Official history of the Canadian Medical Services 1939–45. Ottawa, Cloutier, 1953–56. 2 v.

France

WORLD WAR I

1608
Mignon, Alfred H. A. Le service de santé pendant la guerre 1914–1918. Paris, Masson, 1926–27. 4 v.

Germany

GENERAL

1609
Bauer, Werner. Geschichte der Marine-Sanitätswesens bis 1945. Berlin, Mittler, 1958. 138 p. (Marine-Rundschau, Beiheft 4)

1609.1
Ring, Friedrich. Zur Geschichte der Militärmedizin in Deutschland. Berlin, Deutscher Militärverlag, 1962. 369 p.

FRANCO-PRUSSIAN WAR

1610
Prussia. Kriegs-Ministerium. Medizinal-Abteilung. Sanitäts-Bericht über die deutschen Heere im Kriege gegen Frankreich 1870/71. Berlin, 1884–91. 8 v. in 10.

WORLD WAR I

1611
Germany. Heer. Sanitätsinspektion. Sanitätsbericht über das deutsche Heer (Deutsches Feld- und Besatzungsheer) im Weltkriege 1914/1918. Berlin, Mittler, 1934–38. 3 v. (Deutscher Kriegssanitätsbericht 1914/1918)

1612
Schjerning, Otto von. Handbuch der ärztlichen Erfahrungen im Weltkriege 1914/1918. Leipzig, Barth, 1921–22. 9 v.

WORLD WAR II

1613
U.S. Department of the Air Force. German aviation medicine, World War II. Prepared under the auspices of the Surgeon General, U.S. Air Force. Washington [1950] 2 v.

Great Britain

GENERAL

1614
Johnston, William. Roll of commissioned officers in the medical service of the British Army who served on full pay within the period between the accession of George II and the formation of the Royal Army Medical Corps, 20 June 1727 to 23 June 1898, with an introduction showing the historical evolution of the corps. Ed. by H. A. L. Howell. Aberdeen, University Press, 1917. 638 p.

Brief sketches, citing date of army appointment, campaigns, places of service, and date of death. For better-known figures, includes honorary degrees, hospital connections, achievements in medicine, and chief writings.

1615
Keevil, John J. Medicine and the navy, 1200–1900. Edinburgh, Livingstone, 1957–1963. 4 v.

Comprehensive history of medicine in the British navy. Footnote references throughout, with list of sources at end of each section (v. 1–2) or volume (v. 3–4). v. 3–4 by Christopher Lloyd and Jack L. S. Coulter.

CRIMEAN WAR

1616
Great Britain. Army Medical Department. Medical and surgical history of the British Army which served in Turkey and the Crimea during the war against Russia in the years 1854–56. London, Harrison, 1858. 2 v.

WORLD WAR I

1617
MacPherson, William G. [et al.] Medical services . . . London, H. M. S. O., 1921–24. 11 v. (History of the Great War, based on official documents)

Includes *Medical services, general history* (4 v.); *. . . diseases of the war* (2 v.); *. . . hygiene of the war* (2 v.); *. . . pathology* (1 v.); *. . . surgery of the war* (2 v.)

WORLD WAR II

1618
Cole, Howard N. On wings of healing; the story of the Airborne Medical Services, 1940–1960. Edinburgh, Blackwood, 1963. 225 p.

Quasi official. Chapter 17, Palestine 1945–48; chapter 18, 1947–61

1619
History of the Second World War. United Kingdom Medical Series. Arthur S. MacNalty, ed.-in-chief. London, H. M. S. O., 1952–62. 18 v.

India

GENERAL

1620
Crawford, Dirom G. A history of the In-

dian medical service, 1600–1913. London, Thacker, 1914. 2 v.

1621
—— . Roll of the Indian Medical Service, 1615–1930. London, Thacker, 1930. 710 p.

Brief sketches. Dates of birth and death, military career, and bibliographies. Arrangement chronologic, by localities, with name index.

1622
McDonald, Donald. Surgeons twoe [sic] and a barber, being some account of the life and work of the Indian Medical Service (1600–1947). London, Heinemann, 1950. 295 p.

WORLD WAR II

1623
Combined Inter-Services Historical Section, India and Pakistan. Official history of the Indian Armed Forces in the Second World War, 1939–45. Medical services. Ed. by B. L. Raina. [Calcutta] 1953–61? 4 v?

Japan

RUSSO-JAPANESE WAR

1623.1
Japan. Ministry of War. Meiji sanjushichi-hachi nen sen-eki rikugun eisei shi [Medical history of the army during the Russo-Japanese War of 1904–1905] Tokyo, 1907? 5 v.

WORLD WAR I

1623.2
Japan. Ministry of War. Shiberi shuppei eisei shi [Medical history of the Siberian expedition] Tokyo, Japan, 1924? 6 v.

New Zealand

WORLD WAR I

1624
Carbery, Anderson D. The New Zealand medical service in the Great War, 1914–1918. Auckland, Whitcombe, 1924. 567 p.

WORLD WAR II

1625
New Zealand. Dept. of Internal Affairs. War History Branch. Official history of New Zealand in the Second World War, 1939–45: [Medical history] Wellington, 1954–60. 2 v.

[v. 1] by T. Duncan M. Stout; [v. 2] by T. V. Anson.

Norway

1626
Norske militaerlaeger, 1882–1932. Biografier og billeder. Oslo, Grondahl, 1932. 203 p.

Short biographies and portraits of Norwegian army doctors.

U. S. S. R.

WORLD WAR II

1627
Opyt sovetskoĭ meditsiny v Velikoĭ Otechestvennoĭ Voĭne, 1941–1945 gg. [Experience of Soviet medicine in the Great Patriotic War, 1941–1945] Moskva, Medgiz, 1949–55. 35 v. in 32. Ed. by E. I. Smirnov.

United States

GENERAL

1628
Ashburn, Percy M. History of the Medical Department of the United States Army. Boston, Houghton, 1929. 448 p.

1629
Brown, Harvey E. Medical Department of the United States Army from 1775 to 1873. Washington, Surgeon General's Office, 1873. 314 p.

1630
Henry, Robert S. Armed Forces Institute of Pathology; its first century, 1862–1962. Washington, Department of the Army, Office of the Surgeon General, 1964. 422 p.

1631
Hume, Edgar E. Victories of army medicine; scientific accomplishments of the Medical Department of the United States Army. Philadelphia, Lippincott, 1943. 250 p.

1632
Phalen, James M. Chiefs of the Medical Department, United States Army, 1775–1940; biographical sketches. Carlisle Barracks, Pa., Medical Field Service School, 1940. 158 p. (Army medical bulletin, no. 52)

1633
Roddis, Louis H. A short history of nautical medicine. New York, Hoeber, 1941. 359 p.

General history, with emphasis on maritime medicine in U.S. Navy. Includes chronology (ca. 1000 B.C.–1912) and bibliographic note (p. 351–354). Reprinted from *Annals of medical history*, ser. 3, v. 3, 1941. Supplemented by biographies of U.S. surgeons general in *Military surgeon*, v. 89–92, 1941–42.

1634
U.S. Navy Department. Bureau of Medicine and Surgery. The Dental Corps of the United States Navy; a chronology 1912–1962. Washington, 1962. 132 p.

REVOLUTIONARY WAR

1635
Duncan, Louis C. Medical men in the American revolution, 1775–1783. Carlisle Barracks, Pa., Medical Field Service School, 1931. 414 p. (Army medical bulletin, no. 25)

1636
Owen, William O. Medical Department of the United States Army. Legislative and administrative history during the period of the Revolution, 1776–1786. New York, Hoeber, 1920. 226 p.

MEXICAN WAR

1637
Duncan, L. C. [Medical histories. Pt. 1] Medical history of General Scott's campaign to the City of Mexico in 1847. In Military surgeon 47:436–70, 1920. (Also in Bulletin U.S. Army Medical Department no. 50:61–117, Oct. 1939) [Pt. 2] Medical history of General Zachary Taylor's Army of Occupation in Texas and Mexico, 1845–1847. In Military surgeon 48:76–104, 1921. (Also in Bulletin U.S. Army Medical Department no. 50:26–60, Oct. 1939)

CIVIL WAR

1638
Adams, George W. Doctors in blue; the medical history of the Union Army in the Civil War. New York, Schuman, 1952. 253 p.

1639
Cunningham, H. H. Doctors in gray; the Confederate Medical Service. Baton Rouge, Louisiana State University Press, 1958. 339 p.

1640
Duncan, Louis C. The Medical Department of the United States Army in the Civil War. [Washington, 1914] 1 v. [various pagings]

Collected reprints of articles appearing originally in *Military surgeon*.

1640.1
Maxwell, William Q. Lincoln's fifth wheel: the political history of the United States Sanitary Commission. New York, Longmans, Green, 1956. 372 p.

1641
New York Public Library. Hospital directories of the Civil War of the U.S. Sanitary Commission, 1862–1865, in the New York Public Library. Boston, 1962. 44 v.

1642
U.S. War Department. Surgeon General's Office. The medical and surgical history of the War of the Rebellion (1861–65). Prepared . . . under the direction of Joseph K. Barnes. Washington, 1870–88. 2 pt. in 6 v.

The standard "source" history.

SPANISH AMERICAN WAR

1643
Senn, Nicholas. Medico-surgical aspects of the Spanish American War. Chicago, American Medical Association Press, 1900. 379 p.

1644
[Sternberg, George M.] The work of the Medical Department during the Spanish war. In Report of the Surgeon General of the Army . . . June 30, 1898. Washington, 1898. p. 100–265.

WORLD WAR I

1645
U.S. War Department. Surgeon General's Office. Medical Department of the United States Army in the World War . . . Prepared under the direction of M. W. Ireland. Washington, 1921–29. 15 v. in 17.

WORLD WAR II

1646
U.S. Air Force. Office of the Surgeon General. Medical support of the Army Air Forces in World War II. By Mae M. Link and Hubert A. Coleman. Washington, 1955. 1027 p.

1647
U.S. Department of the Army. Office of the Chief of Military History. United States Army in World War II. The technical services. Washington, 1959– .

Includes volumes on the Medical Department and the Chemical Warfare Service.

1648
——. Office of the Surgeon General. The Medical Department of the United States Army [in World War II]. Washington, 1952– .

1649
U.S. Navy Department. Bureau of Medicine and Surgery. The history of the Medical Department of the United States Navy in World War II. Washington, 1950–53. 3 v. (NAVMED P-5031, P-5021, P-1318)

1650
—. —. The United States Navy Medical Department at war, 1941–1945. [Washington, 1946–] 2 v. in 7.

Cover title: U.S. Navy Medical Department. Administrative history, 1941–45. Mimeographed.

1651
U.S. Office of Scientific Research and Development. Advances in military medicine made by American investigators working under the sponsorship of the Committee on Medical Research. Ed. by E. C. Andrus [et al.]. Boston, Little, Brown, 1948. 2 v. (Its Science and Development in World War II)

POST WORLD WAR II

1652
U.S. Navy Department. Bureau of Medicine and Surgery. The history of the Medical Department of the United States Navy, 1945–1955. [Washington, 1958] 224 p. (NAVMED P-5057)

MUSCULOSKELETAL SYSTEM

Indexes and Abstracts

1653
Arthritis and rheumatic diseases abstracts. Bethesda, 1, 1964– . U.S. National Institute of Arthritis and Metabolic Diseases.

Monthly. Through v. 1, no. 10, 2753 entries, most with abstracts.

1654
Electromyography; international journal of electromyography; abstracts. Louvain. 1, 1961– . University of Louvain. E.M.G. Laboratory.

Quarterly. Abstracts in English, French, and Dutch.

v. 1–2, no. 1, has subtitle: International journal of clinical and experimental electromyography; abstracts of world literature.

1655
Index of rheumatology. New York, 1, 1965– . American Rheumatism Association in cooperation with the National Library of Medicine.

Semimonthly. A recurring bibliography produced by MEDLARS.

1656
Muscular dystrophy abstracts; a service of abstracts from the current medical literature of the world covering muscular dystrophy and areas of basic science pertinent to related disorders. New York, 1, 1957– . Muscular Dystrophy Associations of America, Inc., in cooperation with the Excerpta Medica Foundation.

23–24 issues per year. Approximately 1300 abstracts a year.

1657
World bibliographic index on rheumatic diseases of specialized journals. 1, 1958/59– . In AIR. Archives of Inter-American Rheumatology. (Rio de Janeiro) v. 4, 1961– . Pan-American League against Rheumatism.

3d review, 1962, (AIR v. 8(1–2) Mar.–June, 1965) listed 574 articles from 17 journals. No author index.

2d review, 1960/61 (AIR v. 6(3) Sept. 1963).

Reviews

1658
Rheumatism and arthritis. Review of American and English literature of recent years [1, 1922/23]- . In Annals of internal medicine 8, 1935- .

Irregular. The 16th review (1964) consisted of a selective review of 1215 references. No author index.

v. 1–2 as *The present status of rheumatism and arthritis . . .*; v. 3–7 as *The problem of rheumatism and arthritis . . .*

Recent years published in *Annals of Internal Medicine. Supplement.*

Bibliographies

1659
Khar'kovakaia gosudarstvennaia nauchno-meditsinskaia biblioteka. Revmatizm; bibliografiia otechestvennoĭ literatury, 1934–1953 gg. [Rheumatism; bibliography of national literature, 1934–1953] Khar'kov, 1954. 238 p.

2247 references, including books.

1660
Ryzhkov, Iu. D. [et al.] Sto let izucheniia urovskoĭ Kashina-Beka bolezni; bibliograficheskiĭ ukazatel' otechestvennoĭ literatury [One hundred years of teaching of Kaschin-Beck Urov disease; bibliographic index to national literature] Chita, Urovskaia nauchno-issledovatel'skaia stantsiia, 1958. 59 p.

441 references on osteoarthritis deformans endemica. Includes books, newspaper articles, dissertations, collected works, proceedings, reviews, and bibliographic and archival materials. Contains a chronological index.

1661
Sándor, Róbert. Magyar reumatológiai (balneológiai, fizikoterapiai, bioklimatológiai) bibliográfia (1945–1960) [Bibliography of Hungarian rheumatology (balneology, physical therapy, bioclimatology, 1945–1960)] Budapest, Országos Orvostudományi Könyvtár és Dokumentációs Központ, 1962. 239 p.

Lists 1846 references including books. Covers the literature published in Hungary or by Hungarian authors abroad. Chronological subarrangement. Includes a list of periodicals indexed with abbreviations.

Nomenclature

1662
Ruhl, Mary Jane, and Sokoloff, Leon. A thesaurus of rheumatology. New York, Grune and Stratton, 1965. 182 p.

Prepared by the American Rheumatism Association Literature Analysis Subcommittee. Over 11,000 terms.

Directories

1663
American Rheumatism Association. Directory and by-laws, 1961–1962. New York, 1962.

Alphabetical roster of members with addresses; also includes officers and committees and a geographical listing.

Histories

1664
Copeman, William S. C. A short history of the gout and rheumatic diseases. Berkeley, University of California Press, 1964. 236 p.

Bibliography, including sources: p. 221–227.

Orthopedics

Indexes and Abstracts

CURRENT

1664.1
Archivio "Putti" di chirurgia degli organi di movimento. Firenze, 1, 1951- . Bibliografia, 1950- .

Currently annual. 1962 listed about 950 annotated references from 36 journals. Annotations in Italian. The *Bibliografia* is a separately paged and indexed "supplement" to the *Archivio.*

1950–52, 1 semestre (of two) each year.

NONCURRENT

1665
Abstracts of orthopedic surgery. Washington, 1948–50. U.S. Department of the Army. Office of the Surgeon General.

1950 had in excess of 1300 abstracts.

1666
Bibliografia ortopedica. Bologna, 1–24, 1920–41.

Abstracts in Italian. Includes books.

Published in conjunction with *Chirurgia organi movimento* (not listed)

1667
Jahrbuch für orthopädische Chirurgie. Berlin, 1–4, 1909–12.

1668
Zentralblatt für chirurgische und mechanische Orthopädie; einschliesslich der gesamten Heilgymnastik und Massage. Berlin, 1–13, 1907–19.

Includes books and proceedings of congresses. v. 1 contained about 1000 abstracts.

1669
Zentralblatt für orthopädische Chirurgie und Mechanik. Bern, 1–7, 1884–90.

Reviews

1670
Progress in orthopedic surgery. Chicago, 1940– . American Academy of Orthopaedic Surgeons.

1945 reviewed approximately 890 articles. Reprinted from the *Archives of surgery.*

1671
Seikeigeka saikin no shinpo [Recent advances in orthopedics] Tokyo, 1, 1956– .

1672★
Year book of orthopedics, traumatic and plastic surgery. Chicago, Year Book Medical Publishers, 1902– . (The practical medicine year books)

Abstracts with editorial comment.

1902 as *Pediatrics and orthopedic surgery*; 1903–23, as *Pediatrics . . . orthopedic surgery*; 1940–46 as *Year book of industrial and orthopedic surgery*; 1947–62 as *Year book of orthopedics and traumatic surgery.*

1924–39 as a chapter in no. 2555.

1902–05 as The practical medicine series of year books; 1906–23, The practical medicine series.

Bibliographies

1673
Blencke, August, and Gocht, Hermann. Die orthopädische Weltliteratur . . . 1903–1930. Stuttgart, Enke, 1936. 2 v.

Contains some references earlier than 1903. Includes books, theses.

1674
——. ——. Ergänzungsband, 1931–1935. Bearbeitet von Dr. Erich Witte. Stuttgart, Enke, 1938. 843 p.

Contains some references earlier than 1931. Includes books and theses.

1675
Hoffa, Albert J., and Blencke, August. Die orthopädische Literatur . . . Zugleich Anhang zu . . . Hoffa's Lehrbuch der orthopädischen Chirurgie. Stuttgart, Enke, 1905.

From the earliest literature through 1903. Includes books and theses.

1676
Società italiana di ortopedia e traumatologia. Indice bibliografico italiano di ortopedia e traumatologia. Pagano, 1957. [947] p.

20,000 references from 16 journals from date of founding to 1956. Earliest reference noted was 1880. Includes monographs published since 1907. Detailed classified arrangement. No author index.

At head of title: Cinquantenario della Società italiana di ortopedia e traumatologia (1907–1957).

Histories

1677
Bader, Luigi. Genesi ed evoluzione dell' ortopedia in Italia, dalla chirurgia del medioevo alla chirurgia ortopedica dei nostri giorni. Padova, Editrice liviana, 1962. 814 p.

Biobibliographies from 12th through 19th century (p. 3–166) and bibliography of other works, 1808–1899 (p. 167–174). Accounts of hospitals and other institutions and societies. Periodicals and society publications: p. 707–741. General bibliography: p. 745–759.

1678
Bick, Edgar M. Source book of orthopaedics. 2 ed. Baltimore, Williams & Wilkins, 1948. 540 p.

Pt. 1, p. 1–88, orthopedic surgery before the 19th century; pt. 2, contemporary orthopedic surgery and its recent sources. Not a collection of texts, but a historical survey giving summaries and evaluations of significant contributions. Final chapter on the rise of orthopedic hospitals and institutions. List of 45 orthopedic journals: p. 497–499. References (mainly original works) at ends of chapters. General bibliography: p. 500–501. Preliminary ed. 1933, as *History and source book of orthopaedic surgery*; 1 ed. under present title, 1937.

1679
Half a century of progress in orthopaedic surgery. In Journal of bone and joint surgery 32–B:451–740, 1950.

Chapters by different authors on orthopedic surgery in various countries. Extensive classified list of references for the United States, p. 550–569; shorter lists for other countries.

1680
Rang, Mercer, ed. Anthology of orthopaedics. Edinburgh, Livingstone, 1966. 242 p.

Collection of excerpts in English from all periods, arranged by subjects, with popular biographical notes on the authors. References: p. 233–237.

1680.1
Valentin, Bruno. Geschichte der Fusspflege: Pedicurie, Chiropodie, Podologie. Stuttgart, Thieme, 1966. 103 p.

Includes quacks, podiatry in art. 191 references in footnotes. No index.

1681
——. Geschichte der Orthopädie. Stuttgart, Thieme, 1961. 288 p.

Well rounded history. Bibliographical footnotes.

NEOPLASMS

Indexes and Abstracts

There is no current specialized general index to or abstract of the literature of cancer in English except *Excerpta medica* Sect. 16, which, with *Index Medicus* and other general indexes, must be used to cover the field.

Current

1682
Cancer chemotherapy abstracts. Bethesda, 1, 1960– . Cancer Chemotherapy National Service Center.

Monthly. In 1964 listed more than 3000 references, most with abstracts. About 4700 journals scanned.

1683
Leukemia abstracts. Chicago, 1, 1953– . Sponsored by the Lenore Schwartz Leukemia Foundation; prepared by Research Information Service, John Crerar Library.

Monthly. About 1300 abstracts a year. Minimum time lag 2 months.

1684
Referativnyĭ sbornik: voprosy onkologii [Collection of abstracts: problems of oncology] Moskva, 1, 1964– . Akademiia meditsinskikh nauk.

Abstracts or abridged translations of foreign articles.

1685
Riga. Respublikanskaia nauchnaia meditsinskaia biblioteka. Rak molochnoĭ zhelezy; bibliograficheskiĭ ukazatel' otechestvennoĭ literatury... [Cancer of mammary glands; a bibliographic index to national literature...] Riga, Ministerstvo zdravookhraneniia Latviiskoĭ SSR, 1955/60–

Includes books, dissertations. 429 entries in 1961/63.

Entries in Russian. Title varies slightly.

Noncurrent

1686
Abstracts of Soviet medicine. Cancer Research, 1953–1956. A translation of Sovetskoe Meditsinskoe Referativnoe Obozrenie Onkologiya, v. 5–9. Ed. by H. A. Sissions. Amsterdam, Excerpta Medica Foundation, 1959.

1814 references or abstracts covering the period 1949–55.

1687
Cancer current literature index. New York, 1–2, 1959–60. Excerpta Medica Foundation for the American Cancer Society.

Advanced listing of references later to be abstracted in the Cancer Section of *Excerpta Medica*. 4805 references limited to journal articles and selected congresses.

1688
Carcinogenesis abstracts. Bethesda, 1, 1963–65. National Cancer Institute.

Monthly. Approximately 2300 abstracts a year.

1689
Index analyticus cancerologiae. Paris, 1–

33, 1927–62. Ligue française contre le cancer.

Quarterly. The 1962 volume has 2059 abstracts. Continues no 1690.

1690
Revue analytique des travaux sur le cancer, 1922–26. In Bulletin de l'Association française pour l'étude du cancer, 11–15, 1922–26.

1926 issue had 294 abstracts. Continued by no. 1689.

1691
Zeitschrift für Krebsforschung. Referate. Berlin, 25–55 (1) 1927–1944.

Separately paged supplements to the issues of the *Zeitschrift*. v. 53 listed more than 1100 references, most with abstracts. Includes books and theses.

Reviews

1692★★
Advances in cancer research. New York, 1, 1953– .

Reviews with bibliographies.

1693
Cancer progress. London, 1960– .

Irregular. Review articles with bibliographies.

1694
Current scientific literature review. Cancer immunology abstracts. Philadelphia, Medical Literature, Inc., 1958–61.

1695
Progress in clinical cancer. New York, Grune and Stratton, 1, 1965– .

1696
Progress in experimental tumor research. Fortschritte der experimentellen Tumorforschung. Progrès de la recherche experimentale des tumeurs. Basel, Karger, 1, 1960– .

Annual reviews with bibliographies. In English, German, or French.

1697★
Year book of cancer. Chicago, Year Book Medical Publishers. 1956/57– . (The practical medicine year books)

Abstracts, with editorial comment. Emphasis on clinical aspects.

Bibliographies

1698
American Cancer Society. Medical and Scientific Library. Bibliography on cancer for nurses. New York, 1958. 41 p.

1699
Arutinunov, A. I., and Rudiak, K. E. Opukholi golovnogo i spinnogo mozga; bibliografiia otechestvennoĭ literatury, 1917–1961 gg. [Tumors of cerebrum and spinal cord; a bibliography of the national literature, 1917–1961] Kiev, Gos. medits. izd-vo USSR, 1963. 408 p.

Contains 4591 references, including books and dissertations. Most entries are in Russian.

1700
Bibliografia brasileira de oncologia. Salvador, 1, 1961– . Liga Bahiana contra o Câncer.

v. 1 covers the literature from 1851–1952; v. 2, 1953–60.

1701
Cancer chemotherapy, a bibliography of agents, 1946–1954. Prepared by Bibliography Section, Reference Division, Armed Forces Medical Library. Comp. under the direction of Marjory C. Spencer. Cancer Research 16 (Suppl. 4), 1956.

3704 partly annotated references arranged by agents or groups of agents.

Up-dates no. 1714.

1702
——. ——. Supplement, 1955–1959. Comp. under the direction of Marjory C. Spencer. Cancer Research 25 (Suppl. 36), 1965.

1702.1
Cancer Research Institute, Bratislava. Bibliography of selected contributions of experimental oncology in CSSR, 1964–65. Bratislava, 1966. 87 p.

180 summaries of papers by Czech and foreign authors published in Czech periodicals. The Institute also edited a similar publication covering 1961–63.

1703
Donner Foundation. Index to the literature of experimental cancer research, 1900–1935. Philadelphia, The Foundation, 1948. 1057 p.

1704
Everson, Tilden C., and Cole, Warren H. Spontaneous regression of cancer; a study and abstract of reports in the world medical literature and of personal communications concerning spontaneous regression of malignant disease. Philadelphia, Saunders, 1966. 506 p.

176 abstracts in text; 700 item bibliography at end of volume.

1705
Gesellschaft zur Bekämpfung der Krebs-Krankheiten, Nordrhein-Westfalen. Katalog der Bibliothek der Zentralstelle für Krebsbekämpfung, Düsseldorf. In- und auslädische Krebsliteratur. Erstellt von Arnold Merscheim. Essen, Baedeker [1957] 393 p.

Consists of monographs listed by author or title and serials listed by title.

1706 (not used)

1707
Koenig, Elizabeth. Cancer and virus; a guide and annotated bibliography to monographs, reviews, symposia, and survey articles, with emphasis on human neoplasm, 1950–63. Washington, 1966. 94 p. (Public Health Service. Publication no. 1424)

291 numbered entries.

1708
Mikyška, Jan. Literatura o nádorech; soupis studií ze zahraničních lékařských časopisů v r. 1955 [Literature on tumors; index of studies which appeared in foreign medical journals in 1955] Praha, Státní lékařská knihovna, 1956. 3 pts.

3672 articles from non-Czechoslovak journals, 186 selected books. Titles in original language and Czech. No author index.

1709
National Cancer Association of South Africa. Bibliography on cancer in Africa. Johannesburg, 1963. 106 p.

1889 (earliest reference noted) –1961.

Issued as South African Cancer Bulletin 7(4), Oct.–Dec., 1963. Supplement.

1709.1
——. ——. Supplement. 31 p.

References for 1961–63.

South African Cancer Bull 9(1), Jan.–Mar. 1965. Supplement.

1710
Neubauer, Otto. Bibliography of cancer produced by pure chemical compounds; a survey of the literature up to and including 1947. London, Oxford University Press, 1959. 604 p.

4960 references.

1710.1
Roberts, D. C. Research using transplanted tumours of laboratory animals: a cross referenced bibliography, II. London, Imperial Cancer Research Fund, 1965. 127 p.

588 English language papers received by the Fund, Registry and Information Service for Experimental Tumours, with subject and tumour index.

1711
Rückert, Ernst, and Kleeberg, Heinz. 25 Jahre Krebsforschung im deutschsprachigen Schrifttum. Eine Auswahl von Buch- und Zeitschriftenliteratur aus den Jahren 1931–1955. Berlin, VEB Verlag, Volk und Gesundheit, 1961. 798 p. (Leipzig. Deutsche Bücherei. Sonderbibliographien, 25)

More than 15,000 references.

1712
Selye, Hans. Ovarian tumors bibliography. In Encyclopedia of endocrinology by Hans Selye. Sect: 4. Ovary. Vol. 7, Bibl. Montreal, Richardson, 1946. 427 p.

Author arrangement. Includes books, theses. Earliest reference noted was 1686.

1713★
U.S. National Cancer Institute. A bibliography of the cytologic diagnosis of cancer. Comp. by Erwin F. Hoffman [et al.] Bethesda, Md., 1952. 114 p.

Lists more than 1000 references through 1951. Earliest reference noted was 1853.

1714★
——. An index of tumor chemotherapy; a tabulated compilation of data from the literature on clinical and experimental investigations. By Helen M. Dyer. Washington, 1949. 329 p.

Arrangement by compound or agent with citation to a 2213 item bibliography.

1715★
World Health Organization. Bibliography on the epidemiology of cancer, 1946–1960. Geneva, 1963. 168 p.

Limited to the epidemiology of human cancer. 2671 references. Anatomical site index. Title also in French.

1715.1
——. Inventory of cancer research, as of 31 December 1965. Geneva, 1966. 534, [83] p.

Principally a list of institutions under country arrangement, giving subject of research and principal investigator. In addition has sections: Alphabetical list of investigators, Subject index, Index of institutions by country. Sections referred to as Annexe 1–4.

Nomenclature

1716★
American Cancer Society. Statistics Committee. Manual of tumor nomenclature and coding. Corr. ed. New York, The Society, 1951 [i.e. 1953] 119 p.

Arranged by class, with name list.

1717
Armed Forces Institute of Pathology. Preliminary tumor nomenclature. Washington, 1961. 50 p.

1717.1
International Union Against Cancer. Illustrated tumor nomenclature. Berlin, Springer-Verlag, 1965. 299 p.

273 terms in English, French, Russian, German, Spanish, and Latin. Histological arrangement.

Directories

1718
Cancer services, facilities and programs in the United States. Washington, D.C., [1] 1955– . U.S. Public Health Service. Cancer Control Program.

Geographical arrangement. Data include state advisory groups, summary of legislation, schools of cytotechnology, hospitals and treatment services, funds available, mortality data, registers collecting data on patients. Compiled in 1960 under present title from two earlier publications, *State cancer control programs as planned for fiscal years 1954 and 1955* (PHS Pub. no. 404) and *Cancer services and facilities in the United States*, 1954 (PHS Pub. no. 14).

1962 ed. Public Health Service Publication no. 14 (rev.).

1719
International Union Against Cancer. Facilities for the diagnosis and treatment of cancer throughout the world. [By] George T. Pack [and] Mildred E. Allen. [Basle, 1964?] 76 p.

Listing by country of diagnostic and treatment facilities, including hospitals and clinics; lists other facilities and services and gives statistics on death rates by sex and site.

1720
Koenig, Elizabeth, comp. Russian scientists in cancer-virus research; a bibliodirectory of current studies. New York [1962] 35 p.

71 investigators listed.

1721
U.S. National Cancer Institute. American scientists in cancer-virus research. A biblio-directory of current studies. Comp. by Elizabeth Koenig and Lois Fritz. Bethesda, 1962. 80 p. (Public Health Service. Publication no. 946).

363 investigators listed.

Films

1722
Cancer film guide. Washington, 1961– . U.S. Public Health Service. Prepared for the Cancer Control Branch by the Audiovisual Facility.

1963 ed. contains about 1200 titles.
1961 as *Cancer motion picture guide.*

History

1723
Wolff, Jacob. Die Lehre von der Krebs-

krankheit von den ältesten Zeiten bis zur Gegenwart. Jena, Fischer, 1907–28. 4 v.

Exhaustive, well documented study. Arranged by subject, with analyses of contributions. Footnote references.

NEUROLOGY AND PSYCHIATRY

Indexes and Abstracts

For general questions in psychiatry *Excerpta medica*, Section 8B (no. 9.8) *Psychological abstracts* (no. 2293) and *Index medicus* (no. 11) probably give the most comprehensive coverage.

Current

1724
Abstracts of psychiatry for the general practitioner. Belle Mead, N.J., 1, 1958– . Carrier Clinic.

Quarterly. 120 abstracts per year. Triennial cumulative indexes.

1725
Bibliographie der psychologischen Literatur der sozialistischen Länder aus dem Jahre . . . Berlin, 1, 1958?– . Deutsches Pädagogisches Zentralinstitut.

Annual. Arranged by country: Soviet Union, Czechoslovakia, Bulgaria, Hungary, and East Germany.

1726
Digest of neurology and psychiatry. Hartford, Conn., 1, 1932– . Institute of Living, Hartford.

Monthly. Includes books. About 450 abstracts a year.

Has additional title or subtitle: *Abstracts and reviews of selected literature in psychiatry, neurology and their allied fields.*

Ser. 1–2, 1932–Oct. 1944, as *Abstracts and translations of the science library of the Institute of Living, Hartford.*

1727
Excerpta criminologica. Amsterdam, 1, 1961– . Excerpta Medica Foundation.

Bimonthly. Abstracts. Includes monographs. Includes considerable material from the psychiatric literature as well as specifically criminological sources. About 35 percent of 1961 entries duplicated in *Cumulated index medicus.*

1728
The group psychotherapy literature, 1954– . In International journal of group psychotherapy. New York, 5, 1955– . American Group Psychotherapy Association.

Annual. 1965 listed 199 items with selective review.

1729
Mental health book review index. Flushing, N.Y., 1, 1956– . Council on Research in Bibliography.

Annual. Author or title listing, with titles followed by review sources. No subject index. Each annual lists about 300 books, with 3 or more reviews. Since 1956, 3283 titles have been listed.

Sponsored by the World Federation for Mental Health, etc.

1730
Monthly listings of neuro-psychiatric literature. Cleveland, [1] 1963– . Cleveland State Hospital. Documentation Research Laboratory.

Author arrangement under subdivisions of principal breakdowns: neurology, psychiatry, psychology. Author index in each issue. No annual indexes. Minimum time lag 0 months.

1730.1
Parkinson's disease and related disorders. Citations from the literature. New York, 1963/64– . Parkinson Information Center, Columbia University Medical Library.

Weekly. Annual cumulations.

1731
Psychiatry digest; a summary of the world's psychiatric literature. Northfield, Ill., etc., 15, 1954– .

1965 contained approximately 340 digests. Book reviews listed separately. No annual author or subject indexes.

v. 15–23, 1954–62, as *Journal of clinical and experimental psychopathology and quarterly review of psychiatry and neurology.* Continues no. 1738.

1732
Referátový výběr z psychiatrie a neurologie [Selected abstracts on psychiatry and neurology] Praha, 1, 1951?– . Ústav pro zdravotnickou dokumentaci.

4 times a year. Abstracts in Czech or Slovak of selected articles from foreign periodicals, chiefly in Western languages.

1959 as *Referátový výběr z psychiatrie.*

1733

Zentralblatt für die gesamte Neurologie und Psychiatrie. Berlin, 1, 1910– . Organ des Gesamtverbandes deutscher Nervenärzte.

Currently 4–5 volumes a year in 3 issues and a 4th index issue (much delayed). Recent volumes listed about 1300 references to articles, books, chapters of books, and proceedings of societies, most with abstracts.

Time lag for 1964 rarely less than 8 months.

v. 1, 1910, as *Zeitschrift für die gesamte Neurologie und Psychiatrie. Referate;* v. 2–24, 1911–21, . . . *Referate und Ergebnisse.*

Subtitle: v. 25–87, 1921–38, Referatenteil der Zeitshrift für die gesamte Neurologie und Psychiatrie und Fortsetzung des von E. Mendel begründeten Neurologischen Centralblattes; v. 88–104, 1938–44, without von E. Mendel; v. 105, 1948– , Referatenteil des Archivs für Psychiatrie und Nervenkrankheiten vereinigt mit Zeitschrift für die gesamte Neurologie und Psychiatrie.

Noncurrent

1734

Bericht über die psychiatrische Literatur, 1880–1937. In Allgemeine Zeitschrift für Psychiatrie. Berlin, 37–106, 1881–1939.

The 1939 *Bericht* listed in excess of 1600 references to articles, books and some dissertations, selectively annotated.

Published as a separate issue of the *Zeitschrift* (with v. 54, 1897, called *Literaturheft*).

1735

Jahresbericht Neurologie und Psychiatrie. Berlin, 1–15, 1910–31.

Annual cumulation of references of no. 1733.

v. 1–4, 1910–13, as *Bibliographie über die gesamte Neurologie und Psychiatrie;* v. 5–10, 1921–26, *Jahresbericht über die gesamte . . .*

1736

Jahresbericht über die Leistungen und Fortschritte auf dem Gebiete der Neurologie und Psychiatrie. Berlin, 1–23, 1897–1919.

References listed alphabetically by author and then abstracted or summarized selectively. v. 17, 1913, listed in excess of 12,000 references, including books and theses.

1737

Neurologisches Centralblatt. Referate. Leipzig, 1–40, 1882–1921.

Abstracts of articles, books, theses and proceedings of societies. About 1100 abstracts in v. 21, 1902.

From v. 22–39, 1903–20, contained *Neurologische und psychiatrische Literatur,* 1902–20, a listing of some 2000 references a year, not abstracted but included in the annual author index. Bimonthly through May–June 1914 (v. 33, 1914), semiannual July–Dec. 1914 (v. 34, 1915), quarterly Jan. 1915–20 (v. 34–39, 1915–20).

Merged with no. 1733.

1738

Quarterly review of psychiatry and neurology. Washington, 1–8(1), 1946–Jan. 1953, Apr.–Oct. 1953. Washington Institute of Medicine.

Selected abstracts. Includes book reviews and original articles.

v. 1–7(2), 1946–Apr. 1952, published separately; v. 7(3)–8(1), July 1952–Jan. 1953, in *International record of medicine and general practice clinics,* v. 165(7)–166(1), July 1952–Jan. 1953; Apr.–Oct. 1953 published without voluming in *International record of medicine. . .,* v. 166(4–10), Apr.–Oct. 1953.

v. 6(2), April 1951–53: Incorporating *International record of psychiatry and neurology* (original article section).

1739

Zentralblatt für Nervenheilkunde und Psychiatrie. Leipzig, 1–33, 1878–1910.

v. 17, 1894, had in excess of 600 abstracts or reviews of articles, books, theses, and proceedings of societies.

v. 17, 1894 (June–July) contained *Verzeichniss der neurologischen Literatur für das Quartel 1894* (515 entries), continued in Nov. and Dec. issues as *v. 2 Quartals-Uebersicht der neurologischen Literatur des Auslandes* (724 entries).

v. 1–12, as *Centralblatt für Nervenheilkunde, Psychiatrie und gerichtliche Psychopathologie.*

Continued by no. 1733.

Reviews

1740

Annual survey of psychoanalysis. New York, 1, 1950– .

Reviews with bibliographies. 1956 volume published in 1963. In addition, to reviewing selected monographs, the 1956 volume abstracted from 28 journals.

1741
Current psychiatric therapies. New York, 1, 1961– .

Annual. Supersedes no. 1747.

1742
International review of neurobiology. New York, 1, 1959– .

Annual.

1743
Modern trends in neurology. Washington, etc., ser. 1, 1951– . (Butterworths medical publications. Modern trends series).

Irregular. Includes reviews with bibliographies. Ser. 2 published 1957; ser. 3, 1962.

1744
Progress in biocbernetics. Amsterdam, 1, 1956– .
Progress in biocybernetics. Amsterdam, 1, 1964– .

1745
Progress in neurobiology. London, etc., Cassell, 1, 1956– .

1746★
Progress in neurology and psychiatry; an annual review. New York, 1, 1944/45– .

Reviews with bibliographies.

1747
Progress in psychotherapy. New York, v. 1–5, 1956–60.

Annual review with author and subject indexes. Superseded by no. 1741.

1748
Recent advances in neurology and neuropsychiatry. 7 ed. Ed. by William R. Brain. London, Churchill, 1962. 282 p.

Chapter bibliographies (omitting titles of articles). No overall author index.

1 ed., 1929; 6 ed., 1955. At head of title: Brain and Strauss.

5 ed., 1945, translated into Italian and Rumanian.

1749
Recent progress in psychiatry. London, 1950– .

Irregular. Review articles.

1750
Review of psychiatric progress. In American journal of psychology, 1943– .

Annual. Appears in January issue. Two- to six-page reviews with long bibliographies.

1751
Shinkei kenkyu no shimpo [Advances in neurological science] Tokyo, 1, 1956– .

Quarterly.

1752
Sieshin igaku saikin no shinpo [Recent advances in psychiatry] Tokyo, 1, 1957– .

Irregular.

1753★
Year book of neurology, psychiatry, and neurosurgery. Chicago, Year Book Medical Publishers, 1902– . (The practical medicine year books)

Abstracts, with editorial comment.

1902–06 as *Skin and venereal diseases. Nervous and mental diseases*; 1907–30 as *Nervous and mental diseases*; 1931–32 as *Neurology... psychiatry*; 1933 as *Year book of neurology and psychiatry*; 1934 as *Year book of neurology, psychiatry and endocrinology*.

1902–05 and 1932 as Practical medicine series of year books; 1906–31, Practical medicine series.

Bibliographies

1754
Abderhalden, Emil. Bibliographie der gesamten wissenschaftlichen Literatur über den Alkohol und den Alkoholismus. Berlin, Urban & Schwarzenberg, 1904. 504 p.

1755
Akademiia nauk SSSR. Institut fiziologii im. I. P. Pavlova. Bibliografiia po uslovnym refleksam [Bibliography on conditioned reflexes] Moskva, 1955– .

Pt. 1, 1955, covers 1901–36 and lists 1137 works of 390 authors. Includes a brief review of the field. Pt. 2, 1964, covering 1936–48, contains 1685 references to the publications of 622 authors. Includes books.

1756
——. Sektor seti spetsial'nykh bibliotek. Metodiki issledovaniia vyssheĭ nervnoĭ

deiatel'nosti cheloveka; bibliograficheskiĭ ukazatel' otechestvennoĭ literatury (1900–1960 gg.) [Methods of research in higher nervous activity of man; bibliographic index of national literature (1900–1960)] Moskva, Izd-vo Akademii nauk SSSR, 1963. 91 p.

1269 references. Includes books, chapters of collected works, and reviews of dissertations.

1757
Berlin, Irving N. Bibliography of child psychiatry; with a selected list of films. Washington, American Psychiatric Association, 1963. 94 p. (Its Psychiatric bibliographies no. 1)

Restricted to books and articles in English. Covers mainly the literature from the late 1940's.

1758
California. University. Bureau of Public Administration. Insanity and the criminal law; a bibliography. Berkeley, 1960. 64 p.

Broad jurisdictional and subject classification with author index.

1759
Corsini, Raymond J., and Putzey, Lloyd J. Bibliography of group psychotherapy 1906–1956. Beacon, N.Y., Beacon House, 1957. 75 p. (Psychodrama and Group Psychotherapy Monographs no. 29)

1735 references. Includes books, chapters in books and theses. Arrangement is chronological with alphabetical author listing under year.

Continued by 1772.1

1759.1
Driver, Edwin D. The sociology and anthropology of mental illness; a reference guide. [Amherst] University of Massachusetts Press, 1965. 146 p.

1585 entries, 1956–1963. Includes books, reports, dissertations.

1760
Funkenstein, Daniel H., and Wilkie, George H. Student mental health; an annotated bibliography. London, World Federation for Mental Health [1956] 297 p.

1803 entries, selectively annotated.

1761
Geller, Miriam R. Studies on electroconvulsive therapy 1939–1963; a selected annotated bibliography. Washington, 1966. 413 p. National Clearinghouse for Mental Health Information. (Public Health Service. Publication no. 1447. Bibliography series no. 64)

582 abstracts arranged alphabetically.

1762
——. The treatment of psychiatric disorders with metrazol, 1935–60; a selected annotated bibliography. Bethesda, National Institutes of Health, 1963. 22 p.

Descriptive annotations of controlled studies.

1763
Goldfarb, William. Annotated bibliography of childhood schizophrenia and related disorders as reported in the English language through 1954. New York, Basic Books, 1956. 170 p.

584 items. Arranged alphabetically by principal author. No indexes.

1764
Goncharova, E. E. [et al.] Biokhimiia nervnoĭ sistemy; bibliograficheskiĭ ukazatel' otechestvennoĭ literatury, 1868–1954 [Biochemistry of the nervous system; bibliographic index to the national literature, 1868–1954] Kiev, Izd-vo Akademii nauk Ukrainskoĭ SSR, 1957. 87 p.

Over 700 citations of works by Russian and Soviet authors. Chronological arrangement with subarrangement by author.

1765
Grinstein, Alexander. The index of psychoanalytic writings. New York, International Universities Press, 1956–60. 5 v.

A revision and moderization of no. 1778. Author arrangement. Covers the literature from 1900–52 with some additional material listed in: *Additions and corrections to author index*, v. 5, p. 2739–2802. Lists reviews and abstracts written by authors. Includes works translated. Subject index in v. 5.

1766
Houck. L. Daniel, comp. Bibliography on anxiety states. Nutley, N.J., Roche Laboratories, 1962. 121 p.

Principally the periodical literature 1951–61;

chronologically arranged. Includes briefer sections, Books and nonperiodical literature and Periodical literature prior to 1951.

No author or subject index.

1767

Kiell, Norman, comp. Psychiatry and psychology in the visual arts and aesthetics; a bibliography. Madison, University of Wisconsin Press, 1965. 250 p.

7208 references primarily since and including the 1930's. Includes books, theses. Covers nonmedical and nonpsychological titles. Includes hospital and other forms of medical architecture, personality studies of artists listed under name of artist, physically handicapped and art, tests, projective techniques.

1768

——. Psychoanalysis, psychology and literature; a bibliography. Madison, University of Wisconsin Press, 1963. 225 p.

4460 articles and monographs which deal with literary writing and authors from a psychological point of view. Covers a number of nonmedical sources. Includes sections on the film, comics, journalism, and scriptures.

1769

Kleitman, Nathaniel. Sleep and wakefulness. Rev. ed. Chicago, University of Chicago Press, 1963. 552 p.

A literature review. Bibliography of 4337 numbered items (p. 372–538). Includes books and chapters in books. Arranged by author.

1770

Laehr, Heinrich. Die Literatur der Psychiatrie, Neurologie und Psychologie von 1459–1799. Berlin, Reimer, 1900. 3 v. in 4.

Chronological arrangement. Occasional annotations, descriptive of contents or evaluative. These frequently quoted from Haller (no. 130).

1771

Lewis, Nolan D., and Engle, Bernice, ed. Wartime psychiatry; a compendium of the international literature. New York, Oxford University Press, 1954. 952 p.

Principally some 1150 abstracts of articles and books, 1940–48.

1772

Locke, Norman M. A decade of group psychotherapy; the bibliography for 1950–59. New York, Group Psychotherapy Center, 1960. 48 p.

1014 references from 158 journals. Includes monographs and selected unpublished theses. Author arrangement.

1772.1

Lubin, Bernard and Lubin, Alice W. Group psychotherapy: A bibliography of the literature from 1956 through 1964. East Lansing, Michigan State University Press, 1966. 186 p.

1986 references including books, chapters in books, theses. Author arrangement under year.

Continues 1759.

1773

Menninger, Karl A. A guide to psychiatric books; with some suggested reading lists. 2 ed. New York, Grune & Stratton, 1956. 157 p.

Limited to books in the English language. No annotations.

1774

Mesdag, Maria J. Bibliographie van de werken van nederlandsche schrijvers op he gebied der neurologie en psychiatrie en aanverwante vakken. Amsterdam? 1922–37. 2 pts. in 4 v.

[Pt. 1, v. 1] author list with chronological subarrangement; [pt. 1, v. 2] subject arrangement. Pt. 1 covers 1850–1920 (with a few earlier references); pt. 2 [v. 1–2] covers 1921–34 in identical arrangement. Includes books and theses.

1774.1

Mimosa Frenk Foundation. KWIC index to neurochemistry. Amsterdam, 1961. 123 p.

Title word index of journal literature with author index and address of senior authors. Covers literature from Jan. 1960 to July 1961.

1775

National Society for Crippled Children and Adults. A selective bibliography on cerebral palsy: an author-subject index to literature in the Library of the National Society. Rev. ed. Chicago, 1953. 58 p.

For students and professional workers. Supplemented by no. 2257.

1776

Nevskiĭ, V. A., and Fedotov, D. D. Otechestvennaia nevropatologiia i psikhiatriia XVIII i pervoĭ poloviny XIX veka (1700–1860 gg); bibliograficheskiĭ ukazatel' [National neuropathology and psychiatry of the 18th century and of the first half of the 19th century (1700–1860); bibliographic index] Moskva, Vserossiĭskoe nauch. medits. obschchestvo nevropatologov i psikhiatrov, 1964. 256 p.

Includes scientific, pseudo-scientific and popular works, monographs, textbooks, manuscripts, translations of foreign works by Russian translators (if revised or critically evaluated), articles from collected works, chapters of books, and some reviews of foreign literature. In 2 parts: Pt. 1, 1813 references, 1700–1860, arranged chronologically; pt. 2, 130 references 1861–1962. Geographic index of most important authors.

1777

Reid, Leon L. [et al.] comp. An annotated bibliography of selected references in cerebral palsy, for professional personnel and parents. Pittsburgh, Stanwix House, 1960. 84 p.

603 references from the 1940's to 1959. Includes books, pamphlets. Author arrangement.

1778

Rickman, John. Index psychoanalyticus 1893–1926. London, Hogarth Press and the Institute of Psycho-Analysis, 1928. 276 p. (International Psycho-Analytical Library no. 14)

An author index to all original papers and translations in *Zentralblatt für Psychoanalyse*, 1910–12; *Jahrbuch für Psychoanalyse*, 1909–14; *Zeitschrift für Psychoanalyse*, 1913–26; *Imago*, 1912–26; *International journal of psychoanalysis*, 1920–26; and *Psychoanalytic review*, 1913–26. Also lists monographs and articles on psychoanalysis selected from 38 additional medical journals. 4739 entries. Includes obituaries.

Continued by no. 1765.

1779

Schermerharn, Richard A., ed. Psychiatric index for interdisciplinary research; a guide to the literature, 1950–1961. Washington, U.S. Vocational Rehabilitation Administration, 1964. 1249 p.

Emphasis is on social involvements complicating psychiatric problems. In excess of 28,000 references. Includes books.

1780

Tilton, James R. [et al.] Annotated bibliography on childhood schizophrenia (1955–64). New York, Grune & Stratton, 1966. 144 p.

346 entries from the English language literature, partly annotated. Includes books. Supplement, no. 1763.

1781

Torres Norry, José. Escuelas médicas contemporaneas; clasificación bibliográfica de su teoría y práctica (1900–1953). Buenos Aires, El Ateneo, 1954. 590 p.

Some 8000 references on psychiatry and subclasses, psychosomatic medicine (detailed breakdown by disease, condition or syndrome), psychopharmacology, etc. Relates to "schools" or theories of psychiatry or medicine. Includes books.

Title also in English.

1781.1

U.S. National Clearinghouse for Mental Health Information. The community general hospital as a mental health resource; a selected annotated bibliography. Bethesda, 1966. 38 p. (Public Health Service. Publication no. 1484. Bibliography series no. 66)

References from 1959 to 1966. Author arrangement under subject breakdown. Includes monographs.

1781.2

——. Family therapy; a selected annotated bibliography. Bethesda, 1965 [1966] 30 p.

113 entries beginning with 1953. Includes monographs.

1782

——. A selected bibliography on occupational mental health. Bethesda, 1965. 170 p. (Public Health Service. Publication no. 1338)

1176 partly annotated references from the English language literature mainly 1940's–60's. Includes books, pamphlets. Entries from a large number of nonmedical sources. Prepared by Center for Occupational Mental Health, White Plains, N.Y.

1783

U.S. National Institute of Mental Health. The treatment of psychiatric disorders with insulin, 1936–1960; a selected annotated bibliography. By Miriam R. Geller. Washington, 1962. 33 p. (Public Health Service. Publication no. 941. Bibliography series no. 37)

161 clinical studies. Includes books.

1783.1
U.S. National Institutes of Health. A bibliographic index of evaluation in mental health. Prep. by James K. Dent. Bethesda, 1966. 111 p. (Public Health Service. Publication no. 1545)

Abstracts. Limited to systematic, molar and social assessments in English. Related bibliographies and literature surveys. p. 108–09.

Monographs

1783.2
Arieti, Silvano, ed. American handbook of psychiatry. New York, Basic Books, 1959–66. 3 v.

Covers all aspects of the subject including history. Chapter bibliographies.

Dictionaries

1784
American Psychiatric Association. Committee on Public Information. A psychiatric glossary; the meaning of words most frequently used in psychiatry. 2 ed. Washington, 1964. 79 p.

1785
Choisy, Maryse [et al.] Dictionnaire de psychoanalyse et de psychotechnique. [Paris, 1949–55] 2 v. 1200 p.

v. 2 extracted from *Psyché* (Paris) 1949–55.

Includes biographies. Some entries have bibliographies.

1786★★
Hinsie, Leland E., and Campbell, Robert J. Psychiatric dictionary. 3 ed. New York, Oxford University Press, 1960. 788 p.

Comprehensive dictionary revised to include 2000 new terms and omit 1300 outmoded terms; gives pronunciations of many words; numerous citations to sources.

1787
Kupper, William H. Dictionary of psychiatry and psychology; an illustrated condensed encyclopedia of psychiatry, neurology and psychology. Paterson, Colt Press, 1953. 194 p.

Special features: List of state hospitals for mental disorders, V.A. neuropsychiatric hospitals, etc.

1787.1
Nielsen, John B. Psykiatrisk ordbog. København, Høst, 1963. 138 p.

1788
Porot, Antoine. Manuel alphabétique de psychiatrie clinique et thérapeutique. 3 ed. Paris, Presses Universitaires de France, 1965. 583 p.

Encyclopedic dictionary with signed articles. 1 ed., 1952.

1789
Schmidt, J. E. Narcotics lingo and lore. Springfield, Ill., Thomas, 1959. 199 p.

Almost entirely slang.

1790
Telatin, Luigi. Sindromi neurologiche rare o meno note. Roma, Pozzi, 1950. 420 p.

1791
Telberg, Ira, and Dmitrioff, A. Russian-English glossary of psychiatric terms. New York, Telberg Book Corp., 1964. 86 p.

Equivalent terms, including some nonscientific. P. 60–86: surnames and book titles in Russian and English.

1792
Tuke, D. Hack. A dictionary of psychological medicine. Philadelphia, P. Blakiston, 1892. 2 v. (1477 p.)

Contains much historical material: mental hospitals (by country), eponyms, older terms. Includes French terms, discussion of unusual subjects (fasting mania, etc.)

Nomenclature

1793★
American Psychiatric Association. Committee on Nomenclature and Statistics. Diagnostic and statistical manual: mental disorders. Washington, [1] 1952– .

Officially supported nomenclature of the American Psychiatric Association. 17th printing, 1963.

Directories

1794
American Academy of Neurology. Directory. Minneapolis, 1, 1954– .

1963 ed. lists honorary members, alphabetical list of fellows, active, associate and junior members, with date of election to membership, address.

1795
American Psychiatric Association. Biographical directory of fellows and members. New York, 1, 1941– .

Alphabetical listing by name; geographical index.

1796
——. Calendar of meetings of psychiatric interest. Washington, 1959/64– .

Chronological arrangement of meetings scheduled.

1797
——. List of fellows and members. New York, [1] 1922– .

Alphabetical listing with address, year of election to membership, and indication of certification by the American Boards of Psychiatry and Neurology. Includes some from foreign countries.

Continues *List of members of the American Medico-Psychology Association* (not listed)

1798
——. Committee on Medical Education. A descriptive directory of psychiatric training in the United States and Canada. Washington, 1, 1953– .

General information on certification; main section lists hospitals and other institutions by state and gives address, name of director, hospital statistics, number of residencies, and description of the psychiatric program. 3 ed., 1960.

1 ed. has title: *Psychiatric training in the United States and Canada.*

1799
American Psychoanalytic Association. Roster. New York [1, 195–?]

Alphabetical and geographical listing of members; other information includes officers, lists of affiliate societies and their members, approved training institutions. Published as *Membership roster* until 1957.

1800
Directory for exceptional children. Educational and training facilities describing schools, homes, clinics, hospitals and services for the socially maladjusted, mentally retarded, emotionally disturbed, orthopedically handicapped, cerebral palsied, speech handicapped, brain-injured, epileptic, cardiac, blind, deaf. 4 ed. Boston, Porter Sargent, 1962. 618 p.

Geographical arrangement under subject category. Includes address, director, number of students and staff, rates, and brief description of activities.

1801★
Directory of outpatient psychiatric clinics, psychiatric day-night services and other mental health resources in the United States and territories. Bethesda, Md., 1963– National Institute of Mental Health in cooperation with the National Association for Mental Health, Inc. (Public Health Service. Publication no. 1129)

Lists over 1700 facilities arranged by state and city; gives address, group served, staff.

1802
Directory of resources for mentally ill children in the United States. New York, National Association of Mental Health, 1964. 93 p.

1803
International Psycho-analytical Association. List of members of the regional association, component and affiliate societies. London, [1] 1920?– .

Arranged by country. Lists societies, officers, and members with their organizational affiliation and address. Annual through 1927, then biennial in the *International journal of phychoanalysis* and *Bulletin of the International Psychoanalytical Association.* 1964/65, in the 125th *Bulletin.*

1804
Mental health directory of state and national agencies administering public mental health and related programs.

Bethesda, U.S. National Institute of Mental Health, 1964– .

Arranged by state and including Puerto Rico and the Virgin Islands. Lists state mental health authority, state institutions for the mentally ill, and for the mentally retarded. Includes list of federal penal and correctional institutions, chief social workers in Veterans Administration hospitals, and voluntary organizations.

1805
U.S. National Institute of Mental Health. Register of public and non-public hospitals authorized or recognized for the treatment of mental disorder. Bethesda, 1956. 24 p.

Films

1806
U.S. National Institute of Mental Health. Mental health motion pictures, a selective guide. Washington, 1960. 98 p.

Subject index. Recommended age levels.

1806.1
U.S. Public Health Service. Audiovisual Facility. Atlanta. Neurological and sensory disease film guide, 1966. Washington, 1966. 220 p. (Public Health Service. Publication no. 1033)

1348 entries arranged by subject. Includes bibliographic data, brief description of content, title and distributor listings.

Prepared for the Public Health Service, Neurological and Sensory Disease Service Program.

1807
World Federation for Mental Health. International catalogue of mental health films. 2 ed. London, 1960. 99 p.

Alphabetical title index. Broad subject classification, audience, country or origin, and language.

Histories

Bibliography

1808
Mora, George. The historiography of psychiatry and its development: a re-evaluation. In Journal of the history of the behavioral sciences 1:43–52, 1965.

Reviews literature.

Biography

1809
Haymaker, Webb, ed. The founders of neurology; one hundred and thirty-three biographical sketches prepared for the Fourth International Neurological Congress in Paris . . . with the bibliographical and editorial assistance of Karl A. Baer. Springfield, Ill., Thomas, 1953. 479 p.

Men of 19th and 20th centuries. References at ends of sketches citing publications and biographical and critical studies.

1810
Kolle, Kurt, ed. Grosse Nervenärzte . . . Lebensbilder, in Gemeinschaft mit H. J. de Barahona Fernandes [et al]. Stuttgart, Thieme, 1956–63. 3 v.

65 biographies, each with portrait and bibliography of works.

Psychiatry—General

1811
Ackerknecht, Erwin H. A short history of psychiatry. Tr. by Sulammith Wolff. New York, Hafner, 1959. 98 p.

Compact interpretation of developments from primitive times to early 20th century, with emphasis on leading contributors. Bibliographical comments: p. v-vi. Translation of *Kurze Geschichte der Psychiatrie*, Stuttgart, 1957.

1811.1
Alexander, Franz G., and Selesnick, Sheldon T. The history of psychiatry: an evaluation of psychiatric thought and practice from prehistoric times to the present. New York, Harper & Row, 1966. 471 p.

Primarily on modern period. Notes and bibliography: p. 415–451.

1812
Bromberg, Walter. Man above humanity. A history of psychotherapy. Philadelphia, Lippincott, 1954. 342 p.

From ancient times and primitive societies to the present, stressing British and American developments from the 18th century. Revision of author's *The mind of man*, New York, 1937, which contained classified bibliography (p. 294–307) omitted in revised work. Reprinted as *The mind of man, a history of psychotherapy and psychoanalysis*, New York, Harper, 1959 (Harper Torchbooks, TB 1003).

1813
Friedreich, Johannes B. Versuch einer Literärgeschichte der Pathologie und Therapie der psychischen Krankheiten; von der ältesten Zeiten bis zum neunzehnten Jahrhundert. Würzburg, Strecker, 1830. 655 p.

Description and frequently detailed analyses of important works. Bibliographical footnotes. Full table of contents but no index.

1814
Hunter, Richard A., and Macalpine, Ida. Three hundred years of psychiatry, 1535–1860; a history presented in selected English texts. London, Oxford University Press, 1963. 1107 p.

Includes selections from writings of literary men, philosophers, theologians, and patients as well as physicians, with critical introductions. Mostly British authors. 204 illustrations including facsimiles.

1815
Leibbrand, Werner, and Wettley, Annemarie. Der Wahnsinn; Geschichte der abendländischen Psychopathologie. Freiburg, Alber, 1961. 697 p. (Orbis academicus, II/12)

Concerned with concepts in relation to contemporaneous intellectual developments. Detailed analyses of basic ideas of significant authors from ancient Greece to present time. Bibliographical references and notes: p. 621–681.

1816
Walker, Nigel. A short history of psychotherapy in theory and practice. London, Routledge and Kegan Paul, 1957. 185 p.

Mainly on Freud and after. Brief lists of recommended reading at end of each chapter. Reprinted New York, Noonday Press, 1959.

1817
Whitwell, James R. Historical notes on psychiatry (early times—end of 16th century). London, Lewis, 1936. 252 p.

Chiefly analyses with frequent quotations of various writings, mostly classical, plus section (p. 153–246) of extracts and translations. References throughout.

1818
Zilboorg, Gregory, and Henry, George W. A history of medical psychology. New York, Norton, 1941. 606 p.

Documented history from earliest times. A standard work.

Psychiatry—By Country

FRANCE

1819
Foucault, Michel. Madness and civilization: a history of insanity in the age of reason. Tr. from the French by Richard Howard. New York, Pantheon Books, 1965. 299 p.

Covers 17th and 18th centuries. Notes (by chapters, p. 291–299) include bibliographical references.

1820
Semelaigne, René. Les pionniers de la psychiatrie française avant et après Pinel. Paris, Baillière, 1930–32. 2 v.

Chronologically arranged, beginning with Jacques Dubois (1478–1555). For each author, an extensive list of works (books and articles) or an edition of his works is cited. No other documentation.

GERMANY

1821
Kirchhoff, Theodor, ed. Deutsche Irrenärzte; Einzelbilder ihres Lebens und Wirkens. Berlin, Springer, 1921–24. 2 v.

Biographical studies of 118 psychiatrists, mostly late 18th through early 20th century, with references at end of most studies.

1822
Scholz, Willibald, ed. 50 Jahre Neuropathologie in Deutschland, 1885–1935. Stuttgart, Thieme, 1961. 123 p.

Eight studies by different authors, on single physicians or schools. Bibliography of biographical and critical studies and publications following each study.

GREAT BRITAIN

1823
Jones, Kathleen. Lunacy, law, and conscience, 1745–1845; the social history of the care of the insane. London, Routledge & Paul, 1955. 239 p.

On Great Britain; chiefly public administration. Bibliography: p. 227–234. Documented throughout.

1824
Leigh, Denis. The historical development of British psychiatry. Oxford, Pergamon Press, 1961– .

v. 1, 18th and 19th centuries. General survey and studies of John Haslam, J. C. Prichard, and John Conolly. Bibliography at end of each chapter. "A list of books dealing with psychiatric illness published in English during the eighteenth century": p. 84–93.

PERU

1825
Valdivia Ponce, Oscar. Historia de la psiquiatría peruana. [Lima?] 1964. 293 p.

Surveys successive periods, including pre-Columbian (p. 1–97), with biographical sketches and extensive bibliographies of leading physicians. Classified bibliography of Peruvian psychiatric literature: p. 247–282; bibliography (197 items): p. 287–293.

U.S.S.R.

1826
Wortis, Joseph. Soviet psychiatry. Baltimore, Williams and Wilkins, 1950. 314 p.

Brief survey of earlier Russian psychology and psychiatry, detailed from Pavlov on. Extensive bibliographic references in footnotes. Appendix (p. 239–304) presents selections of translated material, including complete documents and papers.

UNITED STATES

1827
American Psychiatric Association. One hundred years of American psychiatry. New York, Columbia Univ. Press, 1944. 649 p.

17 studies by 13 authors, with an introduction by J. K. Hall. Includes a study by R. H. Shryock on the period before 1844, one by H. E. Sigerist on psychiatry in Europe at the middle of the 19th century, and one by H. A. Bunker on American psychiatric literature, with extensive references, lists of important books and of American periodicals.

1828
Dain, Norman. Concepts of insanity in the United States, 1789–1865. New Brunswick, N.J., Rutgers University Press, 1964. 304 p.

Emphasizes growth and decline of "moral" treatment. References: p. 211–261; classified select bibliography: p. 263–291.

1829
Deutsch, Albert. The mentally ill in America; a history of their care and treatment from colonial times. 2 ed. New York, Columbia University Press, 1949. 555 p.

General survey. Bibliography: p. 520–537, First published 1937.

1830
Hurd, Henry M. [et al.] ed. The institutional care of the insane in the United States and Canada. Baltimore, Johns Hopkins Univ. Press, 1916–17. 4 v.

v. 1: general history; v. 2–3 and the first section of v. 4: history of individual institutions in geographical arrangement; v. 4, p. 337–600: biographies.

1831
Ridenour, Nina. Mental health in the United States; a fifty-year history. Cambridge, Commonwealth Fund, 1961. 146 p.

Survey, undocumented, of organized mental health movement. Sponsored by the New York Association for Mental Health.

Special Topics

1832
Fearing, Franklin. Reflex action: a study in the history of physiological psychology. Baltimore, Williams & Wilkins, 1930. 350 p.

Introductory chapter on the early period; mainly on 17th to early 20th century. Study of ideas in the texts, with numerous quotations. Bibliography (554 references, by author, including sources and secondary works): p. 316–337.

1833
Keele, Kenneth D. Anatomies of pain. Springfield, Ill., Thomas, 1957. 206 p.

From ancient times to the present. Analyses of original works with numerous quotations. References to sources at end of each chapter.

1834
Laín Entralgo, Pedro. Mind and body; psychosomatic pathology; a short history of medical thought. London, Harvill, 1955. 150 p.

Mainly on classical and early Christian thought, with brief treatment of medieval and modern developments. Some bibliographical footnotes. Translation of *Introducción histórica al estudio de la patología psicosomatica*, Madrid, 1950, which was reprinted with minor changes under title: *Enfermidad e pecado*, Barcelona, Toray, 1961. No index in the translation; Spanish editions have name index only.

1835
Liddel, Edward G. T. The discovery of reflexes. Oxford, Clarendon Press, 1960. 174 p.

Chapters on anatomy of nerve cells; electrical phenomena of nerves; pioneer experiments on nervous system; Sherrington and his times. Sources: p. 145–147. Biographical appendix with brief identifications: p. 148–167.

1836
Temkin, Owsei. The falling sickness; a history of epilepsy from the Greeks to the beginnings of modern neurology. Baltimore, Johns Hopkins Press, 1945. 380 p. (Johns Hopkins University. Institute of the History of Medicine. Publications, 1st ser., Monographs. v. 4)

Documented study, with careful analyses of original works, from the ancient Greeks to about 1880. Bibliography (706 items, by author): p. 325–706.

1837
Veith, Ilza. Hysteria: the history of a disease. Chicago, University of Chicago Press, 1965. 328 p.

From ancient Egypt through Freud. Bibliography (including original works): p. 275–286.

1838
Wyss, Dieter. Die tiefenpsychologischen Schulen von den Anfängen bis zur Gegenwart: Entwicklung, Probleme, Krisen. 2 ed. Göttingen, Vandenhoeck & Ruprecht, 1966. 445 p.

Analysis, arranged by persons, schools, and topics, of the theories and practices of psychoanalists as set forth in their works. Begins with Freud. Bibliographical footnotes. 1 ed. 1961.

Brain and Spinal Cord

Indexes and Abstracts

1838.1
Bericht über die Leistungen auf dem Gebiete der Anatomie des Centralnervensystems. Leipzig [1–2]–5, 1901/02–1909/10.

Items listed by author at random under subject with either annotation or selective review following listings.

Also published in no. 39.

Reviews

1839
Progress in brain research. Amsterdam, 1, 1963– .

Irregular. Series of monographs, each on a specific subject such as brain mechanisms, the rhinencephalon and related structures; growth and maturation of the brain; slow electrical processes of the brain; biogenic amines; etc. Articles are in English, German, or French, some with long bibliographies. v. 1–3, 1963; v. 4–11, 1964.

Bibliographies

1839.1
Bickford, Reginald G. [et al.] comp. A KWIC index of EEG literature, and Society proceedings. Amsterdam, Elsevier, 1965. 581 p.

Consists of separate indexes to the general literature and to the abstracts published in the *Society proceedings* section of *Electroencephalography and clinical neurophysiology* v. 1–15, 1949–63. Earliest references noted in the general literature section was 1920.

A publication of the International Brain Research Information Center, Mayo Foundation, Rochester.

1840★
Brazier, Mary A. B., ed. Bibliography of electroencephalography, 1875–1948. [Montreal] International Federation of Electroencephalography and Clinical Neurophysiology. 1950. 178 p. [Electroencephalography and clinical neurophysiology. Supplement no. 1]

Covers normal and disease states.

1841★
Fink, Max. A selected bibliography of electroencephalography in human psychopharmacology, 1951–1962. Amsterdam, Elsevier, 1964. 68 p. (Electroencephalography and clinical neurophysiology. Supplement no. 23)

580 entries, arranged by author, referring to EEG and psychopharmacological studies in humans, in health and sickness, and to reports on compounds distinguished by their psychotropic effects.

Supplements no. 1840.

1842
Kenk, Roman, and Nall, Mabel L. Physiology of the circulation of the brain; an annotated bibliography, 1938–1948. 437 p. (Physiological reviews, v. 32, July 1952. Supplement no. 1)

Strictly pathological or medical information is not included. Author arrangement.

1843
Nall, Mabel L., and Ferguson, Faith C. Physiology of the circulation of the brain; an annotated bibliography. Pt. 2. Report literature, 1938–1952. 148 p. (Physiological reviews, v. 36, July 1956. Supplement no. 2)

Author list. Pt. 2 of no. 1842.

1844
U.S. Veterans Adminsitration. Department of Medicine and Surgery. Medical and General Reference Library. Spinal cord injury; a selected bibliography, 1940–1963. Washington, 1965. 121 p.

3059 entries. Includes books. Covers foreign language material for 1961–63 only.

Supersedes its: *Paraplegia, a classified bibliography of references in English, 1940–1951* (1951) and revisions and enlargements; *Traumatic paraplegia, a selected bibliography* (1957) and supplements (1958–63) (not listed separately)

1844.1
——. ——. Supplement, 1964–1965. Washington, 1966. 38 p.

629 entries.

Nomenclature

1845
Yoshikawa, Tetsuo. Nomina anatomica encephalica. Tokyo, The Author, 1962. 525 p.

Includes separate list of eponyms.

Histories

1846
Davies, John D. Phrenology; fad and science. A 19th century American crusade. New Haven, Yale Univ. Press, 1955. 203 p. (Yale Historical publications. Miscellany, 62)

Studies origins, spread, relationships, and significance of the movement. Documented. Bibliographical note: p. 183–194.

1847
Neuburger, Max. Die historische Entwicklung der experimentellen Gehirn- und Rückenmarksphysiologie vor Flourens. Stuttgart, Enke, 1897. 361 p.

Detailed, documented study from the time of Willis, with some data on earlier periods.

1848
Wellcome Historical Medical Library. The history and philosophy of knowledge of the brain and its functions; an Anglo-American symposium, London, July 15–17, 1957. Oxford, Blackwell, 1958. 272 p.

Series of papers covering topic from antiquity. Most have references at end. Ed. by F. N. L. Poynter.

Hypnosis

Reviews

1849
Annual review of hypnosis literature. New York, 1/2, 1950/51. Society for Clinical and Experimental Hypnosis.

Includes 5 brief review articles with bibliographies; abstracts of 116 articles chiefly from the English language literature.

Directories

1850
American Society of Clinical Hypnosis. Directory. Minneapolis, 1963. 63 p.

Alphabetical listing of members with degree, address, and membership status. Includes Canadian and honorary foreign members. Lists component societies within the United States and affiliated societies abroad.

Mental Deficiency

Special attention is called to nos. 1851, 1854, 1856, and 1857.

Indexes and Abstracts

1851
U.S. National Clearinghouse for Mental Health Information. Mental retardation abstracts. Bethesda, 1, 1964– .

Quarterly. Cumulated annually. 1964 contained 1118 abstracts.

Bibliographies

1852
U.S. Children's Bureau. Galactosemia; a selected bibliography. Comp. by Donough O'Brien. Washington, 1963. [38] p.

96 abstracts from the English language literature.

1853
——. Research relating to mentally retarded children. Washington, 1960. 92 p.

Research reported since 1949. Name index.

1854★
U.S. National Institute of Child Health and Human Development. Supplement to Bibliography of world literature on mental retardation, March 1963–December 31, 1964. By Rick F. Heber and Patrick J. Flanigan. Washington, 1965. 99 p. (Public Health Service. Publication no. 1316)

2372 entries. Supplements no. 1856.

1855
U.S. National Institute of Neurological Diseases and Blindness. Perinatal Research Branch. Abstracts from selected bibliography . . . mental retardation, epilepsy, cerebral palsy, and related subjects. Bethesda, 1962. 96 p.

Detailed critical annotations of 90 periodical articles.

1856★
U.S. President's Panel on Mental Retardation. Bibliography of world literature on mental retardation, Jan. 1940–March 1963. By Rick Heber [et al.] Washington, U.S. Public Health Service, 1963. 564 p.

10,096 entries listed by author. Includes monographs and reports. Covers a number of nonmedical journals, principally in the field of education. Supplemented by no. 1854.

Directories

1857
U.S. Children's Bureau. Clinical programs for mentally retarded children, a listing. Washington, [1] 1958– .

Geographical arrangement. Information includes name of clinic, address, director, ages accepted, hours. 6th listing, 1965.

Histories

1858
Kanner, Leo. A history of the care and study of the mentally retarded. Springfield, Ill., Thomas, 1964. 150 p.

Mainly 19th and 20th centuries. Chiefly factual data. Numerous lists of references throughout.

Psychopharmacology

Indexes and Abstracts

1859
Psychopharmacology abstracts. Bethesda, 1, 1961– . U.S. National Clearinghouse for Mental Health Information.

Monthly. 2718 abstracts in v. 4.

1860
U.S. National Clearinghouse for Mental Health Information. Psychopharmacology handbook. Washington, 1, 1954/59– . (Public Health Service. Publication no. 1006, etc. Bibliography series no. 40, etc.)

v. 1 (rev.)-4, 1954–63, 10,088 abstracts.
Added title: *Animal research in pharmacology;* v. 2. ——. *Central nervous system effects.*
Decennial index [1954–63] Washington, 1966. 457 p.

Bibliographies

1860.1
Sandoz Chemical Works, Inc. Sandoz Pharmaceuticals. Annotated bibliography. Delysid, LSD 25 (d-lysergic acid diethylamide) Hanover, N.J.[1958] 119 p.

381 annotated references; covers 1943–57. Random author arrangement.

1860.2
——. ——. Medical Department. An-

notated bibliography. Addendum. Hanover, N.J. [1] 1959– .

Irregular. Continues no. 1860.1.

Classified index to 1860.1 and to no. 1 of 1860.2 issued as *Catalogue of the literature on Delysid, d-lysergic acid diethylamide or LSD 25*. Hanover, N.J. [n.d.] 18 [ie. 48] p.

1861
U.S. National Clearinghouse for Mental Health Information. Bibliography on clinical psycho-pharmacology, 1958–1960. Bethesda, 1965. 211 p. (Public Health Service. Publication no. 1293. Bibliography series no. 60)

3791 entries. Drug index.

1862 (Not used)

1863
U.S. National Library of Medicine. Psychopharmaca; a bibliography of psychopharmacology, 1952–1957. Comp. by Anne E. Caldwell. Washington, 1958. 258 p. (Public Health Service. Publication no.58. Bibliography series no. 19)

2500 references.

Dictionaries

1864
Un glosario de psycofarmaka; a glossary of psychopharmaka; ein Glossar der Psycho-pharmaka. Philadelphia, Biological and Medical Services, Literary Division, 1963. 202 p.

Lists 5000 equivalents of psychoactive drugs. The first list reads trade name to generic name; the second list, generic name to trade name. Preface in Spanish, English, and German.

1865
Poser, Charles M. International dictionary of drugs used in neurology and psychiatry. Springfield, Ill., Thomas, 1962. 157 p.

Alphabetical lists of generic names and of names of pharmacologic agents with references to generic names; also includes list of chemical designations and list of experimental numbers and names.

Senses and Sense Organs

Indexes and Abstracts

1865.1
Current publications on acoustics. References to contemporary papers on acoustics. In Journal of the Acoustical Society of America 1, 1929– .

Covers physiological and psychological acoustics, noise and noise control, speech communication, mechanical vibration and shock, bioacoustics. Includes research reports, books, theses. Indexes nonmedical sources.

10 years cumulative indexes v. 1–30, 1929–58; 5 years v. 31–35, 1959–63.

1866★
DSH abstracts. Washington, Deafness, Speech and Hearing Publications, Inc., 1, 1960– .

Quarterly. In 1964 more than 1700 abstracts. 275 journals and 16 abstract services regularly searched for relevant items. Indexes a number of journals not indexed in standard medical indexes. Includes books, chapters in books, and government reports.

Bibliographies

1867
Akademiia nauk SSSR. Biblioteka. Fiziologicheskaia akustika: bibliograficheskiĭ ukazatel' sovetskoĭ literatury, 1917–1950 [Physiological acoustics; bibliographical index of Soviet literature, 1917–1950] Izd-vo Akademii nauk SSSR, 1960, 136 p.

1226 references arranged by author. Russian language publications only. Includes books.

1867.1
Fellendorf, George W. ed. Bibliography on deafness; a selected index. The Volta review, 1899–1965; the American annals of the deaf, 1847–1965. Washington, Alexander Graham Bell Assoc. for the Deaf, 1966. 148 p.

Subject arrangement with *Volta review* and *American annals of the deaf* articles listed in turn under subject.

1868
Florida Chemical Research Company, New York. Odors and the sense of smell; a bibliography, 320 B.C.–1947. New York, Airkim Inc., 1952. 342 p.

Includes anatomy and physiology of olfactory system, pathology and perversion of odor perception, body odors, odor detection, odor control, etc.

1869
Fulton, John F. [et al.] A bibliography of visual literature, 1939–1944. Springfield, Ill., Thomas, 1945. 201 p. (Yale Medical Library. Historical Library, Publication no. 11)

Published by the Committee on Medical Research and Development, U.S. Office of Scientific Research and Development; prepared by the Committee on Aviation Medicine of the National Research Council.

3347 entries, exclusive of Supplement.

Supplement, p. 115–201, has separate title page: *A bibliography of visual literature, 1939–1944. Supplement. Unpublished reports on vision from United Nations civilian and military sources.* Compiled by John F. Fulton [et al.] Washington, 1945.

Cover title: *A bibliography of visual literature, 1939–1944, and supplement.*

Some copies issued without *Supplement.*

1870 (not used)

1871
Harvard University. Psycho-Acoustic Laboratory. Bibliography on hearing. Comp. by S. S. Stevens [et al.] Cambridge, Harvard University Press, 1955. 599 p.

10,000 titles arranged alphabetically. Covers 1872–1952.

Includes all entries of: *A bibliography in audition* (1950) (not listed)

1871.1
Pangborn, Rose Marie and Trabue, Ida M. A bibliography of the sense of taste, from 1566 to May 1966. Davis, Calif., 1966. 234 p.

Author list of more than 3000 references. Covers chemoreceptors in general and smell.

1872
U.S. Library of Congress. Reference Department. Visibility, a bibliography. Comp. by Jack Weiner and Morris C. Leikind. Washington, 1952. 90 p.

2008 items, 1925–50.

Dictionaries

1873
Robbins, Samuel D. A dictionary of speech pathology and therapy; with a supplement on phonetic and voice terms. 2 ed. Cambridge, Mass., Sci-Art Publishers, 1963. 128 p.

Alphabetical listing of disorders of speech; definitions adapted from the literature and from unabridged and medical dictionaries.

Directories

1874
American Speech and Hearing Association. Directory. Washington [etc.] 1, 1948– .

Alphabetical list of fellows with brief professional information; includes clinical certification requirements, national officers, affiliated state associations and officers, geographical list of members, clinical certification list, and list of associates.

Published as Annual directory, 1948–1959, in *Journal of speech and hearing disorders* or its supplements. Membership lists published under the society's earlier name, American Speech Correction Association, appeared in the *Journal of speech disorders*, 1937–1947.

1875
Directory of services for the deaf in the United States. Washington, 1966– . Conference of Executives of American Schools for the Deaf and American Instructors of the Deaf.

Lists schools, classes, and clinics in the United States and Canada; also American instructors of the deaf, teacher training centers, international programs, research in progress, publications and films.

Issued annually in the January issue of *American annals of the deaf.*

1876
International directory: schools and organizations for the deaf, 1965. Comp. by Jerome D. Schein and Powrie V. Doctor. Gallaudet College, 1966. 101 p. (Gallaudet Research Publications, Series Internatonal, 1)

Arranged alphabetically by country. For each school and organization gives address only. No entries are provided for the United States and Canada as they are included in no. 1875.

History

1877
Bender, Ruth E. The conquest of deafness: a history of the long struggle to make

possible normal living to those handicapped by lack of normal hearing. Cleveland, Western Reserve University Press, 1960. 208 p.

Primarily a history of education for the deaf since early times. Bibliography (sources and secondary works): p. 183–199.

NOSOLOGY

1878★ ★

American Medical Association. Current medical terminology. 3 ed. Ed. by Burgess L. Gordon. Chicago, 1966. 969 p.

Alphabetized listing of preferred terms, cross references, and a numerical index. Information given includes etiology, symptoms, signs, complications, findings.

1879

American Medical Association. Current procedural terminology. Ed. by Burgess L. Gordon. Chicago, 1966. 172 p.

Terms are listed alphabetically by the names of the therapeutic diagnostic procedures and numerically by the code for each. Terms include procedures of surgery, medicine, obstetrics, psychiatry, roentgenology, clinical laboratory sciences, and physical medicine; also supplementary services such as visits, consultations, examinations, evaluations, and miscellaneous studies.

1880★

International Committee for the Preparation of the Decennial Revision of International Lists of Diseases and Causes of Death. Manual of the international statistical classification of diseases, injuries, and causes of death. Based on the recommendations of the Seventh Revision Conference, 1955, and adopted by the Ninth World Health Assembly under the WHO Nomenclature Regulations. Geneva, World Health Organization, 1957. 2 v.

v. 1, detailed list of 3-digit categories, tabular list of inclusions and 4 digit sub-categories, medical certification and rules for classification, special lists. v. 2, index to categories and tabular list.

6th revision, 1948. 6th and 7th revisions also published in the principal European languages. Introduction in the 6th and 7th revisions contains history of the Committee.

Supersedes no. 1883.

1881★

National Conference on Medical Nomenclature. Standard nomenclature of diseases and operations. 5 ed., by Edward T. Thompson and Adaline C. Hayden. New York, McGraw-Hill. 1961. 964 p.

Published for the American Medical Association.

Arranged as a topographic and etiologic classification. Nomenclature of diseases and nomenclature of operations are listed separately with their code numbers and alphabetic indexes for each are given.

Standard nomenclature of disease, 1 ed., 1933, published under the auspices of the National Conference on Nomenclature of Disease, 2nd, 1935. *Standard nomenclature of diseases and operations* published in 1942 under the auspices of the American Medical Association. *Standard nomenclature of diseases and operations*, 1 ed., 1955; 2 ed., 1958, by Edward T. Thompson and Adaline C. Hayden, published by Physicians' Record Co., Chicago.

1882

Royal College of Physicians, London. The nomenclature of disease. 8 ed. London, H. M. Stationery Office, 1960. 398 p.

The first section gives an etiological classification of disease, which is applied to the body and its systems in the remaining sections. Includes list of eponyms. Omits mnemonics. Irregular.

First published as *The nomenclature of diseases; drawn up by a joint committee appointed by the Royal College of Physicians of London* (*subject to decennial revision*). London, W. J. & S. Goldbourn, 1869. 327 p. Reprinted [in part] by order of the American Medical Association. Philadelphia, Collins, 1869. 99 p.

London edition gives terms in Latin, French, German, and Italian.

1883

U.S. Bureau of the Census. Manual of the international list of causes of death. Washington, 1902–40.

First published as *Manual of international classification of cause of death*; adopted by the United States Census Office for the compilation of mortality statistics for use beginning with the year 1900.

2d revision 1909; 3d revision 1920; 4th revision 1929; 5th 1938(1940). 5th revision includes *Manual of joint causes of death*, 4 ed., 1939.

Successive editions based on revisions by the

International Commission for the Decennial Revision of Nosological Nomenclature.

Some or all editions published in other languages.

Superseded by no. 1880.

1883.1
——. Manual of joint causes of death; showing assignment to the preferred title of the International list of causes of death when two causes are simultaneously reported. 1–3 ed. Washington, 1914–33.

4 ed. published in no. 1883.

1883.2
——. Standard nomenclature of diseases and pathological conditions, injuries, and poisonings for the United States. 1 ed. Washington, 1920. 347 p.

1884
U.S. Dept. of Defense. Disease and injury codes. [Washington] 1963. 1 v. (various pagings) (TB Med 15. NAVMED P-5082. AFM 160–24)

In 6 pts: Diagnosis nomenclature, statistical classification; body parts, statistical classification; diagnosis nomenclature, alphabetic index; body parts, alphabetic index; body part diagnosis codes; external causes of injury, statistical classification.

1885★
U.S. National Center for Health Statistics. International classification of diseases, adapted for indexing hospital records by diseases and operations. Washington, 1962. 2 v. (Public Health Service. Publication no. 719, rev. ed.)

v. 1, Tabular list; v. 2, Alphabetic index. Based on the 7th revision of no. 1880. Changes consist chiefly of addition of fourth-digit codes to provide greater specificity. First published 1959.

1886
U.S. National Institutes of Health. Division of Research Grants. Medical and health related sciences thesaurus. Washington, 1963. 213 p. (Public Health Service. Publication no. 1031)

Contains approximately 12,200 terms. Developed as a staff manual by the compilers of the *Research grants index*.

1887
Woodworth, John M. Nomenclature of diseases. Prepared for the use of the medcial officers of the United States Marine-Hospital Service by the Supervising Surgeon . . . Being the classification and English-Latin terminology of the provisional nomenclature of the Royal College of Physicians, Lond. Washington, 1874. 210 p.

NURSING

Indexes and Abstracts

1888★★
Cumulative index to nursing literature. Glendale, Calif., 1, 1956– . Seventh-Day Adventist Hospital Association.

Quarterly. Cumulated annually. In 1966 indexed 114 journals 75 of which are not *Index medicus* titles. Indexes reviews of books, pamphlets, films.

5 year cumulation, 1956–1960; 3 year cumulation, 1961–1963.

1889
Henderson, Virginia. Nursing studies index; an annotated guide to reported studies, research in progress, research methods and historical materials in periodicals, books and pamphlets in English. v. 3–4, 1950/56–1957/59. Philadelphia, Lippincott, 1963–66. 653, 281 p.

Prepared by Yale University School of Nursing Index Staff. v. 3 published in 1966. v. 1–2 intended to cover the literature 1900–49. A classification for nursing studies, v. 4, p. xiii–xxvi.

1890★★
International nursing index. New York, 1, 1966– . American Journal of Nursing Company in cooperation with the National Library of Medicine.

Quarterly, cumulated annually. Subject section and name section, listing the journal literature. Covers journals not indexed in *Index medicus*. Includes a section *Publications of selected organizations* which lists monographs, pamphlets, reports. Gives price.

Reviews

1891
Simmons, Leo W., and Henderson, Vir-

ginia. Nursing research; a survey and assessment. New York, Appleton, 1964. 461 p.

Reviews the published literature in the fields of occupational orientation, or career dynamics and nursing care.

1892
Yearbook of modern nursing. New York, Putnam, 1956–59.

Reviews of advances or problems in special areas with bibliographies and/or abstracts of relevant articles. Includes review of work of nursing organizations.

Bibliographies

1893
Books for the nurse, 1963–64. Palo Alto, Calif. [etc.] Stacey, 1963. 24 p.

Lists books by subject, with brief bibliographical citation, including price. Also cites forthcoming books.

Kept current by supplements.

1894★★
Catholic Library Association. Hospital Section. Basic book and periodical list for the nursing school and small medical library. Los Angeles, [1] 195?– .

3 ed., 1961, 100 p., contains selected list of books arranged by subject, with publishers, date, and price and alphabetical list of journals with address, frequency, and price.

First published as *Basic book list for libraries in schools of nursing*. Supplement to 3 ed. issued 1963.

Dictionaries

1895
Ballière's nursing dictionary. 16 ed., by Barbara Cape. Baltimore, Williams & Wilkins, 1964. 540 p.

1895.1
Hansen, Helen F. Pocket encyclopedic guide to nursing. New York, Blakiston, 1960. 423 p.

Modified version of the author's encyclopedic guide to nursing; designed to supply the fundamental terminology and subject matter of nursing and the allied medical sciences in encyclopedic form.

1896
Hara, Kirotake [et al.] ed. Kango igaku jiten [Medical dictionary for nurses] Tokyo, Igaku Shoin, 1961. 844 p.

Often with English, German, or Latin equivalent preceding definition; includes eponyms.

1897
Heinemann modern dictionary for nurses. Comp. by Leslie T. Morton and J. J. Abraham. London, Heinemann, 1961. 309 p.

1898
Morten, Honnor. The nurse's dictionary. 25 ed., by P. Jean Cunningham. London, Faber, 1962. 424 p.

Appendixes: practical information on first aid, tests, diets, etc.

1899
Olson, Lyla M., and Dorland, W. A. A reference handbook and dictionary of nursing. Philadelphia, Saunders, 1960. 548 p.

Pt. 1 is a compilation of latest medical terms useful to the nurse; pt. 2 gives information in broad subject categories, such as organizations in the field and addresses, placement agencies, etc.

1900
Pearce, Evelyn C. Medical and nursing dictionary and encyclopedia. 12 ed. London, Faber and Faber, 1958. 557 p.

Chiefly concise definitions, but includes detailed instructions for providing nursing care in a variety of diseases.

1901
Petry, Lucile, ed. The encyclopedia of nursing. Philadelphia, Saunders, 1952. 1011 p.

Dictionary, with some extensive notations. Abbreviations and useful tables included.

1902
Price, Alice L. The American nurses dictionary; the definition and pronunciation of terms in the nursing vocabulary. Philadelphia, Saunders, 1949. 656 p.

Defines approximately 25,000 words. Includes list of abbreviations, prefixes, suffixes, symbols, tables of bones, muscles, etc.

Directories

1903★★
Facts about nursing; a statistical summary. 193?– . American Nurses' Association.

Annual. Includes distribution of nurses, salaries, etc. Mainly U.S.

1904
A list of schools of nursing meeting minimum requirements set by law and board rules in the various states and territories. New York, 1931–43.

Issued 1931–39 by the National League of Nursing Education; 1943 by the Department of Studies, National League of Nursing Education.

1905★★
State-approved schools of professional nursing. New York, 1946– . National League for Nursing.

Compilation of information on schools meeting minimum requirements and those accredited by the National League For Nursing; arranged alphabetically by state and city. Data include type of program, accreditation, educational requirements, enrollment, and graduations and name of dean or director.

1946 ed. as *State-accredited schools of nursing.* 7th ed. 1964.

Continues 1904.

1906
World directory of post-basic and post-graduate schools of nursing. Geneva, World Health Organization, 1, 1965– .

Lists institutions of higher nursing education in 57 countries. For each country, general information on administration, conditions of admission, and curriculum, followed by list of schools with address, year founded, teaching staff, enrollment, course offered, admissions, graduates, and tuition fees.

Histories

The several one-volume textbook histories of nursing intended primarily for nursing students have been omitted.

1907
Abel-Smith, Brian. A history of the nursing profession. London, Heinemann, 1960. 290 p.

Limited to England and Wales, from 1800 onwards. A sociological and economic study of the profession, the struggle for registration, recruitment, and conditions of service. Bibliographical footnotes.

1908
Austin, Anne L. History of nursing source book. New York, Putnam, 1957. 480 p.

Historical and bibliographic introduction for each chapter. References: p. 433–452; bibliography: p. 453–470.

1909
Kernodle, Portia B. The Red Cross nurse in action, 1882–1948. New York, Harper, 1949. 524 p.

Covers work in war and peace, including public health nursing, disaster service, volunteer work. Based in part on official records, national and local, and other documents. Bibliography (sources and secondary works, general and by chapters): p. 479–491.

1910
Nutting, M. Adelaide, and Dock, Lavinia L. A history of nursing. New York, Putnam, 1907–12. 4 v.

Still the most comprehensive history. Bibliography (general and selective): v. 4, p. 323–329.

1911
Roberts, Mary M. American nursing: history and interpretation. New York, Macmillan, 1954. 688 p.

Official history, mostly 20th century. Bibliography with each chapter.

1912
Shryock, Richard H. The history of nursing; an interpretation of the social and medical factors involved. Philadelphia, Saunders, 1959. 330 p.

A critical interpretation of the history of nursing in relation to medicine and to scientific and social conditions. Concludes with a detailed account of nursing in America in the late 19th and 20th centuries.

1913
Stocks, Mary D. A hundred years of district nursing. London, Allen & Unwin. 1960. 229 p.

Public health nursing in Great Britain.

NUTRITION

Indexes and Abstracts

1914
Food science abstracts. London, 1–29,

1929–57. Great Britain. Department of Scientific and Industrial Research.

2655 abstracts in 1957.

v. 1–20, 1929–48, as *Index to the literature of food investigation*.

1915★★
Nutrition abstracts and reviews. Aberdeen, 1, 1931– . Commonwealth Bureau of Animal Nutrition, Rowett Research Institute.

Quarterly. 1964 listed 6995 references, most with abstracts. Indexes approximately 800 titles, many not in *Index Medicus*. Minimum time lag 7 months. Includes methods, chemical composition of foods, physiology of nutrition, diet in health and disease, vitamins, the feeding of animals, book reviews, symposia, proceedings, congress reports, and government reports.

Reviews

1916
Advances in food research. New York, Academic Press, 1, 1948– .

Irregular.

1917
World review of nutrition and dietetics. London, etc., Hafner, 1, 1959– .

Reviews with bibliographies.

Bibliography

1918★
Baker, E. A., and Foskett, D. J. Bibliography of food; a select international bibliography of nutrition, food and beverage technology and distribution 1936–56. New York, Academic Press, 1958. 331 p.

Lists bibliographies, indexes and abstracts, periodicals, and books and journal articles in the various fields. Includes much nonmedical material.

Monographs

1919
American Institute of Biological Sciences. Committee on the Handbook of Biological Data. Standard values in nutrition and metabolism. Philadelphia, Saunders, 1954. 380 p.

Comparative data.

Dictionaries

1920★
Bender, Arnold E. Dictionary of nutrition and food technology. 2 ed. Washington, Butterworths, 1965. 221 p.

Intended for physicians, chemists, and others having a professional interest in food.

1921
Ellis, Rhoda. A dictionary of dietetics. New York, Philosophical Library, 1956. 152 p.

Terms related to diet and diet therapy.

Histories

1922
Becker, Johann H. Versuch einer allgemeinen und besondern Nahrungsmittelkunde. Stendal, Franzen und Grosse, 1810–22. 2 v. in 3.

v. 1: Versuch einer Literatur und Geschichte der Nahrungsmittelkunde. Pts. 1–2: classified bibliography of 7276 works plus unnumbered later editions, translations, commentaries, etc.; includes critical annotations, articles in serials, analytics for parts of books. Pt. 3: history, through 18th century, with accounts of authors and works and references to bibliography. Detailed table of contents but no index.

v. 2, an encyclopedic dictionary, progressed only from A to Brezoles.

1923
Cummings, Richard O. The American and his food; a history of food habits in the United States. Rev. ed. Chicago, University of Chicago Press, 1941. 291 p.

A study of the effect of social and technological forces on the national diet, and a survey of governmental action to improve nutrition. Bibliographical footnotes. 1 ed. 1940.

1924
Drummond, Jack C., and Wilbraham, Anne. The Englishman's food; a history of five centuries of English diet. Revised, with a new chapter by Dorothy Hollingsworth. London, Cape, 1958. 482 p.

Comprehensive history. New edition adds data on World War II and after, but shortens earlier chapters, chiefly by omitting some of the quotations. Bibliographical footnotes. 1 ed. 1939.

1925
Filby, Frederick A. A history of food adulteration and analysis. London, Allen & Unwin, 1934. 269 p.

Thorough history of British developments from the Middle Ages to 1820, with a brief survey to 1930. Includes a chapter on the beginnings of organic analysis of food. 10 appendices of texts and documents. Bibliography: p. 251–265.

1926
Gottschalk, Alfred. Histoire de l'alimentation et de la gastronomie depuis la préhistoire jusqu'à nos jours. Paris, Éditions Hippocrate, 1948. 2 v.

Emphasis on France. Arranged by periods and topics, with references to authors and works and some annotated lists of publications in the text.

1927
Hintze, Kurt. Geographie und Geschichte der Ernährung. Leipzig, Thieme, 1934. 330 p.

Arranged chronologically by locality or group, Egyptian, Babylonian, Hebrew, Greek, Roman, European, Northern, Asian, African, American, Australian. Mainly an ethnological study. Bibliographic references at end of each chapter.

1928
Lusk, Graham. Nutrition. New York, Hoeber, 1933. 142 p. (Clio medica, no. 10.)

Survey from ancient times through the early 20th century. References: p. 125–129. Reprint, New York, Hafner, 1963.

1929
McCollum, Elmer V. A history of nutrition. The sequence of ideas in nutrition investigations. Boston, Houghton Mifflin, 1957. 451 p.

Science of nutrition, chiefly late 19th and 20th centuries. Bibliography with each chapter.

Vitamins

Indexes and Abstracts

1930
Stechow, M., ed. Register der Weltliteratur über Vitamine, und der von ihnen beeinflussten Gebiete soweit aus deutschen Zentralblättern erfassbar. Würzburg, etc., Physica-Verlag, etc., 1943– .

v. 1, 1890–1929; v. 2, 1930–45.

1931
Vitamin abstracts. Chicago, 1, 1947– . Association of Vitamin Chemists.

v. 1–3, 1947–July/Sept 1949, as *Abstracts of vitamin literature.*

Reviews

1932
Ergebnisse der Vitamin- und Hormonforschung. Leipzig, 1–2, 1938–39.

Reviews with bibliographies. Continued in *Vitamine und Hormone.*

1933★★
Vitamins and hormones; advances in research and application. New York, Academic Press, 1, 1943– .

Annual.

Bibliographies

1934
Bibliography of vitamin E. Rochester, N. Y., [1] 1949/50– . Distillation Products Industries, Division of Eastman Kodak Co.

v. [1]–5, 1949/50–1958/60, as *Annotated bibliography of vitamin E.*

1935
Salmonsen, Ella M., comp. Bibliographical survey of vitamins, 1650–1930; with a section on patents by Mark H. Wodlinger. Chicago, Mark H. Wodlinger, 1932. 334 p.

11,338 references arranged chronologically. After 1916, for each year subdivided by type of vitamin. No author index.

1936
Takata, Ryohie, and Katsura, Eisuke, ed. Nippon bitamin bunkenshu, 1884–1960 [Bibliography of vitamin literature in Japan from 1884–1960]. Tokyo? Bitamin 50-shuenen kinen jigyokai, 1962. 1687 p.

Chronological subarrangement. Abstracts are in Japanese. Includes a list of journals abstracted.

Nomenclature

1937
Leitch, Isabella, and Billewicz, W. Z. A scheme for classification of information on

nutrition coded for machine retrieval. Farnham Royal, Eng., Commonwealth Agricultural Bureau, 1963. 227 p. (Commonwealth Bureau of Animal Nurtition, Rowett Research Institute, Bucksburn, Aberdeen, Scotland. Technical communication no. 24).

OBSTETRICS AND GYNECOLOGY

Indexes and Abstracts

Current

1938
Berichte über die gesamte Gynäkologie und Geburtshilfe, sowie deren Grenzgebiete. Berlin, 1, 1923– . Unter dem Protektorat der Deutschen Gesellschaft für Gynäkologie.

Currently 3–5 volumes a year in 3–4 issues and a separate index issue. A recent volume had about 1500 entries from the international literature, most with abstracts. Includes some monographs.

Suspended 1944–51. See also no. 1943.

1939
Gynecology, obstetrics guide. Chicago, Commerce Clearing House, 1963– .

A loose-leaf service consisting of *Current articles*, a list of articles briefly annotated, and *Current abstracts*, articles selected from the *Current articles*. 140 journals abstracted in 1963.

1940★ ★
Obstetrical and gynecological survey. Baltimore, 1, 1946– .

Bimonthly. A recent volume had about 250 abstracts, with editorial comments, mainly from English language periodicals. Includes review articles. Minimum time lag for 1964 4 months.

1941
Rassegna bibliografica della stampa ostetrico-ginecologica. Roma, 1, 1949– .

Bimonthly. 1964 listed 1500 references, most with abstracts. Book reviews listed separately.

1942
Sekai sanfujinka soran [Survey of world obstetrics and gynecology] Tokyo, 1, 1958– .

Monthly. Abstracts 100 Japanese and 74 non-Japanese journals. Text in Japanese; titles of Western works given in the original language.

Noncurrent

1943
Jahresbericht Gynäkologie und Geburtshilfe. Berlin, etc., 1–51, 1887–1937.

Through v. 36, 1922, a review or abstract journal; from v. 37, 1923, references only. Annual cumulation of references of no. 1938.

v. 1–13, 1887–99, as *Jahresbericht über die Fortschritte auf dem Gebiete der Geburtshilfe und Gynäkologie.* v. 14–20, 1900–06, as *Frommel's . . .* v. 21–28, 1907–14, and v. 33–34, 1919–20, as *Jahresbericht über die Fortschritte . . . v.* 35–40, 1921–26, *Jahresbericht über die gesamte Gynäkologie und Geburtshilfe sowie deren Grenzgebiete.* v. 29–32, 1915–18, publication suspended.

v. 37–51, 1923–37, had subtitle: Bibliographisches Jahresregister der Berichte über die gesamte Gynäkologie und Geburtshilfe sowie deren Grenzgebiete.

1944
Obstetrics and gynecology index, 1940–49. Washington, Washington Institute of Medicine, 1949. 375 p.

1945
Quarterly review of obstetrics and gynecology. Washington, 1–10, 1943–52, [Mar. 1953] Washington Institute of Medicine.

Abstracts.

[Mar. 1953] in no. 2541, v. 10(1), 1953, without volume number or date.

v. 9(2), Apr. 1951–[Mar. 1953]: Incorporating the *International record of obstetrics and gynecology* (original article section).

Merged into no. 2541.

Reviews

1946
Modern trends in gynecology. Washington, 3, 1963– . (Butterworths medical publications. Modern trends series)

Irregular. Reviews with bibliographies. Continues no. 1948, in part.

1947.
Modern trends in obstetrics. Washington, 3, 1963– . (Butterworths medical publication. Modern trends series)

Irregular. Reviews with bibliographies. Continues no. 1948, in part.

1948
Modern trends in obstetrics and gynecol-

ogy. London, 1–2, 1950–55. (Butterworths medical publications. Modern trends series)

Reviews with bibliographies. Continued by nos. 1946 and 1947.

1948.1
Recent advances in obstetrics and gynaecology. 11 ed. by John Stallworthy and Gordon Bourne. Boston, Little, Brown, 1966. 438 p.

1 ed., 1926, 10th, 1962.

1949
Sanfujinka saikin no shinpo [Recent advances in obstetrics and gynecology] Tokyo, 1, 1956– .

Triennial.

1950★
Year book of obstetrics and gynecology. Chicago, Year Book Medical Publishers, 1902– . (The practical medicine year books)

Abstracts, with editorial comment.

1902–17, *Obstetrics* and *Gynecology* published in separate volumes; 1918–23 as *Gynecology . . . obstetrics;* 1925–32 *Obstetrics . . . gynecology.*

1902–05 and 1932 as Practical medicine series of year books; 1906–31, Practical medicine series.

Bibliographies

1951
Goszleth, Tibor. Magyar szülészet-nögyógyászati bibliográfia (1926–44, 1945–1960) [Hungarian obstetrico-gynecological bibliography (1926–44, 1945–1960)] Budapest, Országos Orvostudományi Könyvtár és Dokumentációs Központ, 1961. 504, 472 p.

8909 references published in Hungary or by Hungarian authors abroad. Includes books. Chronological subarrangement. Entries in the original language (mostly Hungarian).

1926–44 by J. Bókay.

1952
Kinnunen, Olavi, and Niemineva, Kalevi. The obstetrical and gynaecological literature published in Finland from 1901–1950. Medicina Fennica, 1951. Suppl. 1. 118 p.

1953
Mikhnov, S. D. Sistematicheskiĭ ukazatel' russkoĭ akushersko-ginekologicheskoĭ literatury ot eia vozniknoveniia do 1901 goda [Systematic index of Russian obstetrico-gynecological literature from its origins to 1901] Iur'ev, Mattisen, 1909. 574 p.

In four pts: 1. General works; 2. Gynecology; 3. Obstetrics; 4. Forensic gynecology. Includes some very brief annotations.

1954
Monitore ostetrico-ginecologico. Parte seconda. Recensioni dei lavori italiani di ostetrica e ginecologia, 1928–36. In Monitore. . . 1–9, 1929–37.

1955
Procházková, Marta. Bibliographia Bohemoslovenica gynaecologico-obstetrica atque oncologica annorum 1945–1955. Pragae, Institutum Documentationis Medicae, 1955. 410 p.

In 2 pts: bibliography of obstetrics, p. 1–175; bibliography of oncology, p. 194–389. Includes books. Separate author index for each part.

Dictionaries

1956
Baillière's Midwives' dictionary. Comp. by Vera da Cruz. 4 ed. London, Baillière, Tindall and Cox, 1962. 394 p.

1957
Carter, G. B. [et al.] A dictionary of midwifery and public health. 2 ed. London, Faber and Faber, 1963. 659 p.

Definitions with extended discussion of some subjects. Public health section (p. 533–659) concerns British laws and practice.

1958
Louros, N. K. Obstétrique et gynécologie; glossaire des termes obstétricaux et gynécologiques en français, latin, anglais, russe, allemand, espagnol, italien, grec. Amsterdam, Elsevier, 1964. 444 p.

Lists 2576 terms.

1959
Taber, Clarence W., and Castallo, Mario A. Taber's dictionary of gynecology and obstetrics. Philadelphis, Davis, 1944. 1 v. (various pagings)

Some definitions and descriptions are encyclopedic in scope.

Directories

1960
American College of Obstetricians and Gynecologists. Roll of fellows. Chicago, 195?– .

1961
American directory of obstetricians and gynecologists. Knoxville, Smith, 1, 1954/55– .

Geographical list by state and city; data include birth date and address followed by professional information in code. Name index.

5 ed., 1962/63, by H. H. Jenkins.

1962
Gynäkologen deutscher Sprache, Biographie und Bibliographie. Stuttgart, etc., 1, 1928– .

Alphabetical listing with biographical and professional data and list of publications, some extensive. Includes gynecologists in Austria, Switzerland, and a few elsewhere.

*1 ed. as *Deutscher Gynäkologenkalender*; 2 ed., 1939, as *Deutsches Gynäkologenverzeichnis*; 3 ed., 1960.

1962.1
Royal College of Obstetricians and Gynaecologists. Register of fellows and members. London, 1966– .

Brief professional information. Alphabetical and geographical lists.

Register included in the *Annual report* of the Royal College of Obstetricians and Gynaecologists through 1964.

Histories

1963
American Gynecological Society. Album of the fellows . . . 1876–1930. Floyd Elwood Keene, ed. Philadelphia, Dornan, 1930. 640 p.

Brief biographies with portraits of all the Society's fellows to 1930. living and dead.

1964
Cutter, Irving S., and Viets, Henry R. A short history of midwifery. Philadelphia, Saunders, 1964. 260 p.

A reprint of Cutter's history from *Obstetrics and gynecology*, ed. by Arthur H. Curtis, Philadelphia, 1933, with additions, mainly biobibliographical, by Viets. "Books on the history of midwifery published since 1933" and "A selection of published catalogues. . .": p. 239–242.

1965
Diepgen, Paul. Die Frauenheilkunde der alten Welt. München, 1937. 348 p. (Handbuch der Gynäkologie. 3 ed., by Walter Stoeckel, 1926–37, v. 12, pt. 1)

Bibliography with each section. Includes primitive, Oriental, and American Indian gynecology. Continued by no. 1966.

1966
——. Frau and Frauenheilkunde in der Kultur des Mittelalters. Stuttgart, Thieme, 1963. 242 p.

Bibliographical references at end of each chapter. Continuation of no. 1965.

1967
Dohrn, Rudolf F. A. Geschichte der Geburtshülfe der Neuzeit. Zugleich als dritter Band des Versuches einer Geschichte der Geburtshülfe von Eduard von Siebold. Tübingen, Pietzcker, 1903–04. 2 v.

From 1840 to 1880. Follows the plan of Siebold (no. 1977) but with some subject arrangement and with national histories. Bibliographical references for authors and at ends of sections. Name indexes only.

1968
Fasbender, Heinrich. Geschichte der Geburtshülfe. Jena, Fischer, 1906. 1028 p.

Exhaustive history, with biobibliographical studies of authors, and with surveys of special subjects in the 18th and 19th centuries. Extensive bibliographical references in text and footnotes. Name index only. Reprinted Hildesheim, Olms, 1964.

1969
Fischer, Isidor. Geschichte der Gynäkologie. In Biologie und Pathologie des Weibs, ed. by Josef Halban und Ludwig Seitz. Berlin, Urban & Schwarzenberg, 1924–29. v. 1, p. 1–202.

Survey through 18th century. Classified bibliography: p. 187–202. Not included in the 2 ed. of the work, 1941–45.

1970
Flack, Isaac H. Eternal Eve; the history of gynaecology & obstetrics [by] Harvey Graham [pseud.] London, Heinemann, 1950. 699 p.

Popular survey, brief bibliography. Rcv. ed. London, 1960, 328 p., is much abridged.

1971
Gauss, Carl J., and Wilde, Bernhard. Die deutschen Geburtshelferschulen; Bausteine zur Geschichte der Geburtshilfe. München, Banaschewski, 1956. 333 p.

A survey of the teaching centers and students of 9 founding professors of obstetrics in German-speaking countries from the 18th century to the present. Chronological tables with professors for each teaching center: p. 23–54. Brief biographies: p. 90–326. Bibliography: p. 329–332.

1972
Kerr, John M. Monro, Johnstone, R. W., and Phillips, Miles H., ed. Historical review of British obstetrics and gynaecology, 1800–1950. Edinburgh, Livingstone, 1954. 419 p.

Topical arrangement, with contributions by 19 authors. Bibliographical footnotes. Written as sequel to no. 1979.

1973
La Torre, Felice. L'utero attraverso i secoli da Erofilo ai giorne nostri: storia, iconografia, struttura, fisiologia. Città di Castello, Unione Arti Grafiche, 1917. 831 p.

Preliminary survey tracing development of knowledge and theory, followed by exhaustive history of authors and works, with full analyses and translated passages. Many illustrations, plates, portraits, and facsimiles. References in the text.

1974
Ricci, James V. The development of gynaecological surgery and instruments: a comprehensive review of the evolution of surgery and surgical instruments for the treatment of female diseases from the Hippocratic age to the antiseptic period. Philadelphia, Blakiston, 1949. 594 p.

Comprehensive study. Extensive notes at ends of chapters give bibliographical references and frequent quotations from sources, in the original or in translation. Name index only.

1975
——. The genealogy of gynaecology: history of the development of gynaecology through the ages, 2000 B.C.–1800 A.D. with excerpts from the many authors who have contributed to the various phases of the subject. 2 ed. Philadelphia, Blakiston, 1950. 494 p.

Detailed history with biobibliographical sketches, resumés and excerpts from important works. Extensive references and bibliographies at ends of chapters. Name index only.

1976
——. One hundred years of gynaecology, 1800–1900; a comprehensive review of the specialty during its greatest century, with summaries and case reports of all diseases pertaining to women. Philadelphia, Blakiston, 1945. 651 p.

A closely classified survey of publications, with running historical commentary. Extensive references in footnotes. Includes monographs and articles.

1977
Siebold, Eduard C. J. von. Versuch einer Geschichte der Geburtshülfe. 2 ed. Tubingen, Pietzcker, 1901–02. 2 v.

The classic history. Arranged by period, from ancient Orient to ca. 1840. Primarily accounts of authors and works, with references. Bibliography of general works, v. 1, p. 5–15. Name indexes only. Corrected reprint of 1 ed. (Berlin, 1839–45). Continued by no. 1967.

French translation of Siebold's 1 ed. (*Essai d'une histoire de l'obstétricie*, tr. by F. J. Herrgott, Paris, Steinheil, 1891–93, 3 v.) contains supplementary data. v. 3 covers 1845–ca. 1890.

1978
Speert, Harold. Obstetric and gynecologic milestones; essays in eponymy. New York, Macmillan, 1958. 700 p.

79 essays on 101 gynecologists, with historical accounts, excerpts from sources (in English), biographical sketches, references. Classified arrangement.

1979
Spencer, Herbert R. The history of British midwifery from 1650 to 1800. London, J. Bale, Sons & Danielsson, 1927. 185 p. (Fitzpatrick lectures, 1927)

Biographies of chief writers with lists of works (p. 1–142) followed by topical chapters. Includes list of British lying-in institutions and their staffs. Continued by no. 1972.

1980
Thoms, Herbert K. Chapters in American

obstetrics. 2 ed. Springfield, Ill., Thomas, 1961. 158 p.

From the colonial period through the 19th century; mainly studies of leading contributors. References at ends of chapters.

1981
——, ed. Classical contributions to obstetrics and gynecology. Springfield, Ill., Thomas, 1935. 265 p.

Translated selections from original writings to 1900, arranged by subject, with introductory notes on the authors. Bibliography (histories and biographies): p. 257–259.

1982
——. Our obstetric heritage: the story of safe childbirth. Hamden, Conn., Shoe String Press, 1960. 164 p. (Yale University. School of Medicine. Dept. of the History of Medicine. Publication no. 37)

Survey for the general reader, mainly of key developments from the 16th through the 19th century, with emphasis for the later period on American contributions. Bibliography (secondary works): p. 151–157.

1983
Usandizaga, Manuel. Historia de la obstetricia y de la ginecología en España. Santander [Talleres Aldus] 1944. 361 p.

Through the 18th century, with brief survey of 19th. Includes data on pre-Columbian Spanish America and on Arabic and Jewish authors in Spain. Includes extracts from sources. Checklist of 220 Spanish works and translations from Arabic: p. 289–312. Classified bibliography of 257 secondary works: p. 323–339. Index of Spanish authors, including bibliographic references: p. 313–322.

1984
Vintilă, George D. Istoricul obstetricei si gynecologiei româneşti [History of Rumanian obstetrics and gynecology] Bucureşti, Furnica, 1938. 751 p.

History from the 14th century to 1938, including schools, hospitals, and charitable institutions. Biobibliographies of leading figures: p. 353–444. Annotated bibliographies of theses and academic publications, 1838–1936 (p. 447–540) and of independent publications, 1806–1914 (p. 555–577). Lists of contents of journals, and of society publications and congresses: p. 577–743. References: p. 746–748. No index.

1985
Weindler, Fritz. Geschichte der gynäkologisch-anatomischen Abbildung. Dresden, Zahn & Jaensch, 1908. 186 p.

Careful study, through the 18th century, with valuable illustrations. Sources identified in text. Name index only.

1986
Young, John H. Caesarian section; the history and development of the operation from earliest times. London, Lewis, 1944. 254 p.

Includes extensive lists of references.

OPHTHALMOLOGY

Indexes and Abstracts

Current

1987
Abstracts on military and aviation ophthalmology and visual sciences. Washington, 1, 1953– . Biological Sciences Foundation.

v. 1–5 contain 26,799 abstracts from the earliest literature (ca. 1660) through 1954. Cumulative index to v. 1–5 issued in 1960.

v. 1–2 by Conrad Berens and L. B. Sheppard; v. 3–5 by Berens, Sheppard and J. H. Bickerton.

The literature through 1940 first published in whole or in part under the same title in no. 1994.1, v. 7–8, 1951–52.

1988
Ophthalmic literature. London, 1, 1947– . British Medical Association.

Bimonthly. A recent year listed 5750 entries, most with abstracts.

1989★★
Survey of ophthalmology. Baltimore, 1, 1956– .

Bimonthly. About 250 abstracts of articles a year. Includes review articles and a book review section. Has section: Classics in ophthalmology. Minimum time lag in 1963, 12 months.

1990
Zentralblatt für die gesamte Ophthalmologie und ihre Grenzgebiete. Berlin, 1, 1914– .

Currently 3 to 4 volumes a year in 4 issues and a separate index issue. A recent volume listed about 1500 references, most with abstracts. Includes books.

v. 3–15, 1920–26, had subtitle: Zugleich Referatenteil zu v. Graefes Archiv für Ophthalmologie und Fortsetzung des Michelschen Jahresberichts über die Leistungen und Fortschritte im Gebiete der Ophthalmologie; v. 16, 1926– indicates continuing relationship to von Graefe's Archiv with variation in wording. See also no. 1992.

Noncurrent

1991
Centralblatt für praktische Augenheilkunde. Leipzig, 1–43, 1877–1919.

Monthly. Abstracts of articles, books, proceedings of societies. Includes brief original articles.

1992
Jahresbericht Ophthalmologie. Berlin, etc., 1–65, 1870–1938.

Through v. 54 an annual review or abstract publication, except v. 45–46, pt. 1, 1914–18, which had references only. v. 55–65, references only. Includes books and theses.

v. 1–44, 1870–1913, as *Jahresbericht über die Leistungen und Fortschritte im Gebiete der Ophthalmologie;* v. 45–46, 1914–19, *Nagel-u. Michelscher Jahresbericht Ophthalmologie;* v. 47–53, 1920–26, *Jahresbericht über die gesamte Ophthalmologie.*

v. 47–53, 1920–26, has subtitle: Zugleich bibliographisches Jahresregister des Zentralblattes für die gesamte Ophthalmologie . . . [no. 1990]; v. 54–64, 1927–38, Bibliographisches . . . .

1993
Ophthalmology review [1873–74]–[1877–78] In Archives of ophthalmology and otology (Chicago) 3–7, 1873/74–1878/79.

Selective review of references.

1994
Ophthalmologische Bibliographie. Erlangen, 1863–67, 1870–83.

1870–78 also as *Jahresbericht für Ophthalmologie,* [1]–9.

1864–67 as *Beilageheft zu den klinische Monatsblättern für Augenheilkunde.*

1994.1
Quarterly review of ophthalmology. Washington, 1–8, 1945–52, 1953–60. Washington Institute of Medicine.

Abstracts.

v. 4–5, 1948–49, as *Quarterly review of ophthalmology and allied sciences;* v. 6(1–2), Mar.–June 1950, *Quarterly review of ophthalmology and otorhinolaryngology;* v. 6(3–4), Sept.–Dec. 1950, *Quarterly review of ophthalmology, otorhinolaryngology and bronchoesophagology.*

v. 1–8(2), 1945–June 1952, published separately; v. 8(3–4), Sept.–Dec. 1952, in *International record of medicine and general practice clinics,* v. 165(9, 12), Sept., Dec. 1952; 1953–60 published without voluming in *International record of medicine . . . ,* v. 166–173.

v. 7(1), Mar. 1951–1956: Incorporating *International record of ophthalmology* (original article section).

1995
Regelmässiger Vierteljahresbericht über die Leistungen und Fortschritte der Augenheilkunde, 1878–1923. In Archiv für Augenheilkunde, München, etc., 8–95, 1879–1925.

Selective review of references. Includes books.

1878–80 as *Bericht über die Leistungen und Fortschritte der Augenheilkunde;* 1881–1911 as *Systematischer Bericht über die Leistungen und Fortschritte der Augenheilkunde.*

Some years of the *Systematischer Bericht* have annual t.p. *Bericht über die Leistungen und Fortschritte der Augenheilkunde . . . für Knapp und Schweigger's Archiv für Augenheilkunde* and running title *Bericht über die Fortschritte der Augenheilkunde.*

For an English translation see no. 1996.

1996
Report on the progress of ophthalmology 1878–[1926] In Archives of ophthalmology (Chicago), 8(1)–57(1), 1879–1928.

Selective reviews of references. Includes books.

1881–1911 as *Systematic report on the progress of ophthalmology* in *Arch Ophthal* (*Chicago*) 10(4)–41(6), 1881–1912; 1912–1st and 2nd quarters of 1916 as *Quarterly review of the progress of ophthalmology* in *Arch Ophthal* (*Chicago*) 42(1)–46(2), 1913–17.

1878–1911 a translation into English of no. 1995. 1912– selectively translated from no. 1995 or produced in cooperation with the *Archiv für Augenheilkunde.*

Reviews

1997
Documenta ophthalmologica. Advances in ophthalmology. The Hague, 1, 1938– .

Annual.

1998
Fortschritte der Augenheilkunde. Ad-

vances in ophthalmology. Progrès en ophthalmologie. Basel, 1, 1952– . (Bibliotheca ophthalmologica. Additamenta ad Ophthalmologica, fasc. 36, etc.)

1999
Ganka saikin no shinpo [Recent advances in ophthalmology]. Tokyo, 1, 1955– .

2000
Modern trends in ophthalmology. London, 1, 1940– . (Butterworths medical publications. Modern trends series)

Irregular. Includes reviews with bibliographies. Ser. 2 published 1947; ser. 3, 1955.

2001
Problèmes actuels d'ophthalmologie. Moderne Probleme der Ophthalmologie. Modern problems in ophthalmology. Basel, 1, 1957– . (Bibliotheca opthalmologica. Additamenta ad Ophthalmologica, fasc. 47, etc.)

v. 1, various contributions by world specialists; v. 2, proceedings of the International Colloquium on Photo-coagulation; v. 3, present-day therapy of retinal detachment. Articles in French, German, or English.

2002★
Progress in ophthalmology and otolaryngology. New York, Grune and Stratton, 1, 1946/51.

Supersedes *Ophthalmology in war years* (not listed).

2003
Recent advances in ophthalmology. By Stewart Duke-Elder and Allen J. B. Goldsmith. 4 ed. London, Churchill, 1951. 372 p.

1 ed., 1927; 3 ed., 1934.

2004★
Year book of ophthalmology. Chicago, Year Book Medical Publishers, 1957/58– . (The practical medicine year books)

Abstracts, with editorial comment.

Bibliographies

2005
Ershkovich, E. G., and Shevalev, A. E. Glaukoma; kratkiĭ bibliograficheskiĭ ukazatel' otechestvennoĭ literatury [Glaucoma; a brief bibliographical index to the national literature] Odessa, Odesskoe obl. izd-vo, 1956. 118 p.

86 references in Russian for 1852–1900, and 1200 for 1901–1955. Includes books.

2006
Vári, I., and Betkó, J. A magyar szemészet bibliográfiája (1945–1960) [Hungarian literature on ophthalmology (1945–1960)] Budapest, Országos Orvostudományi Könyvtár és Dokumentációs Központ, 1961. 264 p.

Lists 2019 references, including books. Covers the literature published in Hungry or by Hungarian authors abroad. Chronological subarrangement. Includes a list of periodicals indexed with abbreviations.

2007
Yuge, Tsunekazu, comp. Nippon ganka bunkenshu [Index to Japanese literature in ophthalmology] Tokyo, Kanehara, 1959–61. 3 v.

Abstracts. Covers the literature from as early as 1903 to 1960.

Dictionaries

2008
ABC der Optik; physikalische Optik, optische Instrumente, Spektroskopie, Lumineszenz, Lichttechnick, Elektronenoptik, Photographie, Farbenlehre, physiologische Optik, optische Wahrnehmung. Ophthalmologie, Augenoptik. Ed. by Karl Mutze. Hanau/Main, Verlag Dausien, 1961. 963 p.

Comprehensive dictionary, illustrated.

2009
Alvaro, M. E. [et al.] ed. Lexicon ophthalmologicum: multilingual ophthalmological dictionary. Basel, Karger, 1959. 223 p.

Main section of 2192 terms in English followed by the equivalent in German, Spanish, French, Italian, and Latin; contains sections in each language with numerical reference to numbered term in the English section.

2010
Goldman, Max R. Ophthalmic glossary. Pittsburgh, Rimbach, 1952. 40 p.

Intended for the general practitioner, optometrist, optician, and medical secretary.

2011

Kerney, Ellen. A glossary of French medical terms referable to the eye. New York, Columbia University, Institute of French Studies, 1934. 209 p.

English definitions of French terms; authorities for definitions given.

2012

Schapero, Max [et al.] Dictionary of visual science. Philadelphia, Chilton, 1960. 785 p.

Includes ocular anatomy, physiology, pathology, histology, physiological optics, orthoptics, and visual training. Gives phonetic pronunciations; abbreviations.

Directories

2013

American Academy of Ophthalmology and Otolaryngology. Directory: Alphabetical, geographical official roster, 1964. Rochester, Minn., Custom Printing Inc., 1964. 1 v. (unpaged)

Gives name, address, and specialty for each member.

2014

Concilium Ophthalmologicum. Index ophthalmologicus, in quo recensentur totius mundi artis ophthalmologicae medici institua edita. Leiden, [1] 1930– .

Arranged alphabetically by country. Gives ophthalmological societies, names and addresses of ophthalmologists, schools for the blind and deaf, leading journals in ophthalmology published by each country. 1–3 ed. have title *Indicia ad oculorum morbos medicosque ab oculis pertinentia.* 5 ed., 1958.

Periodicals—Lists

2015

Barr, M. P., and McEwen, W. K. World list of current periodicals in ophthalmology, optics and optometry. In A.M.A. Archives of ophthalmology (Chicago) 63(3):430–72, March 1960.

Separate alphabetical lists for ophthalmology and optometry. Includes annual reports, transactions, proceedings, and congresses. Indexed by country and by abstracting agency.

Histories

2016

Chance, Burton. Ophthalmology. New York, Hoeber, 1939. 240 p. (Clio medica, no. 20).

Survey through the 19th century, including chapters on special subjects. Bibliographical citations in the text. Account of chief historical studies: p. 215–216. Reprinted New York, Hafner, 1962.

2017

Hirschberg, Julius. Geschichte der Augenheilkunde. Leipzig, Engelmann; Berlin, Springer, 1899–1918. 4 v. in 10. (Handbuch der gesamten Augenheilkunde, begrundet von A. Graefe und Th. Saemisch, 2 ed., v. 12–15).

Exhaustive. Covers antiquity through ca. 1875, with a brief summary of later developments. Includes the Orient and America. Historical accounts of periods, countries, and special subjects include full bibliographies; biographical studies include analyses of important contributions and lists of works by and about the authors. v. [4] (Registerband) includes subject and name indexes, and 3 appendices: evolution of terminology; chronology (ca. 2250 B.C.–1850), which also serves as a chronological index; and corrections and additions.

2018

Hubbell, Alvin A. The development of ophthalmology in America, 1800–1870; a contribution to ophthalmologic history and biography. Chicago, American Medical Association, 1908. 197 p.

Survey, with accounts of institutions, societies, education, and journals; biographical sketches; and analyses of publications, with bibliographical data. No index.

2019

James, Robert R. Studies in the history of ophthalmology in England prior to the year 1800. Cambridge, University Press, 1933. 255 p.

Studies of subjects and authors in historical sequence, with extensive extracts from sources and bibliographical descriptions of many of the works.

2020

Magnus, Hugo. Die Augenheilkunde der Alten. Breslau, Kern, 1901. 691 p.

Thorough study, through Paul of Aegina. Extensive bibliographical citations.

2021
Ovio, Giuseppe. L'oculistica di Antonio Scarpa, e due secoli di storia. Napoli, Idelson, 1936. 2 v. (1505 p.)

Detailed analysis of Scarpa and other writers, ca. 1700–1935. Bibliography (3007 references, by author): v. 2, p. 1191–1435.

2022
——. Storia dell'oculistica. v. 1. Cuneo, Ghibaudo, 1951. 1316 p.

Topical arrangement under successive periods, to 1850. Bibliography (2031 items, by author): p. 1199–1292. Index. No more published?

2023
Shastid, Thomas H. Ophthalmology, history of. In Wood, Casey A., ed. The American encyclopedia and dictionary of ophthalmology, Chicago, Cleveland Press, 1913–21, v. 11, 1917, p. 8524–904.

Comprehensive history, from ancient Egypt through the early 20th century. Includes detailed summaries of works, histories of societies, institutions, education, and journals. No index.

2024
Snyder, Charles. A bibliography of the history of ophthalmology. In AMA Archives of ophthalmology 55:397–407. 1956– .

1963/64 (v. 74, 1965, p. 579–592) lists 236 titles, alphabetically by subject. Foreign language titles are translated.

Blind

Bibliographies

2025
American Foundation for the Blind. Books about the blind; a bibliographical guide to literature relating to the blind. By Helga Lende. 2 ed. New York, The Foundation, 1953. 357 p.

4000 annotated book and periodical entries, arranged by subject.

Catalogs

2026
American Foundation for the Blind. Dictionary catalog of the M. C. Migel Memorial Library, New York City. Boston, G. K. Hall, 1966. 2 v.

Directories

2027★
American Foundation for the Blind. Directory of agencies serving blind persons in the United States. New York, 1 [193–?]– .

Arranged geographically; data include name and address of organization, chief administrative officers, functions and area served, also information on general aid, educational, library, and rehabilitation services. 13 ed., 1963. Earlier editions have title: *Directory of activities for the blind in the United States and Canada.*

History

2028
Farrell, Gabriel. The story of blindness. Cambridge, Harvard University Press, 1956. 270 p.

Emphasis on social aspects, care, chiefly 19th and 20th centuries. References (by chapter): p. 249–255.

Optometry

Dictionaries

2029
Atkinson, Thomas G. Oculo-refractive cyclopedia and dictionary. 3 ed. Chicago, Professional Press, 1944. 388 p.

Comprehensive dictionary, with some encyclopedic descriptions.

2030
Hardy, William E. [et al.] A dictionary for opticians and optometrists. London, Hatton Press, 1951. 159 p.

2031
Slutzky, Jerome F. The optometrist's dictionary. Dayton, Ohio, Optometric Press, 1949. 295 p.

Includes abbreviations.

Directories

2032
Blue book of optometrists . . . a register of legally qualified optometrists of the United States, Alaska, Cuba, Hawaii, Puerto Rico, Canada, Mexico. Chicago, 1, 1912– .

Geographical arrangement. Data include optical supply houses and manufacturers, optometric associations, state boards of examiners, laws on practice of optometry, list of optometrists with brief professional information. Also gives list of optometric and optician schools. 27 ed. published by The Professional Press, 1964.

2033
A references list of guild opticians. Washington, D. C., Guild of Prescription Opticians of America, Inc., 1965.

Geographical arrangement by state and city; lists members of the Guild.

OTORHINOLARYNGOLOGY

Indexes and Abstracts

Current

2034
E. E. N. T. digest; a summary of the world's E. E. N. T. & allergy literature. Northfield, Ill., 1, 1938- .

Monthly. 1963 had 1265 abstracts.

v. 1-21(3), 1938-Apr. 1959, as *Digest of ophthalmology and otolaryngology.*

2035
Referátový výběr otorhinolaryngologie [Selected abstracts on otorhinolaryngology] Praha, 1, 1959- . Ústav pro zdravotnickou dokumentaci.

Quarterly. Covers chiefly foreign literature. Entries are in Czech or Slovak first, and the original language with abstracts in Czech or Slovak. Each issue contains between 50 and 70 abstracts. Proceedings of congresses and bibliographies are special features of some issues.

2036
Zentralblatt für Hals-, Nasen- und Ohrenheilkunde sowie deren Grenzgebiete. Berlin, 1, 1922- . Organ der Deutschen Gesellschaft der Hals-Nasen-Ohrenärzte.

3-4 volumes a year, each in 4 to 5 issues with a separate index issue. A recent volume had in excess of 1400 entries from the world literature, most with abstracts. Includes books. Continues no. 2038.

Noncurrent

2037
Bericht über die Leistungen und Fortschritte auf dem Gebiete der Ohrenheilkunke, der Krankheiten der Luftwege und der Grenzgebiete. 1878?-1920. In Zeitschrift für Ohrenheilkunde und für die Krankheiten der Luftwege. München-Wiesbaden, 87-80, 1879?-1921.

Titles of *Bericht* and *Zeitschrift* vary.

2037.1
Bericht über die neueren Leistungen in der Ohrenheilkunde. Leipzig [1]-10, 1888/89-1909/10.

Abstracts. No indexes.

[1-4] as *Bericht über die Leistungen . . .*

Also published as a section of no. 37. Editor Louis Blau.

2038
Internationales Centralblatt für Laryngologie, Rhinologie und verwandte Wissenschaften. Berlin, 1-38, 1884-1922.

v. 19, 1903, listed in excess of 1500 references, most with abstracts. Book reviews and abstracts of proceedings of societies listed separately. Through v. 31, 1915, contained an annual statistical breakdown of references abstracted by country and specialty. Continued by no. 2036.

2039
Jahresbericht Hals- Nasen- und Ohrenheilkunde. Berlin, 1-10, 1922-31.

Cumulation of references of no. 2036.

v. 1, 1922, as *Bibliographie der Hals- . . .* Subtitle: v. 1-5, 1922-26, Zugleich bibliographisches Jahresregister des Zentralblattes für Hals- Nasen- und Ohrenheilkunde, sowie deren Grenzgebiete (Fortsetzung des internationalen Centralblattes für Laryngologie, Rhinologie und verwandte Wissenschaften; v. 6-10, 1927-31, Bibliographisches . . . sowie deren Grenzgebiete.

2040
Otological review. 1873/74-77/78. In Archives of ophthalmology and otology. New York, 4(1)-7(4), 1874-79.

Abstracts.

2040.1
Quarterly review of otorhinolaryngology and bronchoesophagology. Washington, 1-8, 10-12(1), 1942-49, 1951-Feb. 1953, May 1953-55. Washington Institute of Medicine.

Abstracts.

v. 1–2(3), 1942–Sept. 1943, as *Quarterly review of otorhinolaryngology*. In 1950 merged into no. 1994.1; v. 11, 1952, in no. 2541; v. 12(1), Feb. 1953, in *International record of medicine and general practice clinics*, v. 166(2), Feb. 1953; May 1953–55 published without voluming in *International record of medicine . . .*, v. 166(5)–168, May 1953–55.

1951–55; Incorporating the *International record of otorhinolaryngology and bronchoesophagology*.

2041

Report on the progress of otology. 1879–1907. In Archives of otology. New York, 8–37, 1879–1908.

Last report (in *Archives . . .*, v. 37, no. 5), as *Report on the progress in otology and rhinology*.

Reviews

2042

Fortschritte der Hals- Nasen- Ohrenheilkunde. Advances in oto-rhino-laryngology. Progrès en oto-rhino-laryngologie. Basel, 1, 1953– . (Bibliotheca oto-rhino-laryngologica. Supplementa ad Practica-oto-rhino-laryngologica, fasc. 1, etc.)

Text in German, English, or French, with some summaries in all three languages. v. 8–10, 1961, are Rapports du VIIe Congrès international d'oto-rhino-laryngologie.

2043

Jibünkoka saikin no shinpo [Recent advances in otorhinolaryngology] Tokyo, 1, 1956– .

Irregular.

2044

Recent advances in oto-laryngology. 3 ed. By F. Boyes Korkis. London, Churchill, 1958. 438 p.

Chapter bibliographies (omitting titles of articles). No general author index. 1 ed., 1935; 2 ed., 1949.

2045★

Year book of the ear, nose, and throat. Chicago, Year Book Medical Publishers, 1901– . (The practical medicine year books)

Abstracts, with editorial comment.

1901–32 as *The eye, ear, nose and throat*. 1901–05 as Practical medicine series of year books; 1906–32, Practical medicine series.

Bibliographies

2046

Duray, Aladár, and Rózsa, Imre. Magyar fül-orr-gégészeti bibliográfia (1945–1960) [Bibliography of Hungarian otorhinolaryngology (1945–1960)] Budapest, Országos Orvostudományi Könyvtár és Dokumentációs Központ, 1961. 221 p.

2347 references, including books. Covers the literature published in Hungary or by Hungarian authors abroad. Chronological subarrangement. Includes a list of periodicals indexed with abbreviations.

2047

Temkin, Ia. S., ed. Voprosy patogeneza, kliniki i lecheniia glukhoty; sbornik sokrashchennykh perevodov, obzorov i referatov inostrannoĭ periodicheskoĭ literatury [Problems of pathogenesis, clinical aspects and treatment of deafness; a collection of abbreviated translations, reviews and abstracts from the foreign periodical literature] Moskva, Izd-vo inostrannoĭ literatury, 1955. 207 p.

88 selected references from 10 western journals, 1950–54. Titles in Russian and the original language; text in Russian.

Directories

2048

American directory of otolaryngologists and ophthalmologists. Knoxville, Tenn., Smith, 1, 1960/61– .

Brief professional information. Limited to the United States. Arranged by state and city. 2 ed., 1965/66.

2049

International directory of otolaryngology. Philadelphia, 1, 1957– .

2050

The red book of eye, ear, nose and throat specialists. Chicago, Professional Press, 1, 1915– .

Biennial. Listing by state and city; gives professional information and address; includes United States, Canal Zone, Puerto Rico, Virgin Islands, and Canada. 25 ed., 1963.

Histories

2051
Chauveau, Claude. Histoire des maladies du pharynx. Paris, Baillière, 1901–06. 5 v.

Exhaustive history from the classical period through 1875, presenting epitomes of and extensive excerpts (in French) from the sources. Later periods treated by subject. Extensive classified "Index bibliographique" in each volume. Detailed tables of contents but no index.

2052
Feldmann, Harald. Die geschichtliche Entwicklung der Hörprüfungsmethoden. Kürze Darstellung und Bibliographie von den Anfängen bis zur Gegenwart. Stuttgart, Thieme, 1960. 92 p. (Zwanglose Abhandlungen aus dem Gebiet der Hals-, Nasen-, Ohren-Heilkunde, Heft 5)

Bibliography: p. 75–89.

2053
Kassel, Karl. Geschichte der Nasenheilkunde von ihren Anfängen bis zum 18. Jahrhundert. v. 1. Würzburg, Kabitzsch, 1914. 476 p.

Detailed history, with excerpts from sources, through 17th century. Bibliography: p. 469–496. Continued through 19th century in articles in *Zeitschrift für Laryngologie, Rhinologie, Otologie und ihre Grenzgebiete*, v. 7–11, 1914–23, but left incomplete.

2054
Politzer, Adam. Geschichte der Ohrenheilkunde. Stuttgart, Enke, 1907–13. 2 v.

Exhaustive history, to 1911, with analyses of works and extensive bibliographical references. Arranged by period through the 16th century, later by country and subject. Author index.

2055
Stevenson, Robert Scott, and Guthrie, Douglas. A history of oto-laryngology. Edinburgh, Livingstone, 1949. 155 p.

Antiquity through early 20th century. Bibliography: p. 139–146.

2056
Wright, Jonathan. A history of laryngology and rhinology. 2 ed. Philadelphia, Lea & Febiger, 1914. 357 p.

Through the 19th century. Based largely on sources. Extensive bibliographical footnotes.

PARASITOLOGY

Indexes and Abstracts

2057
Helminthological abstracts; a quarterly review of world literature on helminths and their vectors, etc. Farnham Royal, Eng., 1, 1932– .

Prepared by the Commonwealth Bureau of Helminthology. Published by the Commonwealth Agricultural Bureaux.

2500–3000 abstracts per year. Includes books, reports of meetings, dissertations, and many journals not in *Index medicus* (mainly veterinary) or other standard medical indexes.

Reviews

2058
Advances in parasitology. New York, Academic Press, 1, 1963– .

Bibliographies

2059
Akademiia nauk Gruzinskoĭ SSR. Tsentral'naia nauchnaia biblioteka. Bibliografiia po gel'mintam i gel'mintozam cheloveka, zhivotnykh i sel'skokhoziaistvennykh kul'tur v Gruzii (za period s 1865 goda po 1955 god) [Bibliography on helminths and helminthiasis of men, animals and farm cultures in Georgia (from 1865 to 1955)] Tbilisi, 1956. 53 p.

568 entries, including monographs and other printed materials.

2060
Akademiia nauk Kazakhskoĭ SSR. Institut zoologii. Literatura po parazitologii Kazakhstana; referirovannaia bibliografiia po parazitam i parazitarnym bolezniam cheloveka, sel'skokhoziaistvennykh i dikikh zhivotnykh [Literature on parasitology of Kazakstan; annotated bibliography on parasitology and parasitic diseases of men as well as of domestic and wild animals] Alma-Ata, Izd-vo Akademii nauk Kazakhskoĭ SSR, 1957. 311 p.

Author list of 1365 items in Russian, including books, ca. 1860–1957. Includes Latin indexes of parasites and their hosts.

2061
Dimitrova, E., and Pesheva, D. Bibliografiia na bulgarskata khelmintologiia, 1908–1958 [Bibliography of Bulgarian helminthology, 1908–1958] Sofiia, Bulgarska akademiia na naukite, 1961. 86 p.

504 entires, some with brief annotations, in Bulgarian. Includes an index of Latin names of helminths; index of helminths.

2061.1
Fendrych, Miroslav. Bibliografie československé parazitologické literatury do konce roku 1961 [Bibliography of the Czechoslovak literature on parasitology to the end of 1961] Praha Československá akademie věd, 1966. 250 p.

Over 5000 entries on parasitology and allied fields, with special emphasis on natural foci of infection. Includes books. Author arrangement. Limited to works published in Czechoslovakia or by Czechoslovak authors abroad.

2061.2
Kan, Lai-Bing. Parasitic infections of man and animals; a bibliography of articles in Chinese medical periodicals, 1949–64. Hong Kong, Hong Kong University Press, 1966. 119 p.

950 entries, based on 17 Chinese periodicals. Published under the auspices of the Biological Sciences Communication Project, George Washington University.

2062
Kerbabaev, E. B. Bibliografiia po parazitologii Turkmenii (annotirovannaia) [A bibliography on parasitology of Turkmenistan (annotated)] Ashkhabad, Izd-vo Adademii nauk Turkmenskoĭ SSR, 1963. 146 p.

623 references on medical and vetĕrinary parasitology in Russian, 1872–1960. Includes books and handbooks. Brief annotations.

2063
Kiev. Respublikanskaia nauchnaia meditsinskaia biblioteka. Sovetskaia meditsinskaia gel'mintologiia; bibliograficheskiĭ ukazatel' [Soviet medical helminthology; a bibliographic index] Kiev, 1940– .

Pt. 1, 1940/49; pt. 2, 1950/55 (1271 entries), [pt. 3] 1956–60 (in excess of 2500 entries) Comp. F. S. Aronova-Zlatopol'skaia. Includes books. In Russian (Ukrainian).

2064
Pan American Sanitary Bureau. Bibliography of onchocercosis. (Includes selected studies to June 1945). [Washington, 1950] 339 p. (Its Pub. no. 242)

Alphabetical list 1715 references, most with abstracts. Includes books.

2065
Rockefeller Foundation. International Health Board. Bibliography of hookworm disease. New York, 1922. 417 p. (Its Publication no. 11).

5680 references from the earliest publication through 1921. Emphasis is on the social and economic aspects of the disease.

2066
World Health Organization. Bibliography of hookworm disease (ancylostomiasis) 1920–1962. Genève, 1965. 251 p.

4213 entries, arranged by author. Includes books and chapters in books. Title also in French.

Dictionaries

2067
Chebotarev, Roman S., and Ratner, Iuriĭ B. Kratkiĭ parazitologicheskiĭ slovar' [A brief dictionary of parasitology] Minsk, Gos. izd-vo sel'skokhoziaistvennoĭ literatury BSSR, 1962. 320 p.

Contains about 2600 Russian terms with their international equivalents (usually Latin). Includes zoological, biological, chemical, medical, and anatomical terms frequently used in the field of parasitology. Biographical information on Soviet and outstanding foreign parasitologists, living and dead, is given.

Histories

2068
Foster, William D. A history of parasitology. Edinburgh, Livingstone, 1965. 202 p.

From ancient times to ca. 1850. General survey (p. 1–28), followed by chapters on special parasites or groups, and a brief note on later developments. References: p. 193–199.

2069
Hoeppli, Reinhard. Parasites and parasitic infections in early medicine and science. Singapore, University of Malaya Press, 1959. 526 p.

From prehistoric period to ca. 1850; full treatment of the Far East. Extensive bibliographical references for each author. Subject and name indexes.

Entomology

Indexes and Abstracts

2070

Bulletin signalétique d'entomologie médicale et vétérinaire. Paris, 1, 1954– .

Monthly. 3500 abstracts a year. Author, subject, and geographical indexes for each issue. No annual indexes.

2071

Index to the literature of American economic entomology. College Park, Md., etc., 1905/14–59. Entomological Society of America.

Arranged by subjects. Name of insect with author listed under rubric. No author index.

Index to v. 1–11, 1905/14–51, published by the American Association of Economic Entomologists.

2072

Index catalogue to Russian, Central and Eastern European and Chinese literature in medical entomology. College Park, Md., University of Maryland Dept. of Zoology, 1963– .

v. 1, Diptera; v. 2, Ticks; v. 3, Fleas; v. 4, Mites; v. 5, Miscellaneous arthopods; v. 6, Bacterial and spirochaetal diseases. Covers for the most part the period from 1920, although some earlier references are listed. Includes monographs. Author arrangement; no subject index. English translation given for Slavic and Chinese titles.

Reviews

2073

Annual review of entomology. Palo Alto, Calif., 1, 1956– . Annual Reviews, Inc., and the Entomological Society of America.

2074

Review of applied entomology: Series B. Medical and veterinary. London, 1, 1913– .

Monthly. 500–1000 abstracts a year. Monthly author and geographical indexes.

Bibliographies

2075

Index litteraturae entomologicae. Series I. Die Welt-Literatur über die gesamte Entomologie bis inklusive 1863. By Walter Horn and Sigm. Schenkling. Berlin, 1928–29. 3 v. (1426 p.)

Author arrangement.

2075.1

Jellison, William L. and Good, Newell E. Index to the literature of *Siphonaptera* of North America. Washington, 1942. 193 p. (U.S. National Institute of Health. Bulletin no. 178. U.S. Congress. 77th. House Doc. no. 289)

Includes many nonmedical sources. Covers up to July 1, 1939.

2076

Jenkins, D. W. Pathogens, parasites and predators of medically important arthropods; annotated list and bibliography. Geneva, World Health Organization, 1964. 150 p. (World Health Organization Bulletin, v. 30, suppl.)

In two pts: (1) groups of arthropods with parasites and predators listed for each and (2) key to 1781 selected references to articles and books.

Dictionaries

2077

Kéler, Stefan von. Entomologisches Wörterbuch; mit besonderer Berücksichtigung der morphologischen Terminologie. 3 ed. Berlin, Akademie Verlag, 1964? 790 p.

Histories

2078

Bodenheimer, Friedrich S. Materialen zur Geschichte der Entomologie bis Linné. Berlin, Junk, 1928–29. 2 v.

Monumental historical survey, with extensive extracts (in German translation) and summaries of original sources and historical works. Full bibliographical references for each section. From ancient times (including the Far East) to ca. 1750.

2079 (not used.)

PATHOLOGY AND CLINICAL PATHOLOGY

Indexes and Abstracts

Current

2080
Animaux de laboratoire; revue bibliographique. Paris, 1, 1964– . Centre National de la Recherche Scientifique.

Monthly. Approximately 4000 references a year. Arranged by animal; no author index.

2081
Berichte über die allgemeine und spezielle Pathologie. Berlin, 1, 1948– .

Currently 3–4 volumes a year, each in 3 issues and a 4th index issue. Recent volumes had about 1000 abstracts. Since v. 22, 1954/55 the first issue of each volume on "Geschwulstforschung".

Noncurrent

2081.1
ABT; abstracts of bioanalytic technology. Chicago, 1–13(2) 1953–65(June) Council of American Bioanalysts.

Quarterly.

Reviews

2082
Ergebnisse der allgemeinen Pathologie und pathologischen Anatomie. Berlin, 37, 1954– .

2083★
International review of experimental pathology. New York, 1, 1962– .

Annual reviews with bibliographies.

2084
Labstracts; annual sourcebook of laboratory technic. Los Angeles, 1–10, 1954/55–63.

In excess of 1500 references a year from the English language literature, selectively abstracted.

Contains directory of organizations and associations in the United States and Canada related to the field. Gives requirement for membership, number of members, publications, etc.

2085★
Methods in medical research. Chicago, Year Book, 1, 1948– .

Mainly review articles on laboratory techniques, but includes some articles on techniques in surgery or procedures in clinical medicine.

2086
Progress in medical laboratory technique. London, Butterworth, 1, 1962– .

Annual.

2087
Recent advances in clinical pathology. Ser. 4. Ed. by S. C. Dyke. London, Churchill, 1964. 424 p.

Chapter bibliographies (omitting titles of articles). No over-all author index. 1 ed., 1947; ser. 3, 1960.

2088
Recent advances in pathology. 7 ed. Ed. by C. V. Harrison. Boston, Little, 1960. 459 p.

Section bibliographies (omitting titles of articles). No over-all author index. 1 ed., 1932; 6 ed., 1953.

Published in Great Britain by Churchill.

2089★★
Survey of pathology in medicine and surgery. Baltimore, 1, 1964– .

6 times a year. Abstracts, condensations, digests and "capsule reviews." 1400 journals examined.

2090★
Year book of pathology and clinical pathology. Chicago, Year Book Medical Publishers, 1940– (The practical medicine year books)

Abstracts, with editorial comment.

1940–41 as *Year book of pathology and immunology*. Suspended 1942–46.

Bibliographies

2090.1
Cass, Jules S. [et al.] A guide to production, care and use of laboratory animals; an annotated bibliography. 196 p. Federation Proceedings, v. 19, suppl. 6, December 1960.

1512 entries, most with abstracts. Includes books, reports. Chronological arrangement under broad subject headings. Earliest dated reference 1919. Subjects include: normal anatomy, physiology, psychology; diseases, abnormalities, injuries; periodicals of general interest.

2091
Juhász, Jenö. Magyar kórbonctani bibliográfia (1945–1960) [Hungarian bibliography of pathological anatomy (1945–1960)] Budapest, Országos Orvostudományi Könyvtár és Dokumentációs Központ, 1965. 407 p.

3111 entries published in Hungary or by Hungarians abroad in any language. Includes books.

2092
Zweifach, Benjamin W. Annotated bibliography on shock, 1950–1962. Washington, National Academy of Sciences, 1963, 206 p. (National Academy of Sciences-National Research Council. Publication 1182)

944 references listed alphabetically by author. Experimental animal index. Includes human shock.

Dictionaries

2092.1
China (People's Republic) Wei Shêng pu [Ministry of Health] Ping li hsüeh ming tz'ŭ [Glossary of pathological terms] Peking, 1954. 124 p.

Chinese-English, English-Chinese.

Nomenclature

2093★
College of American Pathologists. Committee on Nomenclature and Classification of Disease. Systematized nomenclature of pathology. Chicago, 1, 1965– . Sponsored by American Cancer Society and American Medical Association.

Diseases are coded in 4 categories: topography, morphology, etiology, and function. Includes 4 alphabetical indexes: topography, chemicals and drugs, enzyme disorders, and general.

Directories

2094
College of American Pathologists. Directory. Chicago, 1, 1948– .

Annual. Alphabetical and geographical listing of fellows and members.

Until 1959 issued as *Membership roster*.

Histories

2095
Ackerknecht, Erwin H. History and geography of the most important diseases. New York, Hafner, 1965. 210 p.

Brief survey followed by studies of special diseases. Bibliography: p. 190–193. Translation of *Geschichte und Geographie der wichtigsten Krankheiten*, Stuttgart, 1963.

2096
Bett, Walter R., ed. The history and conquest of common diseases. Norman, University of Oklahoma Press, 1954. 334 p.

References at end of each chapter.

2097
Foster, William D. A short history of clinical pathology; with a chapter on the organization of clinical pathology to the present day, by S. C. Dyke. Edinburgh, Livingstone, 1961. 153 p.

Arranged topically; well documented. References: p. 143–151.

2098
Goldschmid, Edgar. Entwicklung und Bibliographie der pathologisch-anatomischen Abbildung. Leipzig, Hiersemann, 1925. 301 p.

Emphasis on period from 1770 to 1860. Introductory historical sketch, including general references (p. 30–31). Full descriptive bibliography of about 650 illustrated works in chronological sequence, 1517–1925, with supplement including some earlier items. 44 plates, 28 in color. Indexes of authors, artists, publishers and printers, and subjects.

2099
Hecker, Justus F. K. The epidemics of the Middle Ages. Tr. by B. G. Babington. 3 ed. London, Trubner, 1859. 360 p.

Detailed and documented. Chapters on the black death, dancing mania, and sweating sickness. Bibliography (works referred to): p. 313–322. German edition, *Die grossen Volkskrankheiten des Mittelalters*, Berlin, 1865, reprinted Hildesheim, Olms, 1963.

2100
Hirsch, August. Handbook of geographical and historical pathology. Tr. from the 2 Ger. ed. by Charles Creighton. London,

1883–86. 3 v. (New Sydenham Society. Publications, v. 106, 112, 117)

Exhaustive work, with extensive bibliographic references. Traces history and distribution of specific diseases. v. 1: acute infective diseases; v. 2: chronic infective, toxic, parasitic, septic, and constitutional diseases; v. 3: diseases of organs and parts. Translation of *Handbuch der historisch-geographischen Pathologie.*

2101
Krumbhaar, Edward B. Pathology. New York, Hoeber, 1937. 206 p. (Clio medica, no. 19).

Survey. Chronology of "milestones": p. 157–185. Reprinted New York, Hafner, 1962.

2102
Laín Entralgo, Pedro. La historia clínica; historia y teoría del relato patográfico. 2 ed. Barcelona, Salvet, 1961. 668 p.

Documented account, with many illustrative extracts. Greek period to present time.

2103
Long, Esmond R. A history of American pathology. Springfield, Ill., Thomas, 1962. 472 p.

Comprehensive survey. Annotated bibliographic notes, p. 393–427.

2104
——. A history of pathology. [rev. ed.] New York, Dover, 1965. 199 p.

Covers ancient Egypt to the present. Approach mainly biographical, with evaluations of leading authors and contributions. A revised reprint of the Baltimore, 1928, edition with a new appendix on "Recent trends . . . 1929–1963." Bibliography (chronological list of classics): p. 169–170.

2105
——, ed. Selected readings in pathology from Hippocrates to Virchow. Springfield, Ill., Thomas, 1929. 301 p.

2 ed., 1961, adds some 30 new pathologists but cuts older selections substantially.

2106
Major, Ralph H., ed. Classic descriptions of disease; with biographical sketches of the authors. 3 ed. Springfield, Ill., Thomas, 1945. 679 p.

Excerpts in English, with references to the sources, from the Ebers papyrus through the early 20th century. Classified arrangement. Bibliography: p. 657–667. First published 1932.

2107
Sigerist, Henry E. Civilization and disease. Ithaca, N.Y., Cornell University Press, 1943. 255 p.

On disease in relation to civilization, economics, social life, law, history, religion, philosophy, science, literature, art, and music. Bibliographical references at end of each chapter. Reprinted University of Chicago Press, Phoenix Books, 1962.

PEDIATRICS

Indexes and Abstracts

Current

2108★
Child development abstracts and bibliography. Washington, 1, 1927– . Society for Research in Child Development.

3 times a year. v. 38, 1963/64, contained 892 abstracts. Includes books. Emphasis is on psychology, psychiatry, and sociology.

v. 1, 1927, as *Selected child development abstracts currently published in the Journal of Nervous and Mental Disease*, etc.; v. 2–6, 1928–32, as *Child development abstracts and bibliography selected from current issues of the Journal of the American Medical Association*, etc.

v. 1–6, 1927–32, issued by the Committee on Child Development, National Research Council; v. 7–8, 1933–34, edited by the Committee; v. 9, 1935, called Publication of the Committee.

2109
Courrier; revue mensuelle. Paris, 1, 1950– . Centre International de l'Enfance.

10 times a year. Analytical bibliography of 5200 to 5500 references a year from about 866 journals, and an annotated list of recent books in the library of the Center. Annotations for books and articles in French and English. Minimum time lag 3 months.

2110
Pediatrics digest; a summary of the world's pediatrics literature. Northfield, Ill., 1, 1959– .

Monthly. 1964 contained 1266 abstracts. Separate book review section. No author or subject indexes.

2111
Referátový výběr z pediatrie [Selected abstracts on pediatrics] Praha, 1, 1959– . Ústav pro zdravotnickou dokumentaci.

4 issues a year. Covers the foreign literature. Titles in Czech or Slovak and in the original language; abstracts in Czech or Slovak.

2112
Zentralblatt für die gesamte Kinderheilkunde. Berlin, 1, 1911– . Referatenorgan der Deutschen Gesellschaft für Kinderheilkunde

Currently 3–4 volumes a year in 3 issues and a separate index issue. A recent volume listed about 1300 books and articles, most with abstracts.

v. 1–8 as *Zeitschrift für Kinderheilkunde . . . Referate*; v. 9–42, 1920–51 had subtitle: Zugleich Referatentheil der Zeitschrift für Kinderheilkunde. Suspended 1944–51.

See also no. 2113.

Noncurrent

2113
Jahresbericht Kinderheilkunde. Berlin, 1–15, 1911–31.

Cumulation of references of no. 2112; v. 7, 1923, and v. 10–11, 1926–27, also contain review articles.

v. 1–6, 1911–22, as *Bibliographie der gesamten Kinderheilkunde;* v. 7–10, 1923–26, *Jahresbericht über die gesamte Kinderheilkunde.*

v. 1–4, 1911–20, Herausgegeben von der Redaktion des Referatenteil der *Zeitschrift für Kinderheilkunde*; v. 7–15, 1923–31, have subtitle: Bibliographisches Jahresregister des Zentralblattes für die gesamte Kinderheilkunde. Suspended 1914–19.

2114
Quarterly review of pediatrics. Washington, 1–17(2), Feb. 1946–Apr./June 1962. Washington Institute of Medicine.

Abstracts.

v. 6(2)–8, May 1951–53: Incorporating the *International record of pediatrics* (original article section); v. 9–13, 1954–58: Incorporating *International review of pediatrics* (original article section).

2115
Zentralblatt für Kinderheilkunde; eine Monatsschrift für praktische Ärzte. Leipzig, 1–22, 1896–1917.

Includes abstracts. With v. 12(6) divided into German and non-German sections. Also contains reports of proceedings of societies, book reviews, and brief original articles.

Reviews

2116
Actualidad pediátrica; revista de bibliografía internacional. Granada, 1, 1952– .

Monthly. Translations or extended reviews of from 17–20 foreign articles each month. Includes books reviews.

2117
Advances in child development and behavior. New York, Academic Press, 1, 1963– .

2118★★
Advances in pediatrics. New York, Year Book, 1, 1942– .

2119
Modern trends in paediatrics. New York, 1, 1951– . (Butterworths Medical Publications. Modern trends series).

Irregular. Ser. 2 published 1958.

2120
Pediátria anual. Barcelona, 1957(?)– .

2121
Progresos de pediátria y puericultura. Madrid, 1, 1958– .

3 times a year. A recent volume contains around 350 abstracts. Includes proceedings of congresses and original articles. No author index.

2122
Progresos en medicina infantil. Granada, 1956– .

2123
Recent advances in paediatrics. 3 ed. By Douglas Gairdner. London, Churchill, 1965. 349 p.

1 ed., 1954; 2 ed., 1958. 1 ed. translated into Spanish, 1957.

2124
Referata pediátrica; extractos pediátricos mundiales. Madrid, 1, 1961– .

1962 contains 2049 references, most with abstracts. No annual author index.

2125
Shonika saikin no shinpo [Recent advances in pediatrics] Tokyo, 1, 1956– .

Irregular.

2126★
Year book of pediatrics. Chicago, Year Book Medical Publishers, 1902– . (The practical medicine year books)

1902 as *Pediatrics and orthopedic surgery*; 1903–23, *Pediatrics . . . orthopedic surgery*; 1924–32, *Pediatrics*.

1902–05 and 1932 as Practical medicine series of year books; 1906–31, Practical medicine series.

Bibliographies

2127
Bibliography of developmental medicine and child neurology; books and articles received. London, 1962– . Spastics Society. Medical Education and Information Unit. (Developmental medicine and child neurology. Supplement no. 6–7, 9–)

1966 listed 1008 items: 154 books and reports, and 854 articles from 141 journals. Emphasis on pathology (IEM, etc.)

2128
Brackbill, Yvonne, ed. Research in infant behavior: a cross-indexed bibliography. Baltimore, Williams and Wilkins, 1964. 281 p.

1733 author entries arranged at random. Author index. Includes books and chapters in books. Earliest reference noted, 1877. Covers: motor behavior; learning and conditioning; language, vocalization, and communication; cognitive development; social behavior and social variables; emotion and personality development.

2129
John Crerar Library, Chicago. Catalog of the Clifford G. Grulee collection on pediatrics. [Herman H. Henkle, ed.] Chicago 1959. 340 p.

4404 items (1071 are 15th–19th century). Separated by form and century, with detailed subject classification for 20th century. Name and subject indexes.

2130
Meissner, Friedrich L. Grundlage der Literatur der Pädiatrik, enthaltend die Monographien über die Kinderkrankheiten. Leipzig, Fest, 1850. 246 p.

Closely classified checklist of over 7000 works, from the 15th century to 1850, arranged by date under each heading. Includes dissertations. No index.

2131
Nelson, Manfred R., ed. References on prematurity, 1956–1960. [Bethesda] 1961. 165 p.

1295 entries. A few selected articles on postmaturity are included.

2131.1
U.S. Childrens Bureau. Clearinghouse for Research in Childlife. Research relating to children; an inventory of studies in progress. . . Washington, [1] 1948/49– .

Covers: growth and development; personality and adjustment; educational progress; exceptional children; the child in the family; social, economic and cultural influences; health services and surveys; social services and surveys.

Gives brief description of project, principle investigator, etc. Organizations, investigators and subject indexes.

Histories

2132
Caulfield, Ernest J. The infant welfare movement in the eighteenth century. New York, Hoeber, 1931. 203 p.

Devoted to the English movement. References: p. 190–195.

2133
Garrison, Fielding H. Abt-Garrison History of pediatrics. Reprinted from Pediatrics by various authors, v. 1, ed. by Isaac A. Abt [Philadelphia, 1923] With new chapters on the history of pediatrics in recent times by Arthur F. Abt. Philadelphia, Saunders, 1965. 316 p.

Garrison's history (p. 1–170) is a survey from ancient times to the early 20th century, including the Orient, with extracts from the sources and a classified list of about 160 periodicals in chronological sequence. A. F. Abt's supplement covers recent changes and advances in special fields. Bibliographical footnotes.

2134
McCleary, George F. The early history of the infant welfare movement. London, Lewis, 1933. 176 p.

Mainly on the late 19th and early 20th centuries. Many quotations from documents and contemporary works. References in text.

2135
——. The maternity and child welfare movement. London, King, 1935. 227 p.

Describes British movement, from late 19th century. References in text or footnotes.

2136
Peiper, Albrecht. Chronik der Kinderheilkunde. 3 ed. Leipzig, Thieme, 1958. 527 p.

Comprehensive detailed survey, with extensive lists of references for each section. 1 ed. 1951.

2137
Ruhräh, John. Pediatric biographies. Baltimore [1932] 207 p.

49 biographies from Soranus through the younger William Heberden, with facsimiles and extracts from works. Originally published in the *American journal of diseases of children*, v. 35–44, 1928–32. Additional biographies were published in the same journal, v. 45–50, 1933–35.

2138
——. Pediatrics of the past, an anthology. New York, Hoeber, 1925. 592 p.

From Hippocrates through the 18th century. Mainly studies of authors, with bibliographical data, analyses, and extracts from their works. Additional bibliography of pediatric literature (by author, to 1800): p. 564–577.

2139
Still, Sir George F. The history of paediatrics; the progress of the study of the diseases of children up to the end of the XVIIIth century. London, Oxford University Press, 1931. 526 p.

General survey presented chiefly as biobibliographical information on successive major authors, with accounts of works. Appendixes (p. 505–515) list dissertations and other minor writings.

PHARMACY AND PHARMACOLOGY

Indexes and Abstracts

Current

2140 (not used)

2141
Comprehensive bibliography on hospital pharmacy. In American journal of hospital pharmacy (Washington) 8, 1951– .

Irregular. 6th Suppl., 1965, includes over 2000 references published from 1961 to Jan. 1964.

v. 8–14, 1951–57, as *Bulletin of the American Society of Hospital Pharmacists.*

2142
Drug digests from the foreign language literature. Jerusalem, [1] 1965– . Published for the National Library of Medicine and the National Science Foundation by the Israel Program for Scientific Translations.

Monthly. Abstracts of reports on effects of drugs from 52 non-English journals.

No. 1–12, 1965, as *Drug digests.*

2143
Drug information sources. In American journal of pharmacy (Philadelphia) Nov/Dec. 1964– . Special Libraries Association. Science Technology Division. Pharmaceutical Section. Drug Information Sources Committee.

Limited to monographs. Arranged by country. Does not include pharmacopoeias.

2143.1
Gyógyszerészeti és gyógyszer-terápiás dokumentációs szemle [Pharmaceutical and pharmaco-therapy documentation review] Budapest, 1, 1962(?)– . Országos Orvostudományi Könyvtár és Dokumentációs Központ.

Jan.-June 1966 contained 1689 entries.

2144
International pharmaceutical abstracts. Washington, 1, 1964– . American Society of Hospital Pharmacists.

24 times a year. About 6000 abstracts a year covering all aspects of the subject, research, laws and regulations, history, etc.

2145
Pharmaceutical abstracts. Austin, Texas, 1957– . University of Texas. College of Pharmacy.

3–4 times a year. 1963 contained 861 entries listed at random by title, most with abstracts. Includes books, titles of talks, papers presented at meetings.

[v. 1] published as ser. 1–12 (in 12 v.), 1957–60, as *Unpublished abstracts of articles on pharmaceutical subjects*. Issues for 1961– have also numbering for the *Bulletin* of the College of Pharmacy of the University of Texas.

Some volumes have special issue, Pharmacy administration, a random listing of articles by title selectively annotated.

2146
Pharmazeutisches Jahrbuch; Referatesammlung des internationalen pharmazeutischen Schrifttums. Frankfurt, 1957– .

1957 contains about 3000 abstracts; 1958 published in 1963.

2147 (not used)

2148
Register over dansk farmaceutisk litteratur, 1900/37; 1938/45; 1946/60. Copenhagen, 1939; 1950; 1962. 222; 310; 159 p.

Index to: *Archiv for Pharmaci og Chemi, Dansk Tidsskrift for Farmaci, Farmaceutisk Tidende.*

2149
RINGDOC; Derwent pooled pharmaceutical literature documentation: Abstracts journal. London, 1, 1964– .

4–6 issues a month. The abstracts are indexed on separately published cards.

Aug. 29–Nov. 5, 1964, issues had no volume or issue number.

2150
Technique pharmaceutique. Paris, 1954– . Société de Technique Pharmaceutique.

Currently monthly. Gives tables of contents for journals which are grouped into the following classes: pharmaceutics, analytical chemistry, physiology, and miscellaneous. Minimum time lag 1964 2 months. In 1963 listed 667 titles, including a number not in *Index medicus*.

2151★★
Unlisted drugs. New York, 1, 1949– . Special Libraries Association. Science-Technology Division. Pharmaceutical Section.

Reports on about 2000 new names or experimental numbers of investigational drugs each year. Among other brief data cites earliest reference found in the literature.

Noncurrent

2152
Bilten naučne dokumentacije za farmaciju. Bulletin de documentation scientifique pour la pharmacie. Beograd, 1955–61? Jugoslovenski centar za tehničku i naučnu dokumentaciju.

Bimonthly. Citations, annotations and abstracts from about 160 pharmaceutical, medical, and chemical periodicals both domestic and foreign. v. 7, 1961, contains 1961 entries. Titles are given in Serbo-Croatian and in the original language (if different). Table of contents for each issue is in Serbo-Croatian, English, French, and German. No indexes.

2153
Canstatt's Jahresbericht über die Fortschritte in der Pharmacie und verwandten Wissenschaften. Erlangen, etc., 1–10, 1841–50; n.s. 1–15, 1851–65.

Superseded by no. 2154.

2154
Jahresbericht der Pharmazie. Göttingen, 1–77, 1866–1942.

Literature review. Arranged by name of plant, drug or compound.

v. 1–24, 1866–89, as *Jahresbericht über die Fortschritte der Pharmakognosie, Pharmacie und Toxikologie*. Supersedes no. 2153.

2155
Jahresbericht über die Fortschritte der Pharmakotherapie. Strassburg, 1, 1844.

Lists 1867 references, most with abstracts. Published 1885.

2156
Pharmaceutical abstracts. Washington, etc., [1]–13, 1935–47. American Pharmaceutical Association.

Monthly. Includes books, patents.

[v. 1]–5 in *Journal of the American Pharmaceutical Association*, 24–28, 1935–39 (separately paged); v. 6–13 in *Journal of the American Pharmaceutical Association, Scientific edition*, 29–36, 1940–47 (separately paged).

2157
Report on the progress of pharmacy. 1853-1934. In Yearbook of the American Pharmaceutical Association, 1-23, 1912-34.

Abstracts. Includes books.

1853-1911 in *Proceedings of the American Pharmaceutical Association* [v. 6]-59. Annual subject indexes, 1853-1911; annual author and subject indexes, 1912-34. Collective indexes, 1851-1902, 1903-25, issued separately.

2157.1
Year-book of pharmacy; comprising abstracts of papers relating to pharmacy, materia medica, therapeutics, and chemistry contributed to British and foreign journals . . . with Transaction of the British pharmaceutical conference. London, 1864-1927.

Subject but no author index.

Reviews

2158
Advances in chemotherapy. New York, Academic Press, 1, 1964- .

2159★
Advances in drug research. New York, Academic Press, 1, 1964- .

2160
Advances in pharmaceutical sciences. New York, Academic Press, 1, 1964- .

2161★
Advances in pharmacology. New York, Academic Press, 1, 1961- .

2162
Annual review of pharmacology. Palo Alto, Calif., Annual Reviews, Inc., 1, 1961- .

2163
Annual survey of research in pharmacy and proceedings of National conference on pharmaceutical research. Baltimore, 1933/34-1939/40.

2164
Fortschritte der Arzneimittelforschung. Progress in drug research. Progrès des recherches pharmaceutiques. Basel, 1, 1959- .

Articles in English, French or German.

2165★★
Pharmacological reviews. Baltimore, 1, 1949- .

v. 1-2, as supplement to *Journal of pharmacology and experimental therapeutics*; beginning with v. 3, 1951, separate publication.

2166
Progress in medicinal chemistry. Washington, etc., 1, 1961- .

Annual. Surveys of selected topics written by specialists for the chemist, biochemist, pharmacologist, and to a lesser extent, the clinician.

2167
Recent advances in pharmacology. 3 ed., by J. M. Robson and R. S. Stacey. London, Churchill, 1962. 406 p.

Chapter bibliographies (omitting titles of articles). No over-all author index.

2168
Yakugaku saikin no shinpo [Recent advances in pharmacology] Tokyo, 1, 1958- .

Irregular

2168.1★
Year book of drug therapy. Chicago, Year Book Medical Publishers, 1949- . (The practical medicine year books)

Abstracts with editorial comment. The 1963/64 volume has a special section, "Precautions," which indicates the side-effects, actual and potential toxicities, and contraindications of the principal prescription drugs in current use.

Continues no. 2616.1.

Bibliographies

2169
Brazil. Instituto Brasileiro de Bibliografia e Documentacão. Curare; bibliografia Rio de Janeiro, 1957. 386 p.

2956 references.

2170
Chmielinska, Maria. Polska bibliografia zielarstva za okres od poczatku XVI wieku do roku 1940 [Bibliography of Polish pharmacognosy from the beginning of the 16th century to the year 1940] Warszawa, Państwowy Zakład Wydawnictw Lekarskich, 1954. 516 p.

Pt. 1, 246 items through 1800; pt. 2, 5280 items, including books, 1801–1940. Pt. 1 arranged alphabetically by author and keyword; pt. 2 by author only. Includes reproductions of title pages of the oldest imprints.

2171
Evans, A. J., and Train, David. A bibliography of the tabletting of medicinal substances. London, Pharmaceutical Press, 1963. 159 p.

Some 900 references from 131 journals published in 22 countries. Coverage selective for 1935–44, comprehensive for 1945–61.

2172
——. ——. Suppl. 1, Comp. by A. J. Evans. 1964. 59 p.

241 annotated entries.

2173
Guerra, Francisco. Bibliografía de la materia médica mexicana. Cátalogo alfabético según autores de libros, monografías, folletos, tesis recepcionales y artículos en revistas periódicas que se refieren a las propiedades medicinales de las drogas mexicanas. México, Prensa Médica Mexicana, 1950. 423 p.

5357 items. Author list with subject index.

2174
Kelemen, K., and Kelemen, E. Magyar gyógyszertani, gyógyszerterápiás és méregtani bibliográfia (1945–1960) [Bibliography of Hungarian pharmacology, drug therapy and toxicology (1945–1960] Budapest, Országos Orvostudományi Könyvtár és Dokumentációs Központ, 1962. 2 v.

7115 references, including books, to literature published in Hungary and by Hungarian authors abroad. Chronological subarrangement. Includes a list of periodicals indexed.

2175
Liu, Shou-shan, ed. Chung yao yen chiu wen hsien chai yao, 1820–1961. [Abstracts of literature on the study of Chinese drugs, 1820–1961] 1 ed. Peking, 1965. 894 p.

More than 4000 entries, most with abstracts. English-Chinese index. Separate plant and chemical indexes in Latin.

First published 1963.

2176
Lloyd, John U. [et al.] Catalogue of the pharmacopoeias, dispensatories, formularies and allied publications, 1493–1957. In Lloydia; a quarterly journal of biological science 20(1):1–42, March 1957.

Geographic arrangement. Includes homeopathic and military pharmacopeias.

2176.1
Pharmaceutical Manufacturers Association. Washington, D.C. The stability and stability testing of pharmaceuticals; an annotated bibliography, 1939–1963. Washington, 1964. 271 p.

2177
Roche Laboratories. Librium, world-wide bibliography. [n. p.] 1964. 1 v. (various pagings)

830 entries, 1959–64. Alphabetically by year.

2177.1
Sollmann, Torald H. Sollmann bibliographies. Midland, Mich., Dow Chemical Co. [1962?] [763 p.]

Reprints the bibliographies in Sollmann's 5th (1936), 6th (1942) and 8th (1957) ed. of *A manual of pharmacology*.

2177.2
Strieby, I. M., and Spencer, M. C. National and international pharmacopoeias, a checklist. Bulletin of the Medical Library Association 45:410–20, 1957.

Country arrangement.

Revision of the same title in *Bulletin of the Medical Library Association* 40:153–61, 1952.

2177.3
Szabó, Barnabás. Magyar gyógyszerészeti bibliográfia (1945–1960) [Hungarian pharmaceutical bibliography (1945–1960)] Budapest, Országos Orvostudományi Könyvtár és Dokumentaciós Központ, 1966. 239 p.

2508 references. Includes some German titles.

2178
Vitrum Apotekare A. B., Stockholm. A guide to the literature on heparin and anticoagulant therapy in thrombosis. I. Covering the period up to July 1, 1958. Stockholm, Nordiska Bokhandeln, 1959. 159 p.

Chronological under subjects.

2179
Zachert, M. J., and Thomasson, C. L. Bibliography of books and reference works relating to the professional courses in the pharmaceutical curriculum. Pts. 1–2. American journal of pharmaceutical education (Lincoln, Nebr.) 27:266–90, 361–421, 1963.

998 references.

Manuals

2180★
U.S. National Library of Medicine. Drug literature; a factual survey on The nature and magnitude of drug literature. Report prepared for the study of Interagency coordination in drug research and regulation, by the Subcommittee on Reorganization and International Organizations of the Senate Committee on Government Operations. [Washington] 1963. 171 p. (88th Cong., 1st sess. [Senate] Committee print).

Appendix B. Selected list of monographs in pharmacy, p. 57–85; Appendix C. World list of pharmacy periodicals, p. 86–124; Appendix D. Composite list of journals of pharmaceutical interest, p. 125–39; Drug information sources: a world list, p. 140–54.

Dictionaries

2180.1
China (People's Republic) Wei Shêng pu [Ministry of Health] Yao hsüeh ming tz'ŭ ho pien [Glossary of pharmaceutical terms] Peking, 1955. 128 p.

Chinese-English, English-Chinese.

2181
Cooper, John W., and McLaren, Alexander C. Latin for pharmaceutical students; a six months' course of Latin for students of pharmacy and medicine. 5 ed. London, Pitman, 1950. 115 p.

A grammar, but has vocabularies, both Latin-English and English-Latin. Extensive section on prescriptions and their abbreviations.

2182
Gammerman, Adell F., and Semichov, Boris V. Slovar'tibetskolatino-russkikh nazvanii lekarstvennogo rastitel'nogo syr'ia primeniaemogo v tibetskoi meditsine [Tibetan-Latin-Russian dictionary of terms of medical plant raw materials, used in Tibetan medicine] Ulan-Ude, Sibirskoe otdel. Akademii nauk SSSR, 1963. 1 v. (unpaged)

737 terms given first in Latin, then in Russian and in Tibetan with Russian transliteration, with references to the literature for each term. Contains alphabetical indexes of terms in Russian, Tibetan transliterated, original Tibetan, and Buriat-Mongolian; also list of abbreviations.

2183★
Glossary in five languages of principal pharmaceutical terms. Strasbourg, 1962. 144 p.

About 350 terms in alphabetical order in each of five languages: English, French, German, Dutch, and Italian.

Prepared by the Subcommittee of the Public Health Committee (PA) on Pharmaceutical Questions, Council of Europe.

2184
Hunnius, Curt. Pharmazeutisches Wörterbuch. 3 ed. Berlin, Gruyter, 1959. 731 p.

Intended for the practicing pharmacist and the student; predominantly Latin terms followed by explanation in German; includes some chemical formulas.

2185
Scartezzini, Carmelino. Dicionario farmaceutico. Rio de Janeiro, Editora Cientifica [1956] 648 p.

Dictionary of approximately 16,000 terms most frequently used, gives synonymous terms or short definitions.

2186
Steinbichler, Eveline. Steinbichler's Lexikon für die Apothekenpraxis in sieben Sprachen. Mit fünf selbständigen Alphabeten und einer pharmazeutischen Phraseologie. Frankfurt a/M, Govi-Verlag, 1963. 474 p.

3000 to 4000 terms; sections in English, German, French, Spanish, Italian, with Greek and Russian equivalents.

Nomenclature and Lists of Drugs

2187
Drug topics red book. New York, [1] 1897– .

Annual. Alphabetical listing of pharmaceutical items, prices, sizes. List of manufacturers.

2188

Hocking, George M. A dictionary of terms in pharmacognosy and other divisions of economic botany. Springfield, Ill., Thomas, 1955. 284 p.

"An arrangement and explanation of terms which relate to crude drugs . . . with briefer mention of other economic plants and animals." Includes Latin, English, and vernacular names; intended for students and practitioners in the health professions, and those in trade and industry.

2189★★

Marler, E. E. J. Pharmacological and chemical synonyms; a collection of more than 13,000 names of drugs and other compounds drawn from the medical literature of the world. 3 ed. Amsterdam, Excerpta Medica Foundation, 1961. 267 p.

An alphabetical listing of nonproprietary names followed by a list of all known synonyms, chemical and alternative nonproprietary names, and trade names.

2190

Negwer, Martin. Organisch-chemische Arzneimittel und ihre Synonyma; eine tabellarische Übersicht. 3 ed. Berlin, Akademie Verlag, 1966. 1224 p.

Lists 3907 chemicals arranged by formula used in medicine; 26,000 synonyms. Includes therapeutic use.

2191

Niemand, Hans Georg. Arzneimittel synonyma; internationaler Kurzname, Wirkungsrichtung, Handelsname. Berlin, Parey, 1963. 159 p.

Includes an alphabetically arranged list of abbreviated names as well as a subject index to the commercial names of pharmaceutical products.

2192

U.S. National Library of Medicine. Russian drug index. Comp. by Stanley Jablonski. Washington, 1961. 103 p. (Public Health Service. Publication no. 814)

Entries for individual drugs are arranged alphabetically in anglicized form under headings representing broad function groups; index of drug names, synonyms, and cross references. Drugs developed elsewhere but renamed in the Soviet Union are included.

Directories

2193

APhA Directory of pharmacists. Washington, [1] 1964– . American Pharmaceutical Association.

Sect. 1: geographical list of the pharmacists of the United States; sect. 2: alphabetical list with city of practice. Prior to 1945 list of members published in the association's *Journal*; since 1949 issued irregularly as special supplement to *Journal of the American Pharmaceutical Association*. Scientific edition.

2193.1

Association Général des Syndicats Pharmaceutiques. Annuaire général de la pharmacie francaise. Paris, 1932– .

Geographic list of pharmacists for France and colonies. Includes lists of pharmacy journals, schools, laws, associations, etc.

2193.2

Pharmaceutical firms, U.S.A., Canada, Mexico, 1965. 3 ed. Park Ridge, N. J., Noyes Development Corporation, 1965. 91 p.

Alphabetical listing of 500 leading firms. Gives annual sales, divisions, officers, location of plants, etc.

2194

Pharmaceutical Society of Great Britain, London. The annual register of pharmaceutical chemists. London, 1954– .

Alphabetical list giving registration number and date and address. Also company and geographical listings. Continues no. 2195.

2195

——. The registers of pharmaceutical chemists and chemists and druggists. London, 1869?–1953.

Continued by no. 2194.

2196

Pharmaceutical Society of Ireland. Calendar. Dublin, 1875?– .

v. 88, corrected to Dec. 1, 1964. Gives names of staff members of the College of Pharmacy, University of Dublin and of chief officers of the society from its foundation. Alphabetical lists with addresses and registration dates of pharmaceutical chemists, dispensing chemists, registered druggists, and assistant to pharmaceutical chemists.

2196.1
World Health Organization. World directory of schools of pharmacy. Geneva, 1966. 301 p.

Country arrangement. Gives general information on administration of education in pharmacy, conditions of admission, curriculum, examinations, qualifications, license to practice. Occasionally has section on historical information. For individual schools gives year instruction started, numbers on teaching staff, total enrollment, admissions, graduates, annual tuition fee.

Periodicals—Lists

2197★
Andrews, Theodora. World list of pharmacy periodicals. In American journal of hospital pharmacy (Washington) 20:47–84, Feb. 1963.

935 journals listed. Geographic index. Reproduced in no. 2180. Also published as a separate.

2197.1
Biological Sciences Communication Project. George Washington University, Washington, D.C. Pharmacology, toxicology and cosmetic serials; their identification and an analysis of their characteristics. 169 p. (Its Communiqué, 22–65, September 1965)

Title, country, language subject and form (reviews, abstracts, original research) listings.

2197.2
Paris. Université. Faculté de pharmacie. Bibliothèque. Catalogue des périodiques, dressé sous la direction de Gabriel Garnier par Georgette Krehmer et Monique Beulé. 2 ed. Paris, 1961. 553 p.

1 ed., 1954, as *Périodiques et publications de congrès.*

2198
Special Libraries Association. Science Technology Division. Pharmaceutical Section. Union list of periodicals in pharmaceutical libraries. New York, 1952. 189 p.

Gives holdings of 25 pharmaceutical libraries in the United States and Canada.

Histories

Bibliographies

2199
American Institute of the History of Pharmacy. Some pharmaco-historical guidelines to the literature. Three bibliographic essays. Madison, Wis., 1959. 143–172 p.

An introduction to the literature on the history of pharmacy.

Republished from the *American journal of pharmaceutical education*, v. 23, 1959.

2200
Bianchi, V. [et al.] ed. Bibliographia italiana di storia della farmacia. In Minerva farmaceutica 8:89–94, 1959– .

Author list of books and articles of all periods on Italian pharmacy. Numbering continuous: items 2572–2678 in 13:27–29, 1964.

2201
Bouvet, Maurice. Les travaux d'histoire locale de la pharmacie en France des origines à ce jour: répertoire bibliographique. Paris, Société d'histoire de la pharmacie, 1957. 43 p.

Lists about 1000 monographs and articles arranged alphabetically by place names with many cross references, and 27 general and national histories. No index.

2202
Daems, Wilhelmus F., and Vandewiele, L. J. Noord- en zuidnederlandse stedelijke pharmacapeeën. Mortsel-bij-Antwerpen, 1955. 135 p.

Arranged by city, with chronological list (1636–1795) and index of names. Full descriptions of editions. References.

2203
Guitard, Eugène H. Manuel d'histoire de la littérature pharmaceutique; lecons professées à l'Institut d'histoire des sciences de l'Université de Paris et complétées par une biobibliographie pharmaceutique. Paris, Caffin, 1942. 138 p.

World literature to 1600, French literature 1600–1860. "Biobibliographie pharmaceutique": p. 96–135.

2204
Vester, Helmut. Deutsche pharmaziehistorische Bibliographie: 1, Deutsche pharmazeutische Zeitschriftenliteratur u. a., ohne Berücksichtigung der Arbeiten über einzelne Apotheker und Apotheken; 1945–1951. [Stuttgart, 1953] 32 p. (Zur Geschichte der Pharmazie; Beilage zur Deutschen Apotheker-Zeitung. Arbeiten aus Vesters Archiv für Geschichte des deutschen Apothekenwesens)

Classified. Includes articles on general and foreign pharmacy printed in the German periodicals indexed. Author and catchword index. No more published? For the projected v. 3, see no. 2205.

2205
——. Topographische Literatursammlung zur Geschichte der deutschen Apotheken. Stuttgart. 1956–61. 4 v. (474 p.) (Internationale Gesellschaft für Geschichte der Pharmazie. Veröffentlichungen, n. s., v. 9, 14, 17, 19)

In 3 sections: 1. Deutsche Städte und Ortschaften, A-Z (p. 1–411); 2. Deutsche Länder, Provinzen, etc. (v. [4], p. 413–464); 3. Deutsches Reichsgebiet (v. [4], p. 467–474). Under each local entry lists dispensatories, pharmacopeias, registries, ordinances, tariffs, etc., chronologically subarranged and with critical studies; general works, and works on individual pharmacists or apothecaries. Includes publications from the 15th century through 1950; a "Nachtrags- und Ergänzungsband" to include additions and publications from 1950 to 1960 is in preparation. An author bibliography is projected. No index. Originally planned as v. 3 of no. 2204. General references: v. [1], p. x-xii.

Monographs

2206
Adlung, Alfred, and Urdang, Georg. Grundriss der Geschichte der deutschen Pharmazie. Berlin, Springer, 1935. 647 p.

Includes section of brief biographies, and chronologies of legislation, formularies, pharmacopeias, dispensatories, herbals, drugs, etc., with bibliographical references. Name and subject indexes.

2207
Berendes, Julius. Die Pharmacie bei der alten Culturvölkern: historisch-kritische Studien. Halle a. S., Tausch & Grosse, 1891. 2 v. (528 p.)

From antiquity to beginning of the Middle Ages, with survey of Arabic pharmacy through 13th century. Reprinted Hildesheim, Olms, 1963.

2208
Boussel, Patrice. Histoire illustrée de la pharmacie. Paris, Le Prat, 1949. 193 p.

Excellent reproductions, some in color.

2209
Conci, Giulio. Pagine di storia della farmacia. Milano, Edizioni Vittoria, 1934. 351 p.

Emphasis on Italy, through the 18th century. Bibliographical footnotes. Full table of contents, but no index.

2210
Gesellschaft für Geschichte der Pharmazie, Berlin. Chemisch-pharmaceutisches Bio- und Bibliographikon. Ed. by Fritz Ferchl. Mittenwald (Bayern), Nemayer, 1937–38. 2 v. in 1 (603 p.).

Brief biographies with lists of works and editions. Includes anonymous works under initials and titles. Mainly European.

2211
Haas, Hans. Spiegel der Arznei. Ursprung, Geschichte und Idee der Heilmittelkunde. Berlin, Springer, 1956. 256 p.

The development of pharmacology and the history of drugs in relation to pathological and therapeutic doctrines, from ancient times to the present. No bibliography, few references.

2212
Holmstedt, Bo, and Liljestrand, Göran, ed. Readings in pharmacology. New York, Macmillan, 1963. 395 p.

Extracts, in English, with historical introductions and biobibliographical notes on authors. Chiefly 19th and 20th centuries.

2213
Kremers, Edward, and Urdang, Georg. History of pharmacy. Rev. by Glenn Sonnedecker. 3 ed. Philadelphia, Lippincott, 1963. 464 p.

Textbook Emphasis on United States.

2214
Matthews, Leslie G. History of pharmacy in Britain. Edinburgh, Livingstone, 1962. 427 p.

Bibliography: p. 399–409. Also bibliographic footnotes.

2215
Schelenz, Hermann. Geschichte der Pharmazie. Berlin, Springer, 1904. 934 p.

Covers antiquity to 20th century. Documented. Numerous footnote references; bibliography: p. 824–828. Extensive sections of biographies, periodicals, societies, pharmacopeias, etc., legislation, chronologies of medicaments. Reprinted Hildesheim, Olms, 1962.

2216
Shuster, Louis, ed. Readings in pharmacology. Boston, Little, Brown, 1962. 294 p.

19 classical papers, in English or translated, from 1785 to 1957, with introductory remarks and references.

2216.1
Stieb, Ernst W. Drug adulteration; detection and control in nineteenth-century Britain. Madison, University of Wisconsin Press, 1966. 335 p.

Detailed, documented history. Bibliographic notes: p. 221–322.

2217
Trease, George E. Pharmacy in history. London, Baillière, Tindall & Cox, 1964. 265 p.

Mainly Great Britain. Largely factual. References for each chapter.

Antibiotics

Reviews

2218
Antibiotica et chemotherapia: Fortschritte, advances, progrès. Basel, 1, 1954– .

Annual reviews with bibliographies. Articles in English, German or French.

2219 (not used)

2220
Antibiotika-Literaturberichte. Wien, [1957?]– . I. Medizinische Universitätsklinik. Forschungsstelle für Antibiotica.

Annual. Through v. 7, 1962, contains 16,910 references. Arranged by name of antibiotic.

Bibliographies

2221
Elkin, I. I., and Eidel'shtein, S. I. Raboty otechestvennykh avtorov po antibiotikam (1870–1950 gg.) Bibliografiia [Works of national authors on antibiotics (1870–1950). Bibliography] Moskva, Akademiia meditsinskikh nauk SSSR, 1953. 132 p.

About 1300 titles of books and journal articles mostly in Russian but also in other Soviet languages. Covers principally 1944–50.

2222
Lederle Laboratories, New York. Aureomycin bibliography and index. 1951 ed. New York, 1952. 319 p.

3102 references. Author arrangement.

2223
Waksman, Selman A. The literature on streptomycin, 1944–1952. 2 ed. New Brunswick, N.J., Rutgers University Press, 1952. xii, 553 p.

6000 references. Supersedes the 1 ed., 1948.

Dictionaries

2224★
Karel, Leonard, and Roach, Elizabeth S. A dictionary of antibiosis. New York, Columbia University Press, 1951. 373 p.

Lists antibiotics, names of organisms inhibited, and those not affected. Toxicity and experimental clinical data are often given, including surnames of investigators. Extensive bibliography.

Pest Control

Indexes and Abstracts

2225
Pesticides documentation bulletin. Washington, 1, 1965– . U.S. National Agricultural Library.

Biweekly. Keyword arrangement. Includes geographic headings. Author index.

Reviews

2226
Advances in pest control research. New York, Interscience, 1, 1957– .

2227
Residue reviews; residues of pesticides

and other foreign chemicals in foods and feeds. New York, Academic Press, 1, 1962– .

Title also in German.

Bibliographies

2228
Syracuse University Research Corporation. Microbiological and Biochemical Center. Bibliography of organic pesticide publications having relevance to public health and water pollution problems. Prepared for New York State Department of Health, by Patrick R. Dugan, Robert M. Pfister, and Margaret L. Sprague. Syracuse, 1963. 122 p. (New York State Department of Health. Research report no. 10, pt. 2).

950 references, in three separate author lists: 1. Analysis; 2. Effects; 3. General references.

Toxicology

Indexes and Abstracts

2229
Adverse reactions titles. Amsterdam 1, 1966– . Excerpta Medica Foundation.

Arranged under 35 subject headings. 2804 entries in 1966 from approximately 3000 biomedical journals. Minimum time lag 2 months. Author and subject indexes for each issue and annual cumulations.

2229.1
CLUE; foreign clinical literature untoward effects. Philadelphia, International Information Institute, 1, 1966.

Abstracts. Adverse reactions due to drugs, prosthetic devices, cosmetics, pesticides, food additives.

2230
Clin-alert. Louisville, Science Editors, Inc., 1962–

Irregular or semimonthly. Abstracts of articles on drug reactions, with emphasis on the American journal literature. 365 abstracts in 1964. Minimum time lag 1964, 3 weeks. Abstracts listed under drug name and in order of publication.

No author or subject index.

2230.1
F.D.A. clinical experience abstracts. Washington 1, 1963– .

Weekly. Abstracts. Covers currently some 300 serials principally in clinical medicine for significant human data on adverse effects, hazards and efficacy of drugs, devices, and nutrients, and on adverse effects, or hazards of cosmetics, household chemicals, pesticides and food additives. Animal studies on teratogenicity also included.

Arranged alphabetically by main index term. In the case of drugs, by the U.S. adopted or official name if available.

v. 1, 1962–v. 3, no. 3, 1963 as *Adverse effects of drugs, devices, cosmetics;* v. 3, no. 4, 1963–v. 4, 1964 as *Reports in the literature on adverse reactions to drugs and therapeutic devices, cosmetics . . . ;* v. 5–8, 1964 as *MRL journal of literature abstracts;* v. 9, no. 1, Jan. 5, 1965–v. 14, no. 13, June 28, 1966 as *MLB journal of literature abstracts.*

No indexes.

2231
Toxic episodes in children. Amsterdam, 1, 1960– .

Bimonthly. 1965 had 73 abstracts, minimum time lag 1965, 6 months. Abstracts prepared by Excerpta Medica Foundation.

Reviews

2232
Progress in chemical toxicology. New York, Academic Press, 1, 1963– .

2233
Side effects of drugs, as reported in the medical literature of the world. Amsterdam, 1955/56– . Excerpta Medica Foundation.

Classification according to pharmacologic effect of drug. 4 ed., 1963, 356 p.

Bibliographies

2233.1
Arents, George. Tobacco; its history illustrated by the books, manuscripts and engravings in the library of George Arents, Jr., together with an introductory essay, a glossary and bibliographic notes by Jerome E. Brooks. New York, Rosenbach, 1937–52. 5 v.

3386 items, arranged chronologically, from 1507 to 1942, including 1195 dated before 1801 with full bibliographical descriptions and extensive historical notes. Detailed name and subject indexes, v. 5.

Supplemented by no. 2238.1.

2234
Brous, Florence A. Bibliography and survey on lead poisoning, with particular reference to packaging. [n.p.] 1943. 350 p.

Prepared for the Technical Committee of the Packaging Institute.

2235
Gross, Martin. Acetanilid; a critical bibliographic review. New Haven, Conn., Hillhouse Press, 1946. 155 p. (Institute for the Study of Analgesic and Sedative Drugs. Monograph no. 1).

763 references, 1853–1944. Includes books, theses.

2236
——, and Greenberg, Leon A. The salicylates; a critical bibliographic review. New Haven, Conn., Hillhouse Press, 1948. 380 p. (Institute for the Study of Analgesic and Sedative Drugs. Monograph no. 2)

4093 references, 1763–1946. Includes books, theses, and abstracts.

2237
Harmon, Ralph W., and Pollard, Cash B. Bibliography of animal venoms. Gainesville, University of Florida Press, 1948. 340 p.

4157 entries 1875–1946, chronologically arranged.

2238
Larson, P. S. [et al.] Tobacco: experimental and clinical studies; a comprehensive account of the world literature. Baltimore, Williams and Wilkins, 1961. 932 p.

Compiled from more than 6000 articles published in some 1200 journals up to and largely into the year 1959. Review of the literature: p. 1–811; author bibliography: p. 812–921.

2238.1
New York Public Library. Arents Tobacco Collection. Tobacco; a catalogue of the books, manuscripts and engravings acquired since 1942, from 1507 to the present. Comp. by Sarah Augusta Dickson. New York, 1958– .

Supplements no. 2233.1. Pt. 7, issued 1962, covers 1651–1672.

2239
Pierce, Charlie M. Cobalt in biological metabolism: a literature search. 121 p. (U.S. Atomic Energy Commission. TID-3562, April 1961).

972 references from *Chemical abstracts*, Jan. 1955–July 1960. Experimental and clinical.

2240
Russell, Findlay E., and Scharffenberg, Richard S. Bibliography of snake venoms and venomous snakes. West Covina, Calif., Bibliographic Associates, Inc., 1964. 220 p.

9173 items. Earliest reference cited, 1873.

2241
Tompkins, Dorothy Campbell. Drug addiction; a bibliography. Berkeley, University of California, 1960. 130 p.

Approximately 1200 references. Includes pamphlets, reports, books, and newspaper articles relating to the legal, medical, psychological, and regulatory aspects of drug addiction, all published since about 1930.

Supersedes *Narcotics; a list of recent references*, 1959 (not listed).

2242
U.S. National Library of Medicine. Reference Services Division. Bibliography on smoking and health. Prepared for the Surgeon General's Advisory Committee on Smoking and Health by Dorothy Bocker. Washington, 1964. 59 p. (Public Health Service. Publication no. 1124. Bibliography series no. 45)

1066 references, partly annotated, to books and articles. In part supplements the bibliography of no. 2238.

2243
——. ——. Supplement 1963–64. Washington, 1965. 29 p. (Public Health Service. Publication no. 1124. Supplement 1963–1964. Bibliography series no. 45)

374 additional references, continuing the numbering of no. 2242.

Monographs

2244★
National Research Council. Committee on

the Handbook of Biological Data. Handbook of toxicology. Philadelphia, Saunders, 1956–59. 5 v.

v. 1, Acute toxicities of solids, liquids and gases to laboratory animals; v. 2, Antibiotics; v. 3, Insecticides; v. 4, Tranquilizers; v. 5, Fungicides. Data for tables in all volumes were contributed by experts in various areas of the fields represented.

History

2245

Lewin, Louis. Die Gifte in der Weltgeschichte; toxikologische, allgemeinverständliche Untersuchungen der historischen Quellen. Berlin, Springer, 1920. 596 p.

Sections on development in early times; symptoms; antidotes; legislation; poisoning through drugs; unusual methods; suicide; arsenic; famous poisoners; etc. Documented. Bibliographical footnotes.

PHYSICAL EDUCATION AND SPORTS MEDICINE

Indexes and Abstracts

2246

Completed research in health, physical education and recreation. Washington, 1, 1959– . National Education Association. American Association for Health, Physical Education and Recreation.

Annual. Pt. 1, Index; pt. 2, Bibliography; pt. 3, Theses abstracts (abstracts of unpublished Masters' and Doctors' theses).

1965 contained a 491 item bibliography and 466 abstracts of theses.

2247

Index and abstracts of foreign physical education literature. Indianapolis, 1, 1955– . Phi Epsilon Kappa Fraternity.

Includes list of sports medicine, physical education, and sports journals arranged by country.

2248

Nauchnye osnovy fizicheskogo vospitaniia i sporta; referativnyĭ sbornik dissertatsii [Scientific basis of physical education and sports; collection of abstracts of dissertations] Moskva, 1, 1958– . Izd-vo "Fizkul'tura i sport".

v. 1, 160 abstracts; v. 2, 1962, 201 abstracts. Includes medical aspects of sports. Includes only publications of Soviet authors in the Russian language.

Bibliographies

2249

Bibliographie der Sportmedizin und deren Grenzgebiete. Leipzig, 1911/26–1936/53.

Title varies. Editor: Arno Arnold.

v. for 1932/35 issued as *Sportmedizinische Veröffentlichungen*, v. 4. 1936/53 volume, 637 p.

2250

Cyriax, Edgar F. Bibliographia gymnastica medica. London, Wörishofen, 1909. 161 p.

"... an index of literature on the movement cure, in general, with special reference to Ling's medical gymnastics." Covers 1500–1908. Chronological subarrangement.

2251

Tittel, Kurt. Literaturnachweis sportmedizinischer Zeitschriften-veröffentlichungen 1957–1960. Leipzig, 1962. 115 p.

Author list.

Nomenclature

2252

American Medical Association. Committee on the Medical Aspects of Sports. Standard nomenclature of athletic injuries. Chicago, 1966. 157 p.

Alphabetical list of preferred terms giving for each: synonyms, etiology, symptoms, signs, complications, laboratory data, x-ray findings, and pathology. Includes a glossary of terms commonly used in sports medicine, a cross-index of terms, and a list of colloquialisms.

2253 (Not used)

Directories

2254

Who's who in physical culture; list of institutions, research centers, schools, persons and periodicals in sports and physical education. Warszawa, 1, 1960– . Institute for Research in Physical Culture, Warszawa.

2 ed., 1963, lists 856 institutions, with addresses, and names of directors, if available. Organizations index. Includes associations of sports medicine, physical fitness, etc.

1 ed. has title: *List of institutions, research centres, schools, persons and periodicals in the field of physical culture.*

PHYSICAL MEDICINE AND REHABILITATION

Indexes and Abstracts

2255
Brno. Universita. Knihovna. Rehabilitace; soupis článků a publikací o rehabilitaci v československé literatuře let 1945–1956 [Rehabilitation; index to articles and other publications on rehabilitation in the Czechoslovak literature of 1945–1956] Sest L. Kulíková. Brno, 1957. 60 p.

659 references.

2256
Referátový výběr z fysiatrie, balneologie, revmatologie [Selected abstracts on physiatry, balneology and rheumatology] Praha, 1, 1961– . Ústav pro zdravotnickou dokumentaci.

4 issues a year.

2257★
Rehabilitation literature. Chicago, etc., 1, 1940– . National Society for Crippled Children and Adults, Inc.

Monthly. 841 abstracts of the English-language literature in 1964. Includes monographs and reports. Covers those disabled from all causes, including mental.

v. 1–6, 1940–45, as *Bulletin on current literature of interest to crippled children workers;* v. 7–16, 1946–55, *Bulletin on current literature.*

v. 1–6 issued by National Society for Crippled Children of the United States.

2258 (Not used)

Bibliographies

2259
Akademiia nauk SSSR. Sektor seti spetsial'nykh bibliotek. Ul'trazvuk v biologii; bibliografiia otechestvennoĭ i inostrannoĭ literatury za 1950–1962 gg. [Ultrasound in biology; a bibliography of the national and foreign literature, 1950–1962] Moskva, Izd-vo "Nauka", 1964. 182 p.

2503 references. Entries for Chinese and Japanese publications are in the language of their resumés; publications in little-known languages are listed in Russian. Non-Soviet items predominate.

2260★
Graham, Earl C., and Mullen, Marjorie M. Rehabilitation literature, 1950–1955. A bibliographic review of the medical care, education, employment, welfare, and psychology of handicapped children and adults. New York, McGraw-Hill, 1956. 621 p.

Annotates 5214 periodical articles, pamphlets, and books from the English-language literature.

2261
Jankowiak, Józef, and Czabajska, Gabryela. A bibliography of Polish balneology, physical-therapy and climatology from 1945 to 1960. Warsaw, State Medical Publishers, 1962. 58 p.

2261.1
Jordan, H. Zwölf Jahre balneologische und balneobioklimatologische Forschung der DDR im Referat, 1950–1961. Bad Elster, 1965. 146 p.

414 abstracts from German journals (some nonmedical). Random author arrangement.

Dictionaries

2262★
Kamenetz, Herman L. Physiatric dictionary; glossary of physical medicine and rehabilitation. Springfield, Ill., Thomas, 1965. 173 p.

Includes many terms not found in large medical dictionaries; contains abbreviations.

Directories

2263★
Registry of medical rehabilitation therapists and specialists. [St. Louis?] 1, 1954– .

Annual. Address and brief professional information given. 9 ed., 1963 (54 p.).

Sponsored by the American Association for Rehabilitation Therapy. Published by the

Council of the Registry of Medical Rehabilitation Therapists and Specialists.

2264
World directory of physical medicine specialists. Ed. by Sidney Licht. New Haven, Conn., Elizabeth Licht, 1960. 241 p.

Alphabetical listing by country. Gives name and address, and in some cases professional information and photograph.

Histories

2265
Brauchle, Alfred. Naturheilkunde in Lebensbildern. Leipzig, Reclam, 1937. 490 p.

Covers hydrotherapy, massage, diet, healing by suggestion, mainly 19th-20th centuries. Bibliography: p. 476-482. Later versions (*Grosse Naturärzte*, 1944; *Die Geschichte der Naturheilkunde in Lebensbildern*, 1951) are abridged, lack bibliography and index.

2266
Colwell, Hector A. An essay on the history of electrotherapy and diagnosis. London, Heinemann, 1922. 180 p.

From ca. 1700 to the early 20th century. Bibliographical references in text and footnotes.

2267
Coulter, John S. Physical therapy. New York, Hoeber, 1932. 142 p. (Clio medica, no. 7 [i. e. 8])

General survey through the Middle Ages, followed by special chapters on massage and exercise, water, electricity, and radiant energy. Includes brief data on important authors and works. Bibliography (68 references): p. 125-128.

2268
Grasset, Hector. La médecine naturiste à travers les siècles. Histoire de la physiothérapie. Paris, Rousset, 1911. 468 p.

General survey through the 19th century. Many bibliographical citations in text. No index.

PHYSIOLOGY

Indexes and Abstracts

Current

2269
Berichte über die gesamte Physiologie und experimentelle Pharmakologie. (Berichte über die gesamte Biologie. Abt. B) Berlin, 1, 1920- .

Unter Mitwirkung der Deutschen physiologischen Gesellschaft, etc.

Currently 12 volumes or more a year. Each volume in 3 issues and a separate index issue. A recent volume had in excess of 1000 references to books and articles, most with abstracts.

v. 1-2, 1920, as *Berichte über die gesamte Physiologie*. v. 1-15, 1920-23, had subtitle: Zugleich Fortsetzung des Hermann-Weissschen Jahresberichts über die Fortschritte der Physiologie [no. 2271] und des Maly-Andreasch-Spiroschen Jahresberichts über die Fortschritte der Tierchemie oder der physiologischen und pathologischen Chemie [1008] v. 1-34, 1920-26, had subtitle: Neue Folge des Zentralblattes für Biochemie und Biophysik [1011]

Berichte über die gesamte Biologie. Abt. B., v. 35, 1926- .

Continues no. 1008, 1011 and 2271.

For annual cumulation of references see no. 2270.

Noncurrent

2269.1
Bibliographia physiologica. Zurich, etc. 1893/94-1926. Concilium Bibliographicum, Zurich.

Includes books, reports.

1893/94-96 issued without v. number; 1897-98 issued as n.s. v. 1-2; 1905-13 as ser. 3, v. 1-9; 1922-26 as ser. 4.

1905-13 had subtitles: Diario Zentralblatt für Physiologie adnexa; Beiblatt zum Zentralblatt für Physiologie. 1898-1904 said to be in card form. Suspended 1915-22.

See also no. 2272

2270
Jahresbericht Physiologie und experimentelle Pharmakologie. Berlin, 1-18, 1920-37.

Annual cumulation of references of no. 2269.

v. 1, 3, 5, 7, 9, in two parts: pt. 1, Ubersichtsreferate; pt. 2, Bibliographie. The other volumes and from v. 10, 1929, bibliography only.

v. 1-7, 1920-26, as *Jahresbericht über die gesamte Physiologie und experimentelle Pharmakologie, mit vollstandiger Bibliographie*. v. 1-7 has subtitle: Zugleich Fortsetzung des Hermann-Weissschen Jahresberichts über die Fortschritte der animalischen Physiologie und des Maly-Spiro-Andreaschschen Jahresbericht über die Fortschritte der Tierchemie oder der physiologischen, pathologischen und Immuno-chemie und der Pharmakologie. v. 8–18, 1927–37, has subtitle: Bibliographisches Jahresregister der Berichte über die gesamte Physiologie und experimentelle Pharmakologie. Continues nos. 1008, 2271.

2271
Jahresbericht über die Fortschritte der animalischen Physiologie. Stuttgart, 1–22, 1892–1919.

Annual. References listed under subjects by author and then selectively abstracted in order of listing. The 1911 volume lists in excess of 3200 references. Includes some books and theses.

v. 1–20, 1892–1911, as *Jahresbericht über die Fortschritte der Physiologie; Neue Folge des physiologischen Theiles der Jahresberichte von Henle und Meissner, Hofman und Schwalbe, Hermann und Schwalbe.*

Author indexes. General-Register to v. 1–10, 11–20 published separately.

Continued by no. 2269. Continues nos. 859 (Henle & Meissner) and 860 (Hofmann & Schwalbe, Hermann & Schwalbe).

2272
Physiological abstracts. London, 1–22, 1916–37. Physiological Society (Great Britain and Ireland).

v. 22, 1937, contains 4930 entries, most with abstracts. Includes books.

Through v. 9, 1924/25, issued in cooperation with the American Physiological Society, etc. Supplementary and index number to v. 22 dated 1938.

See no. 1007.

2273
Zentralblatt für Physiologie. Leipzig, etc., 1–34, 1887–1921. Organ der Deutschen physiologischen Gesellschaft (from v. 19 (9), 1905)

Abstracts of articles and selected books, theses, and proceedings of societies. Includes original articles.

v. 19–27, 1905–13, have subtitle (varies): mit der *Bibliografia physiologica* als Beiblatt.

See also no. 2269.1

Reviews

2274★
Advances in comparative physiology and biochemistry, New York, 1, 1962– .

v. 2, 1966.

2275
Advances in insect physiology. London, 1, 1963– .

2276★★
Annual review of physiology. Palo Alto, Calif., etc., Annual Reviews, Inc., 1, 1939– .

2277
Ergebnisse der Physiologie, biologischen Chemie und experimentellen Pharmakologie. Berlin, 1, 1902– .

Biennial. Text in German, English, and French.

2278★★
Physiological reviews. Baltimore, 1, 1921– . American Physiological Society.

Quarterly. Review articles with bibliographies. Occasional supplements.

2279
Recent advances in physiology. 8 ed. Ed. by Richard Creese. London, Churchill, 1963. 471 p.

Chapter bibliographies (omitting titles of articles). No over-all author index.

[1 ed] 1925. Editor varies.

Bibliographies

2280
Hill, A.V. Trails and trials in physiology; a bibliography, 1909–1964. Baltimore, Williams and Wilkins, 1965. 374 p.

Pt. 1, 1963 annotated references. Pt. 2, reviews, methods, and further research. Mainly limited to heat production of muscle and nerve.

Dictionaries

2281
Nippon Seiri Gakkai. Ei doku wa taisho seirgaku yogoshu [Technical terms in physiology; English-Japanese, German-Japanese] Tokyo, Nansando, 1960. 239 p.

In two sections: parallel columns of English, Japanese, English.

Histories

2282
Bastholm, Eyvind. The history of muscle

physiology from the natural philosphers to Albrecht von Haller. København, Munksgaard, 1950. 256 p. (Acta historica scientiarum naturalium et medicinalium, v. 7)

With analyses of contributions. Bibliography (154 references): p. 248–253.

2283
Foster, Sir Michael. Lectures on the history of physiology during the sixteenth, seventeenth and eighteenth centuries. Cambridge, University Press, 1901. 310 p.

Development of important themes, with biographical data on the chief contributors and accounts of their work. No bibliography. Reprinted 1924.

2284
Fulton, John F. Physiology. New York, Hoeber, 1931. 141 p. (Clio medica, no. 5)

Bibliography: p. 116–119.

2285
——, ed. Selected readings in the history of physiology. Completed by Leonard G. Wilson. 2 ed. Springfield, Ill., Thomas, 1966. 492 p.

Excerpts from original writings from Aristotle to the 20th century; with historical and biographical introductions and bibliographical references.

2286
Mendelsohn, Everett. Heat and life. The development of the theory of animal heat. Cambridge, Harvard University Press, 1964. 208 p.

Bibliographical footnotes. Selected bibliography (primary sources): p. 185–200.

2287
Rothschuh, Karl E. Entwicklungsgeschichte physiologischer Probleme in Tabellenform. München, Urban und Schwarzenberg, 1952. 122 p.

Chronological surveys in 18 classifications, presenting brief summaries of 2170 discoveries and developments ca. 1600–1920, with dates, names of the scientists, and data concerning original publication. Intended to be used with no. 2288.

2288
——. Geschichte der Physiologie. Berlin, Springer, 1953. 249 p. (Lehrbuch der Physiologie in zusammenhängenden Einzeldarstellungen)

From ancient times through the 19th century. Emphasis for later periods on leading personalities and their schools, with fuller treatment of continental than British or American developments. Selected references (432 items): p. 225–235.

PSYCHOLOGY

Indexes and Abstracts

Current

No. 2292 is one of the outstanding specialized subject indexes. It is regarded as the tool of first choice in searches relating to the psychological literature in all its phases.

2289
Année psychologique. Paris, 1, 1894– .

Currently 2 fascicules a year; each in two sections: 1. Mémoires originaux; 2. Analyses bibliographiques. A recent fascicule listed in excess of 300 references, most with abstracts. Includes books, proceedings of congresses.

2290
Bibliographie der psychologischen Literatur der sozialistischen Länder. Berlin, 1, 1958– . Deutsches Pädagogisches Zentral-institut.

Annual. Country breakdown. Indexes material not in *Psychological abstracts* or medical indexes. Includes monographs, translations.

2291
Documentation sur la psychologie française. Paris, 1, 1957– . Groupe d'études de psychologie de l'Université de Paris.

Each fascicule has varying coverage. Through no. 6, 1963, includes books published from 1746 through about 1960 and articles published from 1843–1960.

[Fasc. 1] as *Dix années de psychologie française.* All fascicules by Dimitri Voutsinas.

2292★
Psychological abstracts. Lancaster, Pa., 1, 1927– . American Psychological Association.

Monthly. 1966 listed 13,622 references, most with abstracts. Indexes a number of journals not normally covered by medical indexes, mainly in the fields of education and business. Includes books, government research reports, obituaries. Indexes but does not abstract *Dissertation abstracts*. Minimum time lag (1966) 2 months.

Monthly through 1953, bimonthly 1954–65.

2293

——. Author index to Psychological index, 1894 to 1935, and Psychological abstracts, 1927 to 1958. Compiled by the Psychology Library, Columbia University. Boston, Hall, 1960. 5 v.

2293.1

—— ——. Suppl. 1, 1959–1963. Boston, Hall, 1965. 863 p.

2293.2

——. Cumulated subject index to Psychological abstracts, 1927–1960. Cumulated by G. K. Hall Co. Boston, Hall, 1966. 2 v.

2294

Psychological bulletin. Lancaster, Pa., 1, 1904– .

Review articles. Includes proceedings of societies and book reviews.

Through v. 35, 1938, had subtitle: Containing the literature section of the *Psychological review* publications (some years have . . . *Psychological review* or . . . psychological publication)

Noncurrent

2295

Psychological book previews. Princeton, 1–2(3), Jan. 1951–July 1952.

Quarterly. Includes brief biographies of the authors.

2296

Psychological index. Princeton, etc., 1–42, 1894–1935.

1935 listed 5927 numbered references. Includes books. From 1911 through 1915 the titles included are for the most part identical with those of no. 2297 for the same period.

Subtitle: no. 1–15, 1894–1908, A bibliography of the literature of psychology and cognate subjects; no. 16–42, 1909–35, An annual bibliography . . .

No. 1–15, 1894–1908, The *Psychological review*, index for [the year] at head of title.

No. 8–15, 1901–08, issued as Bibliographical supplement no. 1–[8] to the *Dictionary of philosophy and psychology*, ed. by J. Mark Baldwin.

Published by the Review Publishing Co., Lancaster, Pa., 1905–10; Psychological Review Co., Lancaster, 1911–20, Princeton, 1921–24; Psychological Review Co. for the American Psychological Association, 1925–35.

2296.1

Tierpsychologische Sammelberichte [1]–5, [1931–37] In Archiv für die Gesamte Psychologie, 89–99, 1933–37.

The fifth report contained 340 annotated references. Includes books. Indexes a number of nonpsychological and nonmedical sources. Author index to fifth report only. Reports no. 1–2 are parts of the general "Literaturberichte".

2297

Verzeichnis des deutschen psychologischen Schriftums 1889–1941. In Zeitschrift für Psychologie und Physiologie der Sinnesorgane. Abt. 1. Zeitschrift für Psychologie. 1–155, 1890–1943.

A total of 93,586 references, 769 to 4547 a year. Indexes some nonpsychological and nonmedical periodicals.

1889–1907, as *Bibliographie der psychophysiologischen Literatur;* 1908–15, as *Bibliographie der deutschen und ausländischen Literatur . . . über Psychologie, ihre Hilfswissenschaften und Grenzgebiete;* 1924–25, as *Bibliographie . . . I. Deutsche Literatur des Jahres . . . über Psychologie, ihre Hilfswissenschaften und Grenzgebiete;* 1926–33, as *Bibliographie der deutschen und ausländischen Literatur des Jahres . . . über Psychologie, ihre Hilfswissenschaften und Grenzgebiete . . . Deutscher Teil.* Footnote indicates that the 1926–32 "ausländischen" part appears in *Archiv für gesamte Psychologie.* However, this part appears in *Archiv* . . . v. 62–79, 1928–31, for only 1926–29 under approximately the same title.

With 1906 the *Zeitschrift* published as Abt. 1 & 2, the bibliography in Abt. 1. Abt. 2. *Zeitschrift für sinnesongane.*

Continued by no. 2314.1.

Not published 1916–23.

Reviews

2298

Advances in experimental social psychology. New York, Academic Press, 1, 1964– .

2299
Advances in the study of behavior. New York, Academic Press, 1, 1965– .

Animal and human behavior.

2300
Annual review of psychology. Palo Alto, Calif., Annual Reviews, Inc., 1, 1950– .

2301
Contemporary psychology; a journal of reviews. Washington, 1, 1956– . American Psychological Association.

Monthly. Book reviews.

2302
Fitzpatrick, William H., and DeLong, Chester W. Soviet medical research related to human stress; a review of the literature. Washington, National Library of Medicine, Scientific Translation Program, 1961. 121 p.

2303
Progress in clinical psychology. New York, Grune & Stratton, 1, 1952– .

Irregular. v. 1 covers 1946–52.

Bibliographies

2304
Applezweig, Mortimer H., comp. Psychological stress and related concepts: A bibliography. 185 p. (Connecticut College, New London, Conn. Department of Psychology. Motivation research project. Technical report no. 7. Office of Naval Research. Project NR 172-228. Contract Nonr 996(02) December 1957).

2611 references listed by author.

Subject-author index issued Jan. 1958.

2305
Bevan, William, and Patton, Rollin M. Selected bibliography: fatigue, stress, bodily change and behavior. 64 p. (WADC technical report 57-125, April 1957)

883 references listed by author. Covers English language literature 1946–56. Includes books, theses, research reports.

2306
Buros, Oscar K., ed. The sixth mental measurements yearbook. Highland Park, N.J., Gryphon Press, 1965. 1714 p.

A classified subject and name index. Attempts to list all commercially available tests—educational, psychological, and vocational—published as separates in English-speaking countries, 1952–58. Contains listings for 1219 tests, 795 critical test reviews, 97 excerpts from reviews of tests and 8001 references for specific tests. Supplements (does not supersede) earlier volumes.

First and second MMY as *The nineteen thirty-eight* and *The nineteen forty mental measurements yearbook.*

Preceded by *Educational, psychological, and personality tests of 1933 and 1934* (44 p.), *1933, 1934 and 1935* (83 p.), and *1936* (141 p.).

See also no. 2307.

2307
——. Tests in print; a comprehensive bibliography of tests for use in education, psychology, and industry. Highland Park, N.J., Gryphon Press, 1961. 479 p.

A publishers, distributors, title, and name index. Serves as a classified index and supplement to no. 2306, First-Fifth.

2308
Daniel, Robert S., and Louttit, Chauncey M. Professional problems in psychology. New York, Prentice-Hall, 1953. 416 p.

Surveys the psychological literature including bibliography. Contains annotated list of reference books (306 items) and list of journals (331 items). Has chapter on psychological organizations.

2309
Emanuilova, E. Katerina. Suvremenna materialisticheska psikhologiia; bibliografski ukazatel, 1948–1956 [Contemporary materialistic psychology; bibliographic index, 1948–1956] Sofiia, Bulgarskata akademiia na naukite, 1959. 231 p.

1603 books and periodical articles by Bulgarian or Russian authors.

2310
Harvard University. The Harvard list of books in psychology. 3 ed. Cambridge, Harvard University Press, 1964. 111 p.

Lists 704 books (304 new; 283 retained from the previous list; and 117 updated as to edition or annotation).

An early version was compiled in 1938 with a supplement in 1944. 1 ed. under the present title, 1949; 2 ed., 1955, with a supplement in 1958.

2311
National Research Council. Research Information Service. Bibliography of bibliographies on psychology, 1900–1927. Comp. by C. M. Louttit. Washington, 1928. 108 p. (Its Bulletin no. 65)

Author listing of 2134 bibliographies and articles and books with references. Some "bibliographies" listed have as few as 2 references. Includes some material dated as early as 1850.

2312
Rand, Benjamin. Bibliography of philosophy, psychology, and cognate subjects. New York, Macmillan, 1905. 2 v. (Baldwin, James M. Dictionary of philosophy and psychology. New York, Macmillan, 1905. v. 3, pts. 1–2)

2313
Stone, Alan A., and Onqué, Gloria C. Longitudinal studies of child personality. Cambridge, Harvard University Press, 1959. 314 p.

Author list of 297 abstracts primarily from the English-language literature, 1923–55. Includes books.

2314
Vernon, David T. A. [et al.] The psychological responses of children to hospitalization and illness; a review of the literature. Springfield, Thomas, 1965. 192 p.

Short term hospitalization. Bibliography p. 167–180.

2314.1
Wellek, Albert, ed. Gesamtverzeichnis der deutschsprachigen psychologischen Literatur der Jahre 1942 bis 1960. Göttingen, Verlag für Psychologie, 1965. 876 p.

15,595 entries arranged by year. Combined author, no subject index. Continues no. 2297.

2314.2
Young, Morris N. Bibliography of memory. Philadelphia, Chilton, 1961. 436 p.

Includes books, theses (some unpublished). Intended as a "definitive" bibliography, including a wide range of closely related material. Covers from the beginning of printing and before (i.e., some manuscripts). Includes memory training, tricks, belles lettres (poems, Proust, inter alia) No subject index.

Dictionaries

2314.3
Černocký, Karel. Psychologický slovník. 2 ed. Hranice, J. Těšík, 1947–8. 2 v. in 1. 526 p.

Czech term followed by equivalent in German, French and English. Terms defined in Czech. Includes bibliographies and biographies.

2315
Dietz, P. A. [et al.] Parapsychologische woordentolk. Den Haag, Leopold, 1956. 99 p.

Contains a list of common terms or phrases in English and French with Dutch equivalents.

2316
Dorsch, Friedrich, ed. Psychologisches Wörterbuch. 7 ed. Hamburg, Meiner, 1963. 552 p.

Inclusive; gives some long definitions and in most cases derivation of word.

1 ed. 1920 by Fritz Giese.

2317
English, Horace B. A comprehensive dictionary of psychological and psychoanalytical terms, a guide to usage. New York, McKay, 1965. 594 p.

2318
Harriman, Philip L. Handbook of psychological terms. Totowa, N.J., Littlefield, Adams, 1965. 222 p.

Primarily for undergraduates.

2319
Hehlmann, Wilhelm. Wörterbuch der Psychologie. 2 ed. Stuttgart, Kröner, 1962. 640 p.

Definitions vary from short to extensive; includes biographical sketches, word derivations, and abbreviations.

2320
Pieron, Henri. Vocabulaire de la psychologie. 3 ed. Paris, Presses Universitaires de France, 1963. 524 p.

Definitions include an occasional English synonym. Contains index of names cited; appendix: lists of French and English abbreviations, symbols used in tests, Greek roots.

2321
Pieter, Józef. Slownik psychologiczny.

Wrocław, Zakład narodowy im. Ossolińskich, 1963. 348 p.

Includes biographies.

2322
Pleasants, Helene. Biographical dictionary of parapsychology, with directory and glossary, 1964–1966. New York, Garrett, 1964. 371 p.

Not limited in time. Includes, for example, Mesmer.

2323
Sandström, Carl I. Psykologisk ordbok; jämte en personförteckning. 6 ed. Stockholm, Almqvist, 1963. 150 p.

List of names includes birth and death dates, when known.

2324
Sury, Kurt von. Wörterbuch der Psychologie. 2 ed. Basel, Schwabe, 1958. 467 p.

2325
Warren, Howard C., ed. Dictionary of psychology. Boston, Houghton, 1934. 371 p.

Includes numerous tables for rapid reference, e.g., on phobias, reflexes, and terms relating to human body and central nervous system, arranged topographically. French and German glossary.

Directories

2326
American Psychological Association. Directory. Washington, 1916– .

Alphabetical and geographical listing. Diplomates and divisional membership lists.

2327
International directory of psychologists, exclusive of the U.S.A. Assen, [1] 1958– . National Academy of Sciences, National Research Council.

Brief biographical and professional data; geographical arrangement.

2328 (not used)

Histories

2329
Boring, Edwin G. A history of experimental psychology. 2 ed. New York, Appleton-Century-Crofts, 1950. 777 p.

Covers from late 17th century. Bibliographical references to each chapter. Reprinted 1957.

2330
Brett, George S. A history of psychology. London, Allen, 1912–21. 3 v.

The classic history, especially for philosophical psychology. Bibliographic references at end of each volume. Author indexes only.

Abridged edition by Richard S. Peters, London, Allen & Unwin, 1953; rev. 1962 (778 p., with chapter on 20th century theories and a bibliography for students, p. 769–772); reprinted Cambridge, Mass., M. I. T. Press, 1965.

2330.1
Dennis, Wayne, ed. Readings in the history of psychology. New York, Appleton-Century-Crofts, 1948. 587 p.

61 selections, in English, from Aristotle to C. L. Hull (1930), mostly 19th and 20th century.

2331
Flugel, John C. A hundred years of psychology, 1833–1933. [3 ed.] Part V: 1933–1963, rev. by Donald J. West. London, Duckworth, 1964. 394 p.

Briefly reviews principal ideas of leading psychologists. Bibliography: p. 359–374. First published 1933.

2332
Herrnstein, Richard J., and Boring, Edwin G., ed. A source book in the history of psychology. Cambridge, Harvard University Press, 1965. 636 p.

116 selection in 15 chapter, mostly before 1900.

2333
Kantor, Jacob R. The scientific evolution of psychology. Chicago, Principia Press, 1963– .

v. 1 covers Hellenic, Roman, Arabic, and scholastic psychology. Bibliography: v. 1, p. 370–378.

2334
Murphy, Gardner. Historical introduction to modern psychology. Rev. ed. New York, Harcourt, Brace, 1949. 466 p.

Detailed history; includes bibliographies.

2335
Rand, Benjamin, ed. The classical psycho-

logists; selections illustrating psychology from Anaxagoras to Wundt. Boston, Houghton Mifflin, 1912. 734 p.

Selections from 43 psychologists, with emphasis on psychological doctrines prior to the experimental movement.

2336
Roback, Abraham A. History of American psychology. New York, Library Publishers, 1952. 426 p.

Especially good for American psychology before 1870.

2337
Schüling, Herman. Bibliographisches Handbuch zur Geschichte der Psychologie: das 17. Jahrhundert. Giessen, Universitätsbibliothek, 1964. xiv, 292 p.

Author catalog of some 2800 17th century publications, including dissertations and analytic entries. Occasional data identifying the authors and annotations concerning contents. References for each citation, and location of copies if known. Abbreviations for bibliographies used: p. viii–xi. Selective classified bibliography on 17th century psychology: p. 282–292. Subject index, and index of authors commented upon or criticized.

2338
Shipley, Thorne, ed. Classics in psychology. New York, Philosophical Library, 1961. 1342 p.

Lengthy selections in English from 37 19th–20th century psychologists and psychiatrists. Biographical data and references for each author. General references: p. 17–18. Name index only.

2339
Watson, Robert I. The great psychologists: from Aristotle to Freud. Philadelphia, Lippincott, 1963. 572 p.

Surveys of successive periods and schools with critical and biographical studies of important psychologists. References: p. 497–558.

2340
Whyte, Lancelot L. The unconscious before Freud. New York, Basic Books, 1960. 219 p.

Traces the concept of unconscious mental processes in European thought from Descartes to Freud, with some account of earlier developments. References at ends of chapters; general bibliography: p. 205–207. Reprinted Anchor Books, Doubleday, 1962.

PUBLIC HEALTH

Indexes and Abstracts

Current

2341
American Medical Association. Archive-Library Department. Index to medical socio-economic literature. Chicago, 1, 1962– .

Annual cumulation of entries in the Department's weekly bulletins. Includes books, theses, pamphlets, and newspaper items, in the English language.

2342★
Bulletin of hygiene. London, 1, 1926– . Bureau of Hygiene and Tropical Diseases.

Monthly. About 4000 abstracts and references a year. Conventional journal coverage; includes monographs. Covers public health, sanitation, occupational hygiene, food and nutrition, mycoses and mycology, communicable diseases (except tropical diseases), bacteriology and immunity. Minimum time lag 3 months.

Published as a complement to the *Tropical diseases bulletin.*

2343
Medical care review. Ann Arbor, 1, 1944– . University of Michigan, School of Public Health, Bureau of Public Health Economics.

Includes articles, or excerpts of articles, from the public press, press releases of institutions. Has section, Other countries.

v. 1–23, 1944–66 as *Public health economics and medical care abstracts.*

2344
Public health engineering abstracts. Washington, 1, 1921– . U.S. Public Health Service.

Monthly. 1964 contained 2228 abstracts. Abstracts selectively a number of titles not normally covered by medical indexes, especially in the fields of atmospheric pollution, sewage, industrial wastes, water supplies. Time lag not less than 4 months.

2345 (Not used.)

2346
Research in public health administration; selected recent abstracts. Baltimore, Johns Hopkins University, 1, 1962– .

Annual. 100–125 abstracts a year.

Noncurrent

2346.1
Bibliographischer Jahresbericht über soziale Hygiene, Demographie und Medizinalstatistik, sowie alle Zweige des sozialen Versicherungswesens. Berlin, etc., 1–[20] 1900/01–1921.

1900–13, Chronicle of events, tables of legislation, abstracts and bibliography; 1914–21 bibliography only.

v. 1–4, 1900/01–4 as *Jahresbericht über die Fortschritte und Leistungen auf dem Gebiete der sozialen Hygiene und Demographie*; v. 5–13, 1905–13 as *Jahresbericht über soziale Hygiene Demographie und Medizinalstatistik, sowie alle Zweige des sozialen Versicherungswesens*. From 1914, under the title above, became part of *Veröffentlichungen aus dem Gebiete der Medizinalverwaltung* (Heft 64, 76, 91, 110, 130, 156, 172).

2347
Hygienische Rundschau. Berlin, 1–32, 1891–1922.

1000–2000 abstracts per volume. Includes books, theses, and annual reports. An occasional Beilage contains reports of proceedings of societies. On occasion, original articles. Continued as no. 2349.

2348
Jahresbericht über die Fortschritte und Leistungen auf dem Gebiete der Hygiene. Braunschweig, 1–31, 1883–1913.

Some 2000 abstracts and discussions per volume. Includes books and reports, summaries of vital statistics by countries, lists of new legislation, new journals, and summaries of proceeding of congresses.

Subtitle: Supplement zur Deutschen Vierteljahreschrift für öffentliche Gesundheitspflege.

2349
Zentralblatt für die gesamte Hygiene, mit Einschluss der Bakteriologie und Immunitätslehre. Berlin, 1–52, 1922–44.

2–3 volumes a year. 2000–2800 abstracts and reviews per volume. Includes books, annual reports, and selected theses. Occasional literature reviews and reports of proceedings of societies.

v. 1–19, 1922–29, as *Zentralblatt für die gesamte Hygiene und ihre Grenzegebiete* (*Fortsetzung der Hygienischen Rundschau*); v. 1–35, 1922–36, published as *Organ der Berliner Gesellschaft fur öffentliche Gesundheitspflege*.

Continues no 2347.

Reviews

2349.1
Year book of public health. Chicago, Year Book Publishers, 1940–41. (The practical medicine year books)

Bibliographies

2350
Freidlin, S. Ia. Bibliografiia sovetskogo zdravookhraneniia za 10 let (1938–1947) [Bibliographies of Soviet public health for 10 years (1938–1947)] Leningrad, Medgiz, 1949. 138 p.

2351
Hanecki, Michał [et al.] Służba zdrowia w Polsce; przegląd ważniejszych prac o organizacji i pokrewnych działach służby zdrowia XIX i XX w. [Health services in Poland; a survey of important works on the organization and related fields of health services in the 19th and 20th centuries] Warszawa, Państwowy Zakład Wydawnictw Lekarskich, 1956. 354 p.

5800 entries, some with brief annotations. Includes books.

2351.1
Industrial Hygiene Foundation of America. An annotated bibliography on noise, its measurement, effects and control. Pittsburgh, 1955. 364 p.

2336 entries, partly annotated. References mainly since the 1920's. Chronological arrangement under subdivisions of: Measurement of sound and noise, Effects of noise, Measurement of hearing loss, Reduction and control of noise.

2352
Merkov, A. M., comp. Sanitarnaia statistika; bibliografiia sovetskoĭ literatury, 1918–1960 gg. [Health statistics; bibliography of Soviet literature, 1918–1960] Moskva, Medgiz, 1963. 359 p.

6522 entries. Includes books, contributions to collected works, congress papers, etc., by Soviet authors in the Russian language.

2353
Minsk. Respublikanskaia gosudarstvennaia nauchnaia meditsinskaia biblioteka. Zdravookhraneniie Belorusskoĭ SSR za sorok let (1919–1958); ukazatel' literatury [Public health in the Belorussian SSR during the forty years (1919–1958); index to literature] Minsk, 1961. 501 p.

Includes monographs, pamphlets, newspaper articles, reviews, collections of scientific works, proceedings of congresses. Annotated. In Russian or Byelorussian.

2354
Pederson, E. B., and Moodie, P. M. The health of Australian aborigines; an annotated bibliography with classification by subject matter and locality. Sydney, Australia, School of Public Health and Tropical Medicine, University of Sydney, 1966. 156 p.

Approximately 1300 references covering 1833 to 1965. Arranged alphabetically with subject and geographic indexes. Includes books, chapters of books, nongovernment and government reports. Covers some nonmedical sources.

2355
Tashkent. Gosudarstvennaia nauchno-meditsinskaia biblioteka. Zdravookhranenie Sovetskogo Uzbekistana; bibliograficheskiĭ ukazatel' literatury (1917–1959) [Public health in Soviet Uzbekistan; bibliographic index to literature (1917–1959] Sost. K. C. Shishova. Tashkent, Medgiz, 1961. 215 p.

2602 entries, books and articles. Geographic index.

2356
U.S. Congress. House. Committee on Ways and Means. Selected list of publications of the committees of the Congress relating to health, medical care, medical facilities, and rehabilitation. Washington, 1961. 71 p.

Covers 1951–60. Arranged by Committee.

Dictionaries

2356.1
China (People's Republic) Wei Shêng pu [Ministry of Health] Kung kung wie shêng hsüch ming tz'ŭ [Glossary of public health terms] Peking, 1956. 95 p.

Russian-Chinese-English, English-Chinese.

2357
Dictionary of water and sewage engineering. Comp. by Fritz Meinck and Helmut Mohle. Amsterdam, Elsevier, 1963. 449 p.

Between 7000 and 8000 terms arranged alphabetically by the German word followed by the English, French, and Italian term. Pt. 2 contains separate indexes in English, French, and Italian with reference to the numbered terms in German.

Directories

2358★
American Public Health Association. Membership directory. New York, etc.. [1] 1946– .

Alphabetical listing gives address, position, section affiliation; geographical listing, names only. 2 ed., 1952; 3 ed., 1962.

2359
Paterson, Robert G. Historical directory of state health departments in the United States of America. Columbus, Ohio Public Health Association, 1939. 68 p.

Arranged by state. Includes chief executives, official names of the departments, and publications issued.

2360
U.S. Public Health Service. Division of General Health Services. Historical roster of state and territorial health officers, 1850–1960. Washington, 1960. 31 p.

Arranged by state. Includes chief executives, official names of the departments, and a brief note on their historical development.

2361
World Health Organization. Regional Office for Europe. Directory of public health laboratories in Europe. Copenhagen, [1] 1962– .

Arranged by country. Gives name of organization, director, address, and activities.

Histories

2362
Charles, Sir John. Research and public

health. London, Oxford University Press, 1961. 114 p. (University of London, Heath Clark lectures, 1959)

Survey from ancient Greece through the 20th century, with consideration of key authors and works. References at end of each chapter.

2363
Rosen, George. A history of public health. New York, MD Publications, 1958. 551 p.

Comprehensive history. Bibliography with each chapter.

2364
Sand, René. The advance to social medicine. London, Staples Press, 1952. 655 p.

General study, including medical profession, hospitals, personal and social hygiene, social anthropology, public health and welfare, industrial and social medicine. Analysis of sources, with extensive footnote references. Classified bibliography: p. 591–599. Translation of *Vers la médecine sociale*, Paris, 1948.

2365
Winslow, Charles-Edward A. The evolution and significance of the modern public health campaign. New Haven, Yale University Press, 1923. 65 p.

Interpretive study.

Austria

2366
Lesky, Erna. Österreichisches Gesundheitswesen im Zeitalter des aufgeklärten Absolutismus. Wien, Rohrer, 1959. 228 p. (Öesterreichische Akademie der Wissenschaften. Philosophisch-historische Klasse. Historische Kommission. Archiv für österreichische Geschichte, v. 122)

Covers Austrian Empire, 1740–90. Based on sources, with references in footnotes.

Germany

2367
Fischer, Alfons. Geschichte des deutschen Gesundheitswesens. Berlin, Herbig, 1933. 2 v.

Comprehensive history through the 19th century. Bibliographical footnotes.

Great Britain

2368
Brand, Jeanne L. Doctors and the state; the British medical profession and government action in public health, 1870–1912. Baltimore, Johns Hopkins Press, 1965. 307 p.

Thorough study. Selective, classified bibliography of sources and secondary works: p. 275–295.

2369
Brockington, Colin Fraser. A short history of public health. 2 ed. London, Churchill, 1966. 240 p.

Mainly on Great Britain since 1800. Bibliography: p. 211–213. 1 ed. 1956.

2370
Frazer, William M. A history of English public health, 1834–1939. London, Baillière, Tindall & Cox, 1950. 498 p.

Competent survey. Bibliographical references in footnotes.

2371
Ross, James S. The national health service in Great Britain; an historical and descriptive study. London, Oxford University Press, 1952. 398 p.

About one third on background before 1948. Based on sources, but lacks bibliography.

Mexico

2372
Alvarez Amezquita, José [et al.] Historia de la salubridad y de la asistencia en México. México, Secretaría de Salubridad y Asistencia, 1960. 4 v.

Comprehensive chronological history including extensive documentary material from pre-Columbian times to 1960, with much information on general medical history. Bibliographies of Mexican physicians and naturalists, 16th century to 1833: v. 3, p. 218–366. v. 4 presents history by locality, and vital statistics. 1922–58. No general index.

New Zealand

2373
MacLean, Francis S. Challenge for health; a history of public health in New Zealand. Wellington, Owen, 1964. 470 p.

References (by chapter): p. 452–458.

Sweden

2374
Kock, Wolfram, ed. Medicinalväsendet i

Sverige, 1813–1962, utgiven med anledning av Kungl. Medicinalstyrelsens 300-års jubileum. Stockholm, Nordiska Bokhandeln, 1963. 764 p.

Covers central medical administration (including Collegium Medicum, 1663–1812), hospitals, mental health, diseases, maternal and child welfare, etc. Summaries in English: p. 695–736.

U.S.S.R.

2375

Barsukov, Mikhail Ivanovich, ed. Ocherki istorii zdravookhraneniia SSSR (1917–1956 gg.) [Essays on the history of public health in the USSR, 1917–1956] Moskva, Medgiz, 1957. 395 p.

Describes development of public health throughout Soviet Union, with chapter on public health before the Revolution. Chronology, 1903–1956: p. 378–390. Bibliography: p. 373–377.

2376

Lotova, E. I. Bibliografiia i obzor osnovnykh rabot po istorii gigieny i sanitarii (1917–1957 gg.) [Bibliography and a review of basic works on the history of hygiene and sanitation (1917–1957)]. Moskva, Institut organizatsii zdravookhraneniia i istorii meditsiny im. N.A. Semashko, 1959. 55 p.

Pt. 1, A review of basic works, p. 6–27. Pt. 2, Bibliography, listing 589 selected books (including dissertations) and articles published in the Soviet Union, in two groups: A., 376 entries on the history of hygiene and sanitation and related fields; B., Personalia, 213 biographies of outstanding workers in the field. Arranged alphabetically by author.

United States

2377

Blake, John B. Public health in the town of Boston, 1630–1822. Cambridge, Harvard University Press, 1959. 278 p. (Harvard historical studies, v. 72)

Detailed study. Footnote references throughout.

2378

Jordan, Philip D. The people's health. A history of public health in Minnesota to 1948. Saint Paul, Minnesota Historical Society, 1953. 524 p.

2379

Means, Richard K. A history of health education in the United States. Philadelphia, Lea & Febiger, 1962. 412 p.

Textbook survey, largely 20th century. References and suggested reading at end of each chapter.

2380

Ravenel, Mazÿck P., ed. A half century of public health. New York, American Public Health Association, 1921. 461 p.

Historical papers on different phases of public health in this country, 1871–1921. No bibliography.

2381

Smillie, Wilson G. Public health: its promise for the future. A chronicle of the development of public health in the United States, 1607–1914. New York, Macmillan, 1955. 501 p.

Survey by periods and topics. Includes chronologies. Appendix (p. 473–487) on pioneers in public health in America, 1610–1925. Bibliographies at ends of chapters.

2382

Straus, Robert. Medical care for seamen; the origin of public medical service in the United States. New Haven, Yale University Press, 1950. 165 p. (Merchant seaman studies, no. 1.)

Includes history of U.S. Marine Hospital Service, with brief accounts of public medical services for seamen in other countries, and other beneficiaries of federal medical services. Bibliographic footnotes.

2383

Williams, Ralph C. The United States Public Health Service, 1798–1950. Washington, Commissioned Officers Association of the United States Public Health Service, 1951. 890 p.

Detailed compilation.

Venezuela

2384

Archila, Ricardo. Historia de la sanidad en Venezuela. Caracas, Impr. Nacional, 1956. 2 v.

Pre-Columbian period to the present. Bibliographical references in footnotes.

Environmental Health

Indexes and Abstracts

2385
APCA Abstracts. Pittsburgh, 1, 1955– . Air Pollution Control Association in cooperation with the U.S. Public Health Service and the Library of Congress.

About 800 abstracts a year from 812 journals.

2386
Water pollution abstracts. London, 1928– . Ministry of Technology.

Monthly. 1965 contained 2069 numbered abstracts. Includes books, private and government research reports, etc. Indexes a number of nonmedical journals.

Through v. 38(3) issued by Department of Scientific and Industrial Research.

Bibliographies

2387
Air pollution bibliography. In Air and water pollution, 2, 1960– .

Papers listed are abstracted in no. 2385.

2388
Bost, E. [et al.] comp. Radioactive-fallout; a bibliography of the world's literature. Washington, 1961. 192 p. (U.S. Atomic Energy Commission. TID-3086)

3507 references arranged by format under subject: reports, journals, miscellaneous (books, congressional hearings, etc.) Through October 1960.

2389
——. ——. Suppl. 1– . (U.S. Atomic Energy Commission. TID-3086, Suppl. 1–)

Suppl. 1, 1525 references, Oct. 1960–Feb. 1962; suppl. 2, 1953 entries, through Dec. 1963.

2390
Cincinnati. University. College of Medicine. Kettering Laboratory of Applied Physiology. Annotated bibliography—the effects of atmospheric pollution on the health of man. [Cincinnati, 1957] 481 p.

790 references.

2391
Levine, Benjamin S. USSR literature on air pollution and related occupational diseases. Washington, U.S. Office of Technical Services, 1960– .

2391.1
U.S. Public Health Service. Carbon monoxide; a bibliography with abstracts. Compiled by Anna Grossmann Cooper. Washington, 1966. 440 p. (Public Health Service. Publication no. 1503. Bibliography series no. 68)

In excess of 983 selected abstracts 1880–1966. Includes books, research reports, legislation. Separate listing: *State, City-county, and interstate reports*, p. 419–26. Geographic index.

Prepared in the Division of Air Pollution.

2392
——. Division of Air Pollution. Air Pollution publications; a selected bibliography, 1955–1963. By Anna Grossmann-Cooper. Washington, 1964. 174 p. (Public Health Service, Publication no. 979. Revised 1964)

Publications by Public Health Service personnel and other persons and organizations receiving Federal air pollution funds. 1029 entries listed by author, title and subject. Contains geographic index for selected studies. Indexes a number of nonmedical journals. Includes state and U.S. Government reports and pamphlets.

Supersedes: . . . *selected bibliography*, 1955–62. (Public Health Service, Publication no. 979)

Incorporates: U.S. Public Health Service. Division of Industrial Hygiene. *Biological aspects of air pollution; an annotated bibliography*, by Harry Heimann and others, Pittsburgh, 1950, 67 p. (not listed separately).

2393
——. ——. Sulfur oxides and other sulfur compounds; a bibliography with abstracts. Comp. by Anna Grossmann Cooper. Washington, 1965. 383 p. (Public Health Service. Publication no. 1093. Bibliography series no. 56)

994 references, 1893–1964. Includes books, chapters in books. Geographic index.

2394
——. Division of Water Supply and Pollution Control. Water pollution control, sewage treatment, water treatment; selected biological references. By William M. Ingram and Kenneth M. Mackenthun. Washington, 1963. 142 p. (Public Health Service. Publication no. 1053. Bibliography series no. 8)

Consists of approximately 1166 references covering 1922–61. Also biological references on industrial waste water, recreational water treatment, organism identification, and aspects of water quality. Includes books and private and government research reports.

2394.1
——. Robert A. Taft Sanitary Engineering Center, Cincinnati. Bibliography on synthetic detergents in water and wastes including analytical methods and physiological effects. Cincinnati, 1964. 91 p.

851 entries arranged by year from 1937.

Directories

2394.2
Governmental air pollution agencies. Directory. Pittsburgh, 1966– . Air Pollution Control Association.

Geographical arrangement. Includes U.S. possessions and Canada.

Published in cooperation with the U.S. Public Health Service.

2395
Organisation for Economic Co-operation and Development. Directorate for Scientific Affairs. Directory of water pollution research laboratories. Paris, 1965. 519 p. (O. E. C. D. Publication no. 18313)

Includes only laboratories and institutions regularly engaging in research of general interest on the pollution of fresh water. For each gives address, director, affiliation, personnel, documentation, special facilities and equipment, and a description of the research program. Arranged by country including Europe (except Albania, East Germany, and Ireland) and North America. No index.

French ed., *Repertoire des laboratoires de recherche sur le pollution des eaux.*

2395.1
U.S. National Referral Center for Science and Technology. A directory of information resources in the United States. Water. Washington, 1966. 248 p.

Includes water pollution, aquatic biology and ecology centers. Gives publications. Includes special libraries and library facilities within centers.

2396
Water pollution control research and training grants. Washington, 1962– . U.S. Public Health Service. Division of Water Supply and Pollution Control. (Public Health Service. Publication no. 1100, etc.)

Occupational Health

Indexes and Abstracts

CURRENT

2397
Industrial hygiene digest. Pittsburgh, 1, 1937– . Mellon Institute. Industrial Hygiene Foundation.

Monthly. 1244 abstracts in 1965, some abstracts evaluative. Indexes a number of nonmedical sources. Includes books, pamphlets.

Subtitle: Industrial health news; literature abstracts. Decennial index, 1955–1964.

2398
Occupational safety and health abstracts. Geneva, 1, 1963– . International Occupational Safety and Health Information Centre (CIS).

About 2000 abstracts a year, reproducing contents of the CIS Service card series. Includes government publications, private and official regulations and standards, etc.

2399
Pneumoconiosis abstracts. London. 1, 1926/38– .

Abstracts of papers published in the *Bulletin of Hygiene.* 1926–

v. 2 covers 1939–50; v. 3 1951–55. v. 1 published in 1953.

2400
U.S. Office of Manpower, Automation and Training. Health and safety aspects of automation and technological change. Washington, 1964. 181 p.

581 entries covering radiation and other occupational hazards. Includes books and reports. No author or subject index.

Subtitle (on cover): A collection of abstracts 1956 to 1962 prepared by the International Labour Office, Geneva, Switzerland.

NONCURRENT

2401
Bibliographie d'hygiene industrielle. Geneva, 1–15, 1923–41. Bureau International du Travail.

v. 14 listed 2620 items. Includes books, theses, government and private reports, and bulletins. Covers a number of nonmedical journals, private and trade publications.

Title and subject headings in French, English, and German through v. 13, 1939; French and English, v. 14–15, 1940–41.

Continued in no. 2402.

2402
Bibliography of occupational medicine. Bibliographie de médecine du travail. Geneva, 1–3, 1948–50. International Labour Office.

Supersedes no. 2401.

Reviews

2403
Modern trends in occupational health. London, 1960– . (Butterworths medical publications. Modern trends series).

Irregular. Reviews the more important general trends, particularly of scientific methods for measuring the working environment and its effects on health. Includes bibliographies.

Bibliographies

2404
Bellingham, Ellen F. [et al.] Bibliography of industrial hygiene 1900–1943; a selected list. Washington, 1945. 95 p. (Public Health Service. Public health bulletin no. 289).

English language literature only. Includes books, government and private reports.

2405
Bibliography of occupational health; occupational health and related publications from the Public Health Service. Washington, 1, 1909/1953– .

No annotations. Includes books, pamphlets, and nonmedical journals. Separate listing of Public Health Service publications.

1909/1953 issue, as Public Health bibliography series, no. 9; second issue covers 1953–57; third issue, 1953–60.

2406
Brno. Universita. Knihovna. Pracovní lékařství; výběr knižní literatury za léta 1948–1958 [Occupational health; selected books from the period of 1948–1958]. Brno, 1959. 52 p.

670 references, about half Czech. Most of the non-Czech literature is in other Slavic languages.

2407
Davis, George G. [et al.] The pneumonokonioses (silicosis): bibliography and laws. Chicago, Industrial Medicine, Inc., 1934–37. 3 v.

Book 1 contains 2768 references covering the period 1555–1933 arranged by period. Books 2–3 contain 396 and 701 abstracts, respectively, covering the literature through 1936. All volumes contain sections on U.S. state laws relating to occupational diseases, etc.

Book 2 has title: *The pneumonokonioses (silicosis) literature and laws of 1934;* Book 3. *The pneumonokonioses (silicosis) literature and laws.*

Books 2–3 have subtitle: International abstracts, extracts and reviews of the pneumonokonioses and their associated diseases and subjects.

2408
Forbes, J.J. [et al.] Review of the literature on dusts. Washington, 1950. 333 p. (U.S. Department of the Interior. Bulletin 478)

Selective bibliography of 657 items. Deals with prevention, control, and economic aspects of pneumoconiosis, silicosis, and related diseases. Revision of Bulletin 400, 1937.

2409
Praha. Ústav hygieny. Bibliographical review of the Czechoslovak literature on communal, school, and food hygiene. Prague, v. 1, 1959– .

Annual. 1961 contains 488 entries. Includes books.

Directories

2410
International Labour Office. International directory of institutions engaged in study, research and other activities in the field of occupational safety and health. Geneva, 1958. 2 v.

Country arrangement.

For each country lists organizations alphabetically. Information given includes address, names of directors, functions, scientific research, publications.

Histories

2411
Hunter, Donald. The diseases of occupations. 3 ed. Boston, Little, Brown, 1962. 1180 p.

Chapters I-IV (p. 1–226) present a historical survey from ancient times to the present. Bibliographical references at end of each chapter. 1 ed., 1955.

2412
Rosen, George. The history of miners' diseases; a medical and social interpretation. New York, Schuman, 1943. 490 p.

Through the 19th century. Author bibliography (261 items, original and secondary): p. 459–476.

2413
Selleck, Henry B., and Whittaker, Alfred H. Occupational health in America. Prepared under the direction of the History Committee of the Industrial Medical Association. Detroit, Wayne State University Press, 1962. 523 p.

Covers the 19th and 20th centuries, with a preliminary survey of English and early American developments. Includes history of the Association. Bibliographical notes, by chapter: p. 469–486.

2414
Teleky, Ludwig. History of factory and mine hygiene. New York, Columbia University Press, 1948. 342 p.

Preliminary survey of industrial hygiene through the 19th century, followed by chapters on special subjects. Bibliography (p. 285–317) includes official and general sources.

Social Welfare

Bibliographies

2414.1
U.S. Department of Health, Education and Welfare. Bureau of Family Services. Abstracts of research and demonstration projects in social welfare and related fields. Washington, 1966. 249 p.

370 projects described. Gives duration of project and publications. Indexes of participating federal agencies, principal investigators, contractors, grantees and subject index.

Directories

2415
American Association of Social Workers: Directory of members. New York, 1952. 200 p.

Approximately 13,500 names, with a geographic list.

Vital Statistics

Indexes and Abstracts

2415.1
Population index. Princeton, 1, 1935– . Princeton University. Office of Population Research and Population Association of America.

Quarterly. 1964 listed in excess of 2700 references, most with abstracts. Includes articles, books, and government publications relating to morbidity, mortality, fertility, demographic factors, and health. Geographical and other indexes.

Bibliographies

2416
Institute of Contemporary Jewry, Jerusalem. Jewish health statistics. Ed. by O. Schmelz, assisted by F. Keidanski. Jerusalem, 1966. 348 p.

3333 entries. Considers physical characteristics, morbidity and health services, in separate chapters for Jews in the diaspora and Jews in Palestine/Israel. Includes books, reports, theses, 19th and 20th centuries.

Complements the Institute's *Jewish demography and statistics, bibliography for 1920–1960* (1961) (not listed)

2416.1
Merkov, A.M. Demograficheskaia statistika (statistika naseleniia); kratkoe posobie dlia vracheĭ [Demographical statistics (population statistics); a brief handbook for physicians] 2 ed. Moskva, Izd-vo "Meditsina", 1965. 215 p.

Includes number and composition of population; birth, mortality, child mortality, and reproduction statistics.

Directories

2416.2
United Nations Educational, Scientific and Cultural Organization. Social Science Clearing House. International repertory of institutions conducting population studies. Paris, 1959. 240 p.

Lists international organizations followed by national arranged by country. Gives name of administrator, chief staff members, if known, activities and publications.

Histories

2417
Greenwood, Major. Medical statistics from Graunt to Farr. Cambridge, University Press, 1948. 73 p. (Fitzpatrick Lectures, 1941 and 1943)

Devoted chiefly to England, 17th to early 19th century. First published in *Biometrika*, v. 32–33, 1941–43.

2418
Westergaard, Harald L. Contributions to the history of statistics. London, King, 1932. 280 p.

Survey of legislation and development of statistical theory and services, 16th–19th centuries. Includes data on population and vital statistics. Bibliographical footnotes. Name index only.

RADIOLOGY

Indexes and Abstracts

Current

2419
La letteratura radiologica italiana; indice bibliografico dei lavori italiani di radiologia. Milano. 1–9, 1895/1920– .

v. 1, covering the literature 1895/1920, contained 1866 entries.

2420
Referátový výběr z roentgenologie [Selected abstracts on roentgenology] Praha, 1, 1954– . Ústav pro zdravotnickou dokumentaci.

About 600–700 abstracts a year. Titles in Czech or Slovak and in the original language. Abstracts are in Czech or Slovak. No subject index.

2421
Voprosy rentgenologii i radiologii. Annotatsii nauchnykh rabot [Problems of roentgenology and radiology. Annotations of scientific works] Moskva, 1, 1958/60– . Gosudarstvennyĭ nauchno-issledovatel'skiĭ rentgeno-radiologicheskiĭ institut.

v. 1, 1962, 360 p., covers 1958–60; v. 2, covering 1961–62, is in preparation. Contains abstracts of monographs (including dissertations) and articles by Soviet authors in the Russian language.

2422
Zentralblatt für die gesamte Radiologie. Berlin, 1, 1926– . Referatenorgan der deutschen Röntgen-Gesellschaft (since v. 9, 1930).

Currently 3–4 volumes a year, 3 issues a volume and a separate index issue. A recent volume listed in excess of 1200 references, most with abstracts. Includes books.

v. 1–7, 1926–30, had subtitle: Zugleich Abteilung B der Zeitschrift für die gesamte physikalische Therapie.

See also no. 2423.

Noncurrent

2423
Jahresbericht Radiologie. Berlin, 1–13, 1926–38.

Annual cumulation of references of no. 2422.

Subtitle: Bibliographisches Jahresregister des Zentralblattes für die gesamte Radiologie.

Reviews

2424
Advances in x-ray analysis. New York, 1, 1960– .

Proceedings of the Annual Conference on Application of X-ray Analysis, 6th– .

2425
Hoshasen igaku saikin no shinpo [Recent advances in radiology] Tokyo, 1, 1959– .

Irregular.

2426
Modern trends in diagnostic radiology. 3d ser. London, Butterworths, 1960. (Butterworths medical publications. Modern trends series)

2427
Progress in radiation therapy. New York, Grune and Stratton, 1958– .

2427.1
Recent advances in radiology. 4 ed. Ed. by Thomas Lodge. London, Churchill, 1964. 346 p.

Chapter bibliographies. No over-all author index.

1 ed., 1931; 3 ed., 1955.

2428★
Year book of radiology. Chicago, Year

Book Medical Publishers, 1932– . (The practical medicine year books)

Abstracts with editorial comment.

Series note added with 1953/54.

2429 (Not used)

Bibliographies

2430
Besio, G. L. Index stratigraphicus: Raccolta di voci bibliografiche sulla stratigrafia dal 1930 al 1959. Genova, Edizioni Universitarie, 1960. 275 p.

Includes books and theses.

2431
Boguslavskiĭ, Ia. M., and Vasil'ev, S. I. Bibliograficheskiĭ spravochnik literatury po liuminestsentnomu analizu v meditsine i biologii (s 1947 g. po iiun 1961) [Bibliographic reference book of literature on luminescent analysis in medicine and biology (from 1947 to June 1961)] Chita, Chitinskiĭ gosudarstvennyĭ meditsinskiĭ institut, 1961. 69 p.

519 entries, including books, dissertations, reviews of dissertations, chapters of books, and periodical articles.

2432
Gocht, Hermann. Die Röntgen-Literatur. Stuttgart, Enke, 1911–36. 15 v.

Covers the literature from 1896 (the earliest citation noted in v. 1) through 1934, with each volume covering one year or more. Includes books, theses.

v. 1 has subtitle: Zugleich Anhang zu Gochts Handbuch der Röntgen-Lehre; with v. 2, Im Auftrag der Deutschen Röntgengesellschaft.

2433 (not used)

2434
Musikka, Sirkka, and Holsti, Lars R. Finnish radiological bibliography, 1896–1963. Helsinki, 1965. 123 p. (Medicina Fennica. Supplementum 2. Finnish Radiological Society. Publications, 2)

Limited to Finnish writers. 1521 entries, including books.

2435
Ujhelyi, Adorján. Magyar radiológiai bibliográfia (1945–1960) [Bibliography of Hungarian radiology (1945–1960)] Budapest, Országos Orvostudományi Könyvtár és Dokumentációs Központ, 1963. 340 p.

2549 references, including books. Covers the literature published in Hungary or by Hungarian authors abroad. Includes a list of periodicals indexed with abbreviations.

2436
Wetterer, Josef, ed. Internationale Radiotherapie; Besprechungwerke auf dem Gebiete der Röntgen-, Curie-, Licht-, und Elektrotherapie. Darmstadt, Wittich, 1926–28. 3 v.

Covers 1925–28. Includes books.

Dictionaries

2437
British Standards Institution. Glossary of terms used in radiology. London, 1955. 82 p. (B.S. 2597:1955)

Short definitions of numbered terms arranged in the following sections: general terms and physics; sources of ionizing radiation; radiography and fluoroscopy; radiotherapy and radiation protection. Index refers to term number.

2438
Deutscher Medizinischer Sprachendienst, München. Termini radiologici: deutsch, english, français, español. München, Urban & Schwarzenberg, 1959. 78 p.

Includes about 1000 words in each language.

2439
Etter, Lewis E. Glossary of words and phrases used in radiology and nuclear medicine. With a section on suggested terminology for roentgenological reports. Springfield, Ill., Thomas, 1960. 203 p.

Prepared for medical secretaries, x-ray technicians, medical students and residents in radiology. Definitions occasionally supported by bibliographic citations; includes abbreviations.

2440
Fossati, Franco. Dizionario tecnico di radiologia: italiano, français, deutsch, english, español. Milano, Wassermann, 1952. 489 p.

Pt. 1: Italian term followed by equivalents in French, German, English, Spanish; pt. 2: 4 sections: French-Italian, German-Italian; English-Italian, Spanish-Italian.

2441
Pompili, Giuseppe. Glossario di medicina nucleare. Torino, Minerva medica, 1961. 285 p.

Full definitions; English equivalent for each term.

2442
Shilling, Charles Wesley. Atomic energy encyclopedia in the life sciences. Philadelphia, Saunders, 1964. 474 p.

More than 1200 definitions. Includes description of corporate bodies.

Directories

2443
American College of Radiology. Membership directory. Chicago, 1964. 191 p.

Alphabetical and geographical listings with addresses. Includes officers, committee and commission members. Before 1957 issued in the College's *Bulletin*; 1957–58 as a separate; after 1958 as a separate number of the *Bulletin*.

2444
American Roentgen Ray Society. Revised membership directory, corrected to March 1, 1965. [Rochester, Minn.] 1965. 127 p.

Alphabetical and geographical listings, with addresses. Includes officers and committee members and list of Caldwell lectures.

2444.1
American Society of Radiologic Technologists. Official roster. Fond du Lac, Wisc., 1964/65– .

Geographic arrangement.

Continues the *Official roster* of the American Society of X-Ray Technicians.

Histories

2445
Bruwer, André J., ed. Classic descriptions in diagnostic roentgenology. Springfield, Ill., Thomas, 1964. 2 v. (2059 p.)

Selections, in English, with brief biographical notes. Bibliographical references. No index.

2446
Glasser, Otto. Wilhelm Conrad Röntgen und die Geschichte der Röntgenstrahlen. 2 ed. Berlin, Springer, 1959. 381 p.

Detailed history of discovery and early period of roentgenology. Bibliography lists 86 items on Röntgen and the discovery, 1044 items on x-rays published in 1896. 1 ed., 1931. English translation, *Wilhelm Conrad Röntgen and the early history of the roentgen rays*, London, John Bale, Sons & Danielsson, 1933, 494 p.

2447
Grigg, Emanuel R. N. The trail of the invisible light: from X-Strahlen to radio-(bio)logy. Springfield, Ill., Thomas, 1965. 974 p. (American lecture series. Publication no. 579)

Contains extensive material, rather disorganized, on personalities, discoveries and "firsts," especially in technology and equipment, terminology, symbols, trademarks, organizations, commercial developments, etc. Bibliography, including list of periodicals, p. 800–864. Indexes of manufacturers, names, and subjects.

2448
Holthusen, Hermann [et al.] ed. Ehrenbuch der Röntgenologen und Radiologen aller Nationen. 2 ed. München, Urban & Schwarzenberg, 1959. 268 p. (Strahlentherapie. Sonderbände, v. 42)

About 350 brief biographies of radiologists who lost their lives directly or indirectly through pioneer work with radium and roentgen rays. Arranged by country.

Nuclear Medicine

Indexes and Abstracts

2448.1
Index radiohygienicus. Praha, 1, 1965– . Institute of Radiation Hygiene.

10 times a year. Covers radiation hygiene and biological effects of ionizing radiation.

Includes books, research reports. All titles given in English. Author and keyword indexes in each issue.

2449★
Nuclear science abstracts. Oak Ridge, Tenn., 1, 1947– . U.S. Atomic Energy Commission.

Semimonthly. In excess of 45,000 abstracts in 1964. Includes journal articles, books, conferences, government and private research.

Reviews

2450★
Annual review of nuclear science. Palo Alto, Calif., Annual Reviews, 1, 1952– .

2451
Progress in atomic medicine. New York, Grune and Stratton, 1, 1965– .

2452
Progress in nuclear energy. Ser. 6, Biological sciences. New York, Pergamon, 1, 1956– .

Edited papers from the Proceedings of the International Conference on the Peaceful Uses of Atomic Energy, 1, 1956– .

2453
Progress in nuclear energy. Ser. 7, Medical sciences. New York, Pergamon, 1, 1956– .

Edited papers from the Proceedings of the International Conference on the Peaceful Uses of Atomic Energy, 1, 1956– .

2454
Progress in nuclear energy. Ser. 12, Health physics. New York, Pergamon, 1, 1959– .

Edited papers of the Proceedings of the International Conference on the Peaceful Uses of Atomic Energy, 2, 1958– .

2454.1
Year book of nuclear medicine. Chicago, Year Book Medical Publishers, 1, 1966– . (The practical medicine year books)

Bibliographies

2454.2
Akademiia nauk SSSR. Sektor seti spetsial'nykh bibliotek. Ukazatel' literatury po primeneniiu radioaktivnykh i stabil'nykh izotopov v biologii za 1950–1958 gg. [Index to literature on the use of radioactive and stable isotopes in biology, 1950–1958] Moskva, 1962. 408 p.

9630 references including books, parts of books, collected works, etc. Comprehensive coverage of Soviet literature; selected non-Soviet items included. Entries are in the original languages.

2454.3
Atomic Bomb Casualty Commission. Bibliography of publications concerning effect of nuclear explosions, 1945–1960. Nagasaki, 1961. 187 p.

2409 references, author arrangement by year. Includes books, chapters in books and some reports.

2455
Kiev. Respublikanskaia nauchnaia meditsinskaia biblioteka. Primenenie radioaktivnykh izotopov v meditsine (Bibliograficheskiĭ ukazatel' otechestvennoĭ literatury za 1940–1945 gg.) [The use of radioactive isotopes in medicine (Bibliographic index of national literature, 1940–1955)] Sost. E. A. Sapozhnikova. Kiev, 1955. 44 p.

Over 400 monographs, collected works, and journal articles, published in the Russian language. No indexes.

2455.1
Uhlmann, W. The determination of radioactive isotopes in urine. Stockholm, 1962. 54, 2, 2 p. (AB Atomenergi. Atom dokumentation. Bibliografi. Bibliography. VDIT-66, November 1962)

164 abstracts (in English) 1950–62, arranged by date. Supersedes VDIT-55, March 1962 (not listed).

2456
U.S. Atomic Energy Commission. Annotated bibliography in radiobiology. Comp. by Sophie V. Stephens and R. D. Boche, Washington, 1953. 360 p. (Its ANL-5111)

2153 abstracts, alphabetical by author. Includes books and research reports. No subject index. Earliest reference cited was 1923.

2456.1
——. Biological effects of ionizing radiation; an annotated bibliography covering the years 1898–1957 . . . Comp. by Marylou Ingram. 2 v. [Oak Ridge, 1966] (Its TID-3097)

12,726 entries most with abstracts. v. 1, abstracts; v. 2, index.

2456.2
——. The effects of radiation and radioisotopes on the life processes; an annotated bibliography. Comp. by Charlie M. Pierce. Oak Ridge, 1963. 3v. (Its TID-3098)

11,944 references, 1958–60, most with annotations. Gives for major zoological classes effects by system or organ. v. 3 contains author and subject index.

2457
——. Physiological studies employing radioisotopes. Compiled by Helen L. Ward.

Oak Ridge, 1965. 284 p. (Its TID-3515 (Supplement 1))

2578 references, 1958–1963, most with annotations.

Supplements 2457.1

2457.1
——. Radioisotopes in animal physiology; a selected list of references. Comp. by J. A. McCormick. Oak Ridge, 1958. 118 p. (Its TID-3515)

2439 references, 1948–57. Broad subject arrangement (therapeutic medicine, clinical research, etc.) Author but no subject index.

2458
——. Nuclear Safety Information Center, Oak Ridge. Indexed bibliography of current nuclear safety literature. Oak Ridge, 1, 1965– .

2459
Wasserman, R. H., and Comar, C. L. Annotated bibliography of strontium and calcium metabolism in man and animals. Washington, 1961. 135 p. (U.S. Department of Agriculture. Agricultural Research Service. Miscellaneous publication no. 821)

REPRODUCTION, FERTILITY, ETC.

Indexes and Abstracts

2460★
Bibliography of reproduction; a classified monthly title list compiled from the world's research literature; vertebrates including man. Cambridge, Eng., 1, 1963– . Reproduction Research Information Service Ltd.

2 volumes a year. v. 1–8 listed some 38,000 references obtained by regularly scanning about 220 journals directly and over 9000 indirectly through *Current contents*, *Index medicus*, etc. Journals scanned include many not in *Index medicus*. Includes books and theses.

2461
Medical gynaecology and fertility abstracts. London, Family Centre, Ltd., 1, 1962– .

Monthly. 1210 abstracts from over 200 journals in 1963.

1961–65 as *Fertility abstracts.*

Reviews

2461.1
Advances in reproductive physiology. London, Logos, [1] 1966– .

Reviews with chapter bibliographies.

2462★
Modern trends in human reproductive physiology. London, 1, Butterworths, 1963– .

Reviews with bibliographies.

2463
Recent advances in sex and reproductive physiology. 3 ed. By J. M. Robson. London, Churchill, 1947. 336 p.

Chapter bibliographies (omitting titles of articles). No over-all author index. 1 ed., 1934; 2 ed., 1940.

2464
U.S. National Institutes of Health. A survey of research on reproduction related to birth and population control, as of January 1, 1963. Washington, 1963. 248 p. (Public Health Service. Publication no. 1066)

Supersedes: A survey . . . as of December, 1962.

Bibliographies

2465
Tietze, Christopher, ed. Bibliography of fertility control, 1950–1965. New York, National Committee on Maternal Health, 1965. 198 p.

1935 references. Covers medical and sociological literature in English, including books, chapters of books and conference papers.

2466
——. Selected bibliography of contraception: 1940–1960. New York, National Committee on Maternal Health, 1960. 76 p. (Its Publication no. 6)

844 references, including books, chapters of books, conference papers. Covers the medical and sociological literature published in the languages of Western Europe. Arranged alphabetically by author.

2467
——. ——. Supplement, 1960–63, New York, National Committee on Maternal Health, 1963. 59 p. (Its Publication no. 18)

Contains 563 references, including some pre-1960 references not in the original bibliography.

2467.1
U.S. Food and Drug Administration. Bureau of Medicine, Washington. Medical Literature Branch abstracts. Reports in the literature on: The problem of safety of the oral contraceptives. 71 p. (MLB bibliography no. 1, November 22, 1965)

Abstracts. Card form. No indexes.

Dictionaries

2468
Dictionnaire de sexologie, sexologia-lexikon; sexologie générale, sexualité, contresexualité, érotisme, erotologie, bibliographie universelle. [Realisé sous la direction de Lo Duca]. Paris, Pauvert, 1962. 566 p.

Histories

2469
Cole, Francis J. Early theories of sexual generation. Oxford, Clarendon Press, 1930. 230 p.

Analysis of important contributions to the study of the spermatozoa, the doctrines of preformation and epigenesis, and fertilization and development. "Literature consulted" (by author, including sources): p. 211–226.

2470
Eversley, David E. C. Social theories of fertility and the Malthusian debate. Oxford, Clarendon Press, 1959. 313 p.

Bibliography (by sections): p. 285–298.

2471
Fryer, Peter. The birth controllers. London, Secker & Warburg, 1965. 384 p.

Preliminary chapter on the "prehistory" of birth control, followed by account of leaders in the movement and their works from the 17th century to the present. References and bibliography: p. 273–371.

2472
Himes, Norman E. Medical history of contraception. New York, Gamut Press, 1963. liii, 521 p.

Comprehensive survey. Bibliography. p. 425–490, alphabetically by author. Reprint of Baltimore, 1936, edition, with new preface by Alan F. Guttmacher tracing developments since 1935.

RESEARCH IN PROGRESS

Inventories of research covering broad fields of medicine and related sciences consisting largely of reference to unpublished material have been listed here. Publications relating to research in progress in a specific field have been listed under subjects.

Indexes and Abstracts

2473★
An inventory of social and economic research in health. Chicago, 1, 1952– . Health Information Foundation.

Describes project, gives sponsor, principal investigator, date final report due.

13 ed., 1964.

2474★
Research grants index. Bethesda, 1961– . U.S. National Institutes of Health. Division of Research Grants. (Public Health Service. Publication no. 925)

Annual. 1963– , in two volumes: v. 1, subject index; v. 2, includes a grant number listing and bibliography (lists works already published under grant), and an alphabetical list of investigators.

2475
U.S. Air Force. Office of Aerospace Research. Air Force research resumés. Washington 1, 1959– .

v. 4, 1964, describes briefly more than 2400 active inhouse and contractual research efforts. Includes basic research in the preclinical sciences, including the behavioral sciences.

1959–62 as *Basic research resumês.*

2476
U.S. Air Force. Office of Scientific Research. Air Force scientific research bibliography. Washington 1, 1950/56– . (AFOSR-700)

Abstracts of research reports. Includes basic research in the preclinical sciences, including the behavioral sciences. v. 4, 1960 published in 1966. Collateral publication in journals noted.

2477
U.S. Atomic Energy Commission. Research and development in progress. Biology and medicine. 1, July 1963– . (TID-4204)

Brief descriptions of work in progress. Indexed by subject, principal investigator, and contracting institution. No. 4 issued April 1966 [527] p.

2478
U.S. Department of Health, Education and Welfare. Grants-in-aid and other financial assistance programs, 1966 ed. Washington, 1966. 527 p.

Supplement to the Department's *Handbook on programs* (not listed).

2478.1
U.S. Public Health Service. Clearinghouse on Current Morbidity Statistics Projects. Sources of morbidity data. Washington, 1–11, 1953–1963.

Annual. Includes mental diseases, injuries. Gives abstract of project, principal investigator, publication plans.

2479
U.S. National Science Foundation. Federal grants and contracts for unclassified research in the life sciences. Washington, 1952–58.

Includes biomedical research sponsored by all Federal agencies.

2480
——. Government-sponsored research projects in psychology, psychiatry, and closely related areas. Washington, 1953–59.

Title varies.

2481
——. Grants and awards for the fiscal year . . . Washington, 1964– .

Listing previously in National Science Foundation, Annual report, no. 2–13, 1952–63.

2482
——. Scientific information activities of Federal agencies. Washington, 1, Oct. 1958– .

Number 29 (NASA) dated Mar. 1965.

2483
U.S. Veterans Administration. Department of Medicine and Surgery. Medical research in the Veterans Administration. Washington, 1957– .

Subject index. Includes author index of articles published by VA investigators.

Descriptive introduction published separately since 1960/61, as *Medical Research in the Veterans Administration. Annual report* (not listed separately).

Bibliographies

2484
U.S. National Institutes of Health. Division of General Medical Sciences. Russian Scientific Translation Program. Medical research in the U.S.S.R. Reviews and reports from western sources; a selected and annotated list of references. Comp. by Elizabeth Koenig. [Bethesda] 1960. 45 p. (Public Health Service. Publication no. 710. Bibliography series no. 28)

199 references, including monographs.

Directories

2485★
New research centers; a periodic supplement to Research centers directory. Detroit, Gale Research 1, 1965– .

Quarterly with cumulative indexes. Updates no. 2486.

2486★
Research centers directory. Detroit, Gale Research, 1, 1960– .

A guide to university-sponsored and other nonprofit research organizations established on a permanent basis and carrying on continuing research programs in agriculture, business, conservation, education, engineering and technology, government, law, life sciences, mathematics, area studies, physical and earth sciences, social sciences, and humanities. Arranged by subject field; information given includes address, director, founding date, principal fields, and publications.

1 ed., 1960, as *Directory of university research bureaus and institutes.* 2 ed., 1965, by Archie M. Palmer and Anthony T. Kruzas.

Updated by no. 2485.

RESPIRATORY SYSTEM

Reviews

2487
Progress in research in emphysema and chronic bronchitis. Basel, Basler Druck- und Verlags Anstalt, 1, 1963- .

Irregular.

Bibliographies

2488
Khar'kovskaia gosudarstvennaia nauchno-meditsinskaia biblioteka. Pnevmokonioz; bibliograficheskiĭ ukazatel' otechestvennoĭ literatury 1918–1954 gg. [Pneumoconiosis; bibliographical index of national literature, 1918–1954]. Khar'kov, 1955. 163 p.

1468 entries. Includes books.

2489
Mandel, William [et al.] Bibliography on sarcoidosis, 1878–1963. Washington, 1964. 229 p. (Public Health Service. Publication no. 1213. Bibliography series no. 51).

3592 entries. At head of cover title: National Library of Medicine.

Directories

2490
American College of Chest Physicians. Membership roster. Chicago [etc.] 1936–59.

1959 ed. lists 6403 members in 89 countries. Geographical arrangement by state and city; United States section followed by other countries in alphabetical order. Address and professional data given. Name index. Issued irregularly. 1936–4? as *Pneumothorax directory*. 1936 ed. issued by the Society under its earlier name, Federation of American Sanataria.

SCIENCE

Indexes and Abstracts

Current

2490.1
Pakistan science abstracts. Karachi, 1, 1961?- Pakistan National Scientific and Technical Documentation Center.

v. 3, 1963 (published in 1966) contained 298 entries, most with abstracts. Includes medicine and basic sciences. Abstracts medical serials not indexed in *Index medicus*.

2490.2
Romanian scientific abstracts. Natural sciences. Bucharest, 1964?- Academy of the Socialistic Republic of Romania. Scientific Documentation Centre.

Monthly. Includes medicine, biology, chemistry. All titles and abstracts in English.

2491
Science citation index. Philadelphia, 1961- . Institute for Scientific Information.

Beginning with 1964, issued quarterly and cumulated annually. 1965 issues indexed 1147 journals (50 per cent medical or paramedical) and all U.S. patents. Cited references include not only articles but books, book reviews, abstracts, reviews, editorials, letters, personal communications, technical notes. Each issue in two parts; Source index (author and anonymous sections) and Citation index (author, anonymous, patent, and acknowledgment sections). See no. 2514.

2491.1
Thailand. National Documentation-Centre. List of scientific reports relating to Thailand. Bangkok, 1, 1964- .

No. 2, 1965 has 2115 entires. Includes books, parts of books, reports, theses. Subject but no author index.

Title also in Thai.

Noncurrent

2491.2
India. National Scientific Documentation Centre. New Delhi. Scientific publications of South and South East Asia. New Delhi, 1–10, 1955–64.

Includes medicine and the basic sciences. Published in cooperation with UNESCO.

Continues 2493.2.

2492
Reuss, Jeremias D. Repertorium commentationum a societatibus litterariis editarum. Gottingae. Dieterich, 1801–21. 16 v.

A classified subject index to learned society publications through the 18th century, with author indexes at the ends of the main sections and outlines of the classification at the front of each volume. Contents: v. 1, natural science (general) and zoology; v. 2, botany and mineralogy; v. 3, chemistry and metallurgy; v. 4, physics; v. 5, astronomy; v. 6, agriculture; v. 7, technology, architecture, military and naval science; v. 8, history; v. 9, philology, literature, art, and music; v. 10–16, medicine and surgery, including (v. 16, pt. 2) veterinary science. Reprinted New York, Franklin, 1961.

2493
Royal Society of London. Catalogue of scientific papers. London, Clay, 1867–1902; Cambridge, University Press, 1914–25. 19 v.

An author index of periodical literature. Covers basic sciences, but little clinical medicine. v. 1–6, ser. 1, 1800–63; v. 7–8, ser. 2, 1864–73; v. 9–11, ser. 3, 1874–83; v. 12, supplement; v. 13–19, ser. 4, 1884–1900. Continued in no. 44.

Ser. 1 includes some material as early as 1771.

2493.1
UNESCO. Science Cooperation Office, Middle East. Cairo. Liste de travaux scientifiques publiés au Moyen-Orient. Le Caire, 1–12? 1948–55?

Includes medicine and basic sciences. Covers Afghanistan, Cyprus, Egypt, Iran, Iraq, Israel, Lebanon, Pakistan, Sudan, Syria, Turkey.

2493.2
UNESCO. South Asia Science Cooperation Office. New Delhi. Bibliography of scientific publications of South Asia (India, Burma, Ceylon) New Delhi 1–12, 1949–54.

Includes medicine and the basic sciences.
Continued by no. 2491.2.

Bibliographies

2493.3
Walford, Albert J. ed. Guide to reference material. 2 ed. v. 1, Science and technology. London, Library Association, 1966. 483 p.

Includes chemistry, anthropological and biological sciences, general biology, botany, zoology, medicine. Annotations.

Dictionaries

2494
Chambers' technical dictionary. Ed. by C. F. Tweney and L. E. C. Hughes. 3 ed. New York, Macmillan, 1958. 1028 p.

Includes medical, biological, and zoological terms.

2495
De Vries, Louis. French-English science dictionary for students in agricultural, biological, and physical sciences; with a revised supplement of terms in aeronautics, electronics, radar, radio, television, atomic energy, nuclear science and technology, and a new guide for translators. 3 ed. New York, McGraw-Hill, 1962. 655 p.

2496
——. German-English science dictionary for students in chemistry, physics, biology, agriculture, and related sciences. New York, McGraw-Hill, 1959. 592 p.

2497
Flood, Walter E. Scientific words; their structure and meaning. New York, Duell, Sloan and Pearce, 1960. 220 p.

Lists about 1150 word elements (roots, prefixes, suffixes) entering into the formation of scientific terms; meaning of each element and its origin given.

2498 (Not used)

Directories

2499★
American men of science; a biographical directory. Ed. by the Jacques Cattell Press. New York, Bowker, etc., 1, 1906– .

11 ed. (7 v., 1965–) contains about 150,000 biographies. Gives address, brief personal data, education, professional data, specialty, and publications. Supplement 1. The physical and biological sciences [A–G] 1966.

1–8 ed. in 1 volume. 9 ed. in three volumes: v. 1, physical sciences; v. 2, biological sciences; v. 3, social and behavioral sciences. 10 ed. in 5 volumes: v. 1–4, physical and biological sciences; v. 5, social and behavioral sciences. 11 ed., v. 1–6, physical and biological sciences; v. 7, social and behavioral sciences.

2500
Chambers' dictionary of scientists. Ed. by A. V. Howard. London, Chambers, 1952. 499 columns.

Brief biographies of both living and dead; includes many physicians.

2501
Directory of British scientists, 1964–65. New York, Bowker, 1964. 2001 p.

Brief professional data.

2502
Murra, Katherine O. International scientific organizations, a guide to their library, documentation, and information services. Washington, Library of Congress, General Reference and Bibliography Division, Reference Department, 1962. 794 p.

Includes organizations in medical and related fields.

2503
National register of scientific and technical personnel in India. New Delhi, 1950–54. India. Council of Scientific and Industrial Research.

v. 2, pts. 1–3, Medical personnel. Alphabetical list of medical graduates, giving birth date, academic qualifications, professional experience and specialization, address, and type of practice. Separate listings for medical licentiates and dentists are included.

2504
Nippon Gakujutsu Shinkokai. Scientific and technical societies in Japan, 1962. Comp. in Scientific Information Section, Higher Education and Science Bureau, Ministry of Education, Japan. Tokyo, Japan Society for the Promotion of Science, 1962. 109 p.

Arranged alphabetically by name under subject field; medical sciences arranged by specialty. Data: address, director, activities, and publications. In English, with name of society repeated in Japanese.

2505
Official year-book of the scientific and learned societies of Great Britain and Ireland. London, Griffin, 1–56, 1884–1939.

Publication suspended 1940–50, then continued by no. 2507.

2506
Polish research guide. Warszawa, 1964– .

Lists academies, universities, colleges, schools, research institutes, museums, research libraries, scientific societies, in all branches of science. Gives address, name of director, and chief staff members. Includes personal name and institution indexes.

Published for the U.S. National Science Foundation on order of the Centralny Instytut Informacji Naukowo-technicznej i Ekonomicznej.

2507
Scientific and learned societies of Great Britain. London, Allen & Unwin, 57, 1951– .

Includes sections on medicine and biology. 61 ed., 1964. Continues no. 2505.

2508★
Scientific and technical societies of the United States and Canada. Washington, National Academy of Sciences, National Research Council, 1, 1927– .

7 ed., 1961, lists 1597 entries for the United States, 239 for Canada. Gives name of president and/or secretary, address, history, purpose, membership, meetings, and publications. Includes medical and related societies. 1–5 ed. as *Handbook of scientific and technical societies and institutions of the United States and Canada.*

2509
Yugoslav scientific research directory. Belgrade, 1964– .

Lists institutes, universities, libraries, and museums in all branches of science. Gives address, founding date, name of director, and chief staff members. Summarizes organization and activities and indicates regular publications. Includes personal name and institution indexes.

Published for the U.S. National Library of Medicine through the National Science Foundation.

Periodicals—Lists

2510
Bolton, Henry C. A catalogue of scientific and technical periodicals, 1665–1895, together with chronological tables and a library check-list. 2 ed. Washington, 1897. 1247 p. (Smithsonian miscellaneous collections, v. 40)

Lists 8603 periodicals with a subject index. Reprinted New York, Johnson Reprint, 1965.

2511
Guide to Latin American scientific and technical periodicals; an annotated list. Washington, 1962. 187 p. Pan American Union, Division of Science Development, and Centro de Documentación Cientifica y Técnica de México.

Lists approximately 1000 journals. The data supplied include title, place of publication, name and address of publication office, frequency, size in centimeters, average number of pages per issue, illustrative materials, and type of reproduction. Includes a geographical index. The appendix is a statistical analysis including publication dates, sponsorship, number by country, editorial policies, language policy, abstracting practices, special sections, coverage by international indexes.

2512
Kokuritsu kokkai toshokan, Tokyo. Directory of Japanese scientific periodicals, 1962; natural sciences, medical sciences and industry. Tokyo, 1962. 229 p.

2513
Midwest Inter-library Center. Rarely held scientific serials in the Midwest Inter-library Center. Chicago, 1963. 197 p. Suppl. 1, 1964. 44 p.

The Midwest Inter-library Center and its member libraries since 1957 have acquired every serial abstracted by *Chemical abstracts* and *Biological abstracts.*

2514
Science Citation Index 1965 guide and journal lists. Philadelphia, Institute for Scientific Information, 1966. 79 p.

1147 journals of which approximately 50 per cent are medical or paramedical. See no. 2491.

2515
U.S. Library of Congress. Science Division. Scientific and technical serial publications, Soviet Union, 1945–1953. Washington, 1954. 118 p. (Monthly list of Russian accessions. Special supplement.)

2033 entries.

2516★
World list of scientific periodicals published in the years 1900–1960. Ed. by Peter Brown and George Burder Stratton. 4 ed. Washington, Butterworths, 1963. 3 v.

Both a bibliography of periodicals relating to science and a union list designed to show at least one location within the United Kingdom. 10,000 of the titles listed in the third edition have been omitted from this one because of their social or commercial character, but the list has grown from 50,000 to 60,000 titles.

Histories

Bibliographies

2517
Critical bibliography of the history of science and its cultural influences. In Isis 1, 1913– .

Classified, generally annotated, bibliography with separate name index for each number. Currently appears annually. A recent number (89th, *Isis* 55:475–605, 1964) contains about 2000 citations.

2518
History of science: an annual review of literature, research and teaching. Cambridge, 1, 1962– .

Each volume contains 8–15 survey articles and essay reviews, 7–15 shorter book reviews, brief notices of books, etc. Emphasis on British research, but intended to be international in scope. Ed. by Alistair C. Crombie and Michael A. Hoskin.

2519
John Crerar Library. A list of books on the history of science. Prepared by A. G. S. Josephson. Chicago, 1911. 297 p. Suppl., 1917, 139 p. 2d Suppl., pts. 1–6, 1942–46.

Classified, with author and subject index. Contents notes. Includes serial publications with analytics for monographs in series and a few articles.

2520
Russo, Franceso. Histoire des sciences et des techniques: bibliographie. Paris, Hermann, 1954. 186 p. (Actualités scientifiques et industrielles, 1204)

Classified bibliography: generalities; history by periods; histories of particular sciences.

2521
Sarton, George. Horus: a guide to the history of science. Waltham, Mass., Chronica Botanica, 1952. 316 p.

Standard guide to the literature. Introductory essays followed by bibliography of all phases of history of science. Frequently includes critical or descriptive notes. Also lists museums, societies, libraries, congresses, etc.

Encyclopedia

2522
Lexikon der Geschichte der Naturwissenschaften; Biographien, Sachwörter und Bibliographien. Mit . . . einer Übersichtstabelle. Von Joseph Mayerhöfer, unter Mitwirkung von E. Bannerth [et al.] Wien, Hollinek, 1959– .

Articles under subjects and under personal and geographical names, usually with extensive bibliographical references. Articles on persons list works and biographical and critical studies. Entries under cities list educational and scientific institutions, academies, and societies, with brief historical data, and also scientists with references to articles. Includes articles on philosophy, mathematics, and technology as well as the natural sciences. In progress.

Monographs

2523
Sarton, George. Introduction to the history of science. Baltimore, Williams & Wilkins, 1927–48. 3 v. in 5. (Carnegie Institution of Washington. Publication no. 376)

Exhaustive reference work covering science and learning in all major European and Oriental civilizations, from Homer to A. D. 1400. Presents surveys of successive periods followed by biographical sketches and bibliographies (editions, translations, critical studies) of persons related to science in its widest sense. Well indexed. General bibliography: v. 3, pt. 2, p. 1872–1911.

2524
Singer, Charles J. [et al.] ed. A history of technology. Oxford, Clarendon Press, 1954–58. 5 v.

Covers early times to late 19th century. Bibliographies at ends of chapters.

2525
Taton, René, ed. Histoire générale des sciences. Paris, Presses universitaires de France, 1957–64. 3 v. in 4.

By a large group of scholars. Bibliographies at ends of chapters or sections. English translation in progress (New York ed.: *History of science*; London ed.: *General history of the sciences*).

2526
Thorndike, Lynn. A history of magic and experimental science. New York, Macmillan, 1923–58. 8 v. (v. 3–8, Columbia University Press)

Summarizes work of hundreds of authors, 1st through 17th centuries. Includes extensive bibliographies and bibliographical footnotes.

2527
Thornton, John L., and Tully, R. I. J. Scientific books, libraries and collectors; a study of bibliography and the book trade in relation to science. 2 ed. London, Library Association, 1962. 406 p.

Describes briefly important books in the history of science, with running commentary on authors and works. Footnote references throughout, including many to critical studies and bibliographies. Bibliography of secondary works, by author, including journal articles, p. 318–373.

SOCIOLOGY

Indexes and Abstracts

2528
The sociology of medicine; a trend report and bibliography. Oxford, Blackwell, 196?. 192 p. (Current sociology, v. 10/11, no. 3, 1961–62)

622 abstracts. Includes books. Prepared for the International Sociological Association, with the support of UNESCO.

Title and other bibliographical data also in French.

Bibliographies

2529
California. University. Institute of Governmental Studies. The offender—a bibliography. Comp. by Dorothy C. Tompkins. Berkeley, 1963. 268 p.

Includes books, chapters in books, reports,

theses from the English-language literature published since 1937. Many nonmedical sources covered. Subject index not exhaustive.

Annotated bibliography of 316 entries, p. 76–187. Unannotated general bibliography arranged by author, p. 188–244. Includes books.

2530 (Not used)

2531
Szabo, Denis. La délinquence juvénile; étiologie et prophylaxie: tendences de la recherche et bibliographie (1945–1960). Amsterdam, North-Holland Pub. Co., 1963. 142 p.

856 annotated references. Includes books. Indexes a number of nonmedical journals. Geographical breakdown.

Added t.p.: Confluence; surveys of research in the social sciences. A series ed. by the International Committee for Social Science Documentation in cooperation with the International Social Science Council and with the support of UNESCO.

2532
U.S. National Clearinghouse for Mental Health Information. Crime and delinquency abstracts. Bethesda, 1, 1963– .

A considerable percentage of the journals, books, and reports indexed are not in standard medical indexes or *Psychological abstracts*.

Contains occasional special bibliographies (Prediction studies in criminology, v. 2, no. 1)

Abstracts included beginning with v. 3.

v. 1–3, 1963–65 as *International bibliography on crime and delinquency*.

With v. 3 *Current projects* section.

Dictionaries

2533
Gould, Julius, and Kolb, William L. A dictionary of the social sciences. Comp. under the auspices of the United Nations Educational, Scientific, and Cultural Organization. New York, Free Press of Glencoe, 1964. 761 p.

2534
Scott, Sir Harold Richard, ed. The concise encyclopedia of crime and criminals. London, Deutsch, 1961. 351 p.

Emphasis on English and American history and current practices of law. Includes medicolegal terms and biographies.

Directories

2535
American Sociological Association. Directory, 1963. Washington, 1963. 178 p.

Alphabetical list of fellows, active, and associate members, with address and current affiliation. Includes geographical listing, student members, and constitution and bylaws.

2536
NASW Directory of professional social workers. New York, [1] 1960– . National Association of Social Workers.

Alphabetical listing of members, giving name, position and employer, address, education, degrees, and section affiliation.

2537
U.S. National Clearinghouse for Mental Health Information. Current projects in the prevention, control, and treatment of crime and delinquency. v. 5, Summer 1964. 432 p. (Public Health Service. Publication no. 1292)

Contains report of 300 projects. With v. 6 continued by no. 2532.

2537.1
U.S. National Referral Center for Science and Technology. A directory of information resources in the United States. Social Sciences. Washington, 1965. 218 p.

Includes health and paramedical information centers.

SURGERY

Indexes and Abstracts

Current

2538★★
International abstracts of surgery. In Surgery, gynecology and obstetrics, Chicago, 16, 1913– . American College of Surgeons.

Monthly, 2 volumes a year. v. 118, Jan.–June 1964, includes 1611 abstracts.

1913–63 issued as a separately paged supplement to *Surgery, gynecology and obstetrics* with identical volume numbers (16–117). With v. 118, 1964, as a section in each issue paged continuously with the journal. Separate author and subject indexes to the abstracts. Minimum time lag 5 months.

2539
International surgical digest; a monthly abstract journal of current literature. Hagerstown, Md., W. F. Prior Co., 1, 1926– .

500–600 abstracts a year, mainly English-language literature. Currently contains a section Drug notes consisting of "Drug warnings".

Some volumes have added title on spine: *Lewis' Practice of surgery* or variation thereof.

2540
Nippon geka seikeigeka chuo zasshi [Japan review of surgery and plastic surgery] Osaka, 1, 1955– .

Abstracts of articles on plastic surgery from 194 Japanese journals.

2541★
Review of surgery. Philadelphia, etc., 1, 1943– .

1964 contained in excess of 600 abstracts. Book reviews listed separately. Beginning with v. 8, 1951, contains original or review articles.

v. 1–8, 1943–51, as *Quarterly review of surgery*; v. 9(1–2), Mar.–June, 1952, incorporated *Quarterly review of otorhinolaryngology and broncho-esophagology* and became *Quarterly review of surgery and surgical specialties*; v. 9(3)–18(1), Sept. 1952--Mar. 1961, incorporated *Quarterly review of obstetrics and gynecology* and became *Quarterly review of surgery, obstetrics and gynecology*; v. 18(2–4), Apr.–Dec. 1961, *Quarterly review of surgery*.

v. 8–10(1), 1951–March 1953: Incorporating the *International record of surgery* (original article section).

Issued 1943–51 by the Washington Institute of Medicine.

2542
Zentralorgan für die gesamte Chirurgie und ihre Grenzgebiete. Berlin, 1, 1913– . Published under supervision of the Deutsche Gesellschaft für Chirurgie.

Currently 3–4 volumes a year, each with 3 issues and a separate index issue. A recent volume had 1170 entries, most with abstracts. Includes books. Minimum time lag 3–4 months.

v. 1–6, 1913–14, as *Zentralblatt für die gesamte Chirurgie und ihre Grenzgebiete*; v. 7–17, 1920–22, had subtitle: Zugleich Fortsetzung des Hildebrand'schen Jahresbericht über die Fortschritte auf dem Gebiete der Chirurgie und des Glassner'schen Jahrbuchs für orthopädische Chirurgie. Suspended June 1914–Mar. 1920 and Apr. 1944–Aug. 1948.

See also no. 2545.

Noncurrent

2543
Abstracts of world surgery, gynaecology and obstetrics. London, 1–11, 1947–52. British Medical Association.

After June 1952 merged with no. 1.

2544
Centralblatt für Chirurgie. 1–70, 1874–1943.

Abstracts.

2545
Jahresbericht Chirurgie. Berlin, 1–43, 1895–1937.

Annual review volumes through v. 33, 1927, except v. 28, 30, 32, 1922, '24, '26, when it included references only. From v. 26–32, 1920–26, included a cumulation of the references abstracted in no. 2542. From v. 33–43, 1927–37, consisted of an annual cumulation of the references abstracted in no. 2542.

v. 1–25 as *Jahresbericht über die Fortschritte auf dem Gebiete der Chirurgie*; v. 26–32, 1920–26, as *Jahresbericht über die gesamte Chirurgie und ihre Grenzgebiete*. v. 26–32, 1920–26, had subtitle: Zugleich Bibliographisches Jahresregister des Zentralorgans für die gesamte Chirurgie und ihre Grenzgebiete, und Fortsetzung des Hildebrand'schen Jahresberichtes über die Fortschritte auf dem Gebiete der Chirurgie und des Glaessnerschen Jahrbuchs für orthopädische Chirurgie. v. 33–43, 1927–37, had subtitle: Bibliographisches Jahresregister des Zentralorgans für die gesamte Chirurgie und ihre Grenzgebiete.

2546 (Note used.)

Reviews

2547★★
Advances in surgery. New York, Interscience, 1–2, 1949.

2548
Advances in surgery. Chicago, Year Book Medical Publisher, 1, 1965– .

2549
Ergebnisse der Chirurgie und Orthopädie. Berlin, 1, 1910– .

2550
Geka kenkyu no shinpo [Recent advances in surgical research] Tokyo, 1, 1957– .

Irregular.

2551
Geka saikin no shinpo [Recent advances in surgery] Tokyo, 1, 1957– .

Biennial.

2552
Modern trends in surgery. Washington, 1, 1962– .

Covers areas of the field in which changes of emphasis are taking place or new techniques developing. Majority of contributors are British. Includes bibliographies.

2553
Progress in surgery. Progrès en chirurgie. Fortschritte der chirurgie. New York, Stechert-Hafner, 1961– .

2554
Recent advances in surgery. Ed. by Selwyn Taylor. 6 ed. London, Churchill, 1964. 438 p.

1 ed., 1928.

2554.1
A review of the literature on burns and trauma. In Medical Services Journal, Canada, v. 9(4), 1954– .

Annual. Selective review followed by bibliography. 1964/65 review listed 601 references. Random author arrangement under subject breakdown. Includes trauma from automobile accidents, sports; site and systems breakdown. No indexes.

v. 9(4)–11, 1954–55, as *A summary of the recent literature on burns and wounds;* v. 12–13, 1956–57, *A review of the literature on burns and wounds.*

v. 9, 1954, *Treatment services bulletin;* v. 10–13, 1955–57, *Canadian services medical journal.*

v. 9, 1954, reviews the literature for 1952/53.

2555★
Year book of general surgery. Chicago, Year Book Medical Publishers, 1901– . (The practical medicine year books)

Abstracts, with editorial comment. Special section: Selected references in surgery.

1901–32 as *General surgery.*

1901–05, 1932 as The practical medicine series of year books; 1906–31 as The practical medicine series.

Bibliographies

2556
Haller, Albrecht von. Bibliotheca chirurgica, qua scripta ad artem chirurgicam facientia a rerum initiis recensentur. Bernae, Haller, 1774–75. 2 v.

Similar in arrangement and method to no. 970. 1903 chapters devoted to individual authors or groups of authors; 39 p. of addenda. Indexes of authors and of anonymous works (by subject).

2557
Vigiliis von Creutzenfeld, Stephan Hieronymus de. Bibliotheca chirurgica in qua res omnes ad chirurgiam pertinentes ordine alphabetico, ipsi vero scriptores, quotquot ad annum usque MDCCLXXIX innotuerunt, ad singulas materias ordine chronologico exhibentur. Vindobonae, Trattner, 1781. 2 v.

Subject bibliography with many works analyzed in detail. Entries generally annotated. Author index.

Manuals

2558
Szulec, J. A. A syllabus for the surgeon's secretary. Detroit, Medical Arts Publishing Co., 1965. 431 p.

Lists laboratory tests and their significance, defines operative terms, lists surgical instruments. For each type of surgery gives anatomical considerations, describes surgical procedures and lists terms. Also lists prefixes and combining forms and abbreviations. Includes a glossary of operative titles. No shorthand.

Directories

2559
American College of Surgeons. Directory. Chicago, 1, 1913– .

Triennial with annual supplements. Gives officers, and geographical and alphabetical lists of fellows with brief professional information including specialty, school attended, societies, and specialty boards to which certified. Cumulative necrology. Issued as *Yearbook*, 1913–52;

2560
Chirurgenverzeichnis. Berlin [etc.], 1, 1920– .

Alphabetical list of surgeons in Germany, Austria, and Switzerland. Biographical and professional data with bibliographies. Includes a list of directors of University surgical clinics in the same countries.

1 ed., 1920, and 2 ed., 1926, have title: *Deutscher Chirurgenkalendar*; 3 ed., 1938, *Deutsches Chirurgen-Verzeichnis*, 4 ed., 1958.

2561
International College of Surgeons. Directory. Chicago, 1, 1960?– .

Gives alphabetical and geographical listing for the United States and other countries. Brief professional information and address.

Histories

2562
Bishop, William J. The early history of surgery, London, Hale, 1960, 192 p.

Covers from prehistory to late 19th century. References "For further reading" at end of each chapter.

2563
Brunn, Walter von. Kurze Geschichte der Chirurgie. Berlin, Springer, 1928. 339 p.

Classified bibliography: p. 309–327.

2564
Davis, Loyal. Fellowship of surgeons. A history of the American College of Surgeons. Springfield, Ill., Thomas, 1960. 523 p.

Narrative history, important for surgery in U.S. in 20th century. No bibliography, few references.

2565
Earle, Arthur Scott, ed. Surgery in America: from the colonial era to the twentieth century. Selected writings. Philadelphia, Saunders, 1965. 280 p.

Papers or extracts from the writings of 24 surgeons to 1900, with brief historical introductions. Selected bibliography (43 items, secondary): p. 271–274.

2566
Gurlt, Ernst J. Geschichte der Chirurgie und ihrer Ausübung: Volkschirurgie, Alterthum, Mittelalter, Renaissance. Berlin, Hirschwald, 1898. 3 v.

Exhaustive history through the 16th century. Contains biographies, bibliographies of authors cited, discussions of their work, and often extracts from their writings. Glossary of terms. Reprinted Hildesheim, Olms, 1964.

2567
Hurwitz, Alfred, and Degensheim, George A. Milestones in modern surgery. New York, Hoeber-Harper, 1958. 520 p.

Selected writings from 19th and 20th centuries, with brief sketches of authors.

2568
Killian, Hans, and Krämer, G. Meister der Chirurgie und die Chirurgenschulen im deutschen Raum: Deutschland, Österreich, deutsche Schweiz. Stuttgart, Thieme, 1951. 231 p.

Brief historical introduction, followed by histories of schools with biographies of professors, mostly 19th and 20th centuries. Bibliography: p. 225–226. Name index only.

2569
Pazzini, Adalberto. Bio-bibliografia di storia della chirurgia. Roma, Edizioni Cosmopolita, 1948. 524 p.

Pt. 1, p. 21–333, biobibliographical notices of 475 surgeons from Hippocrates to Harvey Cushing, arranged by periods and nationalities. Pt. 2, p. 337–494, descriptive author catalog of an exhibition of 289 works. No index.

2570
Plarr, Victor G. Lives of the fellows of the Royal College of Surgeons of England. Rev. by Sir D'Arcy Power . . . W. G. Spencer and G. E. Gask. Bristol, Wright, 1930. 2 v.

Biographies of deceased fellows from the foundation in 1843, in alphabetical order. Some sketches very short, others quite extensive. Include lists of publications, occasional citations of biographical sources. Continued by Sir D'Arcy Power and William R. LeFanu, *Lives of the fellows, 1930–1951*, London, The College, 1953, 889 p.

2571
Power, Sir D'Arcy, ed. A mirror for surgeons; selected readings in surgery. Boston, Little, Brown, 1939. 230 p.

Extracts, with historical notes and citations of sources, from outstanding contributions to surgery, from Arderne to J. Marion Sims. All English or American, except Paré. No index.

2572
Sudhoff, Karl. Beiträge zur Geschichte der Chirurgie im Mittelalter: graphische und textliche Untersuchungen in mittelalterlichen Handschriften. Leipzig, Barth, 1914–18. 2 v. (Studien zur Geschichte der Medizin, v. 10–11/12)

Detailed studies of special aspects. Includes texts in Latin and German.

2573
Thompson, Charles J. S. The history and evolution of surgical instruments. New York, Schuman, 1942. 113 p.

Brief accounts of different types of instruments. No bibliography.

2574
Valle, Rafael H. La cirugía mexicana del siglo XIX. México, Tipográfica Sag, 1942. xcvi, 349 p.

History of surgery, including universities, hospitals, and local history: p. xi-xcvi, with bibliographical references, p. xci-xcvi. Bibliography of books and articles, by author: p. 3–237. Biographical notices: p. 237–280. Chronology 1520–1942: p. 280–293. List of hospitals and scientific societies, with founding dates: p. 294–296.

2575
Zimmerman, Leo M., and Veith, Ilza. Great ideas in the history of surgery. Baltimore, Williams & Wilkins, 1961. 587 p.

Biographical sketches and extensive extracts from works of leading surgeons, from antiquity to present. Bibliography: p. 548–559.

Surgical Specialties

Burns

2576
Blocker, T. G., Jr., and Blocker, Virginia. Burns bibliography, 1952–1962. Galveston, University of Texas, Medical Branch, Dept. of Surgery, [1963] 323 p. (USPHS contract no. 86-62-185, June 25, 1962–June 24, 1963)

933 entries, selectively annotated. Emphasis on civil defence aspects.

Cardiac

2576.1
General Dynamics Corporation. Convair Division. Kardiak Mediterm Bibliography. [n.p., n.d.] 438 p.

Approximately 2500 references relating to research for an artificial heart study program.

2577
Modern trends in cardiac surgery. New York, 1960– . (Hoeber's Modern trends series)

Reviews current practice and future possibilities. Includes bibliographies. All contributors are British.

2578
United Aircraft Corporation. Hamilton Standard Division. Bibliography and references for studies basic to consideration of artificial heart research and development program. Final report. [n.p.] 1966. 125 p. (Report no. SVHSER 3871, Feb. 11, 1966)

1350 references. Entries 1–164 are from the *Trans Amer Soc Artif Intern Organs*, v. 6–11, 1960–65; entries from *Trans* . . . v. 4–5, 1958–59, appear elsewhere throughout the bibliography; entries 854–1195 consist of a MEDLARS search; the remaining entries consist of references from other sources.

To be used in conjunction with Report no. SVHSER 3870 (the text of the final report). Reports submitted to the U.S. National Heart Institute.

Neurosurgery

2579
Zentralblatt für Neurochirurgie. Leipzig, 1, 1936– .

6 numbers a year. Long review articles and abstracts. Suspended 1944–48.

HISTORIES

2580
Sachs, Ernest. The history and development of neurological surgery. New York, Hoeber, 1952. 158 p. (Yale University. School of Medicine. Department of the History of Medicine. Publication no. 29)

From prehistoric to contemporary times. Bibliography (515 items, including sources and secondary works): p. 107–143.

2581
Walker, Arthur Earl, ed. A history of neurological surgery. Baltimore, Williams & Wilkins, 1951. 583 p.

18 chapters by different authors on various phases. Includes some biographical sketches. Bibliography (2371 references to works cited, alphabetical by author): p. 459–561.

Pediatric

2582
Recent advances in paediatric surgery. Ed. by A. W. Wilkinson. Boston, Little, 1963. 306 p.

Chapter bibliographies (omitting titles of articles). No over-all author index.

Published in England by Churchill.

Plastic Surgery

INDEXES AND ABSTRACTS

2582.1
Index of literature on plastic surgery, 1950– . In British journal of plastic surgery (Edinburgh) 4(2), 1951– .

2583★
International abstracts of plastic and reconstructive surgery. In Plastic and reconstructive surgery, 2, 1947– .

2584
Resumenes internacionales de cirugía plástica. In Revista latino americana de cirurgía plástica, 1–4, 1953–59.

Abstracts usually as a separately paged section of the *Revista.* Items not abstracted are listed under the section Temas de cirugia plastica en la literatura mundial.

REVIEWS

2585
Modern trends in plastic surgery. Washington, 1, 1964– .

Irregular. Includes reviews with bibliographies.

2586
Wiederherstellungschirurgie und Traumatologie. Reconstruction surgery and traumatology. Chirurgie repartrice et traumatologie. Basel, Karger, 1, 1953– .

Irregular.

HISTORIES

2587
Maltz, Maxwell. Evolution of plastic surgery. New York, Froben Press, 1946. 368 p.

Survey from antiquity to 1944. Includes biographical sketches with some references to works. Chronology (5000 B.C.–1945): p. 329–359. No bibliography.

2588
Zeis, Eduard. Die Literatur und Geschichte der plastischen Chirurgie. Leipzig, Engelmann, 1863. 299 p. Nachträge. 1864. 52 p.

Classified and annotated bibliography of 2008 items, including monographs, analytic entries, and articles, often citing reviews: p. 1–182. History (mainly 15th–19th centuries): p. 183–290. Index of names and anonymous titles. Supplement includes notes, corrections, and about 150 additional items.

Thoracic

HISTORIES

2589
Meade, Richard H. A history of thoracic surgery. Springfield, Ill., Thomas, 1961. 933 p.

Topical arrangement. Extensive lists of references at ends of chapters.

Transplantation

2590
[Transplantation bibliographies] In Transplantation. Bibliography Section. Baltimore, 1, 1963– .

Bibliographies (most continuing) on special aspects, the latest for each subject being: *Bibliography of tumor transplantation.* Addendum 9. Items 2376–2631 (covering Jan.-Dec. 1964), v. 4(2), 1966; *Bibliography of cartilage transplantation.* Addendum 11. Items 1100–1241 (covering 1963–64), v. 4(2), 1966; *Bibliography of corneal transplantation . . .* Items 2004–2253 (covering 1961–63), v. 3(2), 1965; *Bibliography of lung transplantation.* Items

1-87 (covering 1950-64), v. 3(2), 1965; *Bibliography of kidney transplantation.* Addendum 4. Items 253-427 (covering 1963-64), v. 3(2), 1965; *Bibliography of brephoplastic transplantation.* Addendum 2. Items 185-288 (covering 1955-64), v. 3(4), 1965; *Bibliography of hematopoietic tissue transplantation.* Addendum 2. Items 236-1051 (covering 1960-64), v. 3(6), 1965; *Bibliography of tooth replantation.* Addendum 1. Items 180-215 (covering 1958-62), v. 2(2), 1964; *Bibliography of foreign substance implants in reconstructive surgery.* Addendum 2. Items 2188-2372 (covering 1960-62), v. 2(2), 1964; *Bibliography of liver transplantation.* Addendum 1. Items 68-112 (covering 1959-63), v. 2(3), 1964; *Bibliography of transplantation of chorioallantoic placenta and trophoblast.* Items 1-113 (covering 1893-1962), v. 2(4), 1964; *Bibliography of bone transplantation.* Addendum 6. Items 607-806 (covering 1961-63), v. 2(5), 1964; *Bibliography of parathyroid gland transplantation.* Items 1-88 (covering 1892-1961), v. 1(2), 1963; *Bibliography of recent tissue transplantation literature of the Central and East European countries.* Addendum 3. Items 1-566 (covering 1957-59), v. 1(4), 1963.

Continues bibliographies in *Transplantation bulletin*, 1-30, 1954-62.

v. 21-30, 1958-62, of *Transplantation bulletin* also published in *Plastic and reconstructive surgery and the Transplantation bulletin.*

Traumatic

2591
Bibliografiia sovetskoĭ travmatologii [Bibliography of Soviet traumatology] Leningrad, 1, 1933- .

Irregular. v. 17, 1957, covering the literature for 1948, contains 1518 entries.

2592
Cantor, Paul D., ed. Traumatic medicine and surgery for the attorney. Washington, Butterworths, 1959-64. 10 v.

Contains chapter bibliographies. Subject index to each volume. v. 10, master index, includes popular medical terms with cross-references.

2593
Modern trends in accident surgery and medicine. London, 1959- . (Butterworths medical publications. Modern trends series).

Reviews with bibliographies.

Anesthesia

Indexes and Abstracts

2593.1
Anaesthetic literature. In Anaesthesia (London) 6(2), 1951- .

Quarterly. English language journals only. Annotations.

2594
Anesthesia abstracts. Minneapolis, 1, 1937- .

Currently 2-3 volumes a year each with 250 abstracts selected from approximately 70 journals, mainly English language. Arrangement is alphabetical by author with subject index. Minimum time lag 7 months.

2594.1
Anesthesia digest. Cleveland, 1-8(7), 1950-July 1957.

Monthly. Abstracts. Mainly English language literature.

2595
Referátový výběr z anestesiologie [Selected abstracts on anesthesiology] Praha, 1, 1954- . Ústav pro zdravotnickou dokumentaci.

4 issues a year. Abstracts in Czech or Slovak of selected articles from foreign periodicals, chiefly in western languages.

2596★
Survey of anesthesiology. Baltimore, 1, 1957- .

Bimonthly. 300-400 abstracts a year, mainly English language.

Reviews

2597
Appraisal of current concepts in anesthesiology. St. Louis, Mosby, 1, 1961- .

Chapter bibliographies. No over-all author index. v. 2, 1964.

2598
Modern trends in anesthesia. London, 1, 1958- .

Irregular. Includes reviews with bibliographies. Ser. 2 published 1962.

2599
Recent advances in anesthesia and analgesia. 9 ed. Ed. by C. Langton Hewer. London, Churchill, 1963. 358 p.

Chapter bibliographies (omitting titles of articles). No over-all author index. 1 ed., 1932; 8 ed., 1958.

2600★
Year book of anesthesia. Chicago, Year Book Medical Publishers, 1963/64– . (The practical medicine year books)

Abstracts, with editorial comment. 1901–1962/63 part of no. 2555.

Bibliographies

2601
Harkányi, István. Magyar aneszteziológiai bibliográfia (1945–1960) [Bibliography of Hungarian anesthesiology (1945–1960] Budapest, Országos Orvostudományi Könyvtár és Dokumentációs Központ, 1961. 71 p.

2602
Sadove, Max S., and Wallace, Vernon E. Halothane. Philadelphia, Davis, 1962. 1 v. (various pagings)

Sect. 1, subject review; sect. 2, abstracts on halothane, arranged by author under year, mainly 1956–60.

Directories

2603★
American Society of Anesthesiologists. Directory of members. Chicago, [1] 1942– .

Alphabetical listing with address and very brief professional information; geographical listing. Includes some foreign anesthetists.

2603.1
Frey, Rudolf, and Kronschwitz, H. Verzeichnis der Fachärzte für Anaesthesiologie in Deutschland, Österreich und in der Schweiz. Berlin, Springer, 1966. 229 p.

Brief professional and personal information; includes publications.

Histories

2604
Cole, Frank. Milestones in anesthesia: readings in the development of surgical anesthesia, 1665–1940. Lincoln, University of Nebraska Press, 1965. 290 p.

45 selections, in English, with brief introductions.

2605
Davison, Meredith Henry Armstrong. The evolution of anesthesia. Altrincham, Sherratt, 1965. 236 p.

From antiquity on. Chronology (p. 23–109), followed by chapters on special topics. References in text; no bibliography.

2606
Duncum, Barbara M. The development of inhalation anesthesia, with special reference to the years 1846–1900. London, Cumberlege, Oxford University Press, 1947. 640 p. (Wellcome Historical Medical Museum. Publications. New ser., no. 2)

Thorough study, with ample references in footnotes.

2607
Ellis, Edgar S. Ancient anodynes; primitive anaesthesia and allied conditions. London, Heinemann, 1946. 187 p.

From ancient times through the mid-19th century, including data on primitive cultures, the Orient, and pre-Columbian America; with chapters on special drugs. References (by chapters): p. 168–180.

2608
Faulconer, Albert, and Keys, Thomas E., ed. Foundations of anesthesiology. Springfield, Ill., Thomas, 1965. 2 v.

Selected readings from sources, in English, with brief biographies of authors and citations to original printing. Arranged by topics.

2609
Fulton, John F., and Stanton, Madeline E. The centennial of surgical anesthesia; an annotated catalogue of books and pamphlets bearing on the early history of surgical anesthesia, exhibited at Yale Medical Library, October, 1946. New York, Schuman, 1946. 101 p. (Yale University. School of Medicine. Library. Historical Library. Publication no. 15.)

466 items, including original and secondary works, topically arranged, with historical introductions. Detailed annotations for important works.

2610
Keys, Thomas E. The history of surgical anesthesia, with an introductory essay by

Chauncey D. Leake. New York, Dover, 1963. 193 p.

Survey with extensive references (p. 93–176; 762 items in three sections). 1 ed., 1945.

THERAPEUTICS

Indexes and Abstracts

2610.1
Bibliographies on diseases of medical progress. In Clinical pharmacology and therapeutics, 2(4), 1961– .

Irregular. Selected abstracts from author arranged bibliographies. Currently each bibliography on a special subject: Reactions to tetracycline, Disorders produced by progestational agents, Reactions to phenothiazines and related drugs (1966) No indexes.

v. 2(4), 1961, as *Diseases of medical progress: Progress report;* v. 3(2)–6(6), 1962–65, *Diseases of medical progress: Present status.* Robert H. Moser, compiler.

Keeps current no. 2616.

2610.2
Cahiers de bibliographie thérapeutique française. Paris, 1, 1962– . Centre d'Études de Documentation et de Recherches.

Monthly. Abstracts from (1966) 103 French journals.

2611
Jahrbuch der gesamten Therapie; eine Referatesammlung für die ärztliche Praxis. Berlin, 1953– .

1962 contains about 2000 abstracts from some 180 German-language journals. Special book review section.

2612
Novità terapeutiche. Firenze, 1938– .

Annual. Abstracts.

2613
Progresos de terapéutica clínica. Madrid, 1, 1948– .

Quarterly. Abstracts. Includes original and review articles. No author index.

Reviews

2613.1
Advances in treatment. In Practitioner (Lond), 139, 1937– .

A special number (October). Review of all fields. Not as closely related to the past year as no. 115.

1937–38 as *Advances in diagnosis and treatment.*

2614
Anuario de progresos terapeuticos en medicina interna. Buenos Aires, 1,1947– .

2615
Ergebnisse der physikalisch-diätetischen Therapie. Dresden, 1, 1939– .

Irregular.

2616
Moser, Robert H. Diseases of medical progress. A contemporary analysis of illness produced by drugs and other therapeutic procedures. 2 ed. Springfield, Ill., Thomas, 1964. 543 p.

Literature reviews. Includes radiation-induced and surgically induced diseases. Kept current by no. 2610.1

2616.1
Year book of general therapeutics. Chicago, Year Book Publishers, 1902–48. (The practical medicine year books)

Critical reviews.

1902 as *Materia medica and therapeutics; preventive medicine; climatology; forensic medicine;* 1903–05 . . . *climatology, suggestive therapeutics, forensic medicine;* 1911–15, *Materia medica and therapeutics, preventive medicine, climatology;* 1916, *Materia medica and therapeutics, preventive medicine, climatology;* 1916, *Materia medica and therapeutics . . . preventive medicine;* 1917–23, *Pharmacology and therapeutics . . . preventive medicine;* 1924–32, *General therapeutics.*

1906–10, suspended?

1902–05 and 1932 as Practical medicine series of year books; 1911–31, Practical medicine series.

Continued by no. 2168.1

2617
Yearbook of treatment. London, Cassell, 1884–99.

Subtitle: A critical review for practitioners of medicine and surgery. Merged into no. 121.

Bibliographies

2617.1
Baer, Karl A., and Spencer, Marjory. The

pituitary-adrenocortical function: ACTH, cortisone and related compounds; a bibliography. Washington, 1950. 366 p.

Lists 3447 references.

At head of title: Army Medical Library.

2618
Bethlehem Corporation. Hyperbaric Oxygen Therapy Division. Hyperbaric oxygenation bibliography through December 1963. Bethlehem, Pa., [1964] [7] p.

273 references from 1899. Kept up to date with monthly supplements.

2619
Linde Air Products Company. Bibliography on oxygen therapy. Rev. ed. New York, 1947. 99 p. Suppl. no. 1, 1953. 91 p.

Lists nearly 10,500 articles by author with subject classification indicated.

2619.1
Merck and Co., Inc. Hydrocortisone and cortisone. Rahway, N.J., 1956. 186 p. (Merck service bulletin)

Selected annotated bibliography of 208 entries, mainly from 1953. Includes review chapters with bibliographies.

2620
Skorodinskaia, V.V. [et al.] Bibliograficheskiĭ ukazatel' otechestvennoĭ literatury po tkanevoĭ terapii [Bibliographic index to national literature on tissue therapy] Odessa, Ukrainskiĭ eksper. institut glaznykh bolezneĭ, 1956. 165 p.

Lists 1279 references, from 1933 to Nov. 1955. Includes books. In ten groups; arranged alphabetically by author in 7 groups, chronologically in 3. In Russian.

2621
Vaponefrin inhalation therapy library. Upper Darby, Pa., 1, 1948– .

v. 1 abstracts 108 references covering 1935 through 1948. v. 2, 1948/58, selective review of 365 references.

v. 1 as *Vaponefrin aerosol library.*

2622
Waring, Edward J. Bibliotheca therapeutica; or, Bibliography of therapeutics, chiefly in reference to articles of the materia medica, with numerous critical, historical, and therapeutical annotations, and an appendix containing the bibliography of British mineral waters. London, 1878–79. 2 v. (New Sydenham Society. [Publications] v. 77, 82)

Pt. 1, General treatises (classified). Pt. 2, Articles of materia medica, arranged alphabetically. About 10,000 citations. Indexes of diseases, authors, and subjects.

2623
Williams, Robert L., and Webb, Wilse B. Sleep therapy; a bibliography and commentary. Springfield, Thomas, 1966. 112 p.

761 references, 1950–60.

Dictionaries

2623.1
China (People's Republic) Wei shêng pu [Ministry of Health] Chih liao hsüeh ming tz'ŭ [Glossary of therapeutic terms] Peking, 1954. 77 p.

Chinese-English, English-Chinese.

Histories

2624
Brockbank, William. Ancient therapeutic arts. London, Heinemann, 1954. 162 p. (Fitzpatrick Lectures, 1950–51)

Enema administration, cupping and leeching, counter-irritation, and intravenous injection. References at end of each section.

UROLOGY

Indexes and Abstracts

Current

2624.1
Index to current urological literature. In British journal of urology. 1, 1929– .

First issue as *Index medicus.*

2625★
Urological survey. Baltimore, 1, 1945– .

Bimonthly. About 500 abstracts a year from English-language literature. Occasional collective reviews and book reviews are included.

Noncurrent

2626
Jahresbericht Urologie. Berlin, 1–11, 1921–31.

v. 1–2, 1921–22, v. 4, 1924, v. 6, 1928, contain references and literature reviews, the other volumes references only.

v. 1–6, 1921–28, had subtitle: Zugleich bibliographisches Jahresregister der Zeitschrift für urologische Chirurgie und Fortsetzung des urologischen Jahresberichtes [von Kollmann-Jackoby, v. 2–6]; v. 7–11, 1927–31, Bibliographisches . . . See no. 2629.

Continues no. 2628

2627
Quarterly review of urology. Washington, 1–5, 1946–50. Washington Institute of Medicine.

2628
Urologischer Jahresbericht; einschliesslich der Erkrankungen des männlichen Genitalapparates. Berlin, 1–9, 1905–13.

Annual review. Articles, dissertations, and books, listed by author under subjects and then summarized. v. 3 has about 1500 abstracts.

v. 1–5, 1905–09, as *Jahresbericht über die Leistungen und Fortschritte auf dem Gebiete der Erkrankungen des Urogenitalapparates.*

2629
Zeitschrift für Urologie und Gynäkologie. Referate. Berlin, 7–47, 1921–44.

Includes abstracts of dissertations and books.

v. 7–41, 1921–36, as *Zeitschrift für urologische Chirurgie. Referate.* For annual cumulation of references see no. 2626.

Reviews

2630
Modern trends in urology. London, 1, 1953– . (Butterworths medical publications. Modern trends series.)

2631
Review of urologic surgery, 1919/23–1947/47. In Archives of surgery, 8–60, 1924–50.

88 articles reviewed in v. 60.

The first review as Excerpts from articles on urologic surgery, with comments.

2632★
Year book of urology. Chicago, Year Book Medical Publishers, 1932– . (The practical medicine year books)

Abstracts, with editorial comment. 1932 as *Urology.* Formerly a part of no. 1353. 1932 as Practical medicine series of year books.

Bibliographies

2633
Inasaridze, Georgiĭ Zakharevich. Bibliograficheskiĭ ukazatel' otechestvennoĭ urologii i smezhnykh oblasteĭ za 100 let (1855–1955) [Bibliographical index to the national literature on urology and adjacent fields during 100 years, 1855–1955] Tbilisi, Sabchota Sakartvelo, 1959–62. 4 v.

More than 20,600 references, including books.

2634
Rényi-Vámos, Ference, ed. A magyar urológiai irodalom bibliográfiája [Bibliography of Hungarian literature on urology] Budapest, Orvostudomànyi Dokumentációs Központ, 1959. 386 p.

3567 references, including books, covering 1670–1958. Includes literature published in Hungary or by Hungarian authors abroad. Chronological subarrangement.

Histories

2635
American Urological Association. History of urology. Baltimore, Williams & Wilkins, 1933. 2 v.

A collection of historical papers on various aspects of urology. No index. Useful chiefly for America and for modern history. Lists of references, some extensive, at ends of essays.

2636
Bitschai, J., and Brodny, M. Leopold. A history of urology in Egypt. Cambridge, Mass., Riverside Press, 1956. 122 p.

Emphasis on ancient and medieval periods.

2637
Desnos, Ernest. Histoire de l'urologie. Paris, Doin, 1914. 294 p.

From ancient times through the 19th century. Bibliography: p. 291–294. Separate, from the *Encyclopédie française d'urologie*, v. 1.

2638
Viellard, Camille. L'urologie et les médecines urologiques dans la médecine ancienne. Gilles de Corbeil: sa vie, ses oeu-

vres, son poème des urines. Paris, Rudeval. 1903. 390 p.

Covers antiquity to 18th century, but emphasizes Middle Ages. Bibliography: p. 379–384.

VETERINARY MEDICINE

Entries in this field are more selective than for most other subjects.

Indexes and Abstracts

Current

2639
Accumulative veterinary index; a selective list of publications from the American literature. Arvada, Col., Index Incorporated, 1, 1960/63– .

2640
Index veterinarius. Waybridge, Surrey, 1, 1933– . Commonwealth Bureau of Animal Health.

Quarterly. About 20,000 references a year from nearly 1000 periodicals. Includes books.

2641
Die Veterinärmedizin. Konstance, 1, 1948– .

Bimonthly. Abstracts. Includes books, dissertations.

2642
Veterinary bulletin, Farnham Royal, Eng., etc., 1, 1931– . Prep. by the Commonwealth Bureau of Animal Health.

Monthly. 1962 contained 4450 abstracts. Includes books, book reviews, reports. 1931–47 prepared by the Imperial Bureau of Animal Health.

2643
Was gibt es Neues für den praktischen Tierarzt? Hanover, 1942/48– .

Annual. Abstracts. No author index.

Noncurrent

2644
Jahresbericht Veterinär-medizin. Berlin, 1–71, 1881–1943.

Abstracts.

1–37, 1881–1917, as *Jahresbericht über die Leistungen auf dem Gebiete der Veterinär-Medizin*; 38–47, 1918–27, as *Ellenberger-Schütz Jahresbericht . . . .*

With v. 51(?), 1930(?) had subtitle: Zugleich Referatenteil zum Archiv für wissenschaftliche und praktische Tierheilkunde.

General-Register v. 1–15, 1881–95.

Reviews

2645
Advances in veterinary science. New York, Academic Press, 1, 1953– .

Irregular.

2646
Year book of veterinary medicine. Chicago, Year Book Medical Publishers, 1, 1963– . (The practical medicine year books)

Bibliographies

2647
Internationale veterinärmedizinische Literatur. Berlin, Paul Parey, 1963. 131 p.

1178 references. Title also in English, French, and Italian.

2648
Rühlmann, Dorothee. Bibliographie des deutschsprachigen Schrifttums zur Erforschung und Bekämpfung von anzeigepflichtigen Tierseuchen; eine Zusammenstellung der von 1935–1956 erschienenen Monographien, Dissertationen und Zeitschriftenaufsätze. Leipzig, Hirzel, 1960. 482 p. (Sachsen-Anhalt. Universitäts- und Landesbibliothek, Halle. Schriften zum Bibliotheks-und Büchereiwesen in Sachsen-Anhalte. no. 17)

7111 references.

2649
Schützler, Günther [et al.] Bibliographie der Veterinärmedizin und ihrer Grenzgebiete, 1943–1947. Monographien, Hochschulschriften und Zeitschriftenaufsätze aus Deutschland, Österreich und der Schweiz. Berlin, Trenkel, 1965. 855 p.

About 10,000 entries. Preface contains brief history of veterinary medicine bibliography in Germany.

Dictionaries

2650
Kruger, Gerhard, ed. Veterinarmedizi-

nische Terminologie. 2 ed. Leipzig, Hirzel, 1961. 534 p.

Includes technical terms of anatomy, histology, embryology, and drugs.

2651
Miller, William C., and West, Geoffrey P., ed. Black's Veterinary dictionary. 7 ed. London, Black, 1964. 1017 p.

Inclusive dictionary similar to *Black's Medical dictionary*; has encyclopedic features; includes symptoms, causes, and treatment of diseases; gives derivations of some terms.

2652
Schulz, Herbert E. Vocabularium medicinale polyglotte. Halle/Westf., Deutsches Nomenklatur Archiv, 1963. 1 v. (various pagings)

Lists in parallel columns terms in human and veterinary medicine and dentistry in English, German, Italian, Spanish, and Russian. Emphasis is on veterinary medicine.

2653
Villemin, Martial, comp. Dictionaire des termes vétérinaires et zootechniques. Paris, Vogot Frères, 1963. 352 p.

Concise dictionary of terms.

Nomenclature

2654
U.S. National Cancer Institute. Standard nomenclature of veterinary diseases and operations. 1 ed. rev. Bethesda, Md., 1966. 622 p. (Public Health Service. Publication no. 1466)

Contains code numbers. Classifications by topography, etiology, and operative procedure.

Directories

2655
American Veterinary Medical Association. Directory. Chicago, etc., 1924– .

22 biennial ed., 1966, lists 21,051 veterinarians. Arrangement is geographical with professional data given in code. Also contains information on veterinary medical associations, specialty boards, accredited colleges, digest of veterinary practice acts. Includes Canada and some foreign countries.

1924–37 as *Membership directory*.

2656
The Register of veterinary surgeons, and the supplementary veterinary register. London, Royal College of Veterinary Surgeons, 1884– .

Annual. An alphabetical list of veterinary surgeons, giving date admitted to membership, other academic qualifications. Geographical lists of members in general practice by countries, etc. Sections on government departments, schools, research institutions, and the Royal College of Veterinary Surgeons fellows.

2656.1
Tierärzte Adressbuch für die Deutsche Bundesrepublik und West-Berlin. 5 ed. Hannover, Brucke-Verlag, 1966. 475 p.

Gives organization and members of veterinary institutions and societies. Geographical and name listing of veterinarians.

2657
World directory of veterinary schools. Geneva, [1] 1963– . Published under the auspices of the Food and Agriculture Organization of the United Nations and the World Health Organization.

Arranged alphabetically by country. Gives general information on curriculum, examinations and license, followed by list of schools, with specific information as to enrollment, graduates, and fees.

Periodicals

2658
U.S. National Agricultural Library. Veterinary medical periodicals currently received... Washington, 1963. 10 p. (Library list no. 76)

Lists 136 journals alphabetically by country. Data supplied for each entry include title, publisher, address, frequency, and price.

Histories

2659
Froehner, Reinhard. Kulturgeschichte der Tierheilkunde. Ein Handbuch für Tierärzte und Studierende. Konstanz, Terra Verlag, 1952– .

v. 1, antiquity; v. 2, Germany; v. 3 to be other countries. Extensive biographic and bibliographic data in text.

2660
Leclainche, Emmanuel. Histoire de la médecine vétérinaire. Toulouse, Office du Livre, 1936. 812 p.

General survey through the Renaissance, followed by extensive account of schools, institutions, organizations, etc., general and by country, including U.S. Some references in footnotes and in preface, p. 3–6. Detailed table of contents, but no index.

2661
Merillat, Louis A., and Campbell, Delwin M. Veterinary military history of the United States; with a brief record of the development of veterinary education, practice, organization and legislation. Sponsored by the American Veterinary Medical Association. Chicago, Veterinary Magazine Corp., 1935. 2 v.

Detailed study, with an introductory chapter on general veterinary history. "Veterinary literature" (v. 1. p. 423–448) includes lists of veterinary works by American authors, 1861–1900, of English works published in the U.S., of works translated and published in the U.S., and of popular works; also a survey of veterinary periodicals and society publications. List of army veterinarians, with dates of service: v. 2, p. 977–1129.

2662
Neumann, Louis G. Biographies vétérinaires. Paris, Asselin et Houzeau, 1896. 443 p.

Biobibliographical dictionary. 767 entries.

2663
Schrader, Georg W. Biographisch-literarisches Lexicon der Thierärzte aller Zeiten und Länder, sowie der Naturforscher, Ärzte, Landwirthe, Stallmeister u. s. w., welche sich um die Thierheilkunde verdient gemacht haben. Ed. by Eduard Hering. Stuttgart, Ebner & Seubert, 1863. 490 p.

2001 numbered biobibliographical entries.

2664
Smith, Sir Frederick. The early history of veterinary literature and its British development. London, Baillière, Tindall and Cox, 1919–33. 4 v.

Approach primarily biographical, with accounts of work, bibliographies of writers.

2665
Smithcors, James F. The American veterinary profession. Ames, Iowa State University Press, 1963. 704 p.

Lacks bibliography or documentation.

2666
——. Evolution of the veterinary art; a narrative account to 1850. Kansas City, Mo., Veterinary Medicine Publ. Co., 1957. 408 p.

General survey. Classified bibliography: p. 392–398.

2667
Windisch, Wilhelm. Titelbibliographie der deutschsprachigen Veterinärhistorik, 1900–1957. [München, Uni-Druck, 1957] 144 p.

Classified list of journal articles and monographs. No index.

From the Institut für Staatsveterinärmedizin und Geschichte der Tiermedizin der Tierärztlichen Fakultät der Universität München.

WRITING, PREPARATION OF MANUSCRIPTS, ETC.

Monographs

2668
American Medical Association. Division of Scientific Publications. Style book and editorial manual. Chicago, 1965. 106 p.

2669
Craddock, F. W. Dental writing; notes on the anatomy and pathology of English composition for dentists. Bristol, Wright, 1962. 90 p.

2670
Cross, Louis M. The preparation of medical literature. Philadelphia, Lippincott, 1959. 451 p.

2671
Davidson, Henry A. Guide to medical writing; a practical manual for physicians, dentists, nurses, pharmacists. New York, Ronald, 1957. 338 p.

2671.1
Eshom, Myreta. Medical secretary's manual. New York, Appleton, 1966. 506 p.

Definition of medical terms, with shorthand rendition of terms.

2672
Fishbein, Morris. Medical writing; the technique and art. 3 ed. New York, McGraw-Hill, 1957. 262 p.

2673
Hewitt, Richard M. The physician-writer's book. Philadelphia, Saunders, 1957. 415 p.

2674
Huber, Jack T. Report writing in psychology and psychiatry. New York, Harper, 1961. 114 p.

2675
Klopfer, Walter G. The psychological report; use and communication of psychological findings. New York, Grune and Stratton, 1960. 146 p.

2676
Root, Kathleen Berger, and Byers, Edward E. The medical secretary; terminology and transcription with previews in Gregg shorthand simplified. 2 ed. New York, McGraw-Hill, 1960. 376 p.

Terms, divided by subject, include pronunciation, definition, and shorthand outline. Abbreviations and an index of terminology.

Directories

2676.1
American Medical Writers Association. Washington, D.C. Directory of free-lance writers, editors and researchers. [Washington, 1966] 63 p.

Address and specialty of some 90 persons or services.

ZOOLOGY

Indexes and Abstracts

Current

2677
Bibliografia brasileira de zoologia. Rio de Janeiro, 1, 1950/55– . Instituto de Bibliografia e Documentação.

2280 references in v. 1. Limited to Brazilian publications and publications about Brazil. Covers tropical medicine.

v. 2, 1956/58. v. 1 has *supplemento.*

2678(a)
Index catalogue of medical and veterinary zoology. Authors. Washington, 1902–12. 36 pts. in 4 v. (U.S. Bureau of Animal Industry. Bulletin No. 39)

Covers animal parasites of man and animals. Indexes all literature irrespective of date. Includes books, parts of books, collections, congressional proceedings, documents and theses. Includes material not normally covered by other indexes: i.e., letters to editors; brief remarks in proceedings of meetings; letters and sections in annual reports, etc. Frequently includes reviews listed under author reviewed.

2678(b)
——. Subjects. *Trematoda and Trematode diseases* (U.S. Hygienic Laboratory. Bulletin No. 37, June 1908) 401 p.; *Cestoda and Cestodaria* (Bulletin No. 85, July 1912) 467 p.; *Nematoda, Gordiacea and Acanthocephala and the diseases they cause.* (Bulletin No. 114, June 1920) 886 p.

Arranged alphabetically by scientific name of species of parasites. Gives taxonomic information, hosts and type hosts, body locations, and geographic locality. Complete citation not given; cites author, date and letter for full citation in 2678(a)

2878(c)
—— Key-Catalogue[s]. *Key-Catalogue of the protozoa reported for man* (U.S. Hygienic Laboratory Bulletin No. 140, May 1925) 67 p.; *Key-Catalogue of the worms reported for man* (Bulletin No. 142, Jan., 1926) p. 69–196; *Key-Catalogue of the Crustacea and Arachnoids of importance in public health* (Bulletin No. 148, Apr. 1927) p. 197–289; *Key-Catalogue of insects of importance in public health* (Bulletin No. 150, Mar. 1928) p. 291–408; *Key-Catalogue of parasites reported for primates (monkeys and lemurs) with their possible public health importance* . . . and *Key-Catalogue of primates for which parasites are reported* (Bulletin No. 152, Nov. 1929) p. 409–601; *Key-Catalogue of parasites reported for Chiroptera (bats) with their possible public health importance and The*

confused nomenclature of Nycteribia Lat, 1796 and Spinlurmix Heyden, 1826. (U.S. National Institute of Health Bulletin No. 155, Dec. 1930) p. 603–789; *Key-Catalogue of parasites reported for Insectivora (moles, shrews, etc.) with their possible public health importance* (Bulletin No. 159, June 1931) p. 791–911; *Key-Catalogue of parasites reported for Carnivora (cats, dogs, bears, etc.) with their possible public health importance.* (Bulletin No. 163, Dec. 1934) p. 913–1223.

Index to the literature on the parasites of hosts either referenced independently or listed in 2678a, the reference incomplete in the latter case.

Prefaces to *Key-Catalogues* indicate they are in the order listed above pts. 1–5 of Stiles and Hassall's Host Catalogue, *Index catalogue of medical and veterinary zoology*; pts. 6–8 do not indicate a relationship to the *Index catalogue.*

2678.1

——. Authors. Washington, U.S. Bureau of Animal Industry, 1932–52. 18 pts. in 13 v.

Includes and updates no. 2678(a) Occasional changes in biographical data relating to authors.

2678.2

——. ——. Supplements 1– , U.S. Department of Agriculture, Agriculture Research Service. Washington, 1953– .

Supplements 1–6, include the backlog of each alphabetical letter 1932– as well as all current work (i.e. A-B, A-C, etc. A-Z). With Supplement 7– , 1957– , Authors (A-Z) issued annually.

With Supplement 15, 1965– , *Parasite subject catalogue[s]* covering *Parasites* (divided by taxonomic groups) *Hosts, Treatment,* and *Subject Headings* (i.e. general subjects) are being issued on an annual basis and constitute indexes to the author indexes of the corresponding supplements.

Supplements 1–2, 1953–54, by the Bureau of Animal Industry.

Subject heading section includes geographical sub-headings.

2678.3

——. Subjects. Trematoda and trematode diseases, 1– , 1963– . Department of Agriculture, Agricultural Research Service, Washington, D.C.

Includes and updates U.S. Hygienic Laboratory Bulletin No. 37 and constitutes an index to the trematode entries of pts. 1–18 (2678.1) and Supplements 1–12 (2678.2) of the author indexes.

Incomplete citation; full citation to Author Catalog by author, date, letter.

2679

Zoological record . . . being the records of zoological literature. London, 1, 1864– . Zoological Society of London (from v. 23, 1886).

Currently in 20 sections (published separately). Section 1, Comprehensive zoology; Section 20, List of new generic and subgeneric names recorded; other sections by taxonomic groups.

v. 1–6, 1864–69, as *The record of zoological literature.*

v. 43–51, 1906–14, issued as *International catalogue of scientific literature* 6th–(14th) annual issue. (Section) N, Zoology. These volumes published for the International Council by the Royal Society.

Except for section 20, no indexes.

Noncurrent

2680

Bibliographia zoologica. Leipzig, 1–42, 1896–1933. Concilium Bibliographicum (since v. 31, 1923).

v. 1–42 contain 292,987 references. Arranged by phylum or subphylum.

Subtitle: v. 1–21, 1896–1910, Diario zoologischer Anzeiger adnexa; v. 22–30, 1911–21, Adhuc diario . . . ; v. 31–42, 1923–33, Antea diario . . .

2681

Zentralblatt für Zoologie; allgemeine und experimentelle Biologie. Leipzig, 1–6, 1912–18.

Abstracts chiefly in German and English. No subject index.

Formed by union of nos. 921.1 and 2684.

2682

Zoologisher Bericht. Jena, 1–55, 1922–43/44. Im Auftrage der Deutschen Zoologischen Gesellschaft.

v. 55 contained 1764 entries, most with abstracts. Includes books, dissertations.

2683

Zoologischer Jahresbericht. Berlin, etc., 1879–1913. Zoologische Station zu Neapel.

References listed alphabetically by author under phylum or subject and selectively reviewed.

2684
Zoologisches Zentralblatt. Leipzig, 1–18, 1894–1912.

2685–2686 (Not used)

Reviews

2687
International review of general and experimental zoology. New York, Academic Press, 1, 1964– .

Bibliographies

2688
American Institute of Biological Sciences. Biological Sciences Communication Project. The baboon; an annotated bibliography, with added materials, 1607–1964. San Antonio, Southwest Foundation for Research and Education, 1964. 642 p.

Supersedes George Washington University. Biological Sciences Communication Project. *The baboon; an annotated bibliography, with added selections, 1658–1963.* Pt. 1. San Antonio, Southwest Foundation for Research and Education, 1963. 157 p.

2689
Bibliotheca historico-naturalis. Verzeichnis der Bücher über Naturgeschichte welche in Deutschland, Scandinavien, Holland, England, Frankreich, Italien und Spanien in den Jahren 1700–1846 erschienen sind. By Wilhelm Engelmann, v. 1. Leipzig, Engelmann, 1846. 786 p.

Added t.p. in Latin: Index librorum historiam naturalem spectantium . . . No more published.

2690
Bibliotheca zoologica. Verzeichniss der Schriften über Zoologie welche in den periodischen Werken enthalten und vom Jahre 1846–1860 selbständig erschienen sind; mit Einschluss der allgemein-naturgeschichtlichen, periodischen und palaeontologischen Schriften. Bearbeitet von J. Victor Carus und Wilhelm Engelmann. Leipzig, Engelmann, 1861. 2 v. (2144 p.)

Added t.p.: Bibliotheca Historico-Naturalis. Herausgegeben von Wilhelm Engelmann. Supplement-Band. Enthaltend die in den periodischen Werken aufgenommenen und die vom Jahre 1846–1860 erschienenen Schriften.

2691
Bibliotheca zoologica II. Verzeichniss der Schriften über Zoologie welche in den periodischen Werken enthalten und vom Jahre 1861–80 selbständig erschienen sind; mit Einschluss der allgemein naturgeschichtlichen, periodischen und palaeontologischen Schriften. Bearbeitet von Otto Taschenberg. Leipzig, Engelmann, 1887–1923. 8 v.

2692
Herman, Carlton M. The rabbits as used in disease research; a selected bibliography, including the spontaneous diseases of rabbits. Chicago, U.S. Fish and Wildlife Service, 1942. 519 p.

4859 entries. Chronological arrangement under subject breakdown. Earliest entry 1780. Indexes a number of nonmedical sources.

2693
Magalhaes, Hulda. Bibliography on the golden, Syrian hamster, 1931–1963. [n. p.] 1965. 548 p.

5018 citations arranged chronologically by author.

2694
Mason, Marcus M. Bibliography of the dog. Ames, Iowa State University Press, 1959. 401 p.

12,369 entries arranged alphabetically by author. Covers, principally, literature from 1930's.

2695
Pekas, J. C., and Bustad, L. K. A selected list of references (1960–May 1965) on swine in biomedical research. 149 p. (U.S. AEC. BNWL-115. UC-48, June 1965).

1509 entries

2696
Voss, Hermann. Bibliographie der Menschenaffen (Schimpanse, Orang, Gorilla). Jena, Fischer, 1955. 163 p.

Manuals

2697
Smith, Roger C. Guide to the literature of the zoological sciences. 6 ed. Minneapolis, Burgess, 1962. 231 p.

Dictionaries

2698
Caveness, Fields E. A glossary of nematological terms. [Ibadam, Nigeria] 1964. 68 p.

Includes lists of vernacular names, scientific names, and abbreviations used in nematological literature.

2699
el-Duweini, A. Khalaf. A glossary of zoological terms. Cairo [1958] 170 p.

About 5000 terms. English—Arabic.

2700
Leftwich, A. W. A dictionary of zoology. Princeton, Van Nostrand, 1963. 290 p.

Includes definitions of all principle phyla and classes of animals as well as a large number of orders, suborders, and families.

2701
al-Ma'luf, Amin Fahd. An Arabic zoological dictionary. Cairo, al-Muktataf press, 1932. 271 p.

About 3500 terms. English-Arabic.

2702
Ziegler, Heinrich E. Zoologisches Wörterbuch. 3 ed. Jena, 1925. 786 p.

1 ed., 1907–10.

Nomenclature

2703
Neave, Scheffield A., ed. Nomenclator zoologicus; a list of the names of genera and subgenera in zoology from the tenth edition of Linnaeus, 1758 to the end of 1935. London, Zoological Society of London, 1939–50. 5 v.

Name, number, date, source (journal reference, etc.).

Suppl.: v. 4, p. 713–758. v. 5, 1936–1945, includes further addenda to v. 4.

INDEX

ABC der Optik **2008**
ABT; abstracts of bioanalytic technology **2081.1**
ACTH **2617.1**
AMA medical-health film library **1398**
APCA abstracts **2385, 2387**
APhA directory of pharmacists **2193**
Abadir, F. M. **870**
Abbreviations **195–197**
Abd-El-Malak, Shafik **871**
Abderhalden, Emil **1754**
Abderhalden, Rudolf **245**
Abel-Smith, Brian **1454, 1907**
Abercrombie, Michael **936**
Abnormalities, *see* Congenital Anomalies
Abraham, J. J. **1897**
Abramova, N. D. **1174**
Abstracts, *see* Indexes and Abstracts under subject and geographic headings (e.g., Anatomy, Medicine, Brazil, Germany, etc.)
Abstracts and translations of the science library of the Institute of Living, Hartford **1726**
Abstracts from current urological literature **2624.1**
Abstracts of bacteriology **1541**
Abstracts of Bulgarian scientific literature **73, 912**
Abstracts of chemical papers **1005**
Abstracts of current literature. Aerospace medicine and biology **833**
Abstracts of current literature on venereal disease **1252**
Abstracts of hospital management studies **1433**
Abstracts of Japanese medicine **103**
Abstracts of orthopedic surgery **1665**
Abstracts of psychiatry for the general practitioner **1724**
Abstracts of Soviet medicine **106, 1686**
Abstracts of vitamin literature **1931**
Abstracts of world medicine **1**
Abstracts of world surgery, gynaecology and obstetrics **2543**
Abstracts on military and aviation ophthalmology and visual sciences **1987**
Abt, A. F. **2133**
Abt, I. A. **2133**
Academia Republicii Populare Romîne, Bucharest **2490.2**
Academia Republicii Populare Romîne, Bucharest. Biblioteca **136**
Academia Republicii Populare Romîne, Bucharest. Institutul de Studii Romino-Sovietic **91**
Académie de médecine, Paris **556, 1382**
Academy of Denture Prosthetics. Nomenclature Committee **1306**
Academy of the Hebrew Language, Jerusalem **259**
Acceleration **844, 844.1**
Accidents, *see* Injuries
Accumulative veterinary index **2639**
Acetanilid **2235**
Ackerknecht, E. H. **472, 481, 1194, 1811, 2095**
Acoustics **1865.1**
Actualidad pediatrica **2116**
Actualidades e utilidades médicas **2**
Adams, G. W. **1638**
Adams, Scott **164**
Addiction, Drug **2241**
Adler, J. A. **1474**
Adlung, Alfred **2206**
Admission requirements of American dental schools **1316**
Admission requirements of American medical colleges, including Canada **1367**
Adolescent Psychology **2530**
Adresar zdravstvenih ustanova FNRJ **407**
Adressbuch deutscher Chemiker **1083.1**
Adressen- und Auskunftsbuch über die Kranken-, Heil-, Pflege-, Erziehungs-Wohlfahrts-Anstalten Deutschlands **1440**
Advanced reports from current medical meetings **28.1**
Advances in analytical chemistry and instrumentation **1012**
Advances in applied microbiology **1544**
Advances in biological and medical physics **959**
Advances in botanical research **967**
Advances in cancer research **1692**
Advances in carbohydrate chemistry **1013**
Advances in cardiology **1105**
Advances in cardiopulmonary diseases **1104**
Advances in catalysis and related subjects **1014**
Advances in chemical physics **1015**
Advances in chemotherapy **2158**
Advances in child development and behavior **2117**
Advances in clinical chemistry **1016**
Advances in colloid sciences **1017**
Advances in comparative physiology and biochemistry **2274**
Advances in diagnosis and treatment **2613.1**
Advances in drug research **2159**
Advances in enzyme regulation **1093**
Advances in enzymology and related subjects of biochemistry **1094**
Advances in experimental social psychology **2298**
Advances in fluorine research and dental caries prevention **1280**

Advances in food research **1916**
Advances in genetics **1410**
Advances in gerontological research **1425**
Advances in heterocyclic chemistry **1018**
Advances in immunology **1569**
Advances in inorganic chemistry and radiochemistry **1019**
Advances in insect physiology **2275**
Advances in internal medicine **112**
Advances in lipid research **1020**
Advances in marine biology **922**
Advances in morphogenesis **862**
Advances in ophthalmology **1997, 1998**
Advances in oral biology **1281**
Advances in organic chemistry; methods and results **1021**
Advances in organometallic chemistry **1022**
Advances in oto-rhino-laryngology **2042**
Advances in parasitology **2058**
Advances in pediatrics **2118**
Advances in pest control research **2226**
Advances in pharmaceutical sciences **2160**
Advances in pharmacology **2161**
Advances in protein chemistry **1023**
Advances in reproductive physiology **2461.1**
Advances in surgery **2547, 2548**
Advances in the study of behavior **2299**
Advances in thyroid research **1381**
Advances in treatment **2613.1**
Advances in tuberculosis research **1235**
Advances in veterinary science **2645**
Advances in virus research **1545**
Advances in x-ray analysis **2424**
Adverse effects of drugs, devices, cosmetics **2230.1**
Adverse reactions titles **2229**
Aero Medical Association **849**
Aerospace and Submarine Medicine
  Bibliographies **836–847.1**
  Directories **848**
  Histories **849–850, 1613**
  Indexes and Abstracts **21.5, 833–835, 1987**
Aerospace Medical Association **848**
Ärztliches Handbuch und Ärzteverzeichnis **359**
Ärztliches Jahrbuch für Österreich **345**
Afghanistan
  Indexes and Abstracts **2493.1**
Afonsky, D. **1286**
Africa
  Bibliographies **145.2, 1709, 1709.1**
Agard, W. R. **198**
Agriculture, *see* Botany and Agriculture
Aguirre Beltrán, Gonzalo **608**
Ahern, George **534**
Ahern, M. J. **534**
Aikawa, J. K. **1212**
Aimes, Alexandre **209**
Ainsworth, G. C. **1581**
Air Hygiene Foundation of America **2397**
Air Pollution **2385, 2387, 2390–2392, 2394.2**
Air pollution bibliography **2387**
Air Pollution Control Association **2385, 2394.2**
Airapetian, T. I. **1386**
Akademie der Wissenschaften, Berlin **999**
Akademie-Verlag, Berlin **1081**
Akademiia meditsinskikh nauk SSSR, Moscow **1684, 2221**
Akademiia meditsinskikh nauk SSSR, Moscow. Institut gerontologii i eksperimental'noĭ patologii **1426**
Akademiia nauk Gruzinskoĭ SSR, Tiflis. Tsentral'naia nauchnaia biblioteka **2059**
Akademiia nauk Kazakhskoĭ SSR, Alma-Ata **1161, 1188, 1224**
Akademiia nauk Kazakhskoĭ SSR, Alma-Ata. Institut zoologii **2060**
Akademiia nauk SSSR, Moscow **930, 973**
Akademiia nauk SSSR, Moscow. Biblioteka **318, 1867**
Akademiia nauk SSSR, Moscow. Institut fiziologii im. I. P. Pavlova, **1406.1, 1755**
Akademiia nauk SSSR, Moscow. Institut nauchnoĭ informatsii **21**
Akademiia nauk SSSR, Moscow. Sektor seti spetsial'nykh bibliotek **1756, 2259, 2454.2**
Akademiia nauk URSR, Kiev **1764**
Albert Einstein College of Medicine. Department of Anatomy **1379**
Alchemy, *see* Chemistry and Biochemistry
Alcoholism **1754**
Alexander, F. G. **1811.1**
Alexander Graham Bell Association for the Deaf **1867.1**
Alfaro, Gregorio Aráoz, *see* Aráoz Alfaro, Gregorio
Alkiewicz, Jan **1256**
Allbutt, T. C. **487**
Allen, M. E. **1719**
Allergy
  Bibliographies **151.1**
  Dictionaries **854.1**
  Indexes and Abstracts **851–853, 2034**
  Reviews **854**
Allergy abstracts **851**
Allgemeine medizinische Annalen des Jahres **53, 1800**
Allgemeine medizinische Annalen des Neunzehnten Jahrhunderts **53**
Allgemeine medizinische Zeitung mit Berücksichtigung des neuesten und interessantesten der allgemeine Naturkunde **53**
Allgemeines Repertorium der gesammten deutschen medicinisch-chirurgischen, Journalistik **66**
Allgemeines Repertorium der medizinisch-chirurgischen Journalistik des Auslandes **54**

Almanach général de médecine, de pharmacie pour la France, l'Algerie et les colonies **355**
Almanach général de médecine pour la ville de Paris **355**
Almindelige danske laegeforening **548**
Altitude **839**
Altman, P. L. **931.1, 932, 1126**
Alvarez Amezquita, José **2372**
Alvaro, M. E. **2009**
Amano, K. W. **599**
American Academy of Dental Science **1331**
American Academy of General Practice **385**
American Academy of Neurology **1794**
American Academy of Ophthalmology and Otolaryngology **2013**
American Academy of Orthopaedic Surgeons **1670**
American and Canadian hospitals **1450**
American annals of the deaf **1867.1**
American Association for Health, Physical Education and Recreation **2246**
American Association for Rehabilitation Therapy **2263**
American Association for the Advancement of Science **1522**
American Association for the History of Medicine **650**
American Association of Dental Schools **1316**
American Association of Economic Entomologists **2071**
American Association of Homes for the Aging **1430**
American Association of Medical Clinics **392**
American Association of Social Workers **2415**
American Cancer Society **1687, 2093**
American Cancer Society. Medical and Scientific Library **1698**
American Cancer Society. Statistics Committee **1716**
American Chemical Society **995–998, 1028, 1082, 1086**
American Chemical Society. Committee on Professional Training **1083**
American Chemical Society. Division of Chemical Education **1058**
American Chemical Society. Division of Chemical Literature **1058**
American College of Cardiology **1130**
American College of Chest Physicians **1240, 2490**
American College of Chest Physicians. Council on Postgraduate Medical Education **1104**
American College of Dentists **1317**
American College of Hospital Administrators **1448, 1449**
American College of Obstetricians and Gynecologists **1960**
American College of Physicians **386**
American College of Radiology **2443**
American College of Surgeons **387, 2538, 2559**
American College of Surgeons. Library **1489**
American Dental Association **1268, 1269, 1271, 1308, 1318, 1336**
American dental directory **1318**
American Dermatological Association **1357**
American Diabetes Association **1396**
American directory of obstetricians and gynecologists **1961**
American directory of otolaryngologists and ophthalmologists **2048**
American doctoral dissertations **179**
American encyclopedia and dictionary of ophthalmology **2023**
American Foundation for the Blind **2025–2027**
American Group Psychotherapy Association **1728**
American Gynecological Society **1963**
American Heart Association **1099**
American Homoeopathic Biographical Association **399.1**
American Hospital Association **1435, 1453**
American hospital directory **1453**
American Indians, *see* Indians (American)
American Institute of Biological Sciences **925, 1172, 1173**
American Institute of Biological Sciences. Biological Sciences Communication Project **2688**
American Institute of Biological Sciences. Committee on the Handbook of Biological Data **1919**
American Institute of Medicine **36.2**
American Institute of the History of Pharmacy **2199**
American Instrument Company **1042**
American Journal of Nursing Co. **1830**
American Library Association **1485**
American Medical Association **6, 30, 34, 38, 388, 389, 659, 661, 662, 1398, 1399, 1530, 1878, 1879, 1881, 2093**
American Medical Association. Archive-Library Department **2341**
American Medical Association. Bureau of Legal Medicine and Legislation **1464**
American Medical Association. Committee on the Medical Aspects of Sports **2252**
American Medical Association. Committee on Voluntary Health Agencies **393**
American Medical Association. Council on Medical Education and Hospitals **1370**
American Medical Association. Council on Medical Service **394, 398**
American Medical Association. Division of Scientific Publications **2668**
American Medical Association. Law Department **1465**
American medical directory **389**
American Medical Writers Association **2676.1**
American men of medicine **390**

American men of science **2499**
American Nurses' Association **1903**
American pediatric directory **130**
American Pharmaceutical Association **2156, 2193**
American physicians and surgeons **400**
American Physiological Society **2272, 2278**
American Psychiatric Association **1757, 1795–1797, 1827**
American Psychiatric Association. Committee on Medical Education **1798**
American Psychiatric Association. Committee on Nomenclature and Statistics **1793**
American Psychiatric Association. Committee on Public Information **1784**
American Psychoanalytic Association **1799**
American Psychological Association **2292, 2296, 2301, 2326**
American Public Health Association **1154, 2358, 2380**
American Rheumatism Association **1655, 1663**
American Rheumatism Association. Literature Analysis Subcommittee **1662**
American Roentgen Ray Society **2444**
American Society for Microbiology **1561**
American Society of Anesthesiologists **2603**
American Society of Clinical Hypnosis **1850**
American Society of Hospital Pharmacists **2144**
American Society of Microbiologists **1541, 1547**
American Society of Radiologic Technologists **2444.1**
American Sociological Association **2535**
American Society of X-Ray Technicans **2444.1**
American Speech and Hearing Association **1874**
American Speech Correction Association **1874**
American Trudeau Society **1241**
American Urological Association **2635**
American Veterinary Medical Association **2655, 2661**
Amezquita, José Alvarez, *see* Alvarez Amezquita, José
Anaesthetic Literature **2593.1**
Analgesia **2599**
Analysis, Luminescent **2431**
Analysis, X-ray **2424**
Analytical abstracts **994**
Analytical Chemistry **1012**
Anatomischer Bericht **857**
Anatomische Gesellschaft **857**
Anatomy, *see also* Cytology; Congenital Anomalies; Histology
  Bibliographies **132.1, 149.1, 866–869**
  Dictionaries **259, 870–884, 938**
  Histories **889–892, 895–898, 1973, 1985**
  Indexes and Abstracts **9.1, 27, 44, 855–861**
  Nomenclature **884.1–888**
  Reviews **862–865**
Anatomy, Comparative; History **890**
Anatomy, Pathological **856, 2082, 2091**
Anderson, F. J. **701**
Andreasch, R. **1008**
Andrews, Theodora **2197**
Andrus, E. C. **1651**
Anesthesia
  Bibliographies **2601–2602, 2609–2610**
  Directories **2603, 2603.1**
  Histories **2604–2610**
  Indexes and Abstracts **9.24, 2593.1–2596**
  Reviews **2597–2600**
Anesthesia abstracts **2594**
Anesthesia digest **2594.1**
Anesthesiologists **2603, 2603.1**
Angulo Carpio, M.D. **2415, 2416**
Animal Diseases **2654**
Animal Physiology **2271, 2457.1**
Animal Pox **1572**
Animal Psychology **2296.1**
Animal research in psychopharmacology **1860**
Animals, Laboratory **2080, 2090.1,** *see also* Baboon, Dogs, etc.
Animaux de laboratoire **2080**
Annali di medicina straniera **55**
Annali universali di medicina **41**
Annali universali di medicina e chirurgia **41**
Annata clinica e terapeutica **25**
Année biologique **922.1**
Année endocrinologique **1382**
Année médicale pratique: médicine, obstétrique, spécialités **124**
Année psychologique **2289**
Annotated bibliography of influenza **1172**
Annotated bibliography of medical mycology **1576**
Annotated bibliography of vitamin E **1934**
Annuaire dentaire **1319**
Annuaire des organisations internationales **341**
Annuaire médical **357**
Annuaire médical belge **347**
Annuaire médical egyptien **353**
Annuaire médical et pharmaceutique de la France **356**
Annual international congress calendar **186**
Annual of Czechoslovak medical literature **76**
Annual record of homeopathic literature **56**
Annual reports on the progress of chemistry **1025**
Annual review of biochemical and allied research in India **1026**
Annual review of biochemistry **1027**
Annual review of entomology **2073**
Annual review of hypnosis literature **1849**
Annual review of medicine **114, 115**
Annual review of microbiology **1546**
Annual review of nuclear science **2450**
Annual review of pharmacology **2162**
Annual review of physiology **2276**
Annual review of psychology **2300**
Annual survey of psychoanalysis **1740**

Annual survey of research in pharmacy **2163**
Annuario bibliografico italiano delle scienze mediche ed affini **98**
Annuario medico brasileiro **75**
Annuario medico de Portugal **377**
Anomalies, Congenital, *see* Congenital Anomalies
Anson, T. V. **1625**
Anthrax
Bibliographies **1155.1**
Anthropology
Bibliographies **910–911, 2493.3**
Indexes and Abstracts **9.1. 44, 858.1**
Reviews **909**
Antibiotica et chemotherapia **2218**
Antibiotics
Bibliographies **2221–2223**
Dictionaries **2224**
Indexes and Abstracts **16.3**
Reviews **2218–2220**
Antibiotika-Literaturberichte **2220**
Anuario de medicina y cirugía **40**
Anuario de medicina y cirugía practicas **40**
Anuario de progresos terapeuticos en medicina interna **2614**
Anuario internacional de medicina y cirugía **40**
Anxiety **1766**
Aoyagi, Yasumasa **269**
Apes **2696**
Applezweig, M. H. **2304**
Appraisal of current concepts in anesthesiology **2597**
Aráoz Alfaro, Gregorio **519**
Arber, A. R. **984**
Archer, W. H. **1324, 1335**
Archila, Ricardo **92, 737, 2384**
Archimbaud, Jacques **1505**
Archiv fur Augenheilkunde **1995, 1996**
Archiv fur dïe gesamte Psychologie **2296.1**
Archiva medica belgica **94.1**
Archivio di medicina mutualistica **3**
Archivio "Putti" di chirurgia degli organi di movimento **1664.1**
Arcieri, J. P. **263**
Arents, George **2233.1**
Arents Tobacco Collection **2233.1, 2238.1**
Argentina
Directories **343**
Histories **519–521**
Argentine Republic. Consejo Nacional de Investigaciones Científicas y Técnicas **343**
Arieti, Silvano **1783.2**
Arizona. Histories **676**
Armed Forces Institute of Pathology, *see* U.S. Armed Forces Institute of Pathology
Armed Forces Medical Library, *see* U.S. Armed Forces Medical Library
Armenia. Histories **522**
Army Medical Library, *see* U.S. Army Medical Library
Arnaudov, G. D. **217, 304**
Arnold, Arno **2249**
Aronova-Zlatopol'skaia, F. S. **1115, 2063**
Artelt, Walter **325, 419.1, 437**
Arthopods **2076**
Arthritis, *see* Rheumatic Diseases
Arthritis and rheumatic diseases abstracts **1653**
Artificial Heart **2576.1, 2578**
Arts and Medicine **748–760, 1186, 1201, 1338, 1341, 1680.1, 1767, 1768,** *see also* Caricatures; Illustration, Medical; Portraits; Literature and Medicine; Famous Persons
Artschwager, Ernst **937**
Arutiunov, A. I. **1699**
Aschoff, Ludwig **457**
Ash, Lee **419**
Ashburn, P. M. **1628**
Ashkhabad. Respublikanskaia nauchnaia meditsinskaia biblioteka **1178**
Aslib **180**
Asociación Colombiana de Facultades de Medicina **144.1**
Asociación Odontológica Argentina **1270**
Association des Sociétés Scientifiques Médicales Belges **94.1**
Association Général des Syndicats Pharmaceutiques **2193.1**
Association of American Medical Colleges **1367, 1367.1, 1369**
Association of Military Surgeons of the United States **1601**
Association of Vitamin Chemists **1931**
Atherosclerosis **1114, 1115**
Athletics, *see* Physical Education and Sports Medicine
Atkinson, T. G. **2029**
Atkinson, W. B. **651**
Atomic Bomb Casualty Commission **2454.3**
Atomic Energy, *see* Nuclear Medicine
Atomic Energy Commission, *see* U.S. Atomic Energy Commission
Auerbach, E. F. **707**
Aureomycin **2222**
Austin, A. L. **1908**
Austin, R. B. **169**
Australia
Bibliographies **2354**
Directories **344**
Histories **523–524, 1604–1605**
Australia. Army Medical Services **1604**
Australia in the war of 1939–1945 **1605**
Australian War Memorial **1604, 1605**
Austria
Directories **345–346, 2560, 2603.1**
Histories **525–527, 1375, 2366**

Automation **2400**
Aviation Medicine, *see* Aerospace and Submarine Medicine
Awards, Medical **406, 848, 1367.1**

B.A.S.I.C. **916**
Baas, J. H. **461**
Babington, B. G. **2099**
Baboon **2688**
Bachmann, B. J. **1577**
Bacillus anthracis **1155.1**
Bacteria **1542, 1555, 1551.1, 1551.2,** *see also* Microbiology
Bacteriological reviews **1547**
Bacteriology, *see* Microbiology
Bacteriophage **5.3, 1552**
Bader, Luigi **1677**
Baer, K. A. **1809, 2617.1**
Bagnall, J. S. **1287**
Baillière's midwives' dictionary **1956**
Baillière's nursing dictionary **1895**
Bain, Curtis **1109**
Baker, E. A. **1918**
Baker, J. R. **900**
Baker, W. E. W. **1589**
Bakulev, A. N. **408**
Balassa, B. **1168.1**
Balcázar, J. M. **530**
Baldwin, J. M. **2296, 2312**
Ballistocardiography **1122**
Balneology **1661, 2256, 2261, 2261.1**
Baney, A. M. **1436**
Banga, Jelle **613**
Bantug, J. P. **621**
Barcia Goyanes, J. J. **884.1**
Bariéty, M. J. C. **462**
Barnard, C. C. **1526**
Barnes, J. K. **1642**
Barnhart, J. H. **990**
Baron, D. N. **125**
Barr, M. P. **2015**
Barsukov, M. I. **2375**
Bastholm, Eyvind **2282**
Bates, R. S. **660**
Bauer, Warner **1609**
Baumann, E. D. **614**
Baumgarten's Jahresbericht über die Fortschritte in der Lehre von den pathogenen Mikroorganismen **1542**
Bay, J. C. **970**
Beard, Miriam **805**
Beatriz Cespedes, J. **144.1**
Beccaria, Augusto **425**
Bechet, P. E. **1357**
Becker, J. H. **1922**
Beckham, R. S. **910**
Behavior **2117, 2128, 2299, 2305, 2530**
Behne, A. B. **748**
Beklemishev, N. D. **1161**
Belgium
  Directories **347**
  Indexes and Abstracts **94.1**
  Histories **528–529**
Belgrad. Institute for Military Medical Documentation **93**
Belgrad. Jugoslovenski centar za techničku i naučnu dokumentaciju **2140, 2152**
Bell, H. C. M. **826**
Bellingham, E. F. **2404**
Beltrán, Gonzalo Aguirre, *see* Aguirre Beltrán, Gonzalo
Beltz, R. E. **1045**
Bender, A. E. **1920**
Bender, R. E. **1877**
Benford, R. J. **849**
Bennett, Harry **1064**
Berendes, Julius **2207**
Berens, Conrad **1987**
Berg, Alexander **1586**
Berger, Franz **975**
Bergey's Manual of determinative bacteriology **1558**
Bergman, Emanuel **823**
Bericht über die Fortschritte der Anatomie und Physiologie **858**
Bericht über die Fortschritte der Augenheilkunde **1995**
Bericht über die Leistungen auf dem Gebiete der Anatomie des Centralnervensystems **1838.1**
Bericht über die Leistungen und Fortschritte auf dem Gebiete der Ohrenheilkunde, der Krankheiten der Luftwege und der Grenzgebiete **2037**
Bericht über die Leistungen und Fortschritte der Augenheilkunde **1995, 1996**
Bericht über die neueren Leistungen in der Ohrenheilkunde **2037.1**
Bericht über die psychiatrische Literatur **1734**
Berichte über die allgemeine und spezielle Pathologie **2081**
Berichte über die gesamte Biologie. Abt. A. **914**
Berichte über die gesamte Biologie. Abt. B. **2269**
Berichte über die gesamte Gynäkologie und Geburtshilfe **1938**
Berichte über die gesamte Physiologie **2269**
Berichte über die gesamte Physiologie und experimentelle Pharmakologie **2269**
Berichte über die wissenschaftliche Biologie **914**
Berlin, I. N. **1757**
Berliner Gesellschaft für Öffentliche Gesundheitspflege **2349**
Bernadskiĭ, I. I. **1288**
Bernstein, Seymour **1386.1**

Berolzheimer, D. D. **1049–1051**
Besio, G. L. **2430**
Bethlehem Corporation. Hyperbaric Oxygen Therapy Division **2618**
Betkó, J. **2006**
Bett, W. R. **2096**
Bettmann, O. L. **482**
Beulé, Monique **2197.2**
Bevan, William **2305**
Beverages **1918**
Bianchi, V. **2200**
Bible, *see* Religion and Medicine
Bibliografia brasileira de medicina **72**
Bibliografia brasileira de oncologia **1700**
Bibliografia brasileira de zoologia **2677**
Bibliografia española de historia de la medicina **626**
Bibliografia italiana. Biologia **920**
Bibliografia italiana. Medicina **99**
Bibliografia italiana delle scienze mediche **99.2**
Bibliografia italiana di medicina interna **99.1**
Bibliografia medica italiana **100**
Bibliografia medica portuguese **87.2**
Bibliografia medica venezolana **92**
Bibliografia medico-biologica **101**
Bibliografia ortopedica **1666**
Bibliografia scientifico-tecnica italiana **99, 920**
Bibliograficheskiĭ ukazatel' russkoĭ dermatologii i venerologii **1347**
Bibliograficheskiĭ ukazatel' sovetskoĭ dermatologii i venerologii **1347**
Bibliografiia sovetskoĭ travmatologii **2591**
Bibliographia biotheoretica **915**
Bibliographia genetica **1411**
Bibliographia histochemica **904.2**
Bibliographia italiana di storia della farmacia **2200**
Bibliographia medica **42**
Bibliographia medica belgica **94.1**
Bibliographia medica Čechoslovaca **77**
Bibliographia medica Helvetica **89**
Bibliographia medica latina **26**
Bibliographia neuroendocrinologica **1379**
Bibliographia physiologica **2269.1**
Bibliographia zoologica **2680**
Bibliographical current list of papers, reports, and proceedings of international meetings **187**
Bibliographie anatomique **858.1**
Bibliographie de médecine du travail **2402**
Bibliographie der deutschen und ausländischen Literatur... über Psychologie, ihre Hilfswissenschaften und Grenzgebiete **2297**
Bibliographie der deutschen und ausländischen Literatur... über Psychologie, ihre Hilfswissenschaften und Grenzgebiete... Deutscher Teil **2297**
Bibliographie der gesamten inneren Medizin und ihrer Grenzgebiete **37**
Bibliographie der gesamten Kinderheilkunde **2113**
Bibliographie der Hals- Nasen- und Ohrenheilkunde **2039**
Bibliographie der Haut- und Geschlechtskrankheiten, sowie deren Grenzgebiete **1254**
Bibliographie der psycho-physiologischen Literatur **2297**
Bibliographie der psychologischen Literatur der sozialistischen Länder **2290**
Bibliographie der psychologischen Literatur der sozialistischen Länder aus dem Jahre **1725**
Bibliographie der Sportmedizin und deren Grenzgebiete **2249**
Bibliographie d'hygiène industrielle **2401**
Bibliographie... I. Deutsche Literature des Jahres... über Psychologie, ihre Hilfswissenschaften und Grenzgebiete **2297**
Bibliographie et listes courantes de gastroenterologie **1402**
Bibliographie über die gesamte Neurologie und Psychiatrie **1735**
Bibliographies
  Manuals **136–143**
Bibliographies on diseases of medical progress **2610.1**
Bibliographischer Jahresbericht über soziale Hygiene, Demographie und Medizinalstatistik **2346.1**
Bibliography, Medical **1482–88**
  Histories **434–436**
Bibliography of agriculture **964, 983**
Bibliography of bone transplantation **2590**
Bibliography of brephoplastic transplantation **2590**
Bibliography of cartilage transplantation **2590**
Bibliography of chemical reviews **995**
Bibliography of corneal transplantation **2590**
Bibliography of developmental medicine and child neurology **2127**
Bibliography of foot-and-mouth disease in man **1168.1**
Bibliography of foreign substance implants in reconstructive surgery **2590**
Bibliography of gerontology and geriatrics **1424**
Bibliography of hematopoietic tissue transplantation **2590**
Bibliography of kidney transplantation **2590**
Bibliography of liver transplantation **2590**
Bibliography of lung transplantation **2590**
Bibliography of medical reviews **4, 11**
Bibliography of occupational health **2405**
Bibliography of occupational medicine **2402**
Bibliography of parathyroid gland transplantation **2590**
Bibliography of recent tissue transplantation literature of the Central and East European countries **2590**

Bibliography of reproduction **2460**
Bibliography of reviews in chemistry **995**
Bibliography of systematic mycology **1573**
Bibliography of the genetics of Drosophila **1417**
Bibliography of the history of medicine **414**
Bibliography of the history of medicine in the United States and Canada **650**
Bibliography of the history of ophthalmology **2024**
Bibliography of tooth replantation **2590**
Bibliography of transplantation of chorioallantoic placenta and trophoblast **2590**
Bibliography of tumor transplantation **2590**
Bibliography of vitamin E **1934**
Bibliography on medical education **1365**
Bibliotheca historico-naturalis **2689**
Bibliotheca medica Neerlandica **1492**
Bibliotheca zoologica **2690**
Bibliotheca zoologica II **2691**
Bick, E. M. **1678**
Bickerton, J. H. **1987**
Bickford, R. G. **1839.1**
Biennial review of anthropology **909**
Bierring, Walter **662**
Bilharziasis
  Bibliographies **1156–1160**
Billewicz, W. Z. **1937**
Billings, J. S. **29, 36**
Bilten naučne dokumentacije za farmaciju **2152**
Biochemical and allied research in India **1026**
Biochemical Society **27, 918**
Biochemistry, *see* Chemistry and Biochemistry
Bioclimatology **1661, 2261.1**
Biocybernetics **1744**
Bioelectronics **963**
Bioelectronics directory **963**
Bioelectronics report **963**
Biographies, Medical **446–456, 478**
  Bibliographies **444–445**
  United States **651–658**
  See also Famous Persons
Biographisches Lexikon der hervorragenden Ärzte aller Zeiten und Völker **446**
Biographisches Lexikon der hervorragenden Ärzte der letzten fünfzig Jahre **447**
Biological abstracts **916, 944, 944.1**
Biological Abstracts. Biosciences Information Service **917**
Biological and agricultural index **965**
Biological and Medical Services, Philadelphia **1864**
Biological reviews and biological proceedings of the Cambridge Philosophical Society **923**
Biological reviews of the Cambridge Philosophical Society **923**
Biological Sciences Communication Project. George Washington University, Washington, D.C., **2061.2, 2197.1, 2688**
Biological Sciences Foundation, Washington, D.C. **1987**
Biologie und Pathologie des Weibs **1969**
Biologists **943, 2499**
Biology
  Bibliographies **929, 1048, 2259, 2431, 2454.2, 2493.3**
  Congresses **192.1**
  Dictionaries **216, 242, 286, 293, 936–942, 1418**
  Directories **943**
  Histories **945–957, 1586**
  Indexes and Abstracts **5.5, 5.6, 18.1, 21.2, 27, 44, 74, 101, 912–921.1, 965, 997**
  Manuals **930**
  Monographs **931–935**
  Nomenclature **1081**
  Periodicals **943, 944, 944.1**
  Reviews **922–928**
Biology, Environmental **931.1**
Biology, Marine **922**
Biology, Molecular **961**
Biology, Oral **1281**
Biomedical sciences instrumentation **950**
Biophysics
  Bibliographies **962, 962.1**
  Directories **963**
  Indexes and Abstracts **5.1, 958, 1006, 1011**
  Reviews **959–961**
Biophysikalisches Centralblatt **1006**
Bioresearch titles **920.1**
Biotechnology **846**
Birth Control, *see* Reproduction, Fertility, etc.
Birth defects **902.1**
Birth Defects, *see* Congenital Anomalies
Bishop, W. J. **191, 793, 2562**
Bishop B. P. Museum **258.1**
Bitschai, J. **2636**
Black, W. G. **797**
Black's medical dictionary **240**
Black's veterinary dictionary **2651**
Blagodarnyi, I. A. **1188**
Blair, E. D. **1637**
Blake, J. B. **2377**
Blakiston's illustrated pocket medical dictionary **229**
Blakiston's new Gould medical dictionary **230**
Blanton, W. B. **733**
Blau, Louis **2037.1**
Blehová, E. **1390**
Blencke, August **1673–1675**
Blind
  Bibliographies **2025**
  Catalogs **2026**
  Directories **2027**
  Histories **2028**
Bloch, Iwan **1261**
Blocker, T. G. **2576**
Blocker, Virginia **2576**

Blood **1043, 1108, 1112, 1126, 1128**
Blood Coagulation **1123**
Blood Pressure **1117**
Blood Transfusion **1112**
Bloom, J. H. **565**
Bloomfield, A. L. **128, 1141**
Blue book of optometrists **2032**
Bluff, M. J. **68**
Blunt, Wilfrid **985**
Boalch, D. H. **982.1**
Bochalli, Richard **1244**
Boche, R. D. **2456**
Bocker, Dorothy **1191, 1214, 1222, 1223, 1225, 1579, 1580, 2242**
Bodenheimer, F. S. **845, 2078**
Bogoiavlenskiĭ, N. A. **642**
Boguslavskiĭ, I. M. **2431**
Bojilov, B. **144**
Bókay, J. **1951**
Bolivia, Histories **530**
Bollettino delle scienze mediche **57**
Bollo, L. E. **199**
Bologna. Instituto ortopedico Rizzoli **1494**
Bolton, H. C. **1040, 2510**
Bone Transplantation **2590**
Bonner, T. N. **685, 692, 1373**
Bonser, Wilfred **564**
Bookplates **761**
Books for the nurse, 1963–64 **1893**
Boring, E. G. **2329, 2332**
Borja, Virgilio Paredes, *see* Paredes Borja, Virgilio
Borland, L. R. **1303**
Bosquillon, É. F. M. **471**
Bost, E. **2388, 2389**
Boston. American Academy of Dental Science, *see* American Academy of Dental Science, Boston
Botanical abstracts **916, 966**
Botany and Agriculture
  Bibliographies **132.1, 969–973, 2493.3**
  Dictionaries **938, 975–981**
  Directories **982.1**
  Histories **984–993**
  Indexes and Abstracts **18.1, 44, 964–966**
  Monographs **974**
  Nomenclature **982**
  Periodicals **983**
  Reviews **967–968**
Bottle, R. T. **1059**
Botulism
  Bibliographies **1160.1**
Boucher, C. O. **1307**
Bouillon, Albert **1156**
Bourne, Gordon **1948.1**
Boussel, Patrice **2208**
Bouvet, Maurice **2201**
Bowers, J. Z. **1374**
Brackbill, Yvonne **2128**
Bradford, T. L. **769, 770**
Braier, Léon **290**
Brain, W. R. **1748**
Brain and Spinal Cord
  Bibliographies **1839.1–1844, 1862**
  Indexes and Abstracts **1838.1**
  Nomenclature **1845**
  Reviews **1839**
Brain Circulation **1842, 1843**
Brain Neoplasms **1699**
Braithwaite's retrospect **50**
Brand, J. L. **2368**
Brandon, A. N. **1518**
Brau, Paul **561**
Brauchle, Alfred **2265**
Brazier, M. A. B. **1840**
Brazil
  Bibliographies **143.1, 531, 1157, 1176, 1187, 1192, 1227, 1266, 1700, 2169**
  Histories **531–532, 1187**
  Indexes and Abstracts **72, 95, 2677**
Brazil. Conselho Nacional de Pesquisas. Instituto Brasileiro de Bibliografia e Documentacão **1266**
Brazil. Instituto Brasileiro de Bibliografia e Documentaçâo **1157, 1176, 1192, 1227, 2169, 2677**
Breed, R. S. **1558**
Breitner, Burghard **525**
Brennsohn, Isidorus **554, 555, 605**
Brephoplastic Transplantation **2590**
Bretschneider, Hubert **821**
Brett, G. S. **2330**
Brettauer, Josef **786**
Brim, C. J. **813**
Brislin, J. F. **1289**
British abstracts **27**
British abstracts of medical sciences **918**
British Academy of Forensic Sciences **1470**
British and foreign medical review **58**
British and foreign medico-chirurgical review **59**
British chemical abstracts **1007**
British chemical and physiological abstracts **27**
British Congress on the History of Medicine and Pharmacy **571, 1462**
British Council. Medical Department **151**
British encyclopaedia for medical practice **116**
British Medical Association **1, 1443, 1988, 2543**
British medical book list **151**
British medical dictionary **231**
British pharmaceutical conference **2157.1**
British Postgraduate Medical Federation **126**
British Standards Institution **2437**
Brittain, R. P. **1470**
Brno. Universita. Knihovna **2255, 2406**
Brock, A. J. **497**

Brock, T. D. **1562**
Brockbank, William **2624**
Brockington, C. F. **2369**
Brodman, Estelle **434**
Brodny, M. L. **2636**
Broeckx, Corneille **528**
Bromberg, Walter **1812**
Bronchitis **2487**
Bronchoesophagology **2040.1**
Brooks, J. E. **2233.1**
Brous, F. A. **2234**
Brown, G. H. **569**
Brown, H. E. **1629**
Brown, J. A. C. **232**
Brown, Lawrason **1243**
Brown, Peter **2516**
Browne, E. G. **502**
Brucellosis
  Bibliographies **1161–1163**
Brunn, W. A. L. von **330**
Brunn, Walter von **329, 2563**
Bruno, J. P. **256.1**
Bruwer, A. J. **2445**
Bruzelius, A. J. **635**
Buchanan, R. E. **1559**
Budapest, Országos Orvostudományi Könyvtár és Dokumentációs Központ **80, 151.1, 1112, 1114, 1302, 1354, 1389, 1661, 1951, 2006, 2046, 2091, 2143.1, 2174, 2177.3, 2435, 2601**
Budge, E. A. T. W. **798**
Buley, R. C. **670**
Bulgaria
  Bibliographies **144, 533, 2061, 2309**
  Histories **533**
  Indexes and Abstracts **73, 912**
Bulgarska akademiia na naukite, Sofia **73, 912, 2061, 2309**
Bulgarska akademiia na naukite, Sofia. Tsentralna biblioteka **144**
Bulletin analytique **5**
Bulletin de l'Institut Pasteur **1538**
Bulletin international des services de santé des armées de terre, de mer et de l'air **1590**
Bulletin of hygiene **2342, 2399**
Bulletin on current literature **2257**
Bulletin on current literature of interest to crippled children workers **2257**
Bulletin signalétique **5**
Bulletin signalétique d'entomologie médicale et vétérinaire **2070**
Bulloch, William **1563**
Bundesverband der Deutschen Zahnärzte **1322**
Burch, G. E. **1131**
Burdett's hospitals and charities **1444**
Bureau of Chemical Abstracts **1005, 1007**
Bureau Permanent Interafricain de la Tse-Tse et de la Trypanosomiase **1228**
Burke, R. M. **1245**
Burma
  Indexes and Abstracts **2493.2**
Burns **2554.1, 2576**
Buros, O. K. **2306, 2307**
Burr, C. B. **702**
Burrage, W. L. **653, 654, 698**
Burrow, J. G. **661**
Burrows, E. H. **641**
Busch, D. W. H. **69**
Busch's systematisches Repertorium der gesammten medicinischen Literatur Deutschlands **97**
Bustad, L. K. **2695**
Butler, A. G. **1604**
Butler, S. W. **401**
Butsuri kagaku no shinpo **1039**
Butterworth, Thomas **1355**
Butterworths medical dictionary **231**
Byers, E. E. **2676**
Byoin Yoran **1447**

CBE factors **1048**
C. Canstatt's Jahresbericht über die Fortschitte der gesammten Medicin in allen Ländern **61**
CLUE; foreign clinical literature untoward effects **2229.1**
CME; continuing medical education: medical symposia **1368**
Cabanès, Augustin **749**
Caffaratto, T. M. **904**
Cahiers de bibliographie therapeutique française **2610.2**
Cahn, R. S. **1077**
Caillet, A. L. **799**
Calciati, A. **308**
Calcium Metabolism **2459**
Caldwell, A. E. **1863**
California. Histories **677**
California. University. Bureau of Public Administration **1758**
California. University. Institute of Governmental Studies **2529**
Callahan, L. I. **1065**
Callisen, A. C. P. **60**
Camac, C. N. B. **441**
Cambridge Philosophical Society **923**
Cameron, C. A. **593**
Campbell, A. M. **1200**
Campbell, D. M. **2661**
Campbell, Donald **503**
Campbell, I. R. **1041**
Campbell, J. M. **1290**
Campbell, R. J. **1786**
Canada
  Directories **348, 400, 402, 404, 1316, 1320, 1326, 1328, 1367, 1369, 1437, 1798, 1875, 2027, 2032, 2050, 2193.2, 2508**
  Histories **534–537, 654, 1606–1607**

Periodicals, Lists **2198**
Theses **179**
Canadian Dental Association **1320**
Canadian Hospital Association **1437**
Canadian hospital directory **1437**
Canadian medical directory **348**
Canal Zone
Bibliographies **1597**
Directories **389, 2050**
Cancer, *see* Neoplasms
Cancer chemotherapy **1701**
Cancer chemotherapy abstracts **1682**
Cancer Chemotherapy National Service Center **1682**
Cancer current literature index **1687**
Cancer film guide **1722**
Cancer motion picture guide **1722**
Cancer progress **1693**
Cancer Research Institute, Bratislava **1702.1**
Cancer services and facilities in the United States **1718**
Cancer services, facilities and programs in the United States **1718**
Candille, Marcel **1455**
Canniff, William **535**
Canstatt's Jahresbericht über die Fortschritte der gesammten Medicin in allen Landern **61**
Canstatt's Jahresbericht über die Fortschritte der Staatsarzneikunde **61**
Canstatt's Jahresbericht über die Fortschritte in der Pharmacie und verwandten Wissenschaften **2153**
Cantón, Eliseo **520**
Cantor, P. D. **2592**
Cape, Barbara **1895**
Carbery, A. D. **1624**
Carbohydrates **1013**
Carbon Monoxide **2391.1**
Carcinogenesis **1688**
Carcinogenesis abstracts **1688**
Cardenal Pujals, León **291**
Cardiac Surgery **9.18, 2576.1–2577**
Cardiff, Guillermo Furlong, *see* Furlong Cardiff, Guillermo
Cardiologists **1130**
Cardiovascular abstracts **1099**
Cardiovascular Agents **1120**
Cardiovascular compendium **1100**
Cardiovascular System, *see* Circulatory System
Caricatures **755–760**
Caries, Dental **1287, 1289, 1296**
Carl Christian Schmidt's Jahrbücher **39**
Carlos, A. **147**
Carnegie Institute of Technology, Pittsburgh. Rachel McMasters Miller Hunt Botanical Library **969**
Carnegie Institution of Washington **36, 1591**
Carøe, Kristian **547**
Carrier Clinic, Belle Mead, N. J. **1724**
Carter, G. B. **1957**
Carter, H. R. **1267**
Carter, L. A. **1267**
Cartilage Transplantation **2590**
Carus, J. V. **2690**
Caspari-Rosen, Beate **455**
Cass, J. S. **2090.1**
Cassar, Paul **607**
Castallo, M. A. **1959**
Castelli, Bartolomeo **256.1**
Castiglioni, Arturo **463, 596**
Catalysis **1014**
Catholic Hospital Association of the United States and Canada **201**
Catholic hospital directory **1452**
Catholic hospitals and schools of nursing **1452**
Catholic Library Association. Hospital Section **1894**
Caulfield, E. J. **2132**
Caveness, F. E. **2698**
Celli, Angelo **1195**
Celli-Fraentzel, Anna **1195**
Center for Occupational Mental Health, White Plains, N.Y. **1782**
Center for Occupational Therapy White Plains, N.Y. **109**
Central America
Directories **404**
Central Bureau of Hospital Information, London **1444**
Central Nervous System, *see* Brain and Spinal Cord
Centralblatt für Bakteriologie, Parasitenkunde und Infektionskrankheiten **1539**
Centralblatt für Bakteriologie und Parasitenkunde **1539**
Centralblatt für Chirurgie **2544**
Centralblatt für Nervenheilkunde, Psychiatrie und gerichtliche Psychopathologie **1739**
Centralblatt für praktische Augenheilkunde **1991**
Century of American medicine **663**
Cerebral Palsy **1775, 1777, 1855**
Cerebrovascular bibliography **1101**
Cerebrovascular System **1101**
Černič, Mirko **289**
Černocký, Karel **2314.3**
Československá akademie věd, Praha **1044, 2061.1**
Československá kardiologická společnost, Praha **1111**
Ceylon
Indexes and Abstracts **2493.2**
Chagas' Disease, *see* Trypanosomiasis
Chakraberty, Chandra **581**
Chambers' dictionary of scientists **2500**
Chambers' technical dictionary **2494**
Chance, Burton **2016**
Chapin, W. D. **111**

Charcot, J. M. **754**
Charles, John **2362**
Charles F. Kettering Memorial Hospital, Kettering, Ohio **18.2**
Chauveau, Claude **2051**
Chavez, Ignacio **609**
Chebotarev, R. S. **2067**
Chemical abstracts **995, 996, 1086**
Chemical-biological activities **997**
Chemical Engineering **1063, 1072, 1083**
Chemical Industry **1084**
Chemical reviews **1028**
Chemical Society, London **27, 1000, 1005, 1007, 1025, 1077**
Chemical titles **998**
Chemical who's who **1084**
Chemicals **1075**
Chemicals, Organic **1082**
Chemisch-pharmaceutisches Bio- und Bibliographikon **2210**
Chemisch-pharmaceutisches Central-Blatt **999**
Chemische Gesellschaft in der Deutschen Demokratischen Republik **999**
Chemisches Zentralblatt **999, 1087**
Chemistry and Biochemistry, *see also* Enzymes
  Bibliographies **1040–1051, 2493.3**
  Catalogs **1052–1057**
  Dictionaries **1064–1076**
  Directories **1083–1085**
  Histories **1056, 1088–1092**
  Indexes and Abstracts **7, 21.6, 21.7, 44, 994–1011, 2157.1**
  Manuals **1058–1063**
  Nomenclature **1077–1082**
  Periodicals **1086–1087**
  Reviews **1012–1039**
Chemistry, Analytical **1012**
Chemistry, Biological, *see* Chemistry and Biochemistry
Chemistry, Organic **1009, 1021, 1031, 1035, 1036, 1074, 1079**
Chemistry, Organometallic **1022**
Chemistry, Pharmaceutical **2166**
Chemistry, Physical **1015, 1039, 1072**
Chemists **1083.1, 1084, 1089, 2195**
Chemists, Pharmaceutical **2194, 2195, 2196**
Cheng, Lan Hua **1071**
Chernova, E. N. **318**
Chest and Heart Association (London) **1233**
Chest disease index and abstracts including tuberculosis **1233**
Chest Diseases **1233, 1104**
Chest Physicians **1240, 2490**
Cheu, S. H. **1166**
Chicago Medical Society **686**
Child Development **2108, 2117, 2127**
Child development abstracts and bibliography **2108**
Child development abstracts and bibliography selected from current issues of the Journal of the American Medical Association **2108**
Child, Hospitalized **2314**
Child Psychiatry **1757**
Child Psychology **2313, 2314**
Childhood Schizophrenia **1763, 1780**
Children, Diseases of **16.5**
Children, Exceptional **1800, 1802, 1857, 2131.1**
Chile
  Directories **349**
  Histories **538**
Chile. Servicio National de Salud **349**
Chilean Iodine Educational Bureau **1386.2**
Chimpanzees **2696**
China
  Bibliographies **2061.2, 2175**
  Collections, Periodicals **1504**
  Directories **350**
  Histories **539–541**
  Indexes and Abstracts **74, 919.1, 1004**
Chinchilla, Anastasio **627**
Chinese Academy of Medical Sciences **10**
Chinese medical directory **350**
Chiropodists **367**
Chirurgenverzeichnis **2560**
Chirurgie repartrice et traumatologie **2586**
Chita, RSFSR. Chitinskiĭ institut epidemiologii, mikrobiologii i gigieny **1097**
Chita, RSFSR. Gosudarstvennyĭ meditsinskiĭ institut **2431**
Chmielinska, Maria **2170**
Choi, K. D. **276**
Choisy, Maryse **1785**
Cholera **1139**
  Bibliographies **1164**
  Histories **1153, 1165**
Chopra, R. N. **976**
Choulant, J. L. **415, 416, 429, 889**
Christomopoulos, G. D. **257**
Chromatographic reviews **1029**
Chromatography **1029**
Chromatography, Gas **1047**
Chromatography, Paper **1044**
Ch'uan kuo chung wen ch'i k'an lien ho mu lu **1504**
Chung kuo k'o hsueh wen chai. I hsueh **74**
Chung kuo k'o hsueh wen chai. Sheng wu k'o hsueh **919.1**
Ciferri, Rafaele **1578**
Cincinnati. Academy of Medicine **718**
Cincinnati. University. College of Medicine. Kettering Laboratory of Applied Physiology **1041, 2390**
Circulatory System
  Bibliographies **1111–1125**
  Dictionaries **1128**
  Directories **1130**
  Histories **1131–1137**
  Indexes and Abstracts **9.18, 1099–1103**

Monographs **1126–1127**
Nomenclature **1129**
Reviews **1104–1110**
Citation **1465**
Civil War (U.S.) **1638–1642**
Clairville, A. L. **305–309**
Clapper, R. B. **1418**
Clark, A. S. **458**
Clark, G. N. **566**
Clark, P. F. **458, 1564**
Clarke, E. H. **663**
Clark's directory of southern hospitals **1451**
Classics, Medical **418, 419, 459,** *see also* History of Medicine, Sources
Classification Schemes **1526–1532**
Clay, R. S. **1584**
Cleave, Egbert **771**
Clendening, Logan **442**
Clermont-Ferrand, France. Université. Faculté mixte de médecine et de pharmacie. Bibliothèque **1505**
Cleveland, Ohio
Collections, Periodicals **1506**
Cleveland. Academy of Medicine **715**
Cleveland State Hospital. Documentation Research Laboratory **1730**
Clifford G. Grulee collection on pediatrics **2129**
Climatology **2261**
Clin-alert **2230**
Clinical Pathology, *see* Pathology and Clinical Pathology
Clinical Psychology **2303**
Clinics **392, 1439, 1446**
Clinics, Dermatological **1356**
Clinics, Psychiatric **1801**
Clostridium botulinum **160.1**
Coagulation, Blood **1123**
Cobalt **2239**
Cobb, W. M. **681**
Coccidioidomycosis
Bibliographies **1166, 1166.1**
Coëlho, M. B. **244**
Cole, F. J. **890, 2469**
Cole, Frank **2604**
Cole, H. N. **1618**
Cole, W. H. **1704**
Coleman, H. A. **1646**
Colitis, Ulcerative **1404.1**
Collection Nachet **1587**
College on American Pathologists **2094**
College of American Pathologists. Committee on Nomenclature and Classification of Disease **2093**
Collegium Medicinae Manjurici **36.1**
Colloids **1017**
Colombia
Bibliographies **144.1**
Histories **542**
Indexes and Abstracts **75**
Colorado. Histories **678**
Colorado State Medical Society **678**
Columbia University. Institute of French Studies **2011**
Columbia University. Parkinson Information Center **1730.1**
Columbia University. Psychology Library **2293**
Columbia University. School of Dental and Oral Surgery **1275**
Columbia University. School of Dental and Oral Surgery. Dental Abstracts Society **1275**
Columbia University. School of Dental and Oral Surgery. William Jarvie Society **1273**
Colwell, H. A. **2266**
Colyer, J. F. **1332**
Comar, C. L. **2459**
Combined Inter-Services Historical Section, India and Pakistan **1623**
Commonwealth Agricultural Bureaux **1937, 2057**
Commonwealth Bureau of Animal Health, Weybridge, Eng., *see also* Imperial Bureau of Animal Health, Weybridge, Eng. **2640, 2642**
Commonwealth Bureau of Helminthology, St. Albans, Eng. **2057**
Commonwealth Fund **1388**
Commonwealth Mycological Institute, Kew **1573, 1574, 1576, 1581,** *see also* Imperial Myocological Institute, Kew
Communicable Diseases, General, *see also* Anthrax; Bilharziasis; Botulism; Brucellosis; Cholera, Coccidioidomycosis; Dengue; Filariasis; Foot-and-mouth Disease; Hepatitis, Infectious; Histoplasmosis; Influenza; Leishmaniasis; Leprosy; Leptospirosis; Malaria; Plague; Poliomyelitis; Psittacosis; Rickettsial Diseases; Salmonella; Smallpox; Staphylococcal Infections; Toxoplasmosis; Trypanosomiasis; Tuberculosis; Tularemia; Venereal Diseases; Yellow Fever
Bibliographies **151.1, 1141–1144**
Histories, *see* Epidemiology, Histories
Indexes and Abstracts **10.13, 16.3, 1138–1139, 1539, 1540**
Reviews **1140, 1140.1**
Comparative Physiology **2274**
Completed research in health, physical education and recreation **2246**
Compounds, Heterocyclic **1018, 1078**
Comprehensive bibliography on hospital pharmacy **2141**
Computers **1362**
Comrie, J. D. **240, 567**
Conci, Giulio **2209**
Concilium Ophthalmologicum **2014**
Condensed chemical dictionary **1066**
Conditioned Reflex **1755**
Confederate States of America. Army **1639**
Conference of Executives of American Schools

for the Deaf and American Instructors of the Deaf **1875**
Conference on Application of X-ray Analysis **2424**
Congenital Anomalies
  Bibliographies **2127**
  Directories **903.1**
  Histories **904, 904.1**
  Indexes and Abstracts **9.21, 902.1–903**
Congrès international d'oto-rhino-laryngologie **2042**
Congress of the European Organization for Research on Fluorine and Dental Caries Prevention **1280**
Congresses **186–194, 1368**
Congressos internacionais de medicina tropical e paludismo. 6th, Lisboa, **1142, 1958**
Conn, H. J. **1585**
Connecticut. Histories **679–680**
Connecticut College for Women, New London. Department of Psychology **2304**
Connective Tissue **907**
Contemporary psychology **2301**
Contenau, Georges **491**
Contraception, *see* Reproduction
Cooper, A. G. **2391.1–2393**
Cooper, J. W. **2181**
Cope, Zachary **1408**
Copeman, W.S.C. **568, 1664**
Copenhagen. University. Library. Scientific and Medical Department **78, 1299**
Corbet, W. M. **228**
Cordell, E. F. **696**
Corlett, W. T. **513**
Corneal Transplantation **2590**
Cornelius, A. W. **302**
Cornell University. Graduate School of Business and Public Administration **399**
Corner, G. W. **891**
Corradi, Alfonso **1145**
Correia, Fernando da Silva **1456**
Corsini, R. J. **1759**
Cortisone **2617.1, 2619.1**
Cosmetics **2197.1**
Cosslett, V. E. **1583**
Coulter, J. L. S. **1615**
Coulter, J. S. **2267**
Council for International Organizations of Medical Sciences **342**
Council of American Bioanalysts **2081.1**
Council of Europe. Subcommittee on Pharmaceutical Questions **2183**
Courrier; revue mensuelle **2109**
Court, T. H. **1584**
Court Decisions **1464**
Coury, C. R. **462**
Cousland, P. B. **220**
Cowen, D. L. **710**
Cox, G. J. **1289**
Craddock, F. W. **2669**
Crane, E. J. **1060**
Crawford, D. G. **1620, 1621**
Crawford, Susan **659**
Crawfurd, R. H. P. **1201**
Creese, Richard **2279**
Creighton, Charles **1146, 2100**
Crime and delinquency abstracts **2532**
Crimean War **1616**
Crimes, War **1602**
Criminology **1471, 1474, 1727, 2529, 2532, 2534, 2537**
Crissey, J. T. **1360**
Critical bibliography of the history of science **2517**
Croly, Henry **369**
Crombie, A. C. **2518**
Crookshank, E. M. **1217**
Crosland, M. P. **1086**
Cross, L. M. **2670**
Crowley, C. G. **1291**
Cuba
  Directories **404, 2032**
  Histories **543–544**
  Indexes and Abstracts **96**
Cuba. Ministerio de Salud Publica **22**
Cuboni, E. **1507**
Cummings, R. O. **1923**
Cumulated index medicus **6**
Cumulative index of hospital literature **1435**
Cumulative index to nursing literature **1888**
Cunningham, Eileen **1527**
Cunningham, H. H. **1639**
Cunningham, P. J. **1898**
Curare **2169**
Curran, W. J. **1477**
Current bibliography on allergy and applied immunology **853**
Current chemical papers **1000**
Current contents **7**
Current list of medical literature **28**
Current literature—congenital anomalies **903**
Current literature on venereal disease **1252**
Current literature, poliomyelitis and related diseases **1206**
Current Medical Information, Inc. **1368**
Current medical references **8**
Current psychiatric therapies **1741**
Current publications in gerontology and geriatrics **1424.1**
Current publications on acoustics **1865.1**
Current scientific literature review **1694**
Current tissue culture literature **905**
Current titles from biological journals **920.2**
Current work in the history of medicine **417**
Curtis, A. H. **1964**
Cushing, Harvey **1502**
Cutter, I. S. **1964**
Cybernetics **21.8**

Cyclopedia of medicine, surgery, specialties **409**
Cyclopedia of medicine, surgery and specialties. Review service **117**
Cyprus
Indexes and Abstracts **2493.1**
Cyriax, E. F. **2250**
Cystic fibrosis **1404**
Cystic Fibrosis **1404**
Cytogenetics **1415, 1416, 1419.1**
Cytology
Dictionaries **938, 1419**
Histories **900–902**
Reviews **899**
Czabajska, Gabryela **2261**
Czechoslovakia
Bibliographies **1111, 1702.1, 1955, 2061.1, 2409**
Directories **351**
Histories **545–546**
Indexes and Abstracts **76–77, 2255**
Czechoslovakia. Ministerstvo veřejného zdravotnictví a tělesné výchovy **351**

D.D.S. Digest of dental science **1274**
DSH abstracts **1866**
Da Cruz, Vera **1956**
Daems, W. F. **2202**
Dain, Norman **1828**
Dainton, Courtney **1457**
Daly, L. W. **234**
Dana, C. L. **779**
Dana, Raoul **640**
Daniel, C. F. **1472**
Daniel, R. S. **2308**
Danish Medical Association **78**
Danish medical bulletin. Bibliographical supplement **78**
Dansk Tidsskrift for Farmaci **2148**
Danske Laegestand **547, 548**
Danske sygehus vaesen **1438**
Darlington, C. D. **1420**
Davenport, J. H. **780**
Dávid, József **1112**
David, Théophile **1293**
Davidson, H. A. **2671**
Davies, J. D. **1846**
Davis, D. J. **687**
Davis, G. G. **2407**
Davis, Loyal **2564**
Davis, P. E. **207**
Davison, M. H. A. **2605**
Davy de Virville, Adrien **986**
Davydov, N. N. **977**
Dawes, Ben **946**
Deafness **1866, 1867, 1867.1, 1871, 2047**
Directories **1875, 1876**
Histories **1877**
Deafness, Speech and Hearing Publications, Inc. **1866**
Death, Causes of **1880, 1883, 1883.1**
Debré, A. J. **1327**
Dechambre, Amédée **448**
Deficiency, Mental, *see* Mental Deficiency
Degensheim, G. A. **2567**
Dekker, W. A. L. **225**
Delamare, Jean **241**
Delamare, Valéry **241, 292**
Delaunay, Paul **557, 819**
Del Guercio, L. R. M. **310**
Delinquency, Juvenile **2531, 2532, 2537**
DeLong, C. W. **1095, 2302**
Delprat, C. C. **331**
De Marinis, Tammaro **1494**
Dengue
Bibliographies **1166.2**
Denmark
Bibliographies **145, 145.1**
Directories **352, 1438**
Histories **547–551**
Indexes and Abstracts **78, 2148**
Periodicals **322**
Denmark. Sundhedsstyrelsen **352**
Denmark. Sundhetskollegium **352**
Dennis, Wayne **2330.1**
Dent, J. K. **1783.1**
Dental abstracts **1268, 1275**
Dental Caries **1287, 1289, 1296**
Dental Council of India **1323**
Dental Hygiene Schools **1318**
Dental Hygienists **1320**
Dental Legislation **1926**
Dental Schools, *see* Schools, Dental
Dental Societies **1318–20, 1325–26**
Dental Writing **2669**
Dentistry
Bibliographies **167, 1286–1305**
Collections, Periodicals **1509**
Dictionaries **274, 293, 1306–1315**
Directories **374–382, 1316–1329**
Histories **1331–1346**
Indexes and Abstracts **10, 11, 1268–1278**
Periodicals **1330**
Reviews **1280–1285**
Dentists **346, 352–354, 366, 367, 372, 376, 377, 379, 380, 382, 384, 1317, 1318, 1319, 1320, 1321, 1322, 1323, 1326–1328, 1334, 2503**
Dentists register **1321**
Denton, G. B. **1308**
De Pasquale, N. P. **1131**
De Renzi, Salvatore **597**
Dermatological Clinics **1356**
Dermatologischer Jahresbericht **1348.1**
Dermatologisches Centralblatt **1349**
Dermatologists **1356, 1356.1**
Dermatology
Bibliographies **1256, 1354**
Dictionaries **1355**
Directories **1356**
Histories **1357–1360**

Indexes and Abstracts **9.13, 10.12, 16.11, 1253, 1254, 1347–1350.**
Reviews **1351–1353**
Dermatology and syphilology **1353**
Desnos, Ernest **2637**
Detergents **2394.1**
Deutsch, Albert **1829**
Deutsche Akademie der Naturforscher Leopoldina **420, 443**
Deutsche Botanische Gesellschaft **914**
Deutsche Dermatologische Gesellschaft **1253**
Deutsche Dokumentenstelle für Zahnärztliches Schrifttum, Stuttgart **1330**
Deutsche Gesellschaft für Chirurgie **2542**
Deutsche Gesellschaft für Gerichtliche und Soziale Medizin **1466**
Deutsche Gesellschaft für Geschichte der Medizin, Naturwissenschaft und Technik **419.1–420**
Deutsche Gesellschaft für Geschichte der Medizin und der Naturwissenschaften **420**
Deutsche Gesellschaft für Gyänkologie **1938**
Deutsche Gesellschaft der Hals-Nasen-Ohrenärzte **2036**
Deutsche Gesellschaft für Innere Medizin **13**
Deutsche Gesellschaft für Kinderheilkunde **2112**
Deutsche Gesellschaft für Tuberkulose und Lungenkrankheiten **1232**
Deutsche Gesellschaft für Zahn- Mund- und Kieferheilkunde **1273.1**
Deutsche pharmaziehistorische Bibliographie **2204**
Deutsche Physiologische Gesellschaft **2269, 2273**
Deutsche Röntgengesellschaft **2422**
Deutsche Staatsbibliothek **30.1**
Deutsche Vereningung für Geschichte der Medizin, Naturwissenschaft und Technik **419.1**
Deutsche Zeitschrift für die gesamte gerichtliche Medizin **1466**
Deutsche Zoologischen Gesellschaft **914, 2682**
Deutscher Chirurgenkalender **2560**
Deutscher Gyäkologenkalender **1962**
Deutscher Medizinischer Sprachendienst, München **2438**
Deutsches Chirurgen-Verzeichnis **2560**
Deutsches Gynäkologenverzeichnis **1962**
Deutsches Pädagogisches Zentralinstitut **1725, 2290**
Deutsches zahnärztliches Adressbuch **1322**
Development, Child **2108, 2117, 2127**
Devreesse, Robert **426**
De Vries, Louis **246, 2495, 2496**
Dexter, J. E. **1331**
Dezeimeris, J. E. **449**
Diabetes
Bibliographies **1395**
Directories **1396**
Histories **1397**
Indexes and Abstracts **1392–1394**
Diabetes literature index **1392**
Diabetes-related literature index **1393**
Diabetes research **1394**
Diagnosis
Bibliographies **1362**
Dictionaries **1362.1–1364**
Indexes and Abstracts **1361,**
Diagnostic Radiology **2426**
Diccionario biográfico médico mundial **378**
Diccionario medicobiologico university **291.1**
Dick, E. A. **1582**
Dickson, S. A. **2238.1**
Dictionaire des sciences médicales. Biographie médicale **450**
Dictionaries
By Language
Afrikaans **215**
Arabic **216, 871, 875, 2699, 2701**
Bulgarian **217, 218**
Chinese **220–222, 908.2, 1071, 1307.1, 1362.1, 1554.1, 2092.1, 2180.1, 2356.1, 2623.1**
Czech **876, 2314.3**
Danish **223, 883, 1787.1**
Dutch **224, 228, 2315**
English **195, 197, 210, 212, 229–240, 870, 872, 874, 936, 938, 940, 941, 976, 981, 1064, 1066, 1068, 1069, 1074, 1075, 1193, 1306–1308, 1310, 1311, 1355, 1363, 1418, 1419, 1476, 1479, 1479.1, 1556, 1581, 1582, 1784, 1786, 1787, 1789, 1792, 1864, 1865, 1873, 1895, 1897–1902, 1920, 1921, 1956, 1957, 1959, 2010, 2012, 2029–2031, 2181, 2224, 2262, 2317, 2318, 2322, 2325, 2437, 2439, 2442, 2494, 2497, 2533, 2534, 2651, 2698, 2700**
Finnish **244**
French **209, 241, 242, 878, 880, 939, 978, 1067, 1313.1, 1555, 1785, 1788, 2011, 2320, 2468, 2495, 2653,**
German **213, 214.1, 245–256, 873, 877, 884, 937, 937.1, 975, 980, 1073, 1239, 1312, 1419.1, 1478, 1599.1, 2008, 2077, 2184, 2316, 2319, 2324, 2496, 2650, 2702**
Greek **256.1, 257, 258**
Hawaiian **258.1**
Hebrew **259, 260**
Hungarian **214, 261**
Indonesian **262**
Italian **263–268, 1475, 1790, 2441**
Japanese **269–275, 879, 1364, 1896**
Korean **276**
Latin **277, 278, 875**
Malayan **279**
Norwegian **280**
Polish **211, 281, 282, 2321**

Polyglot **304–317, 854.1, 882, 977, 979, 1076, 1128, 1312.1, 1315, 1474, 1557, 1958, 2009, 2182, 2183, 2186, 2281, 2357, 2438, 2440, 2652**
Portuguese **283, 284, 1309, 1314, 2185**
Russian **285–287, 942, 1065, 1070, 1072, 1791, 2067**
Serbian **288**
Slovenian **289**
Spanish **290–296, 881, 1313, 1419.2**
Swedish **297–299, 2323**
Tagalog **300**
Turkish **301**
Urdu **302**
Zulu **303**
By Subject
Abbreviations **195–197**
Allergy **854.1**
Anatomy **870–884**
Antibiotics **2224**
Biology **936–942**
Botany **975–981**
Chemistry **1064–1076**
Dentistry **1306–1315**
Dermatology **1355**
Diagnosis **1362.1–1364**
Embryology **908.2**
Engineering, Sewage **2357**
Entomology **2077**
Etymology **198–208**
Genetics **1418–1419.2**
Gynecology **1958, 1959**
Hematology **1128**
Histology **877, 878, 908.2**
Legal Medicine **1474–1479**
Malaria **1193**
Medicine **195–317**
Microbiology **1554.1–1557**
Military Medicine **1599.1**
Mycology **1581, 1582**
Neurology **1790**
Nursing **1895–1902**
Nutrition **1920, 1921**
Obstetrics **1956–1959**
Ophthalmology **2008–2012**
Optometry **2029–2031**
Parasitology **2067**
Pathology **2092.1**
Pharmacy **2180.1–2186**
Physiatrics **2262**
Physiology **2281**
Psychiatry **1784–1788, 1791, 1792**
Psychology **2314.3–2325**
Psychopharmacology **1864, 1865**
Public Health **2356.1, 2357**
Radiology **2437–2442**
Science **2494–2497**
Sexology **2468**
Sociology **2533, 2534**
Speech **1873**
Syndromes **209–214.1, 1313.1, 1355, 1790**
Therapeutics **239, 2623.1**
Tuberculosis **1239**
Veterinary Medicine **2650–2653**
Zoology **2698–2702**
Dictionary of American medical biography **654**
Dictionary of water and sewage engineering **2537**
Dictionnaire de sexologie, sexologialexikon **2468**
Dictionnaire encyclopédique des sciences médicales **448**
Dictionnaire historique de la médecine **449**
Dieci anni di bibliografia medica italiana **154**
Diels, Hermann **427**
Diepgen, Paul **457, 464, 1965, 1966**
Diet, Histories, *see* Nutrition, Histories
Diet Therapy **2615**
Dietetics **239, 1917, 1921**
Dietschy, Hans **516**
Dietz, P. A. **2315**
Digest of neurology and psychiatry **1726**
Digest of ophthalmology and otolaryngology **2034**
Digestion **1407**
Diller, Theodore **720**
Dimitrova, E. **2061**
Diotallevi, Lamberto **1297**
Diptera **2072**
Directorio medico mexicano **374.1**
Directorio medico Panameño **375.2**
Directory for exceptional children **1800**
Directory of administrative staff, department chairmen and individual members in medical schools of the United States and Canada **1369**
Directory of approved internships and residencies **1370**
Directory of biological laboratories **1085**
Directory of biomedical institutions in the Union of the Soviet Socialist Republics **383**
Directory of birth defects centers **903.1**
Directory of British scientists **2501**
Directory of Catholic hospitals and allied agencies in the United States and Canada **1452**
Directory of information resources in the United States **395**
Directory of medical and biological research institutes of the USSR **383**
Directory of medical colleges in India **1371**
Directory of medical libraries in the British Isles **1533**
Directory of medical specialists **391**
Directory of outpatient psychiatric clinics, psychiatric day-night services and other mental

health resources in the United States and territories **1801**
Directory of resources for mentally ill children in the United States **1802**
Directory of services for the deaf in the United States **1875**
Directory of university research bureaus and institutes **2486**
Diseases, Animal **2654**
Diseases, Communicable, *see* Communicable Diseases
Diseases, Fungus **1579**
Diseases, Metabolic **1389**
Diseases, Occupational, *see* Occupational Health
Diseases of medical progress: Present status **2610.1**
Diseases of medical progress: Progress report **2610.1**
Diseases, Parasitic, *see* Parasitology
Diseases, Rheumatic, *see* Rheumatic Diseases
Diseases, Rickettsial, *see* Rickettsial Diseases
Diseases, Tropical, *see* Communicable Diseases; Tropical Medicine
Diseases, Venereal, *see* Venereal Diseases
Disney, A. N. 1589
Disorders, Mental **1238, 1783, 1793**
Disorders, Speech **1873**
Dispensatories **2176**
Dissertation abstracts **179, 181**
Distillation Products Industries **1934**
District of Columbia. Histories **681–682**
Dittmer, D. S. **931.1, 932, 1126**
Dittrick, Howard **715**
Diving **836**
Dix années de psychologie française **2291**
Dizionario medico **264**
Dmitrioff, A. **1791**
Dobson, Jessie **872**
Dock, L. L. **1910**
Doctor, P. V. **1876**
Doctoral dissertations accepted by American universities **179**
Documenta cardioangiologica **1102**
Documenta ophthalmologica **1997**
Documentation sur la psychologie française **2291**
Doe, Janet **1485**
Doering, S. J. L. **184**
Doetsch, R. N. **1565**
Dogs **2694**
Dohrn, R. F. A. **1967**
Donáth, Tibor **873**
Donner Foundation **1703**
Dorland, W. A. N. **233, 234, 1899**
Dorsch, Friedrich **2316**
Doull, J. A. **1154**
Downs, W. S. **406, 1084**
Driver, A. H. **744**
Driver, E. D. **1759.1**
Drosophila **1417**
Drug Addiction **2241**
Drug digests **2142**
Drug digests from the foreign language literature **2142**
Drug information sources **2143**
Drug Literature **2180**
Drug Therapy **2155, 2158, 2168.1, 2174, 2218, 2616**
Drug topics red book **2187**
Drugs, Side Effects **2229–2231, 2233**
Drugs, Stability **2176.1**
Drummond, J. C. **1924**
Dry, T. J. **1136**
Drzavna Zalozba Slovenije, Ljubljana **289**
Dubos, Jean **1246**
Dubos, René **1246**
Düsseldorf. Zentralstelle für Krebsbekämpfung. Bibliothek **1705**
Duffy, John **695, 1147**
Dugan, P. R. **2228**
Dujmušić, Stanko **739**
Duke-Elder, Stewart **2003**
Duke University. Medical Center **190.1**
Dumaître, Paule **484**
Dumbleton, C. **942**
Dumesnil, René **483**
Duncan, L. C. **1635, 1637, 1640**
Duncum, B. M. **2606**
Dunglison, Robley **235**
Dunn, L. C. **1421**
Durán, Carlos Martínez, *see* Martínez Durán, Carlos
Durante, M. I. **1309**
Durante Avellanal, Ciro **1309**
Duray, Aladár **2046**
Durham, R. H. **210**
Durling, S. M. (Parker) **757**
Dust **2408**
Duveen, D. O. **1052, 1053**
el-Duweini, A. K. **2699**
Dvinianinov, L. I. **1406.1**
Dvurechenskaia, N. V. **1178**
Dyer, H. M. **1714**
Dyke, S. C. **2087, 2097**
Dyson, G. M. **1061**
Dystrophy, Muscular **1656**
Dzhaparidze-Iosidze, T. B. **166**

E.E.N.T. digest **2034**
Ear, *see* Otorhinolaryngology
Earle, A. S. **2565**
East, C. F. T. **1132**
East, Terence **1109**
East Africa
Bibliographies **145.2**
Eaton, L. K. **1458**

Ebert, Myrl **332**
Eble, Burkard **471**
Economics, Medical **2341, 2343, 2473**
Ecuador
    Bibliographies **146**
    Histories **552–553**
Edelstein, Ludwig **588**
Edling, Carl **635**
Education, Medical and Allied Sciences
    Bibliographies **1365.1, 1366**
    Directories **351, 1367–1372**
    Histories **1373–1378,** *see also* Histories, under various countries
    Indexes and Abstracts **1365**
    Manuals **1366.1**
Education, Medical, Continuing **1368**
Education, Pharmacy **2179**
Education, Physical, *see* Physical Education and Sports Medicine
Education, Psychiatric **1798**
Educational Council for Foreign Medical Graduates **1366.1**
Egypt
    Directories **353**
    Histories, *see* History of Medicine, Ancient; History of Medicine, Arabic
    Indexes and Abstracts **2493.1**
Egypt. Ministry of Education **216**
Egypt. University. Faculty of Medicine **1158**
Eichler, Max **1276**
Eidel'shtein, S. I. **2221**
Electroencephalography **1839.1, 1840, 1841**
Electromyography **1654**
Electromyography **1654**
Electron Microscopy **1583**
Electronics, Medical **958, 962**
Electrophoresis **1042**
Electroshock Therapy **1761**
Electrotherapy **2436**
    Histories **2266**
Elephantiasis **1167**
Elgood, C. L. **591**
Elkin, I. I. **2221**
Ellenberger-Schütz Jahresbericht **2644**
Ellis, E. S. **2607**
Ellis, Rhoda **1921**
Eloy, N. F. J. **451**
Elsevier's Fachwörterbuch der Kriminalwissenschaft in acht Sprachen **1474**
Elsevier's medical dictionary in five languages **311**
Emanuilova, E. K. **2309**
Embryology **9.1, 858.1, 877, 878, 908.1, 908.2, 938**
    Histories **893–894**
Emmerson, J. S. **418**
Emphysema **2487**
Enciclopedia medica italiana **410**
Enciclopedia Salvat de ciencias medicas **411**
Encyclopedia of American associations **396**
Encyclopedia of associations **396**
Encyclopedias **408–413**
Encyclopédie française d'urologie **2637**
Encyklopedie praktického lékaře **412**
Endocarditis **1124, 1125**
Endocrinology, *see also* Diabetes
    Bibliographies **1386–1390**
    Histories **1391**
    Indexes and Abstracts **9.3, 16.1, 1379–1380.**
    Reviews **1381–1385, 1932, 1933**
Engelmann, Wilhelm **149.1, 149.2, 2689, 2690**
Engineering, Chemical **1063, 1072, 1083**
Engineering, Human **847, 1595**
Engineering, Public Health **2344**
Engineering, Sewage **2357**
Engineering, Water **2357**
England, *see* Great Britain
Engle, Bernice **1771**
English, H. B. **2317**
Engström, Einar **297**
Enslin, T. C. F. **149.1**
Entomological Society of America **2071, 2073**
Entomology
    Bibliographies **2075–2076**
    Dictionaries **2077**
    Histories **2078**
    Indexes and Abstracts **2070–2072**
    Reviews **2073–2074**
Entralgo, Pedro Laín, *see* Laín Entralgo, Pedro
Entsiklopedicheskiĭ slovar' voennoĭ meditsiny **1600**
Environment **1048**
Environmental Biology **931.1**
Environmental Health
    Bibliographies **2387–2394.1**
    Directories **2394.2–2396**
    Indexes and Abstracts **2385–2386**
Enzymes
    Bibliographies **1097**
    Nomenclature **1098**
    Reviews **1093–1096**
Epidemics **1143**
    Histories **466, 1145–1147, 2095–2096, 2099–2100**
Epidemiology **10.13, 16.3**
    Histories **1148–1149, 1154–1155,** *see also* Parasitology, Histories; Tropical Medicine, Histories
Epilepsy **1855**
    Histories **1836**
Eponyms
    Bibliography **459**
Eponyms, Anatomy **872**
Equipment **293**
Ergebnisse der allgemeinen Pathologie und pathologischen Anatomie **2082**

Ergebnisse der Anatomie und Entwicklungsgeschichte **863**
Ergebnisse der Biologie **924**
Ergebnisse der Chirurgie und Orthopädie **2549**
Ergebnisse der Enzymforschung **1096**
Ergebnisse der gesamten Tuberkulose- und Lungenforschung **1236**
Ergebnisse der gesamten Tuberkuloseforschung **1236**
Ergebnisse der Hygiene, Bakteriologie, Immunitätsforschung und experimentellen Therapie **1548**
Ergebnisse der Immunitätsforschung, experimentellen Therapie, Bakteriologie und Hygiene **1548**
Ergebnisse der inneren Medizin und Kinderheilkunde **118**
Ergebnisse der medizinischen Grundlagenforschung **119**
Ergebnisse der Mikrobiologie, Immunitätsforschung und experimentellen Therapie **1548**
Ergebnisse der physikalisch-diätetischen Therapie **2615**
Ergebnisse der Physiologie, biologischen Chemie und experimentellen Pharmakologie **2277**
Ergebnisse der Vitamin- und Hormonforschung **1932**
Erivan. Respublikanskaia nauchnomeditsinskaia biblioteka **1386**
Ershkovich, E. G. **2005**
Estonia
    Bibliographies **147**
    Histories **554–555**
Ethnology **5.7**
Etingen, L. E. **1113**
Etter, L. E. **2439**
Etymology **198–208**
Evang, Karl **280**
Evans, A. J. **2171, 2172**
Eversley, D. E. C. **1146, 2470**
Everson, T. C. **1704**
Exceptional Children **1800, 1802, 1857, 2131.1**
Excerpta criminologica **1727**
Excerpta medica **9, 35.1, 319, 886, 1394**
Excerpta Medica Foundation **9, 24, 103, 106, 319, 1656, 1686, 1687, 1727, 2189, 2229, 2231, 2233**
Excerpts from articles on urologic surgery **2631**
Exposés annuels de biochimie médicale **1030**
Eye, *see* Ophthalmology
Eye, ear, nose and throat **2045**
Eycleshymer, A. C. **885**
Eyre, L. B. **950**

F.D.A. clinical experience abstracts **2230.1**
Facts about nursing **1903**
Faidherbe, A. J. **529**
Fairchild, D. S. **690**
Fairley, N. H. **1140.1**
Faller, Adolf **892**
Fallout, Radioactive **2388, 2389**
Family Centre, London **2461**
Family Therapy **1781.2**
Famous Persons **762–768**
Faragó, Lászlo **1354**
Farber, Eduard **1089**
Farmaceutisk Tidende **2148**
Farmhouse, J. C. R. **1142**
Farmhouse, Manuel **1142**
Farrell, Gabriel **2028**
Fasbender, Heinrich **1968**
Fastlicht, Samuel **1292**
Fatigue **2305**
Fats **1038**
Faulconer, Albert **2608**
Fay, H. M. **1184**
Fearing, Franklin **1832**
Feasby, W. R. **1607**
Feces **1046**
Fédération Française des Sociétés de Science Naturelles **922.1**
Federation of American Sanataria **2490**
Federation of American Societies for Experimental Biology **177**
Federation of American Societies for Experimental Biology. Committee on Biological Handbooks **931, 931.1, 932, 1126**
Federation proceedings. Translation supplement **177**
Fedotov, D. D. **1776**
Feeny, Patrick **1185**
Fejgin, Mieczyslaw **211**
Feldmann, Harald **2052**
Fellendorf, G. W. **1867.1**
Fellowships, funds, and prizes available for graduate medical work in the United States and Canada **1371**
Fendrych, Miroslav **2061.1**
Fenner, Friedrich **814**
Ferchl, Fritz **2210**
Ferguson, F. C. **1843**
Ferguson, John **800, 1054**
Ferguson, Mungo **1491**
Fermentation **1044.1, 1543**
Fernandez, Alicia de **320**
Ferreira de Mira, Matias B., *see* Mira, M. B. Ferreira de
Ferrio, Luigi **265**
Fertility, *see* Reproduction
Fertility abstracts **2461**
Fibrinolysis **1123**
Fibrosis, Cystic **1404**
Field, E. J. **874**
Fifield, J. C. **400**
Filariasis
    Bibliographies **1167–1168**
Filby, F. A. **1925**

Filliozat, Jean **582**
Film reference guide for medicine and allied sciences **1400**
Films **374, 1398–1401, 1722, 1757, 1806–1807**
Financial assistance available for graduate study in medicine **1371**
Fink, Max **1841**
Finland
Bibliographies **148–149, 1952, 2434**
Collections, Periodicals **1514**
Directories **354**
Histories **634**
Indexes and Abstracts **79**
Periodicals **322**
Finnish Radiological Society **2434**
First District Dental Society of the State of New York **1305**
Fischer, Alfons **2367**
Fischer, H. W. K. **987**
Fischer, Isidor **447, 1969**
Fishbein, Morris **662, 1208, 2672**
Fishman, A. P. **1133**
Fitzpatrick, W. H. **2302**
Flack, I. H. **1970**
Flanigan, P. J. **1854**
Fleas **2072, 2075.1**
Fleetwood, John **594**
Fletcher, Robert **36**
Flexner, J. T. **664**
Flick, L. F. **1247**
Flies, Tsetse **1229**
Flint's medical and surgical directory of the United States and Canada **402**
Flood, W. E. **200, 2497**
Flores, F. A. **610**
Florida. Histories **683**
Florida Chemical Research Company, New York **1868**
Florkin, Marcel **1098**
Flugel, J. C. **2331**
Fluorine **1041, 1280**
Folk medicine **797–798, 800–802**
Denmark **550**
Great Britain **564**
Lapps **602**
Tibet **637–638**
Fonahn, A. M. **592, 875**
Food **1914, 1916, 1918, 1920**
Histories, *see* Nutrition, Histories
Food and Agriculture Organization of the United Nations **2657**
Food Hygiene **2409**
Food Industry **1072**
Food science abstracts **1914**
Foot-and-Mouth Disease
Bibliographies **1168.1**
Forbes, J. J. **2408**
Foreign Substance Implants **2590**
Forensic Medicine, *see* Legal Medicine
Forensic Science Society, London **1480**
Formularies **2176**
Fortes, Hugo **283**
Fortschritte der Allergielehre **854**
Fortschritte der Arzneimittelforschung **2164**
Fortschritte der Augenheilkunde **1998**
Fortschritte der Chemie organischer Naturstoffe **1031**
Fortschritte der chirurgie **2553**
Fortschritte der experimentellen Tumorforschung **1696**
Fortschritte der Hals- Nasen- Ohrenheilkunde **2042**
Fortschritte der Kardiologie **1105**
Fortschritte der medizinischen Virusforschung **1551**
Fortschritte der Tuberkuloseforschung **1235**
Fortschritte der Zahnheilkunde nebst Literaturarchiv **1278**
Fortún y Foyo, José A. Martínez, *see* Martínez Fortún y Foyo, J. A.
Foskett, D. J. **1918**
Fossati, Franco **2440**
Foster, F. P. **312**
Foster, Michael **2283**
Foster, W. D. **2068, 2097**
Foucault, Michel **508, 1819**
Foundation directory **397**
Fowler, J. E. H. **1311**
Fränkel, G. H. F. **1594**
France
Bibliographies **1293**
Collections, Periodicals **1505**
Directories **355-358, 1319, 1439, 2193.1**
Histories **339, 556–561, 1184, 1459, 1608, 1819–1820, 2201, 2203**
Indexes and Abstracts **858.1, 2292, 2610.2**
Periodicals **339**
France, Bibliothèque Nationale. Département des Imprimés **1490**
France. Centre d'Etudes de Documentation et de Recherches **2610.2**
France. Centre National de la Recherche Scientifique **5, 2080**
France. Ministère de l'Education Nationale. Direction des Bibliothèques et de la Lecture Publique **1520.1**
Francesco, Grete de **805**
Francis, W. W. **1493**
Franco-Prussian War **1610**
Frank, L. F. **735**
Frank, Mortimer **889**
Frari, A. A. **1202**
Frazer, W. M. **2370**
Freeman, S. E. **787**
Freidlin, S. I. **2350**
Frenay, Sister Mary Agnes Clare **201**

Freund, Hugo **1586**
Freund, Jules **562**
Frey, Rudolf **2603.1**
Frick, Karl **1090**
Friedenwald, Harry **774, 775**
Friedreich, J. B. **1813**
Friedrich, W. **69.1**
Fritz, Lois **1721**
Froehner, Reinhard **2659**
Frohn, Wilhelm **1186**
Frommel's Jahresbericht über die Fortschritte auf dem Gebiete der Geburtshilfe und Gynäkologie **1943**
Frost, W. H. **1267**
Fryer, Peter **2471**
Fuels **1072**
Fujikawa, Yu **599, 600**
Fulton, J. F. **435, 837, 850, 1869, 2284, 2285, 2609**
Fungi **1542, 1574, 1581**
Fungus Diseases **1579**
Funkenstein, D. H. **1760**
Furlong Cardiff, Guillermo **521**

Gabriel, H. W. **1363**
Gairdner, Douglas **2123**
Galactosemia **1852**
Galdston, Iago **438, 509**
Gale Research Company **396, 2485, 2486**
Gallaudet College, Washington, D.C. **1876**
Gallot, Émile **947**
Galuzo, I. G. **1224**
Galvan, Antonio **306**
Gammerman, A. F. **2182**
Gandevia, Bryan **523, 524**
Ganis, F. M. **1387**
Ganka saikin no shinpo **1999**
Gantt, W. A. **643**
Garber, S. T. **238**
Garcïa del Real, Eduardo **628**
Garnier, Gabriel **2197.2**
Garnier, Marcel **241, 292**
Garrison, F. H. **333, 419, 444, 465, 889, 1601, 2133**
Gas chromatography abstracts **1001**
Gasiorowski, Ludwik **622**
Gaskell, Eric **1462**
Gastroenterology
- Bibliographies **1406.1, 1407**
- Histories **1408**
- Indexes and Abstracts **36.2, 1402–1404**
- Reviews **1405–1406**

Gastroenterology abstracts and citations **1403**
Gauss, C. J. **1971**
Geist und Kritik der medicinischen und chirurgischen Zeitschriften Deutschlands für Aerzte und Wundärzte **96.1**
Geist und Kritik der medicinischen und chirurgischen Zeitschriften Deutschlands für neunzehnte Jahrhundert **96.1**
Geka kenkyu no shinpo **2550**
Geka saikin no shinpo **2551**
Gelfand, D. P. **383**
Geller, M. R. **1761, 1762, 1783**
Geneeskundig jaarboekje voor Nederland en Rijksdelen Overzee **375**
General Dynamics Corporation. Convair Division **2576.1**
General medicine **127**
General practice clinics **28.1**
General surgery **2555**
General therapeutics **2616.1**
Genetics
- Bibliographies **908.1, 1415–1417.1**
- Dictionaries **938, 1418–1419.2**
- Histories **1420–1423**
- Indexes and Abstracts **5.3, 9.22, 1409**
- Reviews **1410–1414**

Genzel, Peter **937.1**
Geography, Medical **21.1, 21.9, 2345**
George Washington University, Washington, D.C. Biological Sciences Communication Project **2061.2, 2197.1, 2688**
Georgian SSR
- Bibliographies **166, 2059**

Gergeley, János **1114**
Geriatrics **9.20, 1424, 1424.1, 1426–1429**
Germ-free Research **1553–1554**
Germany
- Bibliographies **149.1–150, 1711, 2261.1, 2314.1, 2648–2649**
- Directories **359, 1083.1, 1322, 1356, 1440–1442, 1534, 1962, 2560, 2603.1, 2656.1**
- Histories **329, 338, 562–563, 1186, 1463, 1602, 1609–1613, 1821–1822, 2204–2206, 2367**
- Indexes and Abstracts **66, 96.1, 97, 2297**
- Periodicals **329, 338**
- Theses **181**

Germany. Heer. Sanitätsinspektion **1611**
Germany. Democratic Republic. Dokumentationszentrum für Medizinische Wissenschaftliche Literatur **107**
Germany. Democratic Republic. Ministerium für Gesundheitswesen. Abteilung Wissenschaft **1534**
Germany. Federal Republic. Statistisches Bundesamt **1441**
Germany. Territory under Allied Occupations. U.S. Zone. Military Tribunals **1602**
Gerontology
- Bibliographies **1426–1429**
- Directories **1430**
- Histories **1431–1432**
- Indexes and Abstracts **9.20, 1424, 1424.1**
- Reviews **1425**

Gesamtverband Deutscher Nervenärzte **1733**
Gesellschaft Deutscher Chemiker **1083.1**
Gesellschaft für Geschichte der Pharmazie, Berlin **2210**
Gesellschaft zur Bekämpfung der Krebs-Krankheiten **1705**
Gesundheits Brockhaus **247**
Getz, Bernhard **616**
Gfrörer, Dieter **248**
Ghalioungui, Paul **492**
Ghana
  Bibliographies **150.1**
Gibson, W. C. **453**
Giese, Fritz **2316**
Gilbert, J. B. **649, 762**
Gimlette, J. D. **279**
Gins, H. A. **1218**
Glasgow. University. Hunterian Museum **1491**
Glasgow. University. Library **1055**
Glasser, Otto **2446**
Glaucoma **2005**
Glosario de psycofarmaka **1864**
Gnucheva, V. V. **137, 138, 159**
Gocht, Hermann **1673, 1674, 2432**
Goerke, Heinz **457**
Goiter **1386, 1386.2**
Gold Coast, *see* Ghana
Goldberg, Morris **293, 294**
Goldby, F. **865**
Goldfarb, William **1763**
Goldman, M. R. **2010**
Goldschmid, Edgar **2098**
Goldsmith, A. J. B. **2003**
Goldsmith, W. N. **1352**
Goldstein, M. A. **704**
Goldstein, Miron **493**
Golemanov, Khristo **533**
Goncharova, E. E. **1764**
Good, N. E. **2075.1**
Goodwin, E. J. **705**
Gordon, B. L. **1878, 1879**
Gordon, J. E. **1154**
Gorgas, F. J. S. **1310**
Gorgas Hospital, Ancon, Canal Zone. Medical Library **1597**
Gorillas **2696**
Gorlin, R. J. **212**
Gortvay, György **578**
Goszleth, Tibor **1951**
Gotfredsen, Edvard **473**
Gottfried, Oscar **794**
Gottlieb, David **2530**
Gottschalk, Alfred **1926**
Gould, Julius **2533**
Goulden, W. O. **249**
Gout, history **1664**
Governmental air pollution agencies **2394.2**
Graefe, Alfred **2017**
Graevell's Notizen für praktische Aerzte über die neuesten Beobachtungen in der Medicin **62**
Graham, E. C. **2260**
Graham, Harvey [pseud.], *see* Flack, I. H.
Grainger, T. H. **1566**
Granderye, L. M. **1067**
Granjel, L. S. **439, 626, 629**
Grant, J. **1068**
Grants, Training **2396**
Grapow, Hermann **494**
Grasset, Hector **2268**
Grassick, James **714**
Graubard, Mark **1134**
Gray, Peter **933**
Graziano, E. E. **1362**
Great Britain
  Bibliographies **151, 573, 869, 1290**
  Directories **360–363, 1242, 1321, 1443–1444, 1533, 2194–2195, 2501, 2505, 2507**
  Histories **336, 564–574, 808, 826, 1146, 1205, 1376, 1454, 1457, 1462, 1614–1619, 1814, 1823–1824, 1907, 1913, 1924–1925, 1972, 1979, 2019, 2132, 2135, 2214, 2216.1, 2217, 2368–2371, 2570, 2664**
  Periodicals **336**
  Theses **180**
Great Britain. Airborne Medical Services **1618**
Great Britain. Army Medical Department **1616**
Great Britain. Bureau of Hygiene and Tropical Diseases **1139, 2342**
Great Britain. Dental Board of the United Kingdom **1321**
Great Britain. Department of Scientific and Industrial Research **1914, 2386**
Great Britain. General Council of Medical Education and Registration **1321**
Great Britain. General Dental Council **1321**
Great Britain. General Medical Council **361**
Great Britain. Ministry of Health **1434**
Great Britain. Ministry of Technology **2386**
Great Britain. Sleeping Sickness Bureau **1175, 1177, 1226, 1229**
Great Britain. Tropical Disease Bureau **1175, 1226**
Greece. Histories **1197,** *see also* History of Medicine, Ancient
Green, S. A. **699**
Greenbaum, L. J. **836**
Greenberg, L. A. **2236**
Greene, J. C. **948**
Greenwood, Major **1148, 2417**
Greif, Samuel **1328**
Grigg, E. R. N. **2447**
Grigorash, F. F. **606**
Grinstein, Alexander **1765**
Grmek, M. D. **173, 739, 1431**
Grøn, Fredrik **617**

Grombakh, S. M. **644**
Gross, Martin **2235, 2236**
Gross, S. D. **665, 666**
Grossmann, Anna, *see* Cooper, A. G.
Group Practice **394**
Group Psychotherapy **1728, 1759, 1772**
Group Psychotherapy Center, New York **1772**
Group psychotherapy literature **1728**
Growth **929, 932**
Grundriss der Medizin der alten Ägypter **494**
Guatemala. Histories **575**
Guerini, Vincenzo **1333**
Guerra, Francisco **167, 531, 603, 611, 2173**
Gürson, C. T. **301**
Guía oficial del club médico del Uruguay **406.1**
Guide de la santé et de l'aide sociale **1439**
Guide Rosenwald, médical et pharmaceutique **358**
Guide to Latin American scientific and technical periodicals **2511**
Guidelines for medical school libraries **1481**
Guild of Prescription Opticians of America, Inc. **2033**
Guitard, E. H. **334, 2203**
Gurlt, E. J. **446, 2566**
Guthrie, Douglas **2055**
Guttmacher, A. F. **2472**
Guttmann, W. **255**
Guttstadt, A. **1442**
Guyénot, Émile **949**
Gymnastics, Medical **16.1, 2250**
Gynäkologen deutscher Sprache, Biographie und Bibliographie **1962**
Gynecologists **1960–1962.1**
Gynecology, *see* Obstetrics and Gynecology
Gynecology, obstetrics guide **1939**
Gyógyszerészeti és gyógyszer-terápiás dokumentációs szemle **2143.1**

Haagensen, C. D. **510**
Haan, H. R. M. de **225**
Haas, Hans **2211**
Haberling, Wilhelm **446, 562**
Hackh's chemical dictionary **1068**
Haenel, A. F. **69.1**
Haeser, Heinrich **466, 1143**
Hahn, André **484, 1512**
Hahn, Lucien **141**
Hahon, Nicholas **1567**
Haiti. Histories **576**
Halban, Josef **1969**
Half a century of progress in orthopaedic surgery **1679**
Half-yearly abstract of the medical sciences **63**
Half-yearly compendium of medical science **49**
Halford, F. J. **684**
Hall, G. K. **2293.2**
Haller, Albrecht von **130, 132.1, 866, 970, 2556**
Halothane **2602**
Hamarneh, Sami **504**
Hamer, P. M. **725**
Hammond, E. A. **574**
Hamsters **2693**
Handbook for foreign medical graduates **1366.1**
Handbook of scientific and technical societies and institutions of the United States and Canada **2508**
Handbook to aid in the treatment of Zulu patients **303**
Handbuch der gesamten Augenheilkunde **2017**
Handbuch der Haut- und Geschlechtskrankheiten **1265, 1359**
Handbuch für die Sanitätsberufe Österreichs **346**
Handerson, H. E. **461**
Handicapped **2260**
Handy, E. S. C. **258.1**
Hanecki, Michał **2351**
Hansen, H. F. **1895.1**
Hara, Kirotake **1896**
Harcourt, Raoul d' **514**
Hardy, W. E. **2030**
Hare, E. H. **1378**
Hare, Ronald **1149**
Harkányi, István **2601**
Harmon, R. W. **2237**
Harned, J. M. **202**
Harriman, P. L. **2318**
Harris, C. A. **1310**
Harris, Henry **677**
Harrison, C. V. **2088**
Harrison, Elizabeth **1242**
Harrison, R. J. **865, 874**
Harvard University **2310**
Harvard University. Arnold Arboretum **971.1**
Harvard University. Psycho-Acoustic Laboratory **1871**
Hatfield, E. J. **951**
Hauduroy, Paul **1555**
Hawaii. Histories **684**
Hawelek, Alice **1087**
Hayden, A. C. **1881**
Haymaker, Webb **1809**
Head **212**
Heagerty, J. J. **536**
Health, Environmental, *see* Environmental Health
Health Information Foundation, New York **2473**
Health, Occupational, *see* Occupational Health
Health, Public, *see* Public Health
Health Statistics **2352, 2416–2416.2**
Hearing **1866, 1867, 1875, 1876, 2047**
  Histories **2052**
Heart, *see* Cardiac Surgery; Circulatory System
Heart, Artificial **2576.1, 2578**

Heber, R. F. **1854, 1856**
Hecker, J. F. K. **2099**
Heffter, J. K. **185**
Hehlmann, Wilhelm **2319**
Heimann, Harry **2392**
Hein, W. H. **755**
Heinemann modern dictionary for dental students **1311**
Heinemann modern dictionary for nurses **1897**
Heischkel, Edith **325**
Hektoen, Ludwig **1208**
Helder, M. P. **266**
Hellier, F. F. **1352**
Helminthological abstracts **2057**
Helminthology **1139, 2057, 2059, 2061, 2061.1, 2063**
Hematology **1043, 1108, 1112, 1126, 1128**
Hematopoietic Tissue Transplantation **2590**
Henderson, I. F. **938**
Henderson, Virginia **1889, 1891**
Henderson, W. D. **938**
Henkle, H. H. **2129**
Henle, J. **858**
Henley, Alfred **1042**
Henry, F. P. **721**
Henry, G. W. **1818**
Henry, R. S. **1630**
Heparin **2178**
Hepatitis, Infectious
    Bibliographies **1169**
Heraud, Auguste **978**
Herbals, *see* Botany and Agriculture, Histories
Herber, Otto **876**
Hering, Eduard **2663**
Herman, C. M. **2692**
Hernåndez Morejón, Antonio **630**
Herndon, T. E. **741**
Herrgott, F. J. **1977**
Herringshaw, T. W. **402.1**
Herrlinger, Robert **476**
Herrnstein, R. J. **2332**
Herskowitz, I. H. **1417**
Heterocyclic Compounds **1018, 1078**
Hewer, C. L. **2599**
Hewitt, R. M. **2673**
Hifuka saikin no shinpo **1351**
Hill, A. V. **2280**
Hill, C. F. **1589**
Himes, N. E. **2472**
Hine, M. K. **1294**
Hinsie, L. E. **1786**
Hintze, Kurt **1927**
Hirsch, August **446, 563, 2100**
Hirsch, G. C. **943**
Hirschberg, Julius **2017**
Hirst, L. F. **1203**
Histochemical titles from current literature **905.1**
Histology
    Bibliographies **908–908.1**
    Dictionaries **877, 878, 908.2**
    Indexes and Abstracts **9.1, 858.1, 904.2–906**
    Reviews **907**
Histoplasmosis
    Bibliographes **1170–1171**
History of Medicine **461–486, 1586,** *see also* Art and Medicine; Biography; Classics, Medical; Famous Persons; Folk Medicine; Incunabula; Indians (American); Literature and Medicine; Manuscripts; Medicine, Primitive; Paleopathology; subheading Histories, under countries, states, and special topics
    Ancient **487–498, 810,** *see also* India, Histories
    Arabic **502–507, 591–592**
    Bibliographies **16.7, 414–424, 437, 439–440**
    Chronology **457, 458, 460**
    Medieval **499–501, 741, 827**
    Modern **508–512**
    Sources **441–443, 497, 957, 1135, 1137, 1217, 1360, 1422, 1562, 1565, 1567, 1680, 1814, 1908, 1978, 1981, 2105, 2106, 2137, 2138, 2212, 2216, 2285, 2330.1, 2332, 2335, 2338, 2445, 2565, 2567, 2571, 2575, 2604, 2608**
    Study and Teaching **437–440**
History of science: an annual review **2518**
History of the Second World War. United Kingdom Medical Series **1619**
Hjelt, O. E. A. **148, 634**
Ho, Huai-tê **221**
Hocking, G. M. **2188**
Høeg, L. **883**
Hoeppli, Reinhard **2069**
Hoerr, N. L. **230**
Hoff, E. C. **836, 837**
Hoff, P. M. **838**
Hoffa, A. J. **1675**
Hoffman, E. F. **1713**
Hoffman-Axthelm, Walter **1312**
Hoffmann, Kurt **255**
Holbrook, S. H. **806**
Holländer, Eugen **750, 751, 756, 904.1**
Hollingsworth, Dorothy **1924**
Holmstedt, Bo **2212**
Holsti, L. R. **2434**
Holthusen, Hermann **2448**
Holzmair, Eduard **786**
Homeopathy **56**
    Bibliographies **769**
    Directories **399.1**
    Histories **769–773**
Homes, Mental **1439**
Homes, Nursing **372, 1439**
Homes, Old Age **1430**
Honduras. Histories **577**

Hong Kong
Directories **364**
Hong Kong. Medical and Health Department **364**
Honig, J. M. **1069**
Hookworm Disease **2065, 2066**
Hoolboom-Van Dijck, S. J. M. **226**
Hoptman, Julian **1162**
Hormones **1384, 1932, 1933**
Horn, Walter **2075**
Horus: a guide to the history of science **2521**
Hoseh, M. L. **1070**
Hoseh, Mordecai **383, 1070**
Hoshasen igaku saikin no shinpo **2425**
Hoskin, M. A. **2518**
Hospital abstracts **1434**
Hospital Administration **1433, 1448, 1449**
Hospital atlas **1371.1**
Hospital gazetteer **1443**
Hospital Infections **1221**
Hospital Legislation **1473**
Hospital Libraries **1519**
Hospital literature index **1435**
Hospital periodical literature index **1435**
Hospital progress **1452**
Hospital Psychiatric Departments **1781.1**
Hospital Utilization **1436**
Hospitalized Child **2314**
Hospitals
Bibliographies **1436, 1781.1**
Directories **367, 401, 1242, 1641, 1719**
Australia **344**
Austria **346**
Belgium **347**
Canada **1437**
Czechoslovakia **351**
Denmark **1438**
Egypt **353**
Finland **354**
France **355, 357, 358, 1439**
Germany **1440–1442**
Great Britain **360, 1443–1444**
India **365, 1445–1446**
Ireland **369, 370**
Israel **371.1**
Italy **372**
Japan **374, 1447**
Mexico **374.1**
Netherlands **375**
Portugal **377**
Sweden **379**
Switzerland **380**
Union of South Africa **381**
United States, Institutions **400, 403, 404, 1450–1453, 1718**
United States, Personnel **1448–1449**
Uruguay **406.1**
Yugoslavia **407**
Histories **1454–1463, 1830**
Indexes and Abstracts **1433–1435**
Hospitals; administrators guide issue **1453**
Hospitals; guide issue **1453**
Hospitals; statistics and directory section **1453**
Hospitals, Psychiatric **1800, 1805**
Histories **1830**
Hospitals year book **1444**
Houck, L. D. **1766**
Hovorka, Oskar, Edler von Zderas **801**
Howard, A. V. **2500**
Howe, H. M. **198**
Howell, H. A. L. **1614**
Howell, M. G. **1002**
Hsu, Shan-hsiang **1071**
Huard, P. A. **539**
Hubbell, A. A. **2018**
Huber, J. T. **2674**
Hübotter, Franz **446**
Hughes, Arthur **901**
Hughes, H. H. **150.1**
Hughes, L. E. C. **2494**
Hughes, M. J. **827**
Hughes, T. P. **734**
Human Engineering **847, 1595, 1597.1**
Human engineering bibliographic series **1597.1**
Human engineering bibliography **1595**
Hume, E. E. **1631**
Humphrey, H. B. **988**
Hungarian medical bibliography **80**
Hungary
Bibliographies **151.1, 1112, 1302, 1354, 1389, 1661, 1951, 2006, 2046, 2091, 2174, 2177.3, 2435, 2601, 2634**
Histories **578–580**
Indexes and Abstracts **80–81**
Hunnius, Curt **2184**
Hunter, Donald **2411**
Hunter, R. A. **1814**
Hurd, H. M. **1830**
Hurwitz, Alfred **2567**
Husson, Roger **939**
Hyaluronic Acid **1097**
Hyaluronidase **1097**
Hydrocarbons **1078**
Hydrocortisone **2619.1**
Hygiene **9.17, 16.7, 1539, 2342, 2347–2349**
Hygiene, Food **2409**
Hygiene, Mental **1729, 1760, 1806–1807**
Hygiene, School **2409**
Hygienische Rundschau **2347**
Hygienists, Dental **1320**
Hyperbaric Oxygenation **2618**
Hypnosis
Directories **1850**
Histories **811**
Reviews **1849**
Hysteria, Histories **1837**

I hsueh wen chai **10**
Iason, A. H. **1391**
Ice, John **844.1**
Idel'chik, K. I. **645**
Igaku chuo zasshi. Japana centra revuo medicina **83**
Igaku gencho sakuin **36.1**
Igaku kenkyûsha meibo **373**
Igaku nenkan **374**
Igaku Shoin, Tokyo **373, 1447, 1896**
Ihde, A. J. **1091**
Illinois. Histories **685–687**
Illinois State Medical Society **687**
Illion, Theodor **637**
Illustration, Medical; Histories **481–486, 741–742, 889, 896, 898, 904, 1973, 1985, 2098,** *see also* Art and Medicine; Botany and Agriculture, Histories; Caricatures; Portraits
Imbert, Jean **1459**
Immunity **1209, 1548, 1549**
Immunochemistry **1008**
Immunofluorescence **1571**
Immunology
  Bibliographies **1571–1572**
  Histories **1151**
  Indexes and Abstracts **5.3, 9.4, 853**
  Reviews **1569–1570**
Imperial Bureau of Animal Health, Weybridge, Eng. **2642,** *see also* Commonwealth Bureau of Animal Health, Weybridge, Eng.
Imperial Cancer Research Fund **1710.1**
Imperial Mycological Institute, Kew **1576,** *see also* Commonwealth Mycological Institute, Kew
Inasaridze, G. Z. **2633**
Incunabula **429–433, 1204**
Index analyticus cancerologiae **1689**
Index and abstracts of foreign physical education literature **2247**
Index-catalogue of medical and veterinary zoology **2678, 2678.1, 2678.2**
Index-catalogue of the Library of the Surgeon General's Office, National Library of Medicine **29**
Index catalogue to Russian, Central and Eastern European and Chinese literature in medical entomology **2072**
Index chemicus **1003**
Index der deutschen und ausländischen zahnärztlichen Literatur **1277**
Index der deutschen und ausländischen zahnärztlichen Literatur und zahnärztlichen Bibliographie **1277**
Index der deutschen zahnärztlichen Literatur und zahnärztlichen Bibliographie **1277**
Index litteraturae entomologicae **2075**
Index medicus **11, 36, 326, 1531**
Index medicus. War supplement **1591**
Index medicus danicus **78**
Index medicus novus **43**
Index of current hospital literature **1435**
Index of fungi **1574**
Index of literature on plastic surgery **2582.1**
Index of rheumatology **1655**
Index of the periodical dental literature **1269**
Index radiohygienicus **2448.1**
Index Society **971**
Index to American doctoral dissertations **179**
Index to current urological literature **2624.2**
Index to dental literature **1269**
Index to Indian medical periodicals **82**
Index to medical socioeconomic literature **2341**
Index to original communications in the medical journals of the United States and Canada **111**
Index to the literature of American economic entomology **2071**
Index to the literature of food investigation **1914**
Index universalis **36.1**
Index veterinarius **2640**
Index zur Geschichte der Medizin, Naturwissenschaft und Technik **419.1**
Index zur Geschichte der Medizin und Biologie **419.1**
Indexes, *see* Indexes and Abstracts under subject and geographic headings (e.g., Anatomy, Medicine, Brazil, Germany, etc.)
India
  Directories **365–366, 1323, 1371, 1371.2, 1445–1446, 2503**
  Histories **337, 488, 581–588, 1620–1623**
  Indexes and Abstracts **82, 2493.2**
  Periodicals **337, 1508**
  Reviews **1026**
India. Central Bureau of Health Intelligence **1371**
India. Council of Scientific and Industrial Research **366, 976, 2503**
India. Directorate General of Health Services **1371.2, 1508**
India. Directorate General of Health Services. Central Medical Library **82**
India. Directorate General of Health Services. Ministry of Health **1445, 1446**
India. National Scientific Documentation Centre **2491.2**
Indian dentists register **1323**
Indian medical directory **365**
Indiana. Histories **688–689**
Indiana. University. School of Medicine **1093**
Indiana State Medical Association **689**
Indians (American) **513–518, 1220,** *see also* subheading Histories under Latin America and specific American countries
Indice bibliografico **29.1**

Índice-catálogo médico brasileiro **72**
Indice-catálogo médico Paulista **143.1**
Indice de la literatura dental periódica en castellano y portugués **1270**
Indice de médicos españoles **629**
Indice historico medico español **631**
Indice medico columbiano **75**
Indice medico español **88.1**
Indice terapêutico (Mexico) **374.1**
Indochina. Conseil des Recherches Scientifiques **171**
Indonesia. Histories **589–590**
Indústria Química e Farmacêutica Schering, S. A. **20**
Industrial Hygiene see Occupational Health
Industrial hygiene digest **2397**
Industrial Hygiene Foundation of America, Inc. **2351.1, 2397**
Industrial Medical Association **2413**
Industrial Microbiology **1538.1, 1550**
Industrial microbiology abstracts **1538.1**
Infantile Paralysis, *see* Poliomyelitis
Infants, Premature **2131**
Infection, Staphylococcal, *see* Staphylococcal Infection
Infections, Hospital **1221**
Infections, Lung, Mycotic **1580**
Infections, Rickettsial, *see* Rickettsial Infections
Infections, Salmonella **1214**
Infectious Diseases, *see* Communicable Diseases
Infectious Hepatitis, *see* Hepatitis, Infectious
Influenza
  Bibliographies **1173–1174**
  Indexes and Abstracts **1172**
L'information médicale roumaine **88**
Ingerslev, Vilhelm **549**
Ingram, Marylou **2456.1**
Ingram, W. M. **2394**
Inhalation Therapy **2621**
Injuries **1468, 1880, 1883.2, 1884, 2252, 2554.1, 2592, 2593,** *see also* Surgery, Traumatic
Injury, Spinal Cord **1844**
Inke, Gábor **1482**
Insanity, *see* Mental Disorders
Insect Physiology **2275**
Institut Royal Colonial Belge. Section des Sciences Naturelles et Médicales **1156**
Institute for Research in Biography, Inc., New York **390**
Institute for Scientific Information **7, 2491, 2514**
Institute for the Study of Analgesic and Sedative Drugs **2235, 2236**
Institute of Contemporary Jewry, Jerusalem **2416**
Institute of Hospital Administrators, London **1444**
Institute of Living, Hartford **1726**
Institute of Physics, London **1583**
Institute of Psycho-Analysis, London **1778**
Institute of Radio Engineers. Professional Group on Medical Electronics **962**
Institute of Scientific and Technical Information of China **74, 919.1, 1004**
Instituto Politécnico Nacional de México. Centro de Investigación y de Estudios Avanzados **29.1**
Instrument Society of America **960**
Instrumentation **958, 960, 1012**
Instruments, Surgical; Histories **1974, 2573**
Insulin Therapy **1783**
Intelligenz- Blatt und Bibliographie zum allgemeinen Repertorium der gesammten deutschen medizinisch-chirurgischen Journalistik **66**
Intelligenzblatt der Medizinischen National-Zeitung für Deutschland **53**
Internal Medicine **9.6, 10.1, 13, 16.1, 32, 35, 37, 99.1, 112, 118, 123, 128, 129, 214, 1141, 2614**
Internal medicine digest **11.1**
International abstracts of biological sciences **918**
International abstracts of plastic and reconstructive surgery **2583**
International abstracts of surgery **2538**
International Anatomical Nomenclature Committee **886**
International Association of Agricultural Librarians and Documentalists **982.1**
International bibliography of crime and delinquency **2532**
International Botanical Congress **982**
International Brain Research Information Center, Mayo Foundation, Rochester **1839.1**
International Bureau for Plant Taxonomy and Nomenclature, Utrecht **982**
International catalog of scientific literature **44, 2679**
International Children's Centre, Paris **2109**
International College of Surgeons **2561**
International Colloquium on Photocoagulation **2001**
International Commission for the Decennial Revision of Nosological Nomenclature **1883**
International Committee for Social Science Documentation **2531**
International Committee for the Preparation of the Decennial Revision of International Lists of Diseases and Causes of Death **1880**
International Conference on the Peaceful Uses of Atomic Energy **2452, 2453, 2454**
International Council of Scientific Workers **44**
International Dental Federation **1312.1**
International Dental Federation. Special Commission on Oral and Dental Statistics **1294**

International digest of health legislation **1467**
International directory of otolaryngology **2049**
International directory of psychologists, exclusive of the U.S.A. **2327**
International directory; schools and organizations for the deaf **1876**
International Federation of Electroencephalography and Clinical Neurophysiology **1840**
International Goiter Conference **1381**
International Labour Office **2400, 2401, 2402, 2410**
International medical and surgical survey **36.2**
International medical digest **12**
International nursing index **1890**
International Occupational Safety and Health Information Centre **2398**
International pharmaceutical abstracts **2144**
International Psycho-analytical Association **1803**
International record of internal medicine and dermatology **35**
International record of medicine **35**
International record of medicine and general practice clinics **28.1, 35, 1738, 1994.1, 2040.1**
International record of obstetrics and gynecology **1945**
International record of ophthalmology **1994.1**
International record of otorhinolaryngology and bronchoesophagology **2040.1**
International record of pediatrics **2114**
International record of psychiatry and neurology **1738**
International record of surgery **2541**
International review of connective tissue research **907**
International review of cytology **899**
International review of experimental pathology **2083**
International review of general and experimental zoology **2687**
International review of neurobiology **1742**
International review of pediatrics **2114**
International review of recent advances in medicine **38.1**
International review of the army, navy and air force medical service **1590**
International review of tropical medicine **1140**
International Social Science Council **2531**
International Society for Cell Biology **899**
International Sociological Association **2528**
International surgical digest **2539**
International surveys of recent advances in medicine **38.1**
International Symposium on venereal diseases and the treponematosis. **1252**
International Union Against Cancer **1717.1, 1719**
International Union of Biochemistry **1098**
International Union of Pure and Applied Chemistry **1078**
International Union of Pure and Applied Chemistry. Commission on Codification **1079**
International Union of Pure and Applied Chemistry. Inorganic Chemistry Section **1080**
Internationale Bibliographie der Anatomie des Menschen und Wirbeltiere **855**
Internationale Gesellschaft für Geschichte der Pharmazie **504**
Internationale veterinärmedizinische Literatur **2647**
Internationales Centralblatt für die gesamte Tuberkulose-Literatur **1232**
Internationales Centralblatt für Laryngologie, Rhinologie und verwandte Wissenschaften **2038**
Internationales Centralblatt für Tuberkulose-Forschung **1232**
Internships **1370, 1371.1**
Internships, Dental **1318, 1324**
Inventory of social and economic research in health **2473**
Ionizing Radiation **2456.1**
Iowa. Histories **690–691**
Iowa State Medical Society **691**
Iran
- Bibliographies **152**
- Histories **591–592**
- Indexes and Abstracts **2493.1**

Iraq
- Histories, *see* History of Medicine, Ancient; History of Medicine, Arabic
- Indexes and Abstracts **2493.1**

Ireland
- Directories **367–371, 1242, 1533, 2196, 2505**
- Histories **593–595**
- Theses **180**

Ireland, M. W. **1645**
Irish medical and hospital directory **367**
Irish medical directory **369, 370**
Irish medical directory and hospital year book **367**
Isaev, P. O. **867**
Isché, J. P. **1508.1**
Ishikawa, Mitsuteru **270**
Isotopes **2454.2**
Israel
- Bibliographies **153**
- Directories **371.1**
- Indexes and Abstracts **2493.1**

Israel Medical Association **371.1**
Israel Program for Scientific Translations **2142**
Istituto sieroterapico milanese Serafino Belfanti **1507**
Italy
- Bibliographies **154, 1207, 1676, 1954**

Collections, Periodicals **1507**
Directories **372**
Histories **440, 596–598, 1145, 1195, 1677, 2200, 2209,** *see also* History of Medicine, Ancient
Indexes and Abstracts **98–102, 920.1, 2419**
Italy. Consiglio nazionale delle richerche **920**
Italy. Istituto nazionale per l'assicurazione contro le malattie **3**
Ivanova, A. **287**
Iyengar, M. O. T. **1167, 1168**

JAMA clinical abstracts of diagnosis and treatment **30**
JAMA reference directories **188, 388.1, 397.1**
Jablonski, Stanley **285, 2192**
Jackson, B. D. **971**
Jacobs, M. B. **1556**
Jadassohn, Josef **1265, 1359**
Jadraszko, Sabina **281**
Jaeger, E. C. **203, 940, 941**
Jahrbuch der gesamten Therapie **2611**
Jahrbuch für die Leistungen der gesammten Heilkunde **68**
Jahrbuch für orthopädische Chirurgie **1667**
Jahrbuch für praktische Aerzte **45**
Jahrbucher der in- und ausländischen gesammten Medicin **39**
Jahresbericht Chirurgie **2545**
Jahresbericht der Pharmazie **2154**
Jahresbericht für Ophthalmologie **1994**
Jahresbericht Gynäkologie und Geburtshilfe **1943**
Jahresbericht Hals- Nasen- und Ohrenheilkund **2039**
Jahresbericht innere Medizin **37**
Jahresbericht Kinderheilkunde **2113**
Jahresbericht Neurologie und Psychiatrie **1735**
Jahresbericht Ophthalmologie **1992**
Jahresbericht Physiologie und experimentelle Pharmakologie **2270**
Jahresbericht Radiologie **2423**
Jahresbericht Tuberkuloseforschung **1234**
Jahresbericht über die Ergebnisse der Immunitätsforschung **1549**
Jahresbericht über die Fortschritte auf dem Gebiete der Chirurgie **2545**
Jahresbericht über die Fortschritte auf dem Gebiete der Geburtshilfe und Gynakologie **1943**
Jahresberichte über die Fortschritte der Anatomie und Entwicklungsgeschichte **859**
Jahresbericht über die Fortschritte der Anatomie und Physiologie **860**
Jahresbericht über die Fortschritte der animalischen Physiologie **2271**
Jahresbericht über die Fortschritte der Diagnostik **1361**
Jahresbericht über die Fortschritte der gesammten Medicin in allen Ländern **61**
Jahresbericht über die Fortschritte der Pharmakognosie, Pharmacie und Toxicologie **2154**
Jahresbericht über die Fortschritte der Pharmakotherapie **2155**
Jahresbericht über die Fortschritte der Physiologie **2271**
Jahresbericht über die Fortschritte der Tier-Chemie oder der physiologischen, pathologischen und Immuno-Chemie und der Pharmakologie **1008**
Jahresbericht über die Fortschritte in der Chirurgie und Geburtshülfe in allen Ländern **61**
Jahresbericht über die Fortschritte in der Lehre von den Garungs-Organismen und Enzymen **1543**
Jahresbericht über die Fortschritte in der Lehre von den pathogenen Mikroorganismen umfassend Bacterien, Pilze und Protozoen **1542**
Jahresbericht über die Fortschritte und Leistungen auf dem Gebiete der Hygiene **2348**
Jahresbericht über die Fortschritte und Leistungen auf dem Gebiete der sozialen Hygiene und Demographie **2346.1**
Jahresbericht über die gesamte Chirurgie und ihre Grenzgebiete **2545**
Jahresbericht über die gesamte Gynakologie und Geburtshilfe sowie deren Grenzgebiete **1943**
Jahresbericht über die gesamte innere Medizin und ihre Grenzgebiete **37**
Jahresbericht über die gesamte Kinderheilkunde **2113**
Jahresbericht über die gesamte Neurologie und Psychiatrie **1735**
Jahresbericht über die gesamte Ophthalmologie **1992**
Jahresbericht über die gesamte Physiologie und experimentelle Pharamakologie, mit vollständiger Bibliographie **2270**
Jahresbericht über die gesamte Tuberkuloseforschung und ihre Grenzgebiete **1234**
Jahresbericht über die Leistungen auf dem Gebiete der Veterinär-Medizin **2644**
Jahresbericht über die Leistungen in der Kriegesheilkunde **1592**
Jahresbericht über die Leistungen und Fortschritte auf dem Gebiete der Erkrankungen des Urogenitalapparates **2628**
Jahresbericht über die Leistungen und Fortschritte auf dem Gebiete der Neurologie und Psychiatrie **1736**
Jahresbericht über die Leistungen und Fort-

schritte auf dem Gebiete des Militär-Sanitätswesens **1593**
Jahresbericht über die Leistungen und Fortschritte im Gebiete der Ophthalmologie **1992**
Jahresbericht uber die Leistungen und Fortschritte in der gesammten Medicin **46**
Jahresbericht über die wissenschaftliche Biologie zugleich bibliographisches Jahresregister der Berichte uber die wissenschaftliche Biologie **921**
Jahresbericht über Haut- und Geschlechtskrankheiten, sowie deren Grenzgebiete **1254**
Jahresbericht über soziale Hygiene, Demographie und Medizinalstatistik **2346.1**
Jahresbericht Urologie **2626**
Jahresverzeichnis der deutschen Hochschulschriften **182**
James, R. R. **565, 2019**
Jameson, Eric **807**
Jankowiak, Józef **2261**
Japan
  Bibliographies **847.1, 1936, 2007**
  Collections, Periodicals **1509**
  Directories **373–374, 1447, 1536, 2504**
  Histories **599–601, 1374, 1623.1**
  Indexes and Abstracts **32, 83–84, 103–104, 919, 2540**
  Periodicals **321, 323**
  Periodicals, Lists **2512**
  Reviews **1039**
Japan. Ministry of Education **84**
Japan. Ministry of Education. Higher Education and Science Bureau **2504**
Japan. Ministry of Health and Welfare. Medical Affairs Bureau **1447**
Japan. Ministry of War **1623.1, 1623.2**
Japan. National Diet Library **321**
Japan science review. Biological sciences **919**
Japan science review. Medical sciences **84**
Japan Society for the Promotion of Science **2504**
Japanese hospital directory **1445**
Jaramillo-Arango, Jaime **1196**
Jayne, W. A. **810**
Jeanselme, Edouard **1262**
Jellison, W. L. **2075.1**
Jen min wei shêng ch'u pan shê, Peking **221**
Jenkins, D. W. **2076**
Jenkins, H. H. **1961**
Jeremić, Risto **174**
Jerusalem. S. Syman Public Health Library **153**
Jewish Hospital of Brooklyn. Allergy Division **851**
Jews **2416**
  Histories **774–778**
Jibünkoka saikin no shinpo **2043**
John Crerar Library, Chicago **1683, 2129, 2519**
Johns Hopkins University **2346**
Johns Hopkins University. Institute of the History of Medicine **588, 775, 1836**
Johns Hopkins University. John Work Garrett Library **787**
Johnston, William **1614**
Johnstone, R. W. **1972**
Joint Committee of the Association of American Medical Colleges and the Medical Library Association **1481**
Jolly, Julius **583**
Jones, Kathleen **1823**
Jones, W. H. S. **1197**
Jordan, H. **2261.1**
Jordan, P. D. **2378**
Josephson, A. G. S. **2519**
Jourdan, A. J. L. **450, 471**
Journal of clinical and experimental psychopathology and quarterly review of psychiatry and neurology **1731**
Journal of the chemical society, London **1005**
Journal of the western society of periodontology **1272**
Juhász, Jenö **2091**
Just's botanischer Jahresbericht **968**
Juvenile Delinquency **2531, 2532, 2537**

Kábrt, Jan **313**
Kagan, S. R. **776, 777**
Kagramanian, K. A. **1386**
Kaiser, F. E. **178**
Kala azar bulletin **1175, 1177**
Kamenetz, H. L. **2262**
Kan, Lai-Bing **2061.2**
Kanevskiĭ, L. O. **645**
Kanner, Leo **1858**
Kansas. Histories **692**
Kantor, J. R. **2333**
Karakulov, I. K. **1161**
Karaminova-Tsatcheva, S. D. **144**
Karel, Leonard **2224**
Karpovich, E. A. **286, 1072**
Kashikar, C. G. **583**
Kassel, Karl **2053**
Katō, Katsuji **271**
Katona, András **151.1**
Katsura, Eisuke **1936**
Katz, Jacob **1117**
Kauppi, H. M. **149**
Keele, K. D. **1833**
Keene, F. E. **1963**
Keevil, J. J. **1615**
Keffer, Luiza **1179**
Keidanski, F. **2416**
Keilin, David **902**
Kekkaku bunken no shoroku sokuho **1230**
Kekkaku kenkyu no shinpo **1237**
Kelemen, E. **2174**
Kelemen, K. **2174**

Kéler, Stefan von **2077**
Kellner, Karl **1298**
Kelly, E. C. **459**
Kelly, H. A. **652, 653, 654**
Kemper, G. W. H. **688**
Kenk, Roman **1842**
Kennedy, Catherine **1483**
Kenneth, J. H. **938**
Kentucky. Histories **693–694**
Kentucky. University **911**
Kentucky. University. Medical Center Library **1503**
Kentucky State Medical Association **693**
Kenya
Bibliographies **145.2**
Kerbabaev, E. B. **2062**
Kerney, Ellen **2011**
Kernodle, P. B. **1909**
Kerr, J. M. M. **1972**
Kestner, C. W. **452**
Keys, T. E. **1137, 1483, 2608, 2610**
Khairallah, A. A. **505**
Khalil, M. **1158**
Khanolkar, V. R. **584**
Kharasch, Norman **1009**
Khar'kovskaia gosudarstvennaia nauchno-meditsinskaia biblioteka **1407, 1659, 2488**
Khátir, Munshid **309**
Khrushchev, N. F. **1163**
Kiaer, F. C. **616**
Kibre, Pearl **428**
Kidney Diseases **151.1, 1110**
Kidney Transplantation **2590**
Kiell, Norman **1767, 1768**
Kiev. Respublikanskaia nauchnaia meditsinskaia biblioteka **1043, 1115, 1116, 1169, 1528, 2063, 2455**
Killian, Hans **2568**
Kim, Stephen **1515.1**
Kim, Tu-jong **601.1**
King, Ambrose **1255**
King, L. S. **474, 511**
King, W. H. **772**
Kinnunen, Olavi **1952**
Kirchhoff, Theodor **1821**
Kisch, Bruno **740**
Kiso igaku saikiñ no shinpo **120**
Kita, Hiromasa **373**
Kitay, J. I. **1388**
Klassiker der Medizin **443**
Klebs, A. C. **430, 1204**
Kleeberg, Heinz **1711**
Kleitman, Nathaniel **1769**
Klopfer, W. G. **2675**
Klose, F. A. **69**
Knight, R. L. **1419**
Kobro, Isak **616, 617**
Koch, C. R. E. **1334**
Kock, Wolfram **2374**
Koenig, Elizabeth **1707, 1720, 1721, 2484**
Köves, Péter **1389**
Kokuritsu Kokkai Toshokan, Tokyo **2512**
Kolb, W. L. **2533**
Kolle, Kurt **1810**
Koller, E. K. **1117**
Kondo, Jion **1509**
Kongresszentralblatt für die gesamte innere Medizin und ihre Grenzgebiete **13**
Kopech, G. **905, 908**
Korea, Histories **601.1, 601.2**
Korean War **1598**
Korkis, F. B. **2044**
Kornblitt, Herbert **1470.1**
Kostić, Aleksandar **288, 314**
Krämer, G. **2568**
Kraev, A. V. **1113**
Krankenhaus—Lexikon für das Deutsche Reich **1442**
Krasinski, Cyrill von Corvin **638**
Krauss, A. A. **606**
Krauss, Edith **1534**
Krehmer, Georgette **2197.2**
Kremers, Edward **2213**
Kricker, Gottfried **139, 1484**
Kristensen, Martin **223**
Krogman, W. M. **868**
Kronfeld, Adolf **801**
Kronick, D. A. **333, 335**
Kronschwitz, H. **2603.1**
Krügelstein, F. C. C. **1470.2**
Krüger, Gerhard **877, 2650**
Krumbhaar, E. B. **463, 596, 2101**
Kruzas, A. T. **2486**
Kudlein, Fridolf **476**
Kukainis, I. P. **1041**
Kulíková, L. **2255**
Kupper, W. H. **1787**
Kurth, Wolfram **763**
Kutumbiah, P. **585**

LSD, *see* Lysergic Acid Diethylamide
La, ying, chung wên tui chao i hsüeh ming t'zŭ hui pien **222**
Lääkärit hammaslääkärit, sairaalat **354**
Laboratories **943, 1085**
Laboratories, Forensic Science **1480**
Laboratories in the chemical bio-sciences **1085**
Laboratories, Public Health **2361**
Laboratories, Water Pollution **2395**
Laboratory Animals, **2080, 2090.1** *see also* Baboon, Dogs, etc.
Histories **821**
Labstracts **2084**
Laehr, Heinrich **1770**
Laignel-Lavastine, Maxime **485, 1522**
Laín Entralgo, Pedro **1834, 2102**

Lamb, D. S. **682**
Lang, Hugo **250**
Lange, Wilhelm **763**
Langer, Erich **1356**
Langkavel, B. A. **989**
Lanjouw, Joseph **982**
Lapps. Histories **602**
Larsell, Olof **719**
Larson, P. S. **2238**
Laryngology, *see* Otorhinolaryngology
Lastres, J. B. **618**
Latin America
  Histories **603–604,** *see also* Indians (American)
  Periodicals, Lists **2511**
La Torre, Felice **1973**
Latvia. Histories **605–606**
  Indexes and Abstracts **1685**
Laufer, Heinrich **639**
Laurentian Hormone Conference **1384**
Lauricella, Emanuele **264**
Laval Manriquez, Enrique **538**
Laws **401**
Lead Poisoning **2234**
Leake, C. D. **495, 2610**
Lebanon
  Indexes and Abstracts **2493.1**
Lechevalier, H. A. **1568**
Leclainche, Emmanuel **2660**
Leclerc, Lucien **506**
Lectures on the scientific basis of medicine **126**
Lederle Laboratories, New York **2222**
Lee, W. C. **276**
Lee-Delisle, Dora **261**
LeFanu, W. R. **336, 747, 2570**
Lefebvre, Gustave **496**
Leftwich, A. W. **2700**
Lega Italiana per la Lotta contro la Poliomielite **1207**
Legal Medicine
  Bibliographies **1470–1472**
  Dictionaries **1474–1479**
  Directories **1480**
  Indexes and Abstracts **16.7, 1464–1468**
  Manuals **1473**
  Reviews **1469**
Legislation, Dental **1926**
Legislation, Hospital **1473**
Legislation, Medical **351, 353, 356, 357, 370, 401, 403, 404, 1467**
Legislation, Veterinary **2655**
Leibbrand, Werner **475, 1815**
Leiber, Bernfried **213**
Leigh, Denis **1824**
Leikind, M. C. **1872**
Leipzig. Dutsche Bücherei **1711**
Leishmaniasis **1139**
  Bibliographies **1176–1178**
  Indexes and Abstracts **1175**
Leistungen und Fortschritte der Medizin in Deutschland **68**
Leitch, Isabella **1937**
Lejeune, Fritz **251**
Lemke, Rudolf **752**
Lende, Helga **2025**
Leningrad. Publichnaia biblioteka **137, 138, 159**
Lenore Schwartz Leukemia Foundation **1683**
Lépine, Pierre **242**
Leprosy **1139**
  Bibliographies **1179–1183, 1187**
  Histories **1184–1187**
Leptospirosis
  Bibliographies **1188–1191**
Lesky, Erna **1375, 2366**
Letteratura radiologica italiana **2419**
Leukemia **1683**
Leukemia abstracts **1683**
Leutert, Gerald **887**
Levenberger, Nadia **153**
Levin, V. L. **930**
Levine, B. S. **285, 2391**
Levit, M. M. **321.1**
Levy, Françoise **1455**
Lévy-Valensi, Joseph **558**
Lewin, Louis **2245**
Lewis, N. D. **1771**
Lexicon of English dental terms **1312.1**
Lexikon der Geschichte der Naturwissenschaften **2522**
Leyden. Rijksmuseum voor de Geschiedenis der Natuurwetenschappen **1588**
Librarians, Medical **1535, 1536**
Libraries, Agriculture **982.1**
Libraries, Hospital **1519**
Libraries, Medical
  Bibliographies **1894**
  Catalogs **1489–1502, 2026**
  Classification Schemes **1526–1532**
  Directories **348, 1533–1537**
  Manuals **1481–1488**
  Periodicals, Lists **1504–1517**
  Selection Tools **1518–1525**
Libraries, Nursing **1894**
Libraries, Veterinary **1526**
Library Association. Medical Section **1519, 1533**
Library of Congress, *see* U.S. Library of Congress
Librium **2177**
Libro azul medico mexicano, 1945–46 **374.2**
Licensure **388.1**
Licht, Sidney **2264**
Liddel, E. G. T. **1835**
Liechtenstein
  Directories **380**
Liège. Office international de documentation de médecine militaire **1590**
Lietuviškoji medicininė bibliografija **84.1**

Liga Bahiana contra o Cancer **1700**
Ligue française contre le cancer **1689**
Liljestrand, Göran **2212**
Lincoln's fifth wheel **1640.1**
Linde Air Products Company **2619**
Linguistics **5.7**
Link, M. M. **1646**
Lipenius, Martinus **131**
Lipids **1020, 1038**
Lipinska, Mélina **828**
Lisbon. Instituto de Medicina Tropical **1142**
List of bio-med **322**
List of institutions, research centres, schools, persons and periodicals in the field of physical culture **2254**
List of journals indexed **6, 11** (IM), **28** (CLML), **34** (QCIM), **326** (CIM)
List of periodicals in the World Health Organization Library **1510**
List of schools of nursing **1904**
Literaturarchiv der gesamte Zahnheilkunde **1278**
Literature and Medicine **454, 779–784, 1201–1768,** *see also* Famous Persons
Literature, Drug **2180**
Lithuania
    Indexes and Abstracts **84.1**
Litovskaia meditsinskaia bibliografiia **84.1**
Liu, Shou-shan **2175**
Liver Diseases **1406**
Liver Transplantation **2590**
Livingston, G. A. **1081**
Lloyd, Christopher **1615**
Lloyd, J. U. **2176**
Lloyd, W. E. B. **510**
Locke, N. M. **1772**
Lockheed Missiles and Space Co. **1046, 1362**
Lodge, Thomas **2427.1**
Lo Duca, Giuseppe **2468**
Lohe, Heinrich **1356**
London and provincial medical directory **360**
London medical directory **360**
Long, E. R. **2103, 2104, 2105**
López Piñero, J. M. **632**
Lotova, E. I. **645, 2376**
Louisiana. Histories **695**
Louisiana State Department of Hospitals 1528.1
Louros, N. K. **1958**
Louttit, C. M. **2308, 2311**
Louvain. Université catholique. Laboratoire d'electromyographie **1654**
Louw, J. D. **215**
Lovasy, E. **878**
Lovejoy, E. P. **829**
Lubin, A. W. **1772.1**
Lubin, Bernard **1772.1**
Lüth, Paul **1432**
Lufkin, A. W. **1335**
Luminescent Analysis **2431**
Lung Infections, Mycotic **1580**
Lung Transplantation **2590**
Lungs **1236**
Lusk, Graham **1928**
Luxemberg, *see* Belgium
Lymphatic System **1113**
Lysergic Acid Diethylamide **1860.1, 1860.2**

M. J. Bluff's Uebersicht der Leistungen und Fortschritte der Medicin **68**
MLB journal of literature abstracts **2230.1**
MRL journal of literature abstracts **2230.1**
Macalpine, Ida **1814**
McCleary, G. F. **2134, 2135**
McCluggage, R. W. **1336**
McClung, L. S. **1551.1, 1551.2**
McCollum, E. V. **1929**
McCormack, J. N. **693**
McCormick, J. A. **2457.1**
McCoy, Elizabeth **1551.1, 1551.2**
McDaniel, W. B., 2d **650**
McDonald, Donald **1622**
Macek, Karel **1044**
McElligott, M. G. **295**
McEwen, W. K. **2015**
McGill University **1493**
MacKenna, R. M. B. **1351.1**
Mackenthun, K. M. **2394**
MacKinney, L. C. **499, 741**
McKusick, V. A. **1412, 1417.1**
McLaren, A. C. **2181**
MacLean, F. S. **2373**
Macmillan medical cyclopedia **240**
MacNalty, A. S. **231, 1619**
McNeil, D. R. **1337**
MacPhail, A. **1606**
MacPherson, W. G. **1617**
Madia, Ernesto **1475**
Magalhaes, Hulda **2693**
Magic **798, 799, 801, 803, 2526**
Magnus, Hugo **2020**
Magyar Orvosi bibliografia **81**
Magyary-Kossa, Jyula **579**
Maia, J. de Andrade **72, 143.1**
Major, R. H. **467, 2106**
Major hospital atlas **1371.1**
Malaria **1139**
    Bibliographies **1192**
    Dictionaries **1193**
    Histories **1194–1198**
Malclès, L. N. **140**
Malloch, Archibald **667**
Maloy, B. S. **1476, 1477**
Malta. Histories **607**
Maltz, Maxwell **2587**
al-Ma lūf, Amīn Fahd **2701**
Maly, R. **1008**
Mammary Neoplasms **168.5**

Mandel, William **2489**
Mandelbaum, D. G. **910**
Manget, Jean J. **132**
Manríquez, Enrique Laval, *see* Laval Manríquez, Enrique
Manuscripts, Medieval **425–428, 741**
Manuscripts, Preparation **2668–2676.1**
Marconi, Ruggero **267**
Marie, J. S. F. **1313**
Marine Biology **922**
Marino, Vincenzo **268**
Marler, E. E. J. **2189**
Marshall, M. L. **1485**
Martí-Ibañez, Felix **668**
Martínez Durán, Carlos **575**
Martínez Fortún y Foyo, J. A. **543, 544**
Martinez Sánchez José **1295**
Marvitz, Leif **1338**
Marx, Rudolf **764**
Maryland. Histories **696–697**
Maryland. University. Department of Zoology **2072**
Masie, A. M. **260**
Mason, M. M. **2694**
Massachusetts. Histories **698–700**
Massachusetts. Recess Commission on Hypertension **1117**
Massachusetts Institute of Technology **1010**
Massachusetts Medical Society **698**
Matas, Rudolph **695**
Materia medica and therapeutics, preventive medicine, climatology **2616.1**
Materia medica and therapeutics; preventive medicine; climatology; forensic medicine **2616.1**
Materia medica and therapeutics, preventive medicine, climatology, suggestive therapeutics, forensic medicine **2616.1**
Matheson, N. M. **793**
Matthews, L. G. **2214**
Maxwell, W. Q. **1640.1**
Mayerhöfer, Joseph **2522**
Mazzini, Giuseppe **753**
Mead, K. C. H. **830, 831**
Meade, R. H. **2589**
Means, R. K. **2379**
Medical abbreviations **195**
Medical abstracts **31**
Medical and Chirurgical Faculty, Baltimore **696**
Medical annual; a yearbook of treatment and practitioner's index **121**
Medical Awards **406, 848**
Medical bibliography **93**
Medical Bibliography **1482–88**
Medical books in print **1520**
Medical Care **2343, 2356**
Medical care review **2343**
Medical colleges and training institutions in India **1371.2**
Medical digest **14**
Medical directory (U. K.) **360**
Medical directory for Ireland **371**
Medical directory of Australia **344**
Medical directory of South Africa **381**
Medical Economics **2341, 2343, 2473**
Medical Education, *see* Education, Medical and Allied Sciences
Medical Electronics **958, 962**
Medical electronics and communications abstracts **958**
Medical Geography **21.1, 21.9, 2345**
Medical Gymnastics **16.1**
Medical gynaecology and fertility abstracts **2461**
Medical Historical Research Project. (W.P.A.) Kentucky **694**
Medical intelligencer **64**
Medical Legislation, *see* Legislation, Medical
Medical Librarians **1535–1536**
Medical Libraries, *see* Libraries, Medical
Medical Library Association **327, 1485, 1535**
Medical Library Association. Publication **434**
Medical progress; a review of medical advances **122**
Medical register **361**
Medical register of Ireland **368**
Medical review of reviews **15**
Medical school admission requirements, U. S. A. and Canada **1367**
Medical Schools, *see* Schools, Medical
Medical Secretaries **237, 2558, 2671.1, 2676**
Medical Societies, *see* Societies, Medical
Medical Society of the District of Columbia **682**
Medical Society of the State of New York **190.1**
Medical subject headings **6** (IM), **1530** (QCIM), **1531** (CIM)
Medical survey **38.1**
Medical Technology **16.7, 2079, 2084–2086**
Medical Writing **2668–2676.1**
Medicina fennica **79**
Medicinal Plants, *see* Plants, Medicinal
Medicine
  Bibliographies.
    International **128–135, 2493.3**
    Manuals **136–143**
    Regional and National
      Brazil **143.1, 531**
      Bulgaria **144, 533**
      Colombia **144.1**
      Denmark **145, 145.1**
      Ecuador **146**
      Estonia **147**
      Finland **148–149**
      Georgian SSR **166**

Germany **149.1–150**
Ghana **150.1**
Great Britain **151, 573**
Hungary **151.1**
Iran **152**
Israel **153**
Italy **154**
Mexico **611**
Poland **157**
U. S. S. R. **159–165**
United States **167–170**
Viet-Nam **171–172**
Yugoslavia **173–175**
Catalogs **1057**
Collections, Periodicals **1503, 1505–1517**
Congresses **186–194**
Dictionaries
Abbreviations **195–197**
Etymology **198–208**
Syndromes **209–214**
General Medical **215–317**
Afrikaans **215**
Arabic **216**
Bulgarian **217–218**
Chinese **220–222**
Czech **313**
Danish **223**
Dutch **224–228**
English **229–240**
Finnish **244**
French **241–243**
German **245–256**
Greek **256.1–258**
Hawaiian **258.1**
Hebrew **259–260**
Hungarian **261**
Indonesian **262**
Italian **263–268**
Japanese **269–275**
Korean **276**
Latin **277–278**
Malayan **279**
Norwegian **280**
Polish **281–282**
Polyglot **304–317**
Portuguese **283–284**
Russian **285–287**
Serbian **288**
Slovenian **289**
Spanish **290–296**
Swedish **297–299**
Tagalog **300**
Turkish **301**
Urdu **302**
Zulu **303**
Directories
International
Organizations **341–342**
Physicians **340**
National
Argentina **343**
Australia **344**
Austria **345–346**
Belgium **347**
Canada **348**
Chile **349**
China **350**
Czechoslovakia **351**
Denmark **352**
Egypt **353**
Finland **354**
France **355–358**
Germany **359**
Great Britain **360–363**
Hong Kong **364**
India **365–366**
Ireland **367–371**
Israel **371.1**
Italy **372**
Japan **373–374**
Mexico **374.1–374.3**
Netherlands **375**
New Zealand **375.1**
Panama **375.2**
Poland **376**
Portugal **377**
Spain **378**
Sweden **379**
Switzerland **380**
Union of South Africa **381–382**
U. S. S. R. **383–384**
United States
Physicians **385–391, 400–406**
Organizations **392–399**
Uruguay **406.1, 406.2**
Yugoslavia **407**
Encyclopedias **408–413**
Films **1399, 1400**
Indexes and Abstracts, International **1–71**
Regional and National
Belgium **94.1**
Brazil **72, 95**
Bulgaria **73**
China **74**
Colombia **75**
Cuba **96**
Czechoslovakia **76–77**
Denmark **78**
Finland **79**
Germany **96.1, 97**
Hungary **80–81**
India **82**
Italy **98–102**
Japan **83–84, 103–104**
Lithuania **84.1**
Philippines **85**
Poland **86–87.1**
Portugal **87.2**

Rumania **88**
Spain **88.1**
Switzerland **89**
U. S. S. R. **90–91.1, 106–110**
United States **111**
Venezuela **92**
Yugoslavia **93–94**
Nomenclature **1878, 1886**
Periodicals **318–328, 374, 380, 388, 398, 403**
Reviews **112–127, 2089**
Theses **179–185**
Translations **176–178**, *see also* History of Medicine, Sources
Collections **177**
Directories **178**
Indexes and Abstracts **176**
Medicine, Aerospace, *see* Aerospace and Submarine Medicine
Medicine. History, *see* History of Medicine
Medicine in Art, *see* Art and Medicine; Caricatures; Illustration, Medical; Portraits
Medicine, Internal, *see* Internal Medicine
Medicine, Legal, *see* Legal Medicine
Medicine, Military, *see* Military Medicine
Medicine, Naval **1594, 1615, 1633**
Medicine, Nuclear, *see* Nuclear Medicine
Medicine, Physical, *see* Physical Medicine and Medicine, Primitive **488, 804**, *see also* Indians (American)
Medicine, Social **9.17**
Medicine, Sports, *see* Physical Education and Sports Medicine
Medicine, Traumatic, *see* Injuries; Surgery, Traumatic
Medicine, Veterinary, *see* Veterinary Medicine
Medicinische Bibliographie und Anzeiger zum Centralblatt für die gesamte Medizin **47**
Medicinische Weltliteratur **43**
Medicinska enciklopedija **413**
Medicinska knjiga **94, 175, 288, 314**
Medico-chirurgical review **65**
Medico-chirurgical review and journal of medical science **65**
Medico-chirurgical review and journal of practical medicine **65**
Medico-Chirurgical Society of the District of Columbia **681**
Medicolegal cases **1464**
Meditsinskaia literatura SSR: sistematicheskiĭ ukazatel' knig i zhurnal'nykh stateĭ **90**
Meditsinski entsiklopedichen rechnik **218**
Meditsinskiĭ referativnyĭ zhurnal **16**
Medizin der Sowjetunion und der Volksdemokratien im Referate **107**
Medizinische Jahrbücher für die Čechoslovakische Republik **351**
Medizinische National-Zeitung für Deutschland **53**
Medizinischer Literaturnachweis **30.1**
Medvedeva, S. G. **1188**
Meetings, Psychiatric **1796**
Meffert, Franz **1460**
Meinck, Fritz **2357**
Meissner, F. L. **69, 2130**
Meissner, G. **858**
Mellon, M. G. **1062**
Memory **2314.2**
Mendelsohn, Everett **2286**
Menninger, K. A. **1773**
Mental Deficiency
Bibliographies **1852–1856**
Directories **1857**
Histories **1858**
Indexes and Abstracts **1851**
Mental Disorders **1238, 1757, 1758, 1759.1, 1761–1763, 1766, 1780, 1783, 1793, 1802, 1805**
Histories **1813, 1815, 1819, 1823, 1828–1830, 1837**
Mental health book review index **1729**
Mental health directory of state and national agencies administering public mental health and related programs **1804**
Mental Homes **1439**
Mental Hygiene **1729, 1760, 1783.1, 1806, 1807**
Histories **1831**
Mental Hygiene Services **1800–1802, 1804, 1805, 1857**
Mental Retardation, *see* Mental Deficiency
Mental retardation abstracts **1851**
Merck and Co., Inc. **2619.1**
Merillat, L. A. **2661**
Merkov, A. M. **2352, 2416.1**
Merrill, E. D. **971.1**
Merritt, Webster **683**
Merscheim, Arnold **1705**
Mesdag, M. J. **1774**
Mestler, G. E. **762**
Metabolic Diseases **1389**
Metabolism **1919, 2239**
Metabolism, Calcium **2459**
Methods in medical research **2085**
Methods of biochemical analysis **1032**
Methods of forensic science **1469**
Metrazol Therapy **1762**
Mettler, C. C. **468**
Mettler, F. A. **468**
Mexican War **1637**
Mexico
Bibliographies **611, 1292, 2173**
Directories **404, 374.1–374.3, 2032, 2193.2**
Histories **608–612, 1461, 2372, 2574**
Mexico. Centro de Documentación Cientifica y Técnica **2511**
Mexico. Secretaria de Salubridad y Asistencia **374.3**
Meyboom, Frederika **315**
Meyer, A. W. **893**
Meyer, C. F. **29**

Meyer-Steineg, Theodor **476**
Meyers, M. K. **250**
Michaelis, A. **1419.1**
Michigan. Histories **701–702**
Michigan. University. Bureau of Public Health Economics **2343**
Michigan. University. Cooperative Information Center for Hospital Management Studies **1433**
Michigan Occupational Therapy Association. Special Studies Committee **195**
Michigan State Medical Society **702**
Microbiological Associates **906**
Microbiologists **1561**
Microbiology, *see also* Immunology; Mycology
Bibliographies **1551.1–1554**
Dictionaries **1554.1–1557**
Directories **1561**
Histories **1562–1568** *see also* Microscopy, Histories
Indexes and Abstracts **5.3, 9.4, 16.3, 27, 44, 1538–1543**
Nomenclature **1558–1560**
Reviews **1544–1551**
Microbiology, Industrial **1538.1, 1550**
Microfilm abstracts **181**
Microscopy
Bibliographies **1583, 1583.1**
Histories **1584–1589**
Microscopy, Electron **1583, 1583.1**
Microwaves **962.1**
Midrakh Harefui Jisraeli **371.1**
Midwest Inter-Library Center **2513**
Midwives **375, 377, 1956, 1957**
Migel (M. G.) Memorial Library **2026**
Mignon, A. H. A. **1608**
Mikhnov, S. D. **1953**
Miki, Sakae **601.2**
Mikyška, Jan **1390, 1708**
Military Medical Personnel **356, 403, 1614, 1621, 1626, 1632**
Military Medicine
Bibliographies **1594–1599**
Dictionaries **1599.1**
Encyclopedias **1600**
Histories **1909**
General **1601–1603**
Australia **1604–1605**
Canada **1606–1607**
France **1608**
Germany **1609–1613**
Great Britain **1614–1619**
India **1620–1623**
Japan **1623.1, 1623.2**
New Zealand **1624–1625**
Norway **1626**
U. S. S. R. **1627**
United States **1628–1652**
Indexes and Abstracts **1590–1593, 1987**
Military Psychiatry **1771**
Military Surgery **1591, 1616, 1642–1643**
Miller, Genevieve **650, 1219**
Miller, W. C. **2651**
Mimosa Frenk Foundation **1774.1**
Mineral Waters **401, 2622**
Minerals **1072**
Minerva medicobibliografica **17**
Minsk. Respublikanskaia gosudarstvennaia nauchnaia meditsinskaia biblioteka **2353**
Minton, Richard **1597**
Mira, M. G. Ferreira de **625**
Mises à jour de médecine pratique **18**
Mississippi. Histories **703**
Missouri. Histories **704–705**
Mites **2072**
Mitteilungen zur Geschichte der Medizin, der Naturwissenschaften und der Technik **420**
Mitteilungen zur Geschichte der Medizin und der Naturwissenschaften **420**
Modern problems in ophthalmology **2001**
Modern trends in accident surgery and medicine **2593**
Modern trends in anesthesia **2598**
Modern trends in cardiac surgery **2577**
Modern trends in cardiology **1106**
Modern trends in dental surgery **1282**
Modern trends in dermatology **1351.1**
Modern trends in diagnostic radiology **2426**
Modern trends in endocrinology **1383**
Modern trends in gastro-enterology **1405**
Modern trends in gynecology **1946**
Modern trends in human reproductive physiology **2462**
Modern trends in immunology **1570**
Modern trends in neurology **1743**
Modern trends in obstetrics **1947**
Modern trends in obstetrics and gynecology **1948**
Modern trends in occupational health **2403**
Modern trends in ophthalmology **2000**
Modern trends in paediatrics **2119**
Modern trends in plastic surgery **2585**
Modern trends in surgery **2552**
Modern trends in urology **2630**
Moderne Probleme der Ophthalmologie **2001**
Møller-Christensen, Vilhelm **550**
Mönning, H. O. **215**
Mohle, Helmut **2357**
Molecular Biology **961**
Moll, A. A. **604**
Mommsen-Frankfurt, H. **247**
Moncayo Marques, J. **884.1**
Monge, C. M. **839**
Monitore ostetrico-ginecologico **1954**
Monro, T. K. **454**
Montana. Histories **706**
Monthly abstract of medical sciences **48**
Moodie, P. M. **2354**

Moodie, R. L. **789, 885**
Moortgat, Paul **1313.1**
Mora, George **1808**
Morejón, Antonio Hernández, *see* Hernández Morejón, Antonio
Mori, Masaru **879**
Morphogenesis **862**
Morphology **868, 929, 932, 1426.1**
Morse, W. R. **540**
Morten, Honnor **1898**
Morton, L. T. **419, 1486, 1897**
Moscow. Gosudarstvennaia biblioteka SSSR im. V. I. Lenina **183**
Moscow. Gosudarstvennaia nauchnaia meditsinskaia biblioteka **90, 1118, 1119, 1174, 1529**
Moscow. Gosudarstvennyĭ nauchnoissledovatel' skiĭ rentgenoradiologicheskiĭ institut **2421**
Moser, R. H. **2610.1, 2616**
Mosquitoes **1138.1**
Motherby, George **277**
Moulin, Daniël de **500**
Mráz, Oldřich **1560**
Müller, R. F. G. **586**
Müller, S. **1603**
München. Universität. Institut für Staatsveterinärmedizin und Geschichte der Tiermedizin **2667**
Mukhopādhyāya, Girindranāth **587**
Mullen, M. M. **2260**
Muller, H. J. **1417**
Mullett, C. F. **1205**
Mul'tanovskii, M. P. **160, 287**
Munk, William **569**
Muntner, Süssmann **778**
Muriel de la Torre, Josefina **1461**
Murphy, Gardner **2334**
Murr, C. G. von **132.1**
Murra, K. O. **2502**
Murray, M. R. **905, 908**
Muscular Dystrophy **1656**
Muscular dystrophy abstracts **1656**
Muscular Dystrophy Associations of America, Inc. **1656**
Musculoskeletal System, *see also* Orthopedics
    Bibliographies **1659–1661**
    Directories **1663**
    Histories **2282**
    Indexes and Abstracts **1653–1657**
    Nomenclature **1662**
    Reviews **1658**
Music and Medicine **785**
Musikka, Sirkka **2434**
Mutze, Karl **2008**
Mycology
    Bibliographies **1577–1580**
    Dictionaries **1581–1582**
    Indexes and Abstracts **1573–1574**
    Reviews **1575–1576**
Mycotic Lung Infections **1580**
NASW Directory of professional social workers **2536**
Nachet, Albert **1587**
Nadjmabadi, Mahmoud **152**
Nagel-u. Michelscher Jahresbericht Ophthalmologie **1992**
Naika saikin no shinpo **123**
Nakazawa, Ryōji **1044.1**
Nall, M . L. **1842, 1843**
Nanzando's medical dictionary **272**
Naples. Stazione zoologica **2683**
Narcotics **1789**
National Academy of Sciences **2092**
National Academy of Sciences-National Research Council **1081, 1296, 2092, 2327, 2508**
National Aeronautics and Space Administration, *see* U. S. National Aeronautics and Space Administration
National Agricultural Library, *see* U. S. National Agricultural Library
National Association for Mental Health, Inc. **1801**
National Association for the Prevention of Tuberculosis **1233**
National Association for the Prevention of Tuberculosis and Diseases of the Chest and Heart **1242**
National Association of Mental Health **1802**
National Association of Social Workers **2536**
National Biomedical Sciences Instrumentation Symposium **960**
National Cancer Association of South Africa **1709, 1709.1**
National Cancer Institute, *see* U. S. National Cancer Institute
National Center for Health Statistics, *see* U. S. National Center for Health Statistics
National Clearinghouse for Mental Health Information, *see* U. S. National Clearinghouse for Mental Health Information
National Committee on Maternal Health **2465, 2466**
National Conference on Medical Nomenclature **1881**
National Conference on Nomenclature of Disease, 2d, 1935 **1881**
National Conference on Pharmaceutical Research **2163**
National Cystic Fibrosis Research Foundation **1404**
National Education Association **2246**
National Foundation **902.1–903.1, 1206**
National Foundation for Infantile Paralysis **1208**
National Foundation for Research in Ulcerative Colitis **1401.1**
National Heart Institute, *see* U. S. National Heart Institute
National Institute of Arthritis and Metabolic

Diseases, *see* U. S. National Institute of Arthritis and Metabolic Diseases
National Institute of Child Health and Human Development, *see* U. S. National Institute of Child Health and Human Development
National Institute of Mental Health, *see* U. S. National Institute of Mental Health
National Institute of Neurological Diseases and Blindness, *see* U. S. National Institute of Neurological Diseases and Blindness
National Institutes of Health, *see* U. S. National Institutes of Health
National League for Nursing **1905**
National League of Nursing Education **1904**
National League of Nursing Education. Department of Studies **1904**
National Library of Medicine, *see* U. S. National Library of Medicine
National library of medicine catalog **1531**
National Referral Center for Science and Technology, *see* U. S. National Referral Center for Science and Technology
National register of scientific and technical personnel in India **366, 2503**
National Research Council **934, 1049–1050, 1296**
National Research Council. Chemical-Biological Coordination Center **1081**
National Research Council. Committee on Aviation Medicine **1869**
National Research Council. Committee on Child Development **2108**
National Research Council. Committee on Dental Health **1296**
National Research Council. Committee on the Handbook of Biological Data **1127, 2244**
National Research Council. Division of Medical Sciences **1120**
National Research Council. Division of Medical Sciences. Committee on Aviation Medicine **840**
National Research Council. Food and Nutrition Board **1296**
National Research Council. Research Information Service **2311**
National Research Council of Canada **1287**
National Research Council of Canada. Associate Committee on the Control of Hospital Infections **1221**
National Science Foundation, *see* U. S. National Science Foundation
National Society for Crippled Children and Adults **1775, 2257**
Nauchnaia literatura SSSR; sistematicheskiĭ ukazatel' knig i zhurnal'nykh stateĭ, 1928. Meditsina **108**
Nauchnye osnovy fizicheskogo vospitaniia i sporta **2248**
Naval Medicine **1594, 1615, 1633**
Nazarevskiĭ, N. A. **1426**
Nazarova, M. A. **1119**
Neave, S. A. **2703**
Nebraska. Histories **707**
Neck **212**
Nederlandsche Maatschappij tot Bevordering der Geneeskunst. Bibliotheek **1492**
Needham, Joseph **894**
Neelameghan, Arashanapalai **337**
Negroes. Histories **681**
Negwer, Martin **2190**
Nékám, Lajos **1354**
Nelson, D. R. **841**
Nelson, M. R. **2131**
Nematology **2698**
Nencki, M. V. **1008**
Neoplasm Regression, Spontaneous **1704**
Neoplasm Transplantation **1710.1, 2590**
Neoplasms
  Bibliographies **1698–1715, 1955**
  Directories **1718–1721**
  Films **1722**
  Histories **1723**
  Indexes and Abstracts **9.16, 16.6, 1682–1691**
  Nomenclature **1716–1717.1**
  Reviews **1692–1697**
Neoplasms, Brain **1699**
Neoplasms, Chemotherapy **1682, 1701, 1702, 1714**
Neoplasms, Diagnosis **1713**
Neoplasms, Epidemiology **1715**
Neoplasms, Mammary **1685**
Neoplasms, Ovarian **1712**
Neoplasms, Spinal Cord **1699**
Nervous and mental diseases **1753**
Nervous System, *see* Neurology and Psychiatry
Netherlands
  Bibliographies **1774**
  Collections, Catalogs **1492**
  Directories **375**
  Histories **613–615, 2202**
  Periodicals **331**
Neu, John **1057**
Neubauer, Otto. **1710**
Neuburger, Max **469, 470, 1847**
Neues Repertorium der gesammten deutschen medicinisch-chirurgischen Journalistik **66**
Neueste medizinisch-chirurgische Journalistik des Auslandes **54**
Nuemann, L. G. **2662**
Neureiter, Ferdinand von **1478**
Neurobiology **1742, 1745**
Neurochemistry **1774.1**
Neurologische und psychiatrische Literatur **1737**
Neurologisches Centralblatt **1737**
Neurologists **1794**
Neurology and Psychiatry, *see also* Brain and Spinal Cord; Hypnosis; Mental Deficiency;

Psychopharmacology; Senses and Sense Organs
Bibliographies **1754–1783, 2127**
Dictionaries **1784–1792**
Directories **1794–1805**
Films **1806, 1806.1, 1807**
Histories **752, 1808–1838, 1846–1848, 2052**
Indexes and Abstracts **9.8, 16.9, 1724–1739**
Monographs **1783.2**
Nomenclature **1793**
Reviews **1740–1753**
Neurospora **1577**
Neurosurgery **9.8, 16.4, 1753, 2579**
Histories **2580–2581**
Nevada. Histories **708–709**
Nevada State Medical Society **709**
Neville, H. H. **1073**
Nevskii, V. A. **161, 1776**
New Jersey. Histories **710–711**
New research centers **2485**
New Sydenham Society **71, 2622**
New York. Histories **712–713**
New York. Botanical Garden. **990**
New York (State) Department of Health **2228**
New York Academy of Medicine **712, 1305**
New York Academy of Medicine. Committee on Medicine and the Changing Order **822**
New York Academy of Medicine. History of medicine series **430, 649, 712**
New York Academy of Medicine. Institute on Social and Historical Medicine **438**
New York Academy of Medicine. Library **445, 742, 743**
New York Association for Mental Health **1831**
New York Heart Association **1129**
New York Public Library **1641**
New York Public Library. Arents Tobacco Collection **2238.1**
New York Society of Electron Microscopy **1583.1**
New Zealand
Directories **375.1**
Histories **1624–1625, 2373**
New Zealand. Department of Internal Affairs. War History Branch **1625**
New Zealand Medical Council **375.1**
New Zealand medical register **375.1**
Newburn, L. R. **1294**
Newerla, G. J. **795**
Newman, Charles **1376**
Nguyên-Hii'u **172**
Nichols, J. B. **682**
Nicole, Geneviève **1520.1**
Nielson, J. B. **1787.1**
Niemand, H. G. **2191**
Niemineva, Kalevi **1952**
Nikitin, V. N. **929**
Nippon Gakujutsu Shinkōkai **1044.1, 2504**
Nippon geka seikeigeka chuō zasshi **2540**
Nippon Igaku Toshokan Kyōkai **323**
Nippon igaku toshokanin meibo, Showa 37 nen 10 gatsu genzai **1536**
Nippon iji zasshi sakuin **104**
Nippon naika shōnika chūo zasshi **32**
Nippon Rinshosha, Osaka **270**
Nippon Seiri Gakkai **2281**
Nippon Ishi Gakkai **600.1**
Nissen, Claus **991**
Nixon, P. I. **728–730**
Nobel prize **456**
Noise **1865.1, 2351.1**
Nomenclature **884.1–888, 982, 1077–1082, 1098, 1129, 1308, 1558–1560, 1662, 1716–1717.1, 1793, 1845, 1878–1887, 1937, 2093, 2187–2192, 2252, 2654, 2703**
Norderskiöld, Erik **950**
Norges læger **616**
Norman, Herbert **146**
Norman-Taylor, W. **1144**
Norrie, Gordon **551**
Norris, G. W. **722**
Norske medicinske selskab **616**
Norske militærlæger **1626**
North Dakota. Histories **714**
North Dakota Medical Association **714**
Norway
Histories **616–617, 1626**
Periodicals **322**
Norwood, W.F. **1377**
Nose, *see* Otorhinolaryngology
Nosology **143, 1878–1887**
Notizen für praktische Aerzte über die neuesten Beobachtungen in der Medicin **62**
Nouveau Larousse médical illustré **243**
Novità terapeutiche **2612**
Novokreshchenov, B. V. **1097**
Novye knigi za rubezhom **18.1**
Noyan, Fazil **301**
Noyer, B. **171**
Nuclear Medicine
Bibliographies **2454.2–2459**
Dictionaries **2439, 2441, 2442**
Indexes and Abstracts **9.23, 2448.1, 2449**
Reviews **2450–2454.1**
Nuclear science abstracts **2449**
Nucleic acids **1045**
Nucleic acids **1034, 1045**
Numismatics **786–788**
Nuovo giornale della più recénte letteratura medico-chirurgica d'Europa **67**
Nuremberg Military Tribunals **1602**
Nurses **374.3, 1698**
Nursing
Bibliographies **1893–1894**
Dictionaries **239, 1895–1902**
Directories **1903–1906**
Histories **1907–1913**
Indexes and Abstracts **1888–1890**

Reviews **1891–1892**
Nursing Homes **372, 1439**
Nursing Libraries **1894**
Nursing Schools **348, 1371, 1904–1906**
Nutrition, *see also* Vitamins
Bibliography **1918, 1922**
Dictionaries **1920–1921**
Histories **1922–1929**
Indexes and Abstracts **1914–1915**
Monographs **1919**
Reviews **1916–1917**
Nutrition abstracts and reviews **1915**
Nutting, M. A. **1910**

O'Brien, Donough **1852**
Obstetrical and gynecological survey **1940**
Obstetricians **1960, 1961, 1962.1**
Obstetrics and Gynecology
Bibliographies **133, 149.1, 150, 1951–1955**
Dictionaries **1956–1959**
Directories **1960–1962.1**
Histories **1963–1986, 2135**
Indexes and Abstracts **9.10, 10.7, 16.10, 36.2, 38.1, 1938–1945, 2541, 2543**
Reviews **1946–1950**
Obstetrics and gynecology index **1944**
Occupational Health
Bibliographies **1782, 2391, 2404–2409**
Directories **2410**
Histories **2411–2414**
Indexes and Abstracts **2397–2402**
Reviews **2403**
Occupational safety and health abstracts **2398**
Ocular Refraction **2029**
Oculists **353, 377**
Odessa. Ukrainskiĭ eksperimental'nyĭ institut glaznykh bolezneĭ **2620**
Odontology **1283, 1292, 1309, 1313.1, 1314**
Odors **1868**
Österreichischer Apotheker-Verlag **975**
Official year-book of the scientific and learned societies of Great Britain and Ireland **2505**
Oganesian, L. A. **522**
Ogawa, T. **272**
Ohio. Histories **715–718**
Ohio medical history **716**
Ohio State University. College of Medicine **717**
Olbrich, Gertrud **213**
Old Age Homes **1430**
Oliver, W. H. **1325**
Oliver, Eugène **636**
Olivier, Georges **880**
Ollivier, C. P. **449**
Olpp, Gottlieb **1150**
Olson, L. M. **1899**
Onchocerciasis **2064**
Oncology, *see* Neoplasms
One hundred years of American psychiatry **1827**
Onqué, G. C. **2313**
Operative Surgery **1881, 1885**
Ophthalmic literature **1988**
Ophthalmological review **1993**
Ophthalmological Societies **2014**
Ophthalmologische Bibliographie **1994**
Ophthalmologists **367, 2013, 2014, 2048**
Ophthalmology, *see also* Blind; Optometry
Bibliographies **2005–2007**
Dictionaries **2008–2012**
Directories **2013–2014**
Histories **2016–2024**
Indexes and Abstracts **9.12, 10.9, 16.8, 36.2, 1987–1996, 2034**
Periodicals **2014, 2015**
Reviews **1997–2004**
Opitz, Karl **815**
Oppenheimer, Heinrich **781**
Optician Schools **2032**
Opticians **2033**
Optics **2008, 2015, 2030**
Optometric Schools **2032**
Optometric Societies **2032**
Optometrists **2032**
Optometry
Dictionaries **2029–2031**
Directories **2032–2033**
Periodicals, Lists **2015**
Opyt sovetskoĭ meditsiny v Velikoĭ Otechestvennoi Voine, 1941–1945 gg. **1627**
Oral Biology **1281**
Oral Health **1279**
Oral research abstracts **1271**
Oral Surgeons **1324**
Oral Surgery **1282, 1284**
Oral surgery directory of the world **1324**
Orangutans **2696**
Oregon. Histories **719**
Organic Chemistry, *see* Chemistry, Organic
Organisation for Economic Co-operation and Development. Directorate for Scientific Affairs **2395**
Organizations, International **341, 342**
Organizations, Scientific **2502, 2504–2509**, *see also* Societies
Organometallic Chemistry **1022**
Ornithosis **1209.1, 1209.2**
Orr, H. W. **1489**
Orthodontic directory of America **1325**
Orthodontic directory of the world **1325**
Orthodontists **1325**
Orthopedics
Bibliographies **1673–1676**
Histories **1677–1681**
Indexes and Abstracts **9.9, 16.4, 1664.1–1669**
Reviews **1670–1672, 2549**
Orvostudományi Dokumentációs Központ, Bud-

apest, *see also* Budapest. Országos Orvostudományi Könyvtár és Dokumentációs Központ
Osler, William **431, 477, 1493**
Osol, Arthur **230**
Osteoarthritis **1660**
Otolaryngology, *see* Otorhinolaryngology
Otological review **2040**
Otology, *see* Otorhinolaryngology
Otorhinolaryngologists **2013, 2048–2050**
Otorhinolaryngology, *see also* Deafness
Bibliographies **2046–2047**
Directories **2013, 2048–2050**
Histories **2051–2056**
Indexes and Abstracts **9.11, 10.10, 16.13, 36.2, 2034–2041**
Reviews **2002, 2042–2045**
Ottaviani, Gaetano **896**
Otto, Gustav **605**
Ovarian Neoplasms **1712**
Ovenall, Lynda **1146**
Ovio, Giuseppe **2021, 2022**
Owen, W. O. **1636**
Oxygen **841**
Oxygen Therapy **2619**
Oxygenation, Hyperbaric **2618**
Oya, Zensetsu **273**

Pack, G. T. **1719**
Packaging Institute, New York **2234**
Packard, F. R. **669**
Pagel, J. L. **421, 446, 460, 470, 480**
Pakistan
Histories **1623**
Indexes and Abstracts **2490.1, 2493.1**
Pakistan National Scientific and Technical Documentation Center **2490.1**
Pakistan Science abstracts **2490.1**
Paleopathology **448, 789–792**
Pales, Léon **790**
Palla, Ákos **791**
Palmer, A. M. **2486**
Pamoentjak, K. S. **262**
Panama
Directories **375.2**
Pan-American League Against Rheumatism **1657**
Pan American Sanitary Bureau **2064**
Pan American Union. Division of Science Development **2511**
Pangborn, R. M. **1871.1**
Panýrek, Duchoslav **412**
Papaspyros, N. S. **1397**
Paraguay. Histories **520**
Parapsychology **2315, 2322**
Parasites **2076**
Parasitology, *see also* Entymology
Bibliographies **2059–2066**
Dictionaries **2067**
Histories **2068–2069**
Indexes and Abstracts **10.14, 16.3, 1539, 1540, 2057**
Reviews **2058**
Parathyroid Gland Transplantation **2590**
Pardal, Ramón **515**
Paredes Borja, Virgilio **552**
Paris. Académie de médecine, *see* Académie de médecine, Paris
Paris. Institut de bibliographie **42**
Paris. Université. Faculté de médecine. Bibliothèque **192.1, 1512**
Paris. Université. Faculté de pharmacie. Bibliothèque **2197.2**
Paris. Université. Groupe d'études de psychologie **2291**
Parish, H. J. **1151**
Parker, Sheila M., *see* Durling, S. M. (Parker)
Parkinson's Disease **1730.1**
Parkinson's disease and related disorders **1730.1**
Parma. Ospedale maggiore **1538.2**
Parma. Universitá. Instituto di microbiologia **1538.2**
Parr, Bartholomew **278**
Parr, J. A. **235.1**
Parry, S. C. **316**
Parsons, R. P. **576**
Partington, J. R. **1092**
Partridge, William **1557**
Pasteurella pestis **1199**
Patai, Saul **1074**
Paterson, R. G. **2359**
Pathological Anatomy **856, 2082, 2091**
Pathologists **2094**
Pathology and Clinical Pathology
Bibliographies **2090.1–2092**
Dictionaries **2092.1**
Directories **2094**
Histories **2095–2107**
Indexes and Abstracts **5.4, 9.5, 21.10, 27, 2080–2081.1**
Nomenclature **2093**
Reviews **2082–2090**
Pathology, Clinical, *see* Pathology and Clinical Pathology
Patton, R. M. **2305**
Pauly, Alphonse **422**
Pazzini, Adalberto **440, 598, 820, 2569**
Pearce, E. C. **1900**
Pearsall, Marion **911**
Pedersen, E. B. **2354**
Pediatria anual **2120**
Pediatric Surgery **2582**
Pediatrics **2126, 2133**
Pediatrics
Bibliographies **2127–2131.1**
Histories **753, 2132–2139**
Indexes and Abstracts **9.7, 10.8, 32, 36.2, 2108–2115**
Reviews **118, 2116–2126**

Pediatrics and orthopedic surgery **1672, 2126**
Pediatrics digest **2110**
Peiper, Albrecht **2136**
Pekas, J. C. **2695**
Peking. National Library **1504**
Pennsylvania. Histories **720–722**
Pennsylvania. University. Edgar Fahs Smith Memorial Library **1056**
Penrose, L. S. **1414**
Pepper, O. H. **204**
Perera, Ambrosio **738**
Periodica chimica **1087**
Periodica medica **325**
Periodicals **318–328, 329–339, 374, 374.1 380, 388, 398, 403, 943, 944, 944.1, 983, 1086–1087, 1330, 1504–1517, 1520.1, 2014, 2015, 2193.1, 2197–2198, 2254, 2510–2516, 2658**
Histories **329–339**
Periodontal abstracts **1272**
Periodontology **1272**
Personal injury annual **1468**
Personality **2313**
Perspiration **1046**
Peru. Histories **514, 618–620, 1825**
Pesheva, D. **2061**
Pesonen, Niilo **244**
Pest Control
Bibliographies **2228**
Indexes and Abstracts **2225**
Reviews **2226–2227**
Pesticides **2225, 2227, 2228**
Pesticides documentation bulletin **2225**
Peters, Hermann **486**
Peters, J. A. **1422**
Peters, R. S. **2330**
Petroleum **1072**
Petry, Lucile **1901**
Peyser, Alfred **196**
Pfeiffer, Louis **150**
Pfister, R. M. **2228**
Pflücke, Maxmilian **1087**
Phalen, J. M. **1632**
Pharmaceutical abstracts **2145, 2156**
Pharmaceutical Chemistry **2166**
Pharmaceutical firms, U.S.A., Canada, Mexico **2193.2**
Pharmaceutical Manufacturers Association **2176.1**
Pharmaceutical Society of Great Britain, London **2194, 2195**
Pharmaceutical Society of Ireland **2196**
Pharmaceutisches Central-Blatt **999**
Pharmacies **351, 374.1, 407**
Pharmacists **345–347, 356–358, 365, 372, 374.3, 376, 377, 380, 384, 2193, 2193.1, 2195, 2196**
Pharmacognosy **2170, 2188**
Pharmacological reviews **2165**
Pharmacology, *see* Pharmacy and Pharmacology
Pharmacopoeias **2176, 2177.2**
Pharmacy and Pharmacology, *see also* Antibiotics; Pest Control; Toxicology
Bibliographies **135, 167, 173, 2169–2179**
Catalogs **1054, 1057**
Collections, Periodicals **1509, 1513**
Dictionaries **217, 293, 1314, 2180.1–2186**
Directories **355 358, 374.3, 2193–2196.1**
Histories **755, 2199–2217**
Indexes and Abstracts **10.3, 2140–2157.1**
Manuals **2180**
Nomenclature **2187–2192**
Periodicals **2193.1, 2197–2198**
Reviews **2158–2168**
Pharmacy, Education **2179**
Pharmacy Schools **358, 2193.1, 2196.1**
Pharmazeutisches Jahrbuch **2146**
Phi Epsilon Kappa **2247**
Philately **793–796**
Philippine index medicus **85**
Philippines
Histories **621**
Indexes and Abstracts **85**
Phillips, M. H. **1972**
Phillips, P. C. **706**
Phrenology, Histories **1846**
Physical Chemistry **1015, 1039, 1072**
Physical Culture **73, 2254**
Physical Education and Sports Medicine
Bibliographies **2249–2251**
Directories **2254**
Indexes and Abstracts **2246–2248**
Nomenclature **2252**
Periodicals **2254**
Physical Education Schools **2254**
Physical Medicine and Rehabilitation
Bibliographies **1661, 2259–2261**
Dictionaries **239, 2262**
Directories **2263–2264**
Histories **2265–2268**
Indexes and Abstracts **9.19, 16.1, 2255–2258**
Physical Therapy **16.1, 239, 1661, 2261**
Physicians **340, 343–372, 374.1–388, 389–391, 400–406.2, 2503**
Physicians' basic index **18.2**
Physicians, Chest **1240, 2490**
Physicians' Record Company, Chicago **202, 1450**
Physico-Chemical Society of Japan **1039**
Physiological abstracts **2272**
Physiological Chemistry, *see* Chemistry and Biochemistry
Physiological reviews **2278**
Physiological Society, London **27, 918, 2272**
Physiology
Bibliographies **149.1, 866, 1426.1, 2280**
Dictionaries **938, 2281**
Histories **895, 897, 2282–2288,** *see also* Circulatory System, Histories

Indexes and Abstracts **9.2, 27, 44, 858, 860, 2269–2273**
Reviews **2274–2279**
Physiology, Animal **2271, 2457.1**
Physiology, Comparative **2274**
Physiology, Insect **2275**
Physiotherapists **367**
Pickard, M. E. **670**
Pierce, C. M. **1046, 2239, 2456.2**
Pieron, Henri **2320**
Piéry, Marius **1248**
Pieter, Józef **2321**
Pindborg, J. J. **212, 1338**
Pineal Body **1388**
Piñero, José M. López, *see* López Piñero, J. M.
Pinkhof, H. **227**
Pinto, Pedro **284**
Piper, David **746**
Pittsburgh. University. Graduate School of Public Health. Health Law Center **1473**
Pituitary-adrenocortical Function **2617.1**
Pi y Arsuaga, Joaquim **292**
Placenta Transplantation **2590**
Plague **1139**
Bibliographies **1199, 1202**
Histories **1153, 1200–1205, 2099**
Plants, Medicinal **973, 975, 976, 978, 979, 981, 2182**
Plarr, V. G. **2570**
Plasma Substitutes **1043**
Plastic Surgery, *see* Surgery, Plastic
Playfair, Ernest **469**
Pleasants, Helene **2322**
Ploucquet, W. G. **133**
Pneumoconiosis **2399, 2488**
Pneumoconiosis abstracts **2399**
Pneumology **1231**
Podiatry, Histories **1680.1**
Podmore, Frank **811**
Poisoning, *see* Toxicology
Poland
Bibliographies **157, 1256, 2170, 2261, 2351**
Collections, Periodicals **1517**
Directories **376, 2506**
Histories **622–624**
Indexes and Abstracts **86–87.1**
Poletti, G. B. **1297**
Poliomyelitis
Bibliographies **1207–1209**
Indexes and Abstracts **1206**
Poliomyelitis current literature **1206**
Polish research guide **2506**
Politzer, Adam **2054**
Polk's dental register and directory of the United States and Dominion of Canada **1326**
Polk's medical and surgical directory of the United States **403**
Pollard, C. B. **2237**
Pollitzer, Robert **1164**
Pollution, Air **2385, 2387, 2390–2392**
Pollution, Water **2228, 2386, 2395–2396**
Polska bibliografia lekarska **86**
Pompili, Giuseppe **2441**
Ponce, Oscar Valdivia, *see* Valdivia Ponce, Oscar
Ponteva, E. **244**
Population **2415.1–2416.2**
Population Association of America **2415.1**
Population index **2415.1**
Porot, Antoine **1788**
Portal, Antoine **895**
Portraits **740, 743–747**
Portugal
Bibliographies **1142**
Directories **377**
Histories **625, 1456**
Indexes and Abstracts **87.2**
Portugal. Instituto de Alta Cultura, Centro de Documentaçâo Científica **87.2**
Poser, C. M. **1865**
Postage Stamps, *see* Philately
Postell, W. D. **671, 1487, 1528.1**
Postgraduate Medical Institute **190.1**
Potocko, R. J. **847**
Potter, E. S. **824**
Potter's new cyclopaedia of botanical drugs and preparations **981**
Power, D'Arcy **570, 2570, 2571**
Pox, Animal **1572**
Poynter, F. N. L. **571, 1462, 1501, 1848**
Practical medicine year books **127, 1110, 1285, 1353, 1385, 1672, 1697, 1753, 1950, 2004, 2045, 2090, 2126, 2168.1, 2349.1, 2428, 2454.1, 2555, 2600, 2632, 2646**
Practice, Group **394**
Praha. Institute of Radiation Hygiene **2448.1**
Praha. Institutum documentationis medicae **1955**
Praha. Státní lékařská knihovna **76, 1390, 1521, 1708**
Praha. Státní ústav pro zdravotnickou dokumentační a knihovnickou službu, *see also* Praha. Ústav pro zdravotnickou dokumentaci **77**
Praha. Státní zdravotnické nakladatelstvi **76, 313, 876**
Praha. Ústav hygieny **2409**
Praha. Ústav pro zdravotnickou dokumentaci **19, 1103, 1138, 1231, 1348, 1380, 1732, 2035, 2111, 2256, 2420, 2595,** *see also* Praha. Státní ústav pro zdravotnickou dokumentační a knihovnickou službu
Predoehl, August **1249**
Přehled světove zdravotnické literatury **19**
Preisler, O. C. S. **145**
Premature Infants **2131**
Premuda, Loris **896**
Present status of rheumatism and arthritis **1658**

Pressure, Blood **1117**
Preuss, Julius **816**
Price, A. L. **1902**
Price, J. F. **845**
Princeton University. Office of Population Research **2415.1**
Prinz, Hermann **1339**
Prior (W. F.) Co. **12, 2539**
Pritzel, G. A. **972**
Problem of rheumatism and arthritis **1658**
Problèmes actuels d'ophthalmologie **2001**
Procházková, Marta **1955**
Progrès dans la chimie des substances organiques naturelles **1031**
Progrès de la recherche experimentale des tumeurs **1696**
Progrès de l'exploration de la tuberculose **1235**
Progrès des recherches pharmaceutiques **2164**
Progrès en cardiologie **1105**
Progrès en chirurgie **2553**
Progrès en ophthalmologie **1998**
Progrès en oto-rhino-laryngologie **2042**
Progrès en virologie medicale **1551**
Progresos anuales en la practica medicoquirurgica **33**
Progresos anuales en la practica odontologica **1283**
Progresos de pediatria y puericultura **2121**
Progresos de terapéutica clínica **2613**
Progresos en la practica medicoquirurgica **33**
Progresos en la practica odontologica **1283**
Progresos en medicina infantil **2122**
Progress in allergy **854**
Progress in atomic medicine **2451**
Progress in biocybernetics **1744**
Progress in biophysics and biophysical chemistry **961**
Progress in biophysics and molecular biology **961**
Progress in brain research **1839**
Progress in cardiovascular diseases **1107**
Progress in chemical toxicology **2232**
Progress in clinical cancer **1695**
Progress in clinical psychology **2303**
Progress in drug research **2164**
Progress in experimental tumor research **1696**
Progress in hematology **1108**
Progress in industrial microbiology **1550**
Progress in inorganic chemistry **1033**
Progress in liver diseases **1406**
Progress in medical genetics **1413**
Progress in medical laboratory technique **2086**
Progress in medical virology **1551**
Progress in medicinal chemistry **2166**
Progress in neurobiology **1745**
Progress in neurology and psychiatry **1746**
Progress in nuclear energy **2452–2454**
Progress in nucleic acid research **1034**
Progress in ophthalmology and otolaryngology **2002**
Progress in organic chemistry **1035**
Progress in orthopedic surgery **1670**
Progress in physical organic chemistry **1036**
Progress in psychotherapy **1747**
Progress in radiation therapy **2427**
Progress in research in emphysema and chronic bronchitis **2487**
Progress in stereochemistry **1037**
Progress in surgery **2553**
Progress in the chemistry of fats and other lipids **1038**
Progress in the chemistry of organic natural products **1031**
Progressos da medicina **20**
Proksch, J. K. **1257, 1258, 1263**
Proskauer, Curt **1340, 1341**
Prosthodontics **1306**
Proteins **1023**
Protozoa **1542**
Prussia. Kriegs-Ministerium. Medizinal-Abteilung **1610**
Przegląd piśmiennictwa lekarskiego polskiego **86.1, 87**
Psaltēs, I. A. **258**
Pschyrembel, Willibald **252**
Psittacosis
    Bibliographies **1209.1, 1209.2**
Psychiatric Clinics **1801**
Psychiatric Hospitals **1800, 1805**
    Histories **1830**
Psychiatric Writing **2674**
Psychiatrists **1795, 1797**
Psychiatry, *see* Neurology and Psychiatry
Psychiatry, Child **1757**
Psychiatry digest **1731**
Psychiatry, Education **1798**
Psychiatry, Military **1771**
Psychoanalytical Societies **1803**
Psychoanalysis **1740, 1765, 1768, 1778, 1785, 2317**
Psychoanalysts **1799, 1803**
Psychological abstracts **2292, 2293, 2293.1, 2293.2**
Psychological abstracts. Author index **2293, 2293.1**
Psychological abstracts. Cumulated subject index **2293.2**
Psychological book previews **2295**
Psychological bulletin **2294**
Psychological index **2293, 2293.1, 2296**
Psychological review **2296**
Psychological Tests **2306, 2307**
Psychological Writing **2674–2675**
Psychologists **2326, 2327**
Psychology
    Bibliographies **1303, 1767, 1768, 1770, 2304–2314.2**

Dictionaries **1787, 1792, 2314.3–2325**
Histories **2329–2340**
Indexes and Abstracts **5.7, 1725, 2289–2297, 2480**
Reviews **2298–2303**
Psychology, Adolescent **2530**
Psychology, Animal **2296.1**
Psychology, Child **2313–2314**
Psychology, Clinical **2303**
Psychology, Social **911, 2298**
Psychopharmacology
Bibliographies **1841, 1860.1–1863**
Dictionaries **1864–1865**
Indexes and Abstracts **1859–1860**
Psychopharmacology abstracts **1859**
Psychopharmacology handbooks **1860**
Psychotherapy **1741, 1747, 1761, 1762, 1783, 1788**
Psychotherapy, Group **1728, 1759, 1772, 1772.1**
Public Health, *see also* Environmental Health; Occupational Health; Social Welfare; Vital Statistics
Bibliographies **161, 2228, 2350–2356**
Dictionaries **1957, 2356.1, 2357**
Directories **351, 357, 358, 374, 377, 380, 2358–2361**
Histories **1202, 1913, 1925, 2132, 2134–2135, 2362–2384,** *see also* Epidemiology, Histories
Indexes and Abstracts **9.17, 10.4, 2341–2349**
Public Health Administration **16.7, 2346, 2351**
Public Health Economics **2343**
Public health economics and medical care abstracts **2343**
Public Health Engineering **2344**
Public health engineering abstracts **2344, 2387**
Public Health Officers **2360**
Public Health Officials **344, 353, 356, 358, 365, 372, 1444**
Public Health Schools **348**
Puericulture **2121**
Puerto Rico
Bibliographies **1159**
Directories **389, 1804, 2032, 2050**
Puerto Rico. University. School of Medicine. School of Tropical Medicine. Library **1159**
Purjesz, Béla **214**
Puschmann, Theodor **470, 526, 1378**
Pusey, W. A. **1264, 1358**
Putnam medical dictionary **236**
Putti, Vittorio **1494**
Putzey, L. J. **1759**

Q Fever **1210, 1211**
Quackery. Histories **805–809, 1680.1**
Quartals-Uebersicht der neurologischen Literatur des Auslandes **1739**
Quarterly compendium of medical science **49**
Quarterly cumulative index medicus **34, 1530**
Quarterly cumulative index to current medical literature **38**
Quarterly review of allergy and applied immunology **852**
Quarterly review of American and foreign literature of experimental and applied immunology **851**
Quarterly review of biology **925**
Quarterly review of dermatology and syphilology **1350**
Quarterly review of internal medicine and dermatology **35**
Quarterly review of medicine **35**
Quarterly review of obstetrics and gynecology **1945, 2541**
Quarterly review of ophthalmology **1994.1**
Quarterly review of ophthalmology and allied sciences **1994.1**
Quarterly review of ophthalmology and otorhinolaryngology **1994.1**
Quarterly review of ophthalmology, otorhinolaryngology and bronchoesophagology **1994.1**
Quarterly review of otorhinolaryngology **2040.1**
Quarterly review of otorhinolaryngology and bronchoesophagology **2040.1**
Quarterly review of pediatrics **2114**
Quarterly review of psychiatry and neurology **1738**
Quarterly review of surgery **2541**
Quarterly review of surgery and surgical specialties **2541**
Quarterly review of surgery, obstetrics and gynecology **2541**
Quarterly review of the progress of ophthalmology **1996**
Quarterly review of urology **2627**
Quebbeman, F. E. **676**
Quinan, J. R. **697**
Quinby, Jane **969**
Quoi de nouveau en pratique médicale? **124**
Qvigstad, J. K. **602**

Raach, J. H. **572**
Rabbits **2692**
Radbill, S. X. **761**
Radiation Effects **1387, 2448.1, 2456.1, 2456.2**
Radiation, Ionizing **2456.1**
Radiation Protection **16.7**
Radioactive Fallout **2388, 2389**
Radiobiology **2456**
Radiochemistry **1019**
Radioisotopes **2454.2–2455.1, 2456.2–2457.1**
Radiologists **2443, 2444**
Radiology, *see also* Nuclear Medicine
Bibliographies **2429–2436**
Dictionaries **2437–2442**
Directories **2443–2444.1**
Histories **2445–2448**

Indexes and Abstracts **9.14, 10.15, 16.6, 36.2, 2419–2423**
Reviews **2424–2428**
Radiology, Diagnostic **2426**
Radiotherapy **36.2, 2427, 2436**
Rádl, Emanuel **951**
Radunski, Bernardo **307**
Raettig, Hansjürgen **1209, 1552**
Raige-Delorme, Jacques **449**
Raina, B. L. **1623**
Rakhimov, I. A. **1113**
Ramali, Ahmad **262**
Rand, Benjamin **2312, 2335**
Rang, Mercer **1680**
Rassegna bibliografica della stampa ostetrico-ginecologica **1941**
Rassegna della letteratura medica italiana contemporanea **102**
Rassudova, S. M. **1097**
Ratner, I. B. **2067**
Ravenel, M. P. **2380**
Ravenstein, Adrian **256.1**
Readings, *see* History of Medicine, Sources
Recent advances in anatomy **865**
Recent advances in anesthesia and analgesia **2599**
Recent advances in cardiology **1109**
Recent advances in clinical pathology **2087**
Recent advances in dermatology **1352**
Recent advances in human genetics **1414**
Recent advances in medicine **125**
Recent advances in neurology and neuropsychiatry **1748**
Recent advances in obstetrics and gynaecology **1948.1**
Recent advances in ophthalmology **2003**
Recent advances in oto-laryngology **2044**
Recent advances in paediatric surgery **2582**
Recent advances in paediatrics **2123**
Recent advances in pathology **2088**
Recent advances in pharmacology **2167**
Recent advances in physiology **2279**
Recent advances in radiology **2427.1**
Recent advances in sex and reproductive physiology **2463**
Recent advances in surgery **2554**
Recent advances in tropical medicine **1140.1**
Recent advances in venereology **1255**
Recent book acquisitions of the Army Medical Library **28**
Recent progress in hormone research **1384**
Recent progress in psychiatry **1749**
Recent United States publications **11, 28**
Reconstruction surgery and traumatology **2586**
Reconstructive Surgery, *see* Surgery, Plastic
Record of zoological literature **2679**
Recreation **2246**
Red, G. P. **731**
Red book of eye, ear, nose and throat specialists **2050**
Red Cross **1909**
Redaelli, Piero **1578**
Reed, H. S. **992**
Reeves, Jon **2530**
Referata pediatrica **2124**
Referativnyĭ sbornik: voprosy onkologii **1684**
Referativnyĭ zhurnal **21**
Referátový výběr z anestesiologie **2595**
Referátový výběr z chorob infekčních **1138**
Referátový výběr z dermatovenerologie a příbuzných oborů **1348**
Referátový výběr z endokrinologie **1380**
Referátový výběr z fysiatrie, balneologie, revmatologie **2256**
Referátový výběr z kardiologie **1103**
Referátový výběr z otorhinolaryngologie **2035**
Referátový výběr z patologické anatomie **856**
Referátový výběr z pediatrie **2111**
Referátový výběr z psychiatrie **1732**
Referátový výběr z psychiatrie a neurologie **1732**
Referátový výběr z roentgenologie **2420**
Referátový výběr z tuberkulosy a pneumologie **1231**
Referáty, kritiky, diskuse o nových lékařských knihách ve státních vědeckých knihovnách **1521**
Reference Aids **1523**
Reference list of guild opticians **2033**
References to contemporary papers on acoustics **1865.1**
References to literature of interest to mosquito workers and malariologists **1138.1**
References to literature on mosquitoes and their control **1138.1**
Reflex, Conditioned **1755**
Refraction, Ocular **2029**
Regelmässiger Vierteljahresbericht über die Leistungen und Fortschritte der Augenheilkunde **1996, 1997**
Register of medical practitioners **375.1**
Register of medical practitioners, interns and dentists for the Republic of South Africa **382**
Register of veterinary surgeons, and the supplementary veterinary register **2656**
Register over dansk farmaceutisk litterature **2148**
Registry and Information Service for Experimental Tumours, London **1710.1**
Registry of medical rehabilitation therapists and specialists **2263**
Registry of Medical Rehabilitation Therapists and Specialists. Council **2263**
Rehabilitation, *see* Physical Medicine and Rehabilitation
Rehabilitation literature **2257**

Rehabilitation Therapists **2263**
Reichborn-Kjennerud, Ingjald **617, 802**
Reichs-Medizinal-Kalender für Deutschland **359**
Reichs-Tuberkulose-Ausschuss **1239**
Reicke, Siegfried **1463**
Reid, L. L. **1777**
Reina Valenzuela, José **577**
Religion and medicine **810–820**
Rennert, Helmut **752**
Rényi-Vámos, Ference **2634**
Repertoire des laboratories de recherche sur le pollution des eaux **2395**
Repertorisches Jahrbuch für die Leistungen der gesammten Heilkunde **68**
Report on the progress of ophthalmology **1966**
Report on the progress of otology **2041**
Report on the progress in otology and rhinology **2041**
Report on the progress of pharmacy **2157**
Reports in the literature on adverse reactions to drugs and therapeutic devices, cosmetics **2230.1**
Reproduction
  Bibliographies **2465–2467.1**
  Dictionaries **2468**
  Histories **2469–2472**
  Indexes and Abstracts **2460–2461**
  Monographs **932**
  Reviews **2461.1–2464**
Reproduction Research Information Service, Ltd. **2460**
Research. Histories **821–822**
Research centers directory **2485, 2486**
Research, Germ-free **1553–1554**
Research grants index **2474**
Research in Progress
  Bibliographies **1144, 1715.1, 2131.1, 2414.1, 2484**
  Directories **343, 1083, 1875, 2485–2486, 2506, 2509**
  Indexes and Abstracts **2473–2483**
Research in public health administration **2346**
Research Support **2396, 2478, 2479, 2481**
Researchers **373, 1084, 1720, 1721, 2414.1, 2676.1**
Residencies **1370, 1371.1**
Residencies, Dental **1318, 1324**
Residencies, Psychiatric **1798**
Residue reviews **2227**
Respiratory System
  Bibliographies **2488–2489**
  Directories **2490**
  Histories **902, 1134**
  Indexes and Abstracts **9.15, 10.6, 1233**
  Reviews **2487**
Respiratory Tract Diseases **10.6, 2037,** *see also* Tuberculosis
Resumenes internacionales de cirugia plastica **2584**
Resumptio genetica **1409**
Retrospect of medicine **50**
Retrospect of practical medicine and surgery **50**
Reuss, J. D. **2492**
Review of allergy **852**
Review of allergy and applied immunology **852**
Review of American chemical research **1010**
Review of applied entomology **2074**
Review of applied mycology **1575**
Review of medical and veterinary mycology **1576**
Review of medicine, surgery and obstetrics-gynecology **38.1**
Review of physical chemistry of Japan **1039**
Review of psychiatric progress **1750**
Review of surgery **2541**
Review of the current American and foreign literature of experimental and applied immunology **851**
Review of the literature on burns and trauma **2554.1**
Review of urologic surgery **2631**
Reviews, *see* Reviews under subject and geographic headings (e.g., Medicine, Radiology, India, Japan, etc.)
Revista de referate din literatura sovietică de specialitate **91**
Revista de resumenes **22**
Revolutionary War (U.S.) **167, 1635–1636**
Revue analytique des travaux sur le cancer, 1922–26 **1690**
Revue des sciences médicales en France et à l'étranger **51**
Revue international des services de santé des armées de terre, de mer et de l'air **1590**
Rheumatic Diseases **1653, 1655, 1657–1659, 1661–1662**
  Histories **1664**
Rheumatism and arthritis **1658**
Rhinology, *see* Otorhinolaryngology
Ricci, J. V. **1974–1976**
Richards, D. W. **1133**
Richards, R. T. **732**
Richer, P. M. L. P. **754**
Richter, Paul **1359**
Richter, W. M. von **646**
Rickettsial Diseases **1139**
  Bibliographies **1210–1211.2**
  Histories **1212–1213**
Rickman, John **1778**
Ridenour, Nina **1831**
Riecke, Erhard **1356.1**
Rieger, Rigomar **1419.1**
Riesman, David **501**

Riga. Respublikanskaia nauchnaia meditsinskaia biblioteka **1685**
Ring, Friedrich **1609.1**
RINGDOC **2149**
Rippa, B. K. **545**
Ristić, V. K. **175**
Ritterbush, P. C. **952**
Roach, E. S. **2224**
Roback, A. A. **2336**
Robbins, S. D. **1873**
Roberts, D. C. **1710.1**
Roberts, Ffrangcon **205**
Roberts, M. M. **1911**
Robertson, H. F. **1363**
Robledo, Emilio **542**
Robson, J. M. **2167, 2463**
Roche Laboratories **2177**
Rochester. University. Atomic Energy Project **1387**
Rockefeller Foundation. International Health Board **2065**
Rockefeller Institute for Medical Research. Medical Electronics Center **962**
Rocky Mountain medical journal **190.1**
Rocky Mountain Spotted Fever
  Bibliographies **1211**
  Histories **1212**
Roddis, L. H. **1633**
Rodiakin, N. F. **1178**
Rodríguez, María T. Santander, *see* Santander Rodríguez, M. T.
Rodríguez Rivero, P. D. **881**
Rodriquez, L. A. **516**
Roentgenology, *see* Radiology
Roger, Jacques **953**
Rogers, F. B. **164**
Rohde, E. S. **993**
Rolando, L. **146**
Roloff, W. **1239**
Roma sanitaria **372**
Romanian Scientific Abstracts. Natural Sciences **2490.2**
Romei Braconi, L. **1128**
Roos, Charles **765, 1598**
Rooseboom, Maria **1588**
Root, K. B. **2676**
Rose, Arthur **1066**
Rose, Elizabeth **1066**
Rosen, George **455, 672, 2363, 2412**
Rosenbaum, Julius **415**
Rosenberg, C. E. **1165**
Roshem, Julien **1248**
Ross, J. S. **2371**
Rossiĭskiĭ, D. M. **647**
Rossiĭskiĭ meditsinskiĭ spisok **384**
Roster of executives of state medical associations **398**
Rothe, I. V. **142**
Rothschuh, K. E. **2287, 2288**
Roversi, A. S. **1507**
Rowett Research Institute, Aberdeen **1915, 1937**
Royal College of Obstetricians and Gynaecologists **1962.1**
Royal College of Physicians, London **362, 363, 566, 569, 744–746, 1882, 1886.1**
Royal College of Physicians, London. Library **1495**
Royal College of Physicians of Edinburgh. Library **1496**
Royal College of Physicians of Ireland **595**
Royal College of Surgeons in Ireland **593**
Royal College of Surgeons of England **747, 2570**
Royal College of Veterinary Surgeons, London **2656**
Royal Medical and Chirurgical Society of London. Library **1497**
Royal Microscopical Society **1589**
Royal Society of London **44, 2493, 2679**
Royal Society of Medicine, London **1497**
Rózsa, Imre **2064**
Rudiak, K. E. **1699**
Rückert, Ernst **1711**
Rühlmann, Dorothee **2648**
Ruhe, D. S. **1401**
Ruhl, M. J. **1662**
Ruhräh, John **599, 2137, 2138**
Ruiz Torres, Francisco **296**
Rumania
  Histories **1984**
  Indexes and Abstracts **88, 2490.2**
Rumania. Board of Health. Documentation Center **88**
Rumania. Medical Publishing House **88**
Rumanian medical review **88**
Rusinov, N. V. **1528**
Ruskin, Arthur **1135**
Russell, F. E. **2240**
Russell, G. W. **679**
Russell, K. F. **573, 869**
Russell, P. F. **1198**
Russell Sage Foundation, New York **397**
Russia. Ministerstvo vnutrennykh diel. Meditsinskiĭ departament **384**
Russia (U.S.S.R.) Ministerstvo zdravookhraneniia **16**
Russian-English biological dictionary **942**
Russo, D. R. **689**
Russo, Francesco **2520**
Russo-Japanese War **1623.1**
Růžička, Karel **162**
Ryzhkov, I. D. **1660**

Sachs, Ernest **2580**
Sachs, J. J. **68**
Sacklén, J. F. **635**

Sadove, M. S. **2602**
Saemisch, Theodor **2017**
Saigon. Service de Documentation **172**
Saints. Histories **820**
Salicylates **2236**
Saliva **1286, 1301**
Sallander, Hans **1500**
Salmonella **1217–1220**
    Bibliographies **1214–1216**
Salmonella Infections **1214**
Salmonsen, E. M. **1208, 1935**
Samaniego, J. J. **553**
Samion-Contet, Janine **192.1, 484, 1512**
Sanatoria **1242, 1446**
Sanborn, W. R. **1571**
Sánchez Granjel, Luis, *see* Granjel, L. Sánchez
Sanchez-Monge y Parellada, Enrique **1419.2**
Sand, René **2364**
Sándor, Róbert **1661**
Sandoz Chemical Works, Inc. Sandoz Pharmaceuticals **1860.1, 1860.2**
Sandström, C. I. **2323**
Sanfujinka saikin no shinpo **1949**
Sanitariums **400**
Sanitation **16.7, 2342, 2344, 2357, 2394**
Santander Rodríguez, M. T. **627, 629**
Santos, Lycurgo de Castro **532**
São Paulo (State) Departamento de Profilaxia da Lepra. Biblioteca **1179, 1180, 1181**
São Paulo (State) Departamento de Profilaxia da Lepra. Biblioteca e Documentacâo **1182**
Sapozhnikova, E. A. **2455**
Sarcoidosis **2489**
Sarton, George **432, 2521, 2523**
Satō, Kazuo **274**
Saunders, J. B. de C. M. **489**
Scartezzini, Carmelino **1314, 2185**
Schaller, Anton **882**
Schapero, Max **2012**
Scharffenberg, R. S. **1045, 2240**
Schein, J. D. **1876**
Schenkling, S. S. **2075**
Schermerharn, R. A. **1779**
Schiaffino, Rafael **736**
Schistosomes **1156, 1159**
Schistosomiasis, *see* Bilharziasis
Schizophrenia, Childhood **1763, 1780**
Schjerning, Otto von **1612**
Schlenz, Hermann **2215**
Schmelz, O. **2416**
Schmid-Daberkow, Gertrud **1599.1**
Schmidt, H. J. **1330**
Schmidt, Ingeborg **842, 843**
Schmidt, J. E. **1479–1789**
Schmidt's Jahrbücher der in- und ausländischen gesammten Medicin **39**
Schoen, Ernest **979**
Schoen, Max **785**
Schönbauer, Leopold **527**
Schoemaker, D. **885**
Schoenewald, F. S. **235**
Schönfeld, Walther **832**
Scholarships **1367, 1367.1**
Scholderer, Victor **431**
Scholz, Willibald **1822**
School Health **1760, 2246, 2409**
Schools, Dental **1316, 1318–1320, 1324–1326, 1329, 1371**
Schools, Dental Hygiene **1318**
Schools, Medical **342, 344, 346, 348, 353, 355, 357, 358, 360, 365, 372, 374, 374.1, 380, 381, 389, 401, 403, 407, 1367, 1369, 1371, 1371.2, 1372, 1453**
Schools, Nursing **348, 1371, 1904–1906**
Schools, Optician **2032**
Schools, Optometric **2032**
Schools, Pharmacy **357, 2193.1, 2196.1**
Schools, Physical Education **2254**
Schools, Public Health **348**
Schools, Veterinary **2655–2657**
Schoute, Dirk **589, 590**
Schoute, G. J. **227**
Schrader, G. W. **2663**
Schüling, Hermann **2337**
Schuettler, C. L. **1042**
Schützler, Günther **2649**
Schullian, D. M. **785**
Schulte, B. P. M. **615**
Schulz, H. E. **2652**
Schumacher, Joseph **498, 1395**
Schuurmans Stekhoven, Willem **228**
Schwalbe, G. **859**
Schwartz, J. C. **405**
Schweizerisches medizinisches Jahrbuch **380**
Science **1500**
    Dictionaries **2494–2497**
    Directories **2499–2509**
    Histories **5.7, 2517–2527**
    Indexes and Abstracts **2490.1–2493.2**
    Periodicals **2510–2516**
    Selection Tools **1522, 1524**
Science abstracts of China. Biological sciences **919.1**
Science abstracts of China. Chemistry and chemical technology **1004**
Science abstracts of China. Medicine **74**
Science books **1522**
Science citation index **2491, 2514**
Science Council of Japan **84**
Scientific and learned societies of Great Britain **2507**
Scientific and technical societies of the United States and Canada **2508**
Scientific basis of medicine **126**
Scientific Literature, Inc., Philadelphia **1401.1**
Scientific meetings, describing future meetings

of technical, scientific, medical and management organizations and universities **189**
Scientific Societies **2504–2505, 2507–2508**
Scientists **2499, 2500, 2501, 2503**
Scotland, *see* Great Britain
Scott, H. H. **1152**
Scott, H. R. **2534**
Scrub Typhus **1211.1, 1211.2**
Seaborn, Edwin **537**
Secher, K. I. A. **223**
Secretaries, Medical **237, 2558, 2671.1, 2676**
Seibutsu kagaku saikin no shinpo **926**
Seikeigeka saikin no shinpo **1671**
Seitner, P. G. **1081**
Seitz, Ludwig **1969**
Sekai sanfujinka soran **1942**
Selected child development abstracts **2108**
Selection Tools **1518–1525**
Selesnick, S. T. **1811.1**
Selleck, H. B. **2413**
Semelaigne, René **1820**
Semichov, B. V. **2182**
Senn, Nicholas **1643**
Senses and Sense Organs, *see also* Blind
  Bibliographies **1867–1872**
  Dictionaries **1873**
  Directories **1874–1876**
  Films **1806.1**
  Indexes and Abstracts **1865.1, 1866**
Seppala, Arvo **1514**
Šercer, Ante **413**
Serology **9.4**
Servicio Científico de Publicaciones Medicas del Uruguay **406.2**
Seventh-Day Adventist Hospital Association **1888**
Sewage Engineering **2357**
Sewage Treatment **2394**
Sex **2463, 2468**
Selye, Hans **1121, 1712**
Shafer, H. B. **673**
Sharaf, Mohammed **216**
Shastid, T. H. **2023**
Shelley, W. B. **1360**
Shellhase, L. J. **1596**
Sheppard, L. B. **1987**
Shevalev, A. E. **2005**
Shika kokugeka saikin no shinpo **1284**
Shilling, C. W. **2442**
Shinkei kenkyu no shinpo **1751**
Shipley, Thorne **2338**
Shishova, K. C. **2355**
Shock, N. W. **1424.1, 1427–1429**
Shock **2092**
Shock Therapy **1761, 1762, 1783**
Shonika saikin no shinpo **2125**
Short, Arthur **817**
Shryock, R. H. **512, 674, 674.1, 822, 1912**
Shuster, Louis **2216**
Side Effects, Drugs **2229–2231, 2233**
Side effects of drugs **2233**
Siebold, E. C. J. von **1967, 1977**
Sieshin igaku saiken no shinpo **1752**
Sigerist, H. E. **478, 488, 675, 2107**
Signeur, A. V. **1047**
Silicosis **2407**
Silva, Fernando da Correia, *see* Correia, Fernando da Silva
Simmons, L. W. **1891**
Simpson, R. R. **782**
Singer, C. J. **479, 889, 897, 954, 2524**
Siphonapters **2075.1**
Sirks, M. J. **955**
Sissons, H. A. **1686**
Skarzyński, Bolesław **623**
Skin and venereal diseases **1353**
Skin and venereal diseases. Nervous and mental diseases **1353, 1753**
Skinner, H. A. **206**
Skorodinskaia, V. V. **2620**
Sleep **1769**
Sleep Therapy **2623**
Sleeping Sickness, *see* Trypanosomiasis
Sleeping sickness bulletin **1226**
Sliosberg, A. **311**
Slutzky, J. F. **2031**
Smallpox **1572**
  Histories **1217–1220**
Smedt, Marc de **1471**
Smell **1868**
Smillie, W. G. **1154, 2381**
Smirnov, J. I. **1627**
Smith, Austin **234**
Smith, Brian Abel, *see* Abel-Smith, Brian
Smith, D. B. **1491**
Smith, Frederick **2664**
Smith, G. I. **207**
Smith, R. C. **2697**
Smithcors, J. F. **2665, 2666**
Smithsonian Institution **518, 971.1, 1040**
Smoking **2233.1, 2238, 2238.1, 2242, 2243**
Snakes **2240**
Snell, C. T. **1075**
Snell, F. D. **1075**
Snell, W. H. **1582**
Snowman, Jacob **818**
Snyder, Charles **2024**
Snyder, R. G. **844, 844.1**
Sobecka, Z. **1076**
Social Medicine, *see* Public Health
Social Psychology **911, 2298**
Social Sciences **2533**
Social Welfare
  Bibliographies **2414.1**
  Directories **2415**
Social Work, Army **1597**

Social Workers **2415, 2536**
Sociedad Venezolana de Historia de la Medicina **881**
Società italiana di ortopedia e traumatologia **1676**
Società medico-chirurgica di Bologna **57**
Societas Medicorum Fennica Duodecim **149**
Société de technique pharmaceutique **2150**
Société des sciences médicales de Tunisie **640**
Société d'histoire de la pharmacie. Paris **2201**
Societies, Dental **1318–1320, 1325, 1326**
Societies, Medical **344, 345, 348, 356, 358, 360, 370–372, 374, 374.1, 375, 380, 389, 397.1, 398, 399, 401, 403, 1453**
  Histories **337, 339, 566, 570, 593, 595, 659, 661, 662**
Societies, Ophthalmological **2014**
Societies, Optometric **2032**
Societies, Psychoanalytical **1803**
Societies, Scientific **2504–2505, 2507–2508**
  Histories **660**
Societies, Veterinary **2655, 2656.1**
Society for Clinical and Experimental Hypnosis **1849**
Society for Research in Child Development **2108**
Society of American Bacteriologists **1561**
Society of Analytical Chemistry **994**
Society of Biological Chemists, India **1026**
Society of Chemical Industry **27, 1007**
Sociologists **2535**
Sociology
  Bibliographies **911, 2529–2532**
  Dictionaries **2533–2534**
  Directories **2535–2537.1**
  Indexes and Abstracts **5.7, 2528**
Sociology of medicine **2528**
Sørensen, E. C. **883**
Sokół, Stanisław **624**
Sokoloff, Leon **1662**
Sokolov, E. I. **1118**
Sollmann, T. H. **2177.1**
Solotorovsky, M. **1568**
Somolinos d'Ardois, Germán **612**
Sonnedecker, Glenn **2213**
Sourkes, T. L. **456**
South Carolina. Histories **723–724**
South Carolina Medical Association **723, 724**
South Pacific
  Bibliographies **1144, 1168**
  Directories **344**
South Pacific Commission **1167, 1168**
Southwest Foundation for Research and Education, San Antonio **2688**
Souza-Araujo, H. C. **1187**
Sovetskaia literatura po meditsine **90**
Sovetskie knigi po meditsine **91.1**
Sovetskoe meditsinskoe referativnoe obozrenie **109**
Sovetskoe meditsinskoe referativnoe obozrenie. Onkologiia **1686**
Sozinskey, T. S. **825**
Space Flight **845**
Space Medicine, *see* Aerospace and Submarine Medicine
Space Technology Laboratories. Technical Library **845**
Spain
  Bibliographies **1295**
  Directories **378**
  Histories **439, 626–632, 1983**
  Indexes and Abstracts **88.1**
Spain. Consejo Superior de Investigaciones Cientificas. Instituto Jose Celestino Mutis de Farmacognosia **1415, 1416**
Spain. Instituto Nacional de Investigaciones Agronomicas **1419.1**
Spanier, L. M. **1515**
Spanish American War **1643–1644**
Spastics Society, London. Medical Education and Information Unit **2127**
Special Libraries Association **178, 189**
Special Libraries Association. Science Technology Division. Pharmaceutical Section **2143, 2151, 2198**
Spector, W. S. **934**
Speech **1866**
Speech Disorders **1873**
Speert, Harold **1978**
Spencer, H. R. **1979**
Spencer, M. C. **1701, 1702, 2177.2, 2617.1**
Spinal Cord, *see* Brain and Spinal Cord
Spinal Cord Injury **1844**
Spinal Cord Neoplasms **1699**
Spiro, K. **1008**
Spis fachowych pracowników słuzby zdrowia **376**
Spisok meditsinkikh vracheĭ **384.1**
Sportmedizinisch Veröffentlichungen **2249**
Sports **2248, 2254**
Sports Medicine, *see* Physical Education and Sports Medicine
Sprague, M. L. **2228**
Sprengel, Kurt **134, 135, 471**
Sprengel, K. P. J. **471**
Sprengel, Wilhelm **471**
Squires, H. C. **633**
Stacey, R. S. **2167**
Stageman, Anne **1436**
Stallworthy, John **1948.1**
Standard medical directory of North America **404**
Stanton, I. A. **237**
Stanton, M. E. **2609**
Staphylococcal Infection
  Bibliographies **1221–1223**
State-accredited schools of nursing **1905**

State-approved schools of professional nursing **1905**
State cancer control programs **1718**
Statistics, Vital, *see* Vital Statistics
Stearn, A. E. **1220**
Stearn, E. A. W. **1220**
Stechow, M. **1930**
Stedman, T. L. **235, 238, 1479.1**
Steen, E. B. **197**
Steinbichler, Eveline **2186**
Stephens, S. V. **2456**
Stereochemistry **1037**
Stern, N. S. **129**
Sternberg, G. M. **1644**
Sternfeld, Alfred **1298**
Steroids **1078, 1386.1**
Steudel, Johannes **419.1, 443**
Steuer, R. O. **489**
Stevens, S. S. **1871**
Stevenson, Alan **969**
Stevenson, L. G. **456**
Stevenson, R. S. **766, 2055**
Stich, Virginia **1597**
Sticker, Georg **1153, 1265**
Stieb, E. W. **2216.1**
Still, G. F. **2139**
Stocks, M. D. **1913**
Stoeckel, Walter **1965**
Stomatology **16.12, 1273, 1288, 1302, 1304, 1313.1**
Stomatology references **1273**
Stone, A. A. **2313**
Stone, E. P. **517**
Stone, R. F. **655**
Stony Brook Foundation, Inc. **925**
Storer, H. R. **788**
Storer, Malcolm **788**
Stotz, E. H. **1098**
Stout, T. D. M. **1625**
Stratigraphy **2430**
Stratton, G. B. **2516**
Straus, Robert **2382**
Strean, L. P. **1355**
Streeter, E. C. **889**
Streptomycin **2223**
Stress **2302, 2304, 2305**
Strickland, W. N. **1577**
Strieby, I. M. **2177.2**
Striker, Cecil **718**
Strömgren, H. L. **1299, 1342, 1343**
Strontium Metabolism **2459**
Stroppiana, Luigi **796**
Strugger, Siegfried **980**
Stubbe, Hans **1423**
Student Health **1760, 2246**
Students **453**
Students, Foreign **1366.1**
Students, Graduate **1367, 1367.1**
Stümke, Hans **193**
Stupanus, Emanuel **256.1**
Sturtevant, W. C. **518**
Subject Headings **1529, 1530, 1531**
Submarine Medicine, *see* Aerospace and Submarine Medicine
Sudan
    Histories **633**
    Indexes and Abstracts **2493.1**
Sudhoff, Karl, **338, 420, 433, 443, 476, 480, 889, 1204, 1344, 2572**
Sudhoffs Klassiker der Medizin **443**
Suid-Afrikaanse Akademie vir Wetenskap en Kuns **215**
Sulfur **2393**
Summarium des neuesten aus der gesammten Medicin **69.1**
Summarium des neuesten aus der in- und ausländischen Medicin zum Gebrauche praktischer Aerzte **69.1**
Summarium des neuesten und wissenwurdigsten aus der gesammten Medicin zum Gebrauche für practischen Aerzte und Wundärzte **69.1**
Suomalainen Lääkäriseura Duodecim **79**
Suomen lääketieteellinen bibliografia **149**
Surgeon General's Advisory Committee on Smoking and Health **2242**
Surgeons **349, 353, 357, 364, 374.3, 387, 390, 400, 402, 402.1, 403, 405, 2559, 2560, 2561**
Surgeons, Oral **1324**
Surgeons, Veterinary **2656**
Surgery, *see also* Anesthesia; Orthopedics
    Bibliographies **132.1, 133, 149.1, 150, 167, 2556–2557**
    Dictionaries **239, 293**
    Directories **357, 364, 374.3, 399.1, 402, 402.1, 403, 405, 2559–2561**
    Encyclopedias **409**
    Films **1399**
    Histories **895, 1408, 2562–2575**
    Indexes and Abstracts **9.9, 10.2, 16.4, 33, 36.2, 38.1, 40, 41, 54, 59, 65–67, 70, 71, 96.1, 2538–2545**
    Manuals **2558**
    Reviews **117, 2090, 2547–2555**
Surgery, Cardiac **9.18, 2576.1–2577**
Surgery, Military **1591, 1616, 1642, 1643**
Surgery, Neurological, *see* Neurosurgery
Surgery, Operative **1881, 1885**
Surgery, Oral **1282, 1284**
Surgery, Pediatric **2582**
Surgery, Plastic
    Bibliography **2588**
    Histories **2587–2588**
    Indexes and Abstracts **2540, 2582.1–2584**
    Reviews **1672, 2585–2586**
Surgery, Reconstructive, *see* Surgery, Plastic
Surgery, Thoracic **9.15, 2589**
    Histories **2589**

Surgery, Traumatic **16.4, 1672, 1676, 2586, 2591–2593**, *see also* Injuries
Surgical Specialties **2576–2593**
Survey of anesthesiology **2596**
Survey of bioelectronic approaches to the study of behavior **963**
Survey of biological progress **927**
Survey of ophthalmology **1989**
Survey of pathology in medicine and surgery **2089**
Surveys and abstracts **116**
Sury, Kurt von **2324**
Svensk läkare-matrikel **635**
Svenska läkaresällskapet **635**
Svenska tandläkare **1326.1**
Svenska tandläkare i ord och bild **1326.2**
Sveriges lakäre-historia **635**
Sweat **1046**
Sweden
  Directories **379, 1326.1, 1326.2**
  Histories **634–635, 2374**
  Periodicals **322**
Sweden. Medicinalstyrelsen **379, 2374**
Swine **2695**
Switzerland
  Directories **380, 2560, 2603.1**
  Histories **636**
  Indexes and Abstracts **89**
Sydney. University. School of Public Health and Tropical Medicine **2354**
Symbols, Medical **823–825**
Symptomatology **275, 1364**
Syndromes **209–214.1, 1313.1, 1355, 1790**
Synthesis microbiologica **1538.2**
Synthetic Organic Chemical Manufacturers Association **1082**
Syphilis, *see* Veneral Diseases
Syracuse University Research Corporation. Microbiological and Biochemical Center **2228**
Syria
  Indexes and Abstracts **2493.1**
Systematic report on the progress of ophthalmology **1995, 1996**
Systematischer Bericht über die Leistungen und Fortschritte der Augenheikunde **1995, 1996**
Systematisches Repertorium der gesammten medicinischen Literatur Deutschlands **97**
Sytamco, J. R. **300**
Szabó, Barnabás **2177.3**
Szabo, Denis **2531**
Szulec, J. A. **2558**

Tabanelli, Mario **490**
Taber, C. W. **239, 1959**
Tablets, Pharmacy **2171, 2172**
Tabulae biologicae **935**
Tadzhik. S. S. R. Ministerstvo zdravookhraneniia **161**
Taft, Jonathan **1300**
Takata, Ryohie **1936**
Talbot, C. H. **574**
Tanganyika
  Bibliographies **145.2**
Taschenberg, Otto **2691**
Tashkent. Gosudarstvennaia nauchno-meditsinskaia biblioteka **2355**
Tasmania
  Directories **344**
Tasnádi-Kubacska, Andras **791**
Taste **1871.1**
Taton, René **2525**
Taylor, A. E. **236**
Taylor, N. B. **236, 238**
Taylor, Selwyn **2554**
Tbilisskiĭ gosudarstvennyĭ meditsinskiĭ institut **166**
Tchernichowsky, S. **260**
Teah, B. A. **1553, 1554**
Technique pharmaceutique **2150**
Technology **2510, 2511, 2515**
  Histories **2524**
Technology, Medical **16.7, 2079, 2084–2086**
Telatin, Luigi **1790**
Telberg, Ira **1791**
Teleky, Ludwig **2414**
Temkin, I. S. **2047**
Temkin, Owsei **1836**
Tennessee. Histories **725**
Tennessee State Medical Association **725**
Teratology, *see* Congenital Anomalies
Terra, Paul de **1315**
Tests, Psychological **2306–2307**
Tews, R. M. **1483**
Texas. Histories **728–731**
Texas. University. College of Pharmacy **2145**
Texas. University. Graduate School of Biomedical Sciences at Houston **190.1**
Texas. University. Medical Branch. Department of Surgery **2576**
Texas Christian University. Institute of Behavioral Research **963**
Texas Medical Association **729**
Thacher, James **656**
Thailand
  Indexes and Abstracts **2491.1**
Thailand. National Documentation Centre **2491.1**
Therapeutics
  Bibliographies **2618–2623**
  Dictionaries **239, 2623.1**
  Histories **2624**
  Indexes and Abstracts **25, 30, 2157.1, 2610.1–2613**
  Nomenclature **1879**
  Reviews **121, 1548, 2613.1–2617**
Therapeutics, Psychiatric **1741, 1762, 1783, 1788**

Therapists, Rehabilitation **2263**
Therapy, Diet **2615**
Therapy, Drug *see* Drug Therapy
Therapy, Family **1781.2**
Therapy, Inhalation **2621**
Therapy, Oxygen **2619**
Therapy, Physical **16.1, 239, 1661, 2261**
Therapy, Shock **1761, 1762, 1783**
Therapy, Sleep **2623**
Therapy, Tissue **2620**
Theses **179–185**
Thimm, C. A. **1229**
Thomasson, C. L. **2179**
Thompson, C. J. S. **803, 808, 2573**
Thompson, E. T. **1881**
Thompson, L. **406**
Thoms, H. K. **680, 1980–1982**
Thomson, H. W. **279**
Thomson, W. A. R. **240**
Thoracic Surgery **9.15, 2589**
Thorndike, Lynn **428, 2526**
Thornton, J. L. **423, 2527**
Thorpe, B. L. **1334**
Throat **2034, 2036, 2039, 2042, 2045**
Thrombohemorrhage **1121**
Thrombosis **2178**
Thyroid Gland **1381**
Tibet. Histories **637–639**
Ticks **2072**
T'ien, Li-chih **221**
Tierärzte Adressbuch für die Deutsche Bundesrepublik und West-Berlin **2656.1**
Tierpsychologische Sammelberichte **2296.1**
Tietze, Christopher **2465, 2466**
Tilton, J. R. **1780**
Tischner, Rudolf **773**
Tissue, Connective **907**
Tissue Culture **905, 906, 908**
Tissue Culture Association **908**
Tissue culture bibliography **906**
Tissue Therapy **2620**
Tittel, Kurt **2251**
Tobacco **2233.1, 2238, 2238.1, 2242, 2243**
Tomaszewski, Wiktor **282**
Tompkins, D. C. **2241, 2529**
Tooth Replantation **2590**
Top, F. H. **1154**
Torres Norry, José **1781**
Torsuev, N. A. **1183**
Tovell, Ann **524**
Toverud, Guttorm **1296**
Towarzystwo Lekarskie Warszawskie **86.1**
Toxic episodes in children **2231**
Toxicology
  Bibliographies **151.1, 2174, 2234–2243**
  Histories **2245**
  Indexes and Abstracts **5.2, 9.2, 21.4, 2147, 2229–2231**
  Monographs **2244**
  Periodicals **2197.1**
  Reviews **2232–2233**
Toxicology, Child **2231**
Toxoplasmosis
  Bibliographies **1224–1225**
Trabue, I. M. **1871.1**
Train, David **2171**
Training Grants **2396**
Transfusion, Blood **1112**
Translation supplement **177**
Translations **176–178, 418,** *see also* History of Medicine, Sources
Translators and translations **178**
Transplantation **2590**
[*Transplantation bibliographies*] **2590**
Trauma, *see* Injuries
Traumatic Surgery, *see* Surgery, Traumatic
Traumatology, *see* Surgery, Traumatic
Travaux d'histoire locale de la pharmacie en France . . . répertoire bibliographique **2201**
Trease, G. E. **2217**
Treatment, *see* Therapeutics
Trelles y Govín, C. M. **96**
Trenkov, K. I. **140.1**
Treue, Wilhelm **767**
Triepel, Hermann **884**
Trophoblast Transplantation **2590**
Tropical diseases bulletin **1139**
Tropical Medicine **1139, 1140, 1140.1, 1142, 1144,** *see also* Communicable Diseases
  Histories **1150, 1152**
Trypanosomiasis **1139**
  Bibliographies **1227–1229**
  Indexes and Abstracts **1226**
Tsentral'nyĭ meditsinskiĭ zhurnal **110**
Tsentral'nyĭ referativnyĭ meditsinskiĭ zhurnal **110**
Tsetse Flies **1229**
Tsoukas, A. G. **258**
Tsusaki, Takamichi **373**
Tsutsugamushi Disease **1211.1, 1211.2**
Tuberculosis
  Bibliographies **1238**
  Dictionaries **1239**
  Directories **1240–1242**
  Histories **1243–1250**
  Indexes and Abstracts **9.15, 10.6, 16.2, 1230–1234**
  Reviews **1235–1237**
Tuberculosis index and abstracts of current literature **1233**
Tuberculosis index and digest of current literature **1233**
Tuberculosis index including chest diseases **1233**
Tuke, D. H. **1792**
Tularemia
  Bibliographies **1251**

Tully, R. I. J. **2527**
Tunisia. Histories **640**
Turkey
  Indexes and Abstracts **2493.1**
Tweney, C. F. **2494**
Tyler, A. F. **707**
Typhus **1211.1, 1211.2**
  Histories **1213**

UNESCO, *see* United Nations Educational, Scientific and Cultural Organization
Uebersicht der vorzüglichsten Ergebnisse aus der medicinischen Literatur des Auslandes **68**
Uganda
  Bibliographies **145.2**
Uhlmann, W. **2455.1**
Ujhelyi, Adorjań **2435**
Ulcerative Colitis **1404.1**
Ulcerative colitis abstracts **1404.1**
Ultraschall in Medizin und Grenzgebieten **2258**
Ultrasonics **2258**
Ultrasonics **2258, 2259**
Ultrasons **2258**
Underwood, E. A. **479, 1146**
Underwood, F. I. **703**
Unger, L. H. **69**
Unghváry, László **214.1**
Union of American Biological Societies **916**
Union of International Associations **186, 187**
Union of South Africa
  Directories **381–382**
  Histories **641**
U.S.S.R., *see also* Armenia; Estonia; Latvia
  Bibliographies **159–162, 164, 165, 846, 867, 929, 973, 1043, 1097, 1113, 1115–1116, 1118–1119, 1161–1163, 1169, 1174, 1178, 1183, 1188, 1288, 1406.1, 1407, 1426–1426.1, 1659–1660, 1699, 1756, 1764, 1867, 1953, 2005, 2060, 2062–2063, 2221, 2302, 2309, 2350, 2352–2353, 2355, 2391, 2455, 2484, 2488, 2591, 2620, 2633**
  Directories **383–384.1, 1720**
  Histories **642–648.1, 1627, 1826, 2375–2376**
  Indexes and Abstracts **90–91.1, 106–110, 1347, 1686, 2421**
  Manuals **1488**
  Nomenclature **2192**
  Periodicals **318, 321.1**
  Periodicals, Lists **2515**
  Reviews **1095**
United Aircraft Corporation. Hamilton Standard Division **2578**
United Nations Educational, Scientific and Cultural Organization **2491.2, 2528, 2531, 2533**
United Nations Educational, Scientific and Cultural Organization. Science Cooperation Office, Middle East **2493.1**
United Nations Educational, Scientific and Cultural Organization. Social Science Clearing House **2416.2**
United Nations Educational, Scientific and Cultural Organization. South Asia Science Cooperation Office **2493.2**
United Nations. Food and Agriculture Organization, *see* Food and Agriculture Organization of the United Nations
United Nations. Library **1510**
United States
  Bibliographies **167–170, 1290, 1599, 2639**
  Collections, Periodicals **1503, 1515–1516**
  Directories **188, 385–406, 1083, 1130, 1240–1241, 1316–1318, 1326–1328, 1367, 1369–1371.1, 1430, 1448–1453, 1535, 1561, 1663, 1718, 1721, 1794–1795, 1797–1802, 1804–1805, 1850, 1857, 1874–1875, 1903–1905, 1960–1961, 2013, 2027, 2032–2033, 2048, 2050, 2094, 2193, 2193.1, 2263, 2326, 2358–2360, 2395.1, 2415, 2443–2444, 2490, 2499, 2508, 2535–2536, 2537.1, 2559, 2603, 2655**
  Directories, Individuals **385–391, 400–406, 1130, 1317–1318, 1448–1449, 1535, 1561, 1663, 1794–1795, 1797, 1799, 1850, 1874, 1960–1961, 2013, 2032–2033, 2094, 2193, 2263, 2326, 2358, 2360, 2415, 2443–2444, 2490, 2499, 2535–2536, 2559, 2603, 2655**
  Directories, Institutions **1083, 1316, 1367, 1430, 1450–1453, 1800–1802, 1804–1805, 1857, 1875, 1904–1905, 2027**
  Directories, Organizations **392–399, 2193.1, 2395.1, 2485–2486, 2537.1**
  Histories **332, 649–675, 769, 771–772, 776, 806, 809, 822, 849, 988, 1147, 1154, 1165, 1194, 1331, 1334, 1336, 1337, 1345, 1357, 1373, 1377, 1458, 1564, 1628–1652, 1827–1831, 1846, 1911, 1923, 1963, 1980, 2018, 2103, 2336, 2377–2383, 2413, 2564, 2565, 2661, 2665,** *see also* Indians (American); under names of individual states
  Indexes and Abstracts **111, 1010, 2071**
  Manuals **1473**
  Periodicals **332, 2198, 2513**
  Presidents **764–765, 768**
  Theses **179, 181**
U.S. Air Force. Office of Aerospace Research **2475**
U.S. Air Force. Office of Scientific Research **2476**
U.S. Air Force. Office of the Surgeon General **1646**
U.S. Armed Forces Institute of Pathology **1630, 1717**
U.S. Armed Forces Medical Library **28, 29, 1498, 1701, 1702,** *see also* U.S. Army. Surgeon General's Office. Library; U.S. Army

Medical Library; U.S. National Library of Medicine
U.S. Army. Chemical-Biological-Radiological Agency. Biological Laboratories **1170, 1171, 1189, 1190, 1209.1, 1571**
U.S. Army. Chemical Corps **1155.1, 1160.1, 1166.1, 1166.2, 1171, 1190, 1199, 1209.2–1211.1, 1251, 1572**
U.S. Army. Human Engineering Laboratories **1597.1**
U.S. Army. Medical Department **1628, 1629, 1631, 1632, 1636, 1640, 1644, 1645, 1648**
U.S. Army. Surgeon General's Office. Library **30,** *see also* U.S. Armed Forces Medical Library; U.S. Army Medical Library; U.S. National Library of Medicine
U.S. Army Air Forces **1646**
U.S. Army Medical Library **28, 29, 34, 1498, 2617.1,** *see also* U.S. Armed Forces Medical Library; U.S. Army. Surgeon General's Office. Library; U.S. National Library of Medicine
U.S. Atomic Energy Commission **2449, 2456–2457.1, 2477**
U.S. Atomic Energy Commission (series) **2239, 2388, 2389, 2456–2457.1, 2695**
U.S. Atomic Energy Commission. Nuclear Safety Information Center, Oak Ridge **2458**
U.S. Bureau of American Ethnology **518**
U.S. Bureau of Animal Industry **2678, 2678.1, 2678.2**
U.S. Bureau of the Census **1883–1883.2**
U.S. Children's Bureau **1852, 1853, 1857**
U.S. Children's Bureau. Clearinghouse for Research in Childlife **2131.1**
U.S. Congress. House. Committee on Ways and Means **2356**
U.S. Congress. Senate. Committee on Government Operations **2180**
U.S. Defense Documentation Center **1362**
U.S. Department of Agriculture. Agricultural Research Service **2459**
U.S. Department of Commerce. Clearinghouse for Federal Scientific and Technical Information **176,** *see also* U.S. Department of Commerce. Office of Technical Services
U.S. Department of Commerce. Office of Technical Services **176, 2391,** *see also* U.S. Department of Commerce. Clearinghouse for Federal Scientific and Technical Information
U.S. Department of Defense **1884**
U.S. Department of Health, Education and Welfare **2478**
U.S. Department of Health, Education and Welfare. Bureau of Family Services **2414.1**
U.S. Department of the Air Force **1613**
U.S. Department of the Air Force. Surgeon General **1613**
U.S. Department of the Army. Office of the Chief of Military History **1647**
U.S. Department of the Army. Office of the Surgeon General **1630, 1648, 1665**
U.S. Department of the Army. Surgeon General's Office **1629**
U.S. Department of the Interior **2408**
U.S. Federal Advisory Council on Medical Training Aids **1400**
U.S. Federal Aviation Agency. Civil Aeromedical Research Institute **844**
U.S. Fish and Wildlife Service **2692**
U.S. Food and Drug Administration. Bureau of Medicine **2467.1**
U.S. Library of Congress **1498, 2385**
U.S. Library of Congress. Aerospace Technology Division **962.1, 1048**
U.S. Library of Congress. General Reference and Bibliography Division **190, 2502**
U.S. Library of Congress. Reference Department **1872**
U.S. Library of Congress. Science and Technology Division **835, 1301**
U.S. Library of Congress. Science Division **944.1, 2515**
U.S. Marine-Hospital Service **1886.1**
U.S. Medical Field Service School, Carlisle Barracks, Pa. **1632, 1635**
U.S. National Aeronautics and Space Administration **834**
U.S. National Aeronautics and Space Administration. Scientific and Technical Information Division **847, 1122**
U.S. National Agricultural Library **964, 974, 983, 2225, 2658**
U.S. National Cancer Institute **1688, 1713, 1714, 1721, 2654**
U.S. National Center for Health Statistics **1885**
U.S. National Clearinghouse for Mental Health Information **1761, 1781.1, 1781.2, 1782, 1851, 1859, 1860, 1861, 2532, 2537**
U.S. National Heart Institute **2578**
U.S. National Heart Institute. Committee on Thrombolytic Agents **1123**
U.S. National Institute of Arthritis and Metabolic Diseases **1392, 1403, 1653**
U.S. National Institute of Child Health and Human Development **1854**
U.S. National Institute of Mental Health **1783, 1801, 1804–1806**
U.S. National Institute of Neurological Diseases and Blindness. Joint Council Subcommittee on Cerebrovascular Disease **1101**
U.S. National Institute of Neurological Diseases and Blindness. Perinatal Research Branch **1855**
U.S. National Institutes of Health **168, 1095, 1162, 1762, 1783.1, 1860, 2464**

U.S. National Institutes of Health. Division of General Medical Sciences. Russian Scientific Translation Program **2484**
U.S. National Institutes of Health. Division of Research Grants **1886, 2474**
U.S. National Library of Medicine **4, 6, 11, 28, 29, 164, 169, 176, 177, 326, 414, 757, 1045, 1123, 1191, 1214, 1222, 1223, 1225, 1269, 1365.1, 1498, 1499, 1515, 1515.1, 1523, 1531, 1532, 1537, 1863, 2142, 2180, 2192, 2489, 2509,** *see also* U.S. Armed Forces Medical Library; U.S. Army. Surgeon General's Office. Library; U.S. Army Medical Library
U.S. National Library of Medicine. Medical Literature Analysis and Retrieval System **1123, 1365, 1392, 1655, 1890, 2578**
U.S. National Library of Medicine. Reference Division **1579, 1580, 1598**
U.S. National Library of Medicine. Reference Services Division **1524, 2242, 2243**
U.S. National Library of Medicine. Scientific Translation Program **2302**
U.S. National Referral Center for Science and Technology **395, 2395.1, 2537.1**
U.S. National Science Foundation **194, 2142, 2479–2482, 2506, 2509**
U.S. Navy. Dental Corps **1634**
U.S. Navy. Medical Department **1649, 1650, 1652**
U.S. Navy Department. Bureau of Medicine and Surgery **836, 1634, 1649, 1650, 1652**
U.S. Navy Department. Office of Naval Research **836, 1301, 1595**
U.S. Office of Manpower, Automation and Training **2400**
U.S. Office of Scientific Research and Development **1651**
U.S. Office of Scientific Research and Development. Committee on Medical Research **1651**
U.S. Office of Scientific Research and Development. Committee on Medical Research and Development **1869**
U.S. President's Panel on Mental Retardation **1856**
U.S. Public Health Service **170, 171, 1537, 1722, 1856, 2344, 2383, 2385, 2391.1, 2394.2, 2405**
U.S. Public Health Service. Audiovisual Facility, Atlanta **1722, 1806.1**
U.S. Public Health Service. Cancer Control Branch **1722**
U.S. Public Health Service. Cancer Control Program **1718**
U.S. Public Health Service. Clearinghouse on Current Morbidity Statistics Projects **2478.1**
U.S. Public Health Service. Communicable Disease Center **1400**
U.S. Public Health Service. Communicable Disease Center. Venereal Disease Branch **1252**
U.S. Public Health Service. Division of Air Pollution **2391.1, 2392, 2393**
U.S. Public Health Service. Division of Chronic Diseases **1124, 1125**
U.S. Public Health Service. Division of Dental Public Health and Resources **1303**
U.S. Public Health Service. Division of General Health Services **2360**
U.S. Public Health Service. Division of Hospital and Medical Facilities **1436**
U.S. Public Health Service. Division of Industrial Hygiene **2392**
U.S Public Health Service. Division of Special Health Services **1252**
U.S. Public Health Service. Division of Special Health Services. Veneral Disease Program **1252**
U.S. Public Health Service. Division of Water Supply and Pollution Control **2394, 2396**
U.S. Public Health Service. Neurological and Sensory Disease Service Program **1806.1**
U.S. Public Health Service. Robert A. Taft Sanitary Engineering Center, Cincinnati **2394.1**
U.S. Sanitary Commission **1640.1, 1641**
U.S. Veterans Administration. Department of Medicine and Surgery **2483**
U.S. Veterans Administration. Department of Medicine and Surgery. Medical and General Reference Library **1525, 1844**
U.S. Veterans Administration. Library Division. Special Service. Department of Medicine and Surgery **1516**
U.S. Veterans Administration. Medical and General Reference Library **1238, 1599**
U.S. Vocational Rehabilitation Administration **1779**
U.S. Walter Reed Army Institute of Research **1596**
U.S. War Department. Surgeon General's Office **1642, 1645**
University Microfilms, Inc. **179, 181**
Unlisted drugs **2151**
Unpublished abstracts of articles on pharmaceutical subjects **2145**
Unseld, D. W. **254**
Uppsala. Universitet. Bibliotek **1500**
Urdang, Georg **2206, 2213**
Urine **1046, 2455.1**
Urological survey **2625**
Urologischer Jahresbericht **2628**
Urology
    Bibliographies **2633–2634**
    Histories **2635–2638**
    Indexes and Abstracts **16.4, 36.2, 2624.1–2629**
    Reviews **2630–2632**
Uruguay
    Directories **406.1, 406.2**

Histories **520, 736**
Usandizaga, Manuel **1983**
Utah. Histories **732**
Utilization, Hospital **1436**
Utkin, L. A. **973**
Uvarov, E. B. **1065**

Vaccination, *see* Smallpox
Vaccinia **1572**
Vachnadze, E. A. **166**
Vail', V. S. **161**
Valach, Vladislav **313**
Valdivia Ponce, Oscar **1825**
Valdizán, Hermilio **619, 620**
Valentin, Bruno **1680.1, 1681**
Valenzuela, José Reina, *see* Reina Valenzuela, José
Valle, R. H. **2574**
Vályi, Edit **1302**
van der Merwe, F. Z. **215**
Vandewiele, L. J. **2202**
Van Ingen, Philip **712**
Van Luik, James **1063**
Van Nostrand chemist's dictionary **1069**
Vaponefrin aerosol library **2621**
Vaponefrin inhalation therapy library **2621**
Vári, I. **2006**
Variola, *see* Smallpox
Vasil'ev, K. G. **606**
Vasil'ev, S. I. **2431**
Veillon, E. **317, 878**
Veith, Ilza **1837, 2575**
Velez, Edwin **306**
Velez Boza, Fermin **908.1**
Venereal Diseases
Bibliographies **1256–1259, 1354**
Directories **1260**
Histories **1261–1265**
Indexes and Abstracts **9.13, 16.11, 36.2, 1252–1254, 1347–1350**
Reviews **1255**
Venezuela
Bibliographies **908.1**
Histories **737–738, 2384**
Indexes and Abstracts **92**
Periodicals **320**
Venezuela. Ministerio de Sanidad y Asistencia Social **92**
Venice. Istituto per la Collaborazione Culturale **264**
Venoms **2237, 2240**
Vernon, D. T. A. **2314**
Verzeichnis der deutschen Ärzte und Heilanstalten **359**
Verzeichnis des deutschen psychologischen Schriftums 1889–1941 **2297**
Verzeichniss der neurologischen Literatur **1739**
Veszprémí, István, *see* Weszprémí, István
Vester, Helmut **2204, 2205**
Veterans **1599**
Veterinärmedizin **2641**
Veterinarians **352, 374.1, 374.3, 380, 384, 2655, 2656, 2656.1**
Veterinary bulletin **2642**
Veterinary Legislation **2655**
Veterinary Libraries **1526**
Veterinary Medicine
Bibliographies **167, 171, 173, 2647–2649**
Dictionaries **293, 2650–2653**
Directories **352, 374.1, 374.3, 380, 384, 2655–2657**
Histories **2659–2667**
Indexes and Abstracts **2639–2644**
Nomenclature **2654**
Periodicals **2658**
Reviews **2645–2646**
Veterinary Schools **2655–2657**
Veterinary Societies **2655, 2656.1**
Veterinary Surgeons **2656**
Veth, Cornelis **758**
Vibration **844, 844.1**
Viellard, Camille **2638**
Vierordt, Hermann **424, 446**
Viet-Nam
Bibliographies **171–172**
Viet-Nam. Centre National de la Recherche Scientifique **172**
Viets, H. R. **436, 700, 1964**
Viewpoints in biology **928**
Vigiliis von Creutzenfeld, S. H. de **2557**
Villemin, Martial **2653**
Vil'shanskaia, M. L. **1118, 1174**
Vinař, Josef **546**
Vintilă, G. D. **1984**
Virchow, R. **46**
Virgin Islands
Directories **389, 1804, 2050**
Virginia. Histories **733–734**
Virology **16.3, 1551**
Viruses **5.3, 1545, 1707**
Visibility **1872, 1987**
Vision **1869, 1987, 2012**
Visser, C. **228**
Vital notes on medical periodicals **327**
Vital Statistics
Bibliographies **2352, 2416, 2416.1**
Directories **2416.2**
Histories **2417–2418**
Indexes and Abstracts **2415.1, 2478.1**
Vitamin abstracts **1931**
Vitamin B 12 **1078**
Vitamin E **1934**
Vitamins
Bibliographies **1934–1936**
Indexes and Abstracts **1930–1931**
Nomenclature **1937**
Reviews **1932–1933**
Vitamins and hormones **1933**

Vitrum Apotekare A. B., Stockholm **2178**
Vivisection. Histories **821**
Vogt, Helmut **759**
Volkmann, Herbert **255**
Volta review **1867.1**
Voluntary Health Agencies **393**
Voprosy rentgenologii i radiologii **2421**
Voss, Hermann **2696**
Voutsinas, Dimitri **2291**
Vü-Văn-Nguyên **172**

W. Roths Jahresbericht über die Leistungen und Fortschritte auf dem Gebiete des Militär-Sanitätswesens **1593**
Waga kuni ni okeru koku igaku bunken mokuroku **847.1**
Wain, Harry **208**
Waksman, S. A. **1250, 2223**
Walder., M. R. **709**
Walford, A. J. **2493.3**
Walker, A. E. **2581**
Walker, A. S. **1605**
Walker, E. H. **971.1**
Walker, M. R. **708**
Walker, Nigel **1816**
Wallace, V. E. **2602**
Waller, Erik **1500**
Wallis, George **277**
Walsh, J. J. **713**
Walter Reed Army Institute of Research, *see* U.S. Walter Reed Army Institute of Research
Wang, Chi-min **541**
War Crimes **1602**
Ward, H. L. **2457**
Waring, E. J. **2622**
Waring, J. I. **723, 724**
Warren, H. C. **2325**
Warsaw. Centralny Instytut Informacji Naukowo-Technicznej i Ekonomicznej **2506**
Warsaw. Centrum Wyszkolenia Sanitarnego. Biblioteka **86**
Warsaw. Główna Biblioteka Lekarska **86, 87, 1517**
Warsaw. Institute for Research in Physical Culture **2254**
Warsaw. Lekarsky Instytut Naukovo-Wydawniczy **155**
Warsaw. Państwowy Zakład Wydawnictw Lekarskich **87.1, 211, 281, 376, 2170, 2351**
Was gibt es Neues für den praktischen Tierarzt? **2643**
Was gibt es Neues in der Medizin? **23**
Washington Institute of Medicine **28.1, 35, 38.1, 1350, 1738, 1945, 1994.1, 2040.1, 2114, 2541, 2627**
Wasserman, C. S. **399**
Wasserman, Paul **399**
Wasserman, R. H. **2459**
Watanabe, Yoshitaka **275, 1364**
Water Engineering **2357**
Water Pollution **2228, 2386, 2394.1, 2395, 2395.1, 2396**
Water pollution abstracts **2386**
Water Pollution Control **2394**
Water pollution control research and training grants **2396**
Water Treatment **2394**
Watson, I. A. **657**
Watson, R. I. **2339**
Weatherhead, L. D. **812**
Webb, W. B. **2623**
Weber, A. **760**
Weber, A. G. **1304**
Wegner, R. N. **898**
Wehmer, Carl **325**
Weichardt, Wolfgang **1548**
Weightlessness **844, 844.1**
Weinberger, B. W. **1305, 1345, 1346**
Weindler, Fritz **1985**
Weiner, Jack **1872**
Welfare, Social **2415**
Wellcome Historical Medical Library **417, 564, 574, 607, 741, 1501, 1848**
Wellcome Historical Medical Museum **567, 2606**
Wellek, Albert **2314.1**
Wells, Calvin **792**
Wernich, Albrecht **446**
Wernstedt, W. E. **298**
West, C. J. **1049–1050**
West, D. J. **2331**
West, G. P. **2651**
Westergaard, H. L. **2418**
Western Society of Periodontology **1272**
Weszprémi, István **580**
Wetterer, Josef **2436**
Wettley, Annemarie **1815**
What goes on **190.1**
Whitfield, R. N. **703**
Whitney, W. N. **601**
Whittaker, A. H. **2413**
Whitwell, J. R. **1817**
Who's important in medicine **390**
Who's who among physicians and surgeons **405**
Who's who in American dentistry **1327**
Who's who in American medicine **1925, 406**
Who's who in dentistry **1328**
Who's who in physical culture **2254**
Whyte, L. L. **2340**
Wickes, Stephen **711**
Widdess, J. D. H. **595**
Widner, E. M. **1041**
Widstrand, Axel **635**
Wiederherstellungschirurgie und Traumatologie **2586**
Wiklund, K. B. **602**

Wilbraham, Anne **1924**
Wildberg, C. F. L. **1472**
Wilde, Bernhard **1971**
Wilke, Georg **804**
Wilken-Jensen, Knud **854.1**
Wilkie, G. H. **1760**
Wilkinson, A. W. **2582**
Williams, A. S. **1081**
Williams, Harley **1242**
Williams, R. C. **2383**
Williams, R. L. **2623**
Williams, S. W. **658**
Willius, F. A. **1136, 1137**
Wilson, L. G. **2284**
Windisch, Wilhelm **2667**
Winslow, C. E. A. **1154, 1155, 2365**
Winther, Mathias **145.1**
Wisconsin, Histories **735**
Wisconsin. University **1215, 1216**
Wisconsin. University. Library **1057**
Wissenschaftliche Uebersicht der gesammten medicinisch-chirurgischen Literatur **70**
Wickersheimer, Ernest **339, 559, 560**
Wistrand, A. H. **635**
Witkowski, G. J. **783**
Witt, F. H. **1341**
Witte, Erich **1674**
Wodlinger, M. H. **1935**
Woerdeman, M. W. **888**
Wold, K. C. **768**
Wolff, Jacob **1723**
Wolstenholme, Gordon **746**
Women in Medicine, Histories **826–832**
Wong, Ming **539**
Wood, C. A. **1493, 2023**
Woodworth, J. M. **1887**
World bibliographic index on rheumatic diseases of specialized journals **1657**
World directory of dental schools **1329**
World directory of medical schools **1372**
World directory of physical medicine specialists **2264**
World directory of post-basic and post-graduate schools of nursing **1906**
World directory of veterinary schools **2657**
World Federation for Mental Health **1729, 1760, 1807**
World Health Organization **1160, 1164, 1259, 1260, 1329, 1366, 1372, 1467, 1715, 1880, 1906, 2066, 2076, 2196.1, 2657**
World Health Organization. Expert Committee on Malaria. Drafting Committee on Revision of Malaria Terminology **1193**
World Health Organization. Library **1510**
World Health Organization. Regional Office for Europe **2361**
World list of scientific periodicals **2516**
World Medical Association **328**
World Medical Association. U.S. Committee **340**
World medical periodicals **328**
World review of nutrition and dietetics **1917**
World War I **1604, 1606, 1608, 1611, 1612, 1617, 1623.2, 1624, 1645**
World War II **1605, 1607, 1612–1613, 1618, 1623, 1625, 1627, 1646–1651, 1918**
World-wide abstracts of general medicine **24**
Wortis, Joseph **1826**
Wren, R. C. **981**
Wren, R. W. **981**
Wrete, Martin **299**
Wright, Jonathan **2056**
Wright, M. H. **1524**
Writing, Dental **2669**
Writing, Preparation of Manuscripts, etc.
    Directories **2676.1**
    Monographs **2668–2676**
Writing, Psychiatric **2674**
Writing, Psychological **2674, 2675**
Wu, Lien-Teh **541**
Wüstenfeld, Ferdinand **507**
Wykaz oryginalnych prac lekarskich polskich za czas od r. 1831 do 1890 włacznie **157**
Wyss, Dieter **1838**

X-ray Analysis **2424**

Yakugaku saikin no shinpo **2168**
Yale University. School of Medicine. Department of the History of Medicine (series) **167**
Yale University. School of Nursing. Index Staff **1889**
Yale University. Yale Medical Library. Historical Library **837, 838, 1502, 1869**
Yaws **1259**
Yearbook of anesthesia **2600**
Yearbook of cancer **1697**
Yearbook of cardiovascular and renal diseases **1110**
Yearbook of dentistry **1285**
Yearbook of dermatology **1353**
Yearbook of dermatology and syphilology **1353**
Yearbook of drug therapy **2168.1**
Yearbook of endocrinology **1385**
Yearbook of endocrinology, metabolism and nutrition **1385**
Yearbook of general surgery **2555**
Yearbook of general therapeutics **2616.1**
Yearbook of industrial and orthopedic surgery **1672**
Yearbook of medicine **127**
Yearbook of medicine, surgery, and their allied sciences **71**
Yearbook of modern nursing **1892**
Yearbook of neurology and psychiatry **1753**

Yearbook of neurology, psychiatry and endocrinology **1385, 1753**
Yearbook of neurology, psychiatry, and neurosurgery **1753**
Yearbook of nuclear medicine **2454.1**
Yearbook of obstetrics and gynecology **1950**
Yearbook of ophthalmology **2004**
Yearbook of orthopedics and traumatic surgery **1672**
Yearbook of orthopedics, traumatic and plastic surgery **1672**
Yearbook of pathology and clinical pathology **2090**
Yearbook of pathology and immunology **2090**
Yearbook of pediatrics **2126**
Yearbook of pharmacy **2157.1**
Yearbook of public health **2349.1**
Yearbook of radiology **2428**
Yearbook of the ear, nose, and throat **2045**
Yearbook of treatment **2617**
Yearbook of urology **2632**
Yearbook of veterinary medicine **2646**
Yearsley, P. M. **784**
Yellow Fever **1139**
  Bibliographies **1166.2, 1266**
  Histories **1267**
Yoshikawa, Tetsuo **1845**
Young, James **1054**
Young, James H. **809**
Young, John H. **1986**
Young, M. N. **2314.2**
Young, Thomas **143**
Yuge, Tsunekazu **2007**
Yugoslav scientific research directory **2509**
Yugoslavia
  Bibliographies **173–175**
  Directories **407, 2509**
  Histories **739**
  Indexes and Abstracts **93–94**

Zabludovskiĭ, P. E. **648**
Zachert, M. J. **2179**
Zagreb. Leksikografski zavod FNRJ **413**
Zamkova, Z. N. **140.2, 165, 1488**
Zasukhina, D. N. **1224**
Zaunick, Rudolph **420, 443**
Zbor liječnika Hrvatske, Zagreb **739**
Zdravotnická ročenka československá **351**
Zee, Zai-Ziang **1017**
Zeis, Eduard **2588**
Zeitschrift für die gesamte Neurologie und Psychiatrie. Referate **1733**
Zeitschrift für Kinderheilkunde **2112**
Zeitschrift für Krebsforschung. Referate **1691**
Zeitschrift für Urologie und Gynäkologie **2629**
Zeitschrift für urologische Chirurgie **2629**
Zensetsu, Kōchi **601**
Zentralblatt für allgemeine und experimentelle Biologie **921.1, 2681**
Zentralblatt für Bakteriologie, Parasitenkunde, Infektionskrankheiten und Hygiene **1539**
Zentralblatt für Bakteriologie, Parasitenkunde und Infektionskrankheiten **1540**
Zentralblatt für Biochemie und Biophysik **1011**
Zentralblatt für chirurgische und mechanische Orthopädie **1668**
Zentralblatt für die gesamte Chirurgie und ihre Grenzegebiete **2542**
Zentralblatt für die gesamte Hygiene **2349**
Zentralblatt für die gesamte Hygiene und ihre Grenzegebiete **2349**
Zentralblatt für die gesamte innere Medizin und ihre Grenzgebiete (Kongresszentralblatt) **13**
Zentralblatt für die gesamte Kinderheikunde **2112**
Zentralblatt für die gesamte Neurologie und Psychiatrie **1733**
Zentralblatt für die gesamte Ophthalmologie und ihre Grenzgebiete **1990**
Zentralblatt für die gesamte Radiologie **2422**
Zentralblatt für die gesamte Tuberkuloseforschung **1232**
Zentralblatt für die gesamte Zahn- Mund- und Kieferheilkunde **1273.1**
Zentralblatt für die medizinischen Wissenschaften **52**
Zentralblatt für Hals- Nasen- und Ohrenheilkunde **2036**
Zentralblatt für Haut- und Geschlechtskrankheiten **1253, 1254**
Zentralblatt für Kinderheilkunde **2115**
Zentralblatt für Nervenheilkunde und Psychiatrie **1739**
Zentralblatt für Neurochirurgie **2579**
Zentralblatt für normale Anatomie und Mikrotechnik **861**
Zentralblatt für normale und pathologische Anatomie mit Einschluss der Mikrotechnik **861**
Zentralblatt für orthopädische Chirurgie und Mechanik **1669**
Zentralblatt für Physiologie **2273**
Zentralblatt für Zoologie **2681**
Zentralorgan für die gesamte Chirurgie **2542**
Zetkin, Maxim **256**
Zeuch, L. H. **687**
Ziegler, H. E. **2702**
Zilboorg, Gregory **1818**
Zimmer, H. R. **588**
Zimmerman, L. M. **2575**
Zimmermann, Walter **956**
Zino, Elena **267**
Zinsser, Hans **1213**
Zirkle, Conway **955**
Zmeev, L. F. **648.1**
Zoological record **2679**
Zoological Society of London **2679, 2703**

Zoologischer Bericht **2682**
Zoologischer Jahresbericht **2682**
Zoologisches Zentralblatt **2681, 2684**
Zoology
    Bibliographies **2493.3, 2688–2696**
    Dictionaries **938, 2698–2702**
    Indexes and Abstracts **44, 2677–2684**
    Manuals **2697**
    Nomenclature **2703**
    Reviews **2685–2687**
Zuckerman, Solly **957**
Zweifach, B. W. **2092**

FOR REFERENCE USE ONLY